Duchenne Muscular Dystrophy

Advances in Therapeutics

NEUROLOGICAL DISEASE AND THERAPY

Advisory Board

Louis R. Caplan, M.D.
Professor of Neurology
Harvard University School of Medicine
Beth Israel Deaconess Medical Center
Boston, Massachusetts

John C. Morris, M.D.
Friedman Professor of Neurology
Co-Director, Alzheimer's Disease Research Center
Washington University School of Medicine
St. Louis, Missouri

Bruce Ransom, M.D., Ph.D.
Warren Magnuson Professor
Chair, Department of Neurology
University of Washington School of Medicine
Seattle, Washington

Kapil Sethi, M.D.
Professor of Neurology
Director, Movement Disorders Program
Medical College of Georgia
Augusta, Georgia

Mark Tuszynski, M.D., Ph.D.
Associate Professor of Neurosciences
Director, Center for Neural Repair
University of California–San Diego
La Jolla, California

1. Handbook of Parkinson's Disease, *edited by William C. Koller*
2. Medical Therapy of Acute Stroke, *edited by Mark Fisher*
3. Familial Alzheimer's Disease: Molecular Genetics and Clinical Perspectives, *edited by Gary D. Miner, Ralph W. Richter, John P. Blass, Jimmie L. Valentine, and Linda A. Winters-Miner*
4. Alzheimer's Disease: Treatment and Long-Term Management, *edited by Jeffrey L. Cummings and Bruce L. Miller*
5. Therapy of Parkinson's Disease, *edited by William C. Koller and George Paulson*
6. Handbook of Sleep Disorders, *edited by Michael J. Thorpy*
7. Epilepsy and Sudden Death, *edited by Claire M. Lathers and Paul L. Schraeder*
8. Handbook of Multiple Sclerosis, *edited by Stuart D. Cook*
9. Memory Disorders: Research and Clinical Practice, *edited by Takehiko Yanagihara and Ronald C. Petersen*
10. The Medical Treatment of Epilepsy, *edited by Stanley R. Resor, Jr., and Henn Kutt*
11. Cognitive Disorders: Pathophysiology and Treatment, *edited by Leon J. Thal, Walter H. Moos, and Elkan R. Gamzu*
12. Handbook of Amyotrophic Lateral Sclerosis, *edited by Richard Alan Smith*
13. Handbook of Parkinson's Disease: Second Edition, Revised and Expanded, *edited by William C. Koller*
14. Handbook of Pediatric Epilepsy, *edited by Jerome V. Murphy and Fereydoun Dehkharghani*
15. Handbook of Tourette's Syndrome and Related Tic and Behavioral Disorders, *edited by Roger Kurlan*
16. Handbook of Cerebellar Diseases, *edited by Richard Lechtenberg*
17. Handbook of Cerebrovascular Diseases, *edited by Harold P. Adams, Jr.*
18. Parkinsonian Syndromes, *edited by Matthew B. Stern and William C. Koller*
19. Handbook of Head and Spine Trauma, *edited by Jonathan Greenberg*
20. Brain Tumors: A Comprehensive Text, *edited by Robert A. Morantz and John W. Walsh*
21. Monoamine Oxidase Inhibitors in Neurological Diseases, *edited by Abraham Lieberman, C. Warren Olanow, Moussa B. H. Youdim, and Keith Tipton*
22. Handbook of Dementing Illnesses, *edited by John C. Morris*
23. Handbook of Myasthenia Gravis and Myasthenic Syndromes, *edited by Robert P. Lisak*
24. Handbook of Neurorehabilitation, *edited by David C. Good and James R. Couch, Jr.*
25. Therapy with Botulinum Toxin, *edited by Joseph Jankovic and Mark Hallett*
26. Principles of Neurotoxicology, *edited by Louis W. Chang*

27. Handbook of Neurovirology, *edited by Robert R. McKendall and William G. Stroop*
28. Handbook of Neuro-Urology, *edited by David N. Rushton*
29. Handbook of Neuroepidemiology, *edited by Philip B. Gorelick and Milton Alter*
30. Handbook of Tremor Disorders, *edited by Leslie J. Findley and William C. Koller*
31. Neuro-Ophthalmological Disorders: Diagnostic Work-Up and Management, *edited by Ronald J. Tusa and Steven A. Newman*
32. Handbook of Olfaction and Gustation, *edited by Richard L. Doty*
33. Handbook of Neurological Speech and Language Disorders, *edited by Howard S. Kirshner*
34. Therapy of Parkinson's Disease: Second Edition, Revised and Expanded, *edited by William C. Koller and George Paulson*
35. Evaluation and Management of Gait Disorders, *edited by Barney S. Spivack*
36. Handbook of Neurotoxicology, *edited by Louis W. Chang and Robert S. Dyer*
37. Neurological Complications of Cancer, *edited by Ronald G. Wiley*
38. Handbook of Autonomic Nervous System Dysfunction, *edited by Amos D. Korczyn*
39. Handbook of Dystonia, *edited by Joseph King Ching Tsui and Donald B. Calne*
40. Etiology of Parkinson's Disease, *edited by Jonas H. Ellenberg, William C. Koller and J. William Langston*
41. Practical Neurology of the Elderly, *edited by Jacob I. Sage and Margery H. Mark*
42. Handbook of Muscle Disease, *edited by Russell J. M. Lane*
43. Handbook of Multiple Sclerosis: Second Edition, Revised and Expanded, *edited by Stuart D. Cook*
44. Central Nervous System Infectious Diseases and Therapy, *edited by Karen L. Roos*
45. Subarachnoid Hemorrhage: Clinical Management, *edited by Takehiko Yanagihara, David G. Piepgras, and John L. D. Atkinson*
46. Neurology Practice Guidelines, *edited by Richard Lechtenberg and Henry S. Schutta*
47. Spinal Cord Diseases: Diagnosis and Treatment, *edited by Gordon L. Engler, Jonathan Cole, and W. Louis Merton*
48. Management of Acute Stroke, *edited by Ashfaq Shuaib and Larry B. Goldstein*
49. Sleep Disorders and Neurological Disease, *edited by Antonio Culebras*
50. Handbook of Ataxia Disorders, *edited by Thomas Klockgether*
51. The Autonomic Nervous System in Health and Disease, *David S. Goldstein*

52. Axonal Regeneration in the Central Nervous System, *edited by Nicholas A. Ingoglia and Marion Murray*
53. Handbook of Multiple Sclerosis: Third Edition, *edited by Stuart D. Cook*
54. Long-Term Effects of Stroke, *edited by Julien Bogousslavsky*
55. Handbook of the Autonomic Nervous System in Health and Disease, *edited by C. Liana Bolis, Julio Licinio, and Stefano Govoni*
56. Dopamine Receptors and Transporters: Function, Imaging, and Clinical Implication, Second Edition, *edited by Anita Sidhu, Marc Laruelle, and Philippe Vernier*
57. Handbook of Olfaction and Gustation: Second Edition, Revised and Expanded, *edited by Richard L. Doty*
58. Handbook of Stereotactic and Functional Neurosurgery, *edited by Michael Schulder*
59. Handbook of Parkinson's Disease: Third Edition, *edited by Rajesh Pahwa, Kelly E. Lyons, and William C. Koller*
60. Clinical Neurovirology, *edited by Avindra Nath and Joseph R. Berger*
61. Neuromuscular Junction Disorders: Diagnosis and Treatment, *Matthew N. Meriggioli, James F. Howard, Jr., and C. Michel Harper*
62. Drug-Induced Movement Disorders, *edited by Kapil D. Sethi*
63. Therapy of Parkinson's Disease: Third Edition, Revised and Expanded, *edited by Rajesh Pahwa, Kelly E. Lyons, and William C. Koller*
64. Epilepsy: Scientific Foundations of Clinical Practice, *edited by Jong M. Rho, Raman Sankar, and José E. Cavazos*
65. Handbook of Tourette's Syndrome and Related Tic and Behavioral Disorders: Second Edition, *edited by Roger Kurlan*
66. Handbook of Cerebrovascular Diseases: Second Edition, Revised and Expanded, *edited by Harold P. Adams, Jr.*
67. Emerging Neurological Infections, *edited by Christopher Power and Richard T. Johnson*
68. Treatment of Pediatric Neurologic Disorders, *edited by Harvey S. Singer, Eric H. Kossoff, Adam L. Hartman, and Thomas O. Crawford*
69. Synaptic Plasticity : Basic Mechanisms to Clinical Applications, *edited by Michel Baudry, Xiaoning Bi, and Steven S. Schreiber*
70. Handbook of Essential Tremor and Other Tremor Disorders, *edited by Kelly E. Lyons and Rajesh Pahwa*
71. Handbook of Peripheral Neuropathy, *edited by Mark B. Bromberg and A. Gordon Smith*
72. Carotid Artery Stenosis: Current and Emerging Treatments, *edited by Seemant Chaturvedi and Peter M. Rothwell*
73. Gait Disorders: Evaluation and Management, *edited by Jeffrey M. Hausdorff and Neil B. Alexander*

74. Surgical Management of Movement Disorders (HBK), *edited by Gordon H. Baltuch and Matthew B. Stern*
75. Neurogenetics: Scientific and Clinical Advances, *edited by David R. Lynch*
76. Epilepsy Surgery: Principles and Controversies, *edited by John W. Miller and Daniel L. Silbergeld*
77. Clinician's Guide To Sleep Disorders, *edited by Nathaniel F. Watson and Bradley Vaughn*
78. Amyotrophic Lateral Sclerosis, *edited by Hiroshi Mitsumoto, Serge Przedborski and Paul H. Gordon*
79. Duchenne Muscular Dystrophy: Advances in Therapeutics, *edited by Jeffrey S. Chamberlain and Thomas A. Rando*

Duchenne Muscular Dystrophy
Advances in Therapeutics

edited by

Jeffrey S. Chamberlain
University of Washington
Seattle, Washington, U.S.A.

Thomas A. Rando
Stanford University
Palo Alto, California, U.S.A.

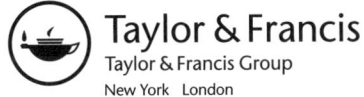

Taylor & Francis
Taylor & Francis Group
New York London

Published in 2006 by
Taylor & Francis Group
270 Madison Avenue
New York, NY 10016

© 2006 by Taylor & Francis Group, LLC

No claim to original U.S. Government works
Printed in the United States of America on acid-free paper
10 9 8 7 6 5 4 3 2 1

International Standard Book Number-10: 0-8247-2325-2 (Hardcover)
International Standard Book Number-13: 978-0-8247-2325-5 (Hardcover)
Library of Congress Card Number 2005056854

This book contains information obtained from authentic and highly regarded sources. Reprinted material is quoted with permission, and sources are indicated. A wide variety of references are listed. Reasonable efforts have been made to publish reliable data and information, but the author and the publisher cannot assume responsibility for the validity of all materials or for the consequences of their use.

No part of this book may be reprinted, reproduced, transmitted, or utilized in any form by any electronic, mechanical, or other means, now known or hereafter invented, including photocopying, microfilming, and recording, or in any information storage or retrieval system, without written permission from the publishers.

For permission to photocopy or use material electronically from this work, please access www.copyright.com (http://www.copyright.com/) or contact the Copyright Clearance Center, Inc. (CCC) 222 Rosewood Drive, Danvers, MA 01923, 978-750-8400. CCC is a not-for-profit organization that provides licenses and registration for a variety of users. For organizations that have been granted a photocopy license by the CCC, a separate system of payment has been arranged.

Trademark Notice: Product or corporate names may be trademarks or registered trademarks, and are used only for identification and explanation without intent to infringe.

Library of Congress Cataloging-in-Publication Data

Duchenne muscular dystrophy : advances in therapeutics / edited by Jeffrey S. Chamberlain, Thomas A. Rando.
  p. ; cm. -- (Neurological disease and therapy ; 79)
Includes bibliographical references and index.
ISBN-13: 978-0-8247-2325-5 (hardcover : alk. paper)
ISBN-10: 0-8247-2325-2 (hardcover : alk. paper)
  1. Duchenne muscular dystrophy--Treatment. I. Chamberlain, Jeffrey S. II. Rando, Thomas A. III. Series.
  [DNLM: 1. Muscular Dystrophy, Duchenne--therapy. WE 559 D8279 2005]

RJ482.D78D82 2005
616.7'4806--dc22   2005056854

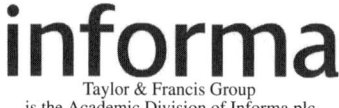

Taylor & Francis Group
is the Academic Division of Informa plc.

Visit the Taylor & Francis Web site at
http://www.taylorandfrancis.com

Preface

Duchenne muscular dystrophy is a disease with both ancient and modern significance. It has likely been present in humans since the emergence of the species. The phenotype may have been recognized and recorded in ancient cave drawings, and the clinical and hereditary patterns were described in the medical literature a century and a half ago. Its modern significance lies in the fact that it was the first hereditary disorder whose genetic basis was identified by positional cloning in the molecular biology revolution of the late 20th century. Duchenne muscular dystrophy is among the most prevalent genetic disorders of childhood, it is the most common inherited disease in terms of new genetic mutations, and it is a lethal disease. Still, none of these factors have resulted in any major advances in treatment and it remains, to this day, an incurable and nearly untreatable condition. Corticosteroids provide temporary benefit, but with unacceptable side effects for long-term use. Physical therapy and prosthetics optimize muscle function but have no impact on disease progression. Assisted ventilation can prolong survival. However, even in combination, the prognosis for a boy diagnosed with Duchenne muscular dystrophy remains grim and the disease is almost as devastating today as it was when described by Edward Meryon in England and Guillaume Duchenne in France in the mid 19th century.

Nevertheless, hope persists and investigators relentlessly pursue therapeutic breakthroughs for the treatment of Duchenne muscular dystrophy and related disorders. As an X-linked recessive, single gene defect, the promise of gene therapy looms large. As a disease that may share common pathophysiological mechanisms with a plethora of related muscular dystrophies, the hope of pharmacological therapy that would be beneficial to all such disorders remains high. As a disease with progressive tissue degeneration, the emerging field of regenerative medicine offers optimism.

This book is intended to provide a summary on the state-of-the-art of current experimental approaches to treatments for Duchenne muscular dystrophy that are under active investigation. The clinical, genetic, and pathophysiological aspects of the disease are reviewed in the context of emerging therapeutic modalities. Next, the importance of accurate detection is highlighted by chapters on principles of diagnostic modalities and advances in molecular diagnostics. These fundamental considerations are then followed by chapters on advances in experimental therapeutics. Challenges to the development of treatments for Duchenne muscular dystrophy are emphasized, and guiding principles of therapeutics are laid out. The chapters on individual therapeutic modalities are divided, somewhat arbitrarily, into sections on pharmacological interventions, therapy based on principles of regenerative medicine, and last but not least, gene therapy. The authors have written these chapters within a historical context and with an eye to the future. Ultimately, these emerging therapeutics will need to be tested in human clinical trials, which for cell and gene therapy require navigating a large number of regulatory issues that vary from one country to another. As such, therapeutic advances will depend not only on scientific progress, but also on coordinated efforts of investigators, clinicians, ethicists, and policy makers. We hope that this book will be of interest to students of muscular dystrophies, whether they be clinicians or scientists, whose interests are directed to the ultimate challenge—finding a treatment and, finally, a cure for Duchenne muscular dystrophy and all other muscular dystrophies.

Jeffrey S. Chamberlain
University of Washington School of Medicine
Seattle, Washington, U.S.A.

Thomas A. Rando
Stanford University School of Medicine
Stanford, California, U.S.A.

Contents

Preface .... *iii*
Contributors .... *xiii*
Introduction .... *xvii*

SECTION I: DUCHENNE MUSCULAR DYSTROPHY BACKGROUND

1. **Clinical Overview of Duchenne Muscular Dystrophy** *1*
   Richard T. Moxley III
   Historical Background 1
   Clinical Manifestations 4
   Diagnosis 9
   Treatment 13
   Questions and Opportunities Related to Future Treatment for DMD 16
   References 18

2. **The Functional Biology of Dystrophin: Structural Components and the Pathogenesis of Duchenne Muscular Dystrophy** *21*
   Eijiro Ozawa
   Keynotes on the Pathogenesis of Duchenne Muscular Dystrophy 21
   Sarcolemmal and Cytoskeletal Architectures Related to DMD 24
   Structural Defects in DMD 33

Transverse Fixation System: The Structural Basis for a
  Mechanical Hypothesis of DMD Pathogenesis 38
What Induces the Degenerative Processes
  in DMD? 41
Epilogue 46
References 47

3. **The Functional Biology of Dystrophin: Associated
   Signaling Pathways and Potential Targets
   for Therapeutic Intervention** *55*
   Gayle Smythe, Steven J. Winder, and Thomas A. Rando
   Introduction 55
   Dystrophin Domains and Protein Interactions 57
   Cellular Signaling Pathways Associated with
     the DAPC 61
   Conclusions 67
   References 68

SECTION II: DIAGNOSTIC CONSIDERATIONS

4. **Duchenne Muscular Dystrophy and Becker Muscular Dystrophy:
   Diagnostic Principles** *77*
   *H. B. Ginjaar, J. T. den Dunnen, E. Bakker, and
   G. J. B. van Ommen*
   Introduction 77
   Confirmation Diagnosis of DMD/BMD 78
   Prenatal Diagnosis 83
   Concluding Remarks 84
   References 86

5. **Mutation Detection** *91*
   Thomas W. Prior
   Gene Studies 91
   Molecular Diagnostics 94
   Point Mutation Detection in the Dystrophin Gene 101
   Conclusions 103
   References 103

6. **Protein Studies in Duchenne Muscular Dystrophy** *105*
   Kathryn North and Sandra Cooper
   Background 105

Methodological Approach to Protein Diagnosis of
    Dystrophinopathies 112
References 118

SECTION III: CURRENT THERAPEUTICS

7. Medical Management of Duchenne Muscular Dystrophy *123*
Roula Al-Dahhak and John T. Kissel
Introduction 123
Corticosteroids 126
Other Agents 135
Summary and Conclusions 140
References 141

8. Rehabilitation Management of Duchenne Muscular Dystrophy *149*
Craig M. McDonald, Gregory T. Carter, Jay J. Han, and Joshua O. Benditt
Introduction 149
Initial Rehabilitation Evaluation 150
Evaluating Disease Progression 154
Rehabilitation Management 154
The Role of Exercise 167
Improving Functional Mobility 169
References 170

9. Orthopedic Interventions in the Management of Duchenne Muscular Dystrophy: A Review of Current Practice and Clinical Outcomes *177*
Irwin M. Siegel and John D. Hsu
Introduction 177
Biomechanics 177
Management 179
Stage I: Diagnosis Until 8 to 9 Years of Age 180
Fractures 183
Stage II: 9 to 12 Years of Age 184
Lower Extremity Surgery 184
Compartment Syndrome 187
Talipes Equinovarus 188
Stage III: Full-Time Sitting 189

Scoliosis 191
Summary 197
References 197

SECTION IV: EXPERIMENTAL THERAPEUTICS

10. **Therapeutic Principles and Challenges in Duchenne Muscular Dystrophy** *201*
    Dominic J. Wells
    Introduction 201
    Animal Models 202
    Gene Therapeutic Approaches to DMD 205
    Pharmacological Therapeutic Approaches
      to DMD 211
    Potential Problems in Translating Laboratory Studies
      into Clinical Treatments 214
    Conclusions 216
    References 217

11. **Experimental Pharmacologic Therapies in Duchenne Dystrophy: Current Clinical Trials** *227*
    Shannon L. Venance and Robert C. Griggs
    Introduction 227
    Preclinical Studies 232
    Active Clinical Trials 233
    Future Directions 238
    IGF-I 240
    Conclusions 241
    References 241

12. **Utrophin: The Intersection Between Pharmacological and Genetic Therapy** *251*
    Kelly J. Perkins and Kay E. Davies
    Introduction 251
    The Utrophin Gene and Protein 252
    Animal Models 254
    Promoter Studies of Utrophin 255
    Other Effectors of Utrophin Upregulation 263
    Utrophin-Based Therapeutic Strategies 263
    Conclusions 267
    References 267

13. Regenerative Therapy *279*
J. E. Morgan, Karima Brimah, C. A. Collins, and
T. A. Partridge
Introduction 279
Hypothetical Mechanisms 280
Regeneration of Skeletal Muscle from
    Muscle Precursor Cells 281
Growth Factors as Regenerative Therapy for
    Myopathic or Aged Muscles 283
Stem Cells in Skeletal Muscle 285
Conclusions 286
References 287

**14. Cellular Mediated Delivery: The Intersection Between
Regenerative Medicine and Genetic Therapy** *295*
K. Liadaki, F. Montanaro, and L. M. Kunkel
Introduction 295
Muscle Cells Available for Therapy of DMD 296
Delivery Methods 298
Intramuscular Transplants of Myoblasts 299
Donor Cell Selection 301
Muscle Side Population Cells 302
Other Muscle-Derived Cells Available for Cell-Mediated
    Therapy of DMD 303
Nonmuscle-Derived Cells Participating in
    Muscle Repair 306
Stem Cells Derived from Dorsal Aorta
    (Mesangioblasts) 307
BM-Derived Cells with Myogenic Potential 308
Mesenchymal Stem Cells 309
Skin 309
Conclusions 310
References 311

**15. Oligonucleotide-Mediated Exon Skipping and Gene Editing
for Duchenne Muscular Dystrophy** *319*
Carmen Bertoni and Thomas A. Rando
Introduction 319
AONs 320

Oligonucleotide-Mediated Gene Editing 326
Other Technologies 335
Conclusions 337
References 337

16. The Intravascular Delivery of Naked DNA for Treating Duchenne Muscular Dystrophy *343*
Jon A. Wolff and Hans Herweijer
Introduction 343
Plasmid DNA Delivery 345
Intravascular Delivery of Naked Plasmid DNA 348
mdx Mouse Studies 353
Future Prospects 358
References 359

17. Adenoviral-Mediated Gene Therapy *363*
Laura Goldberg and Paula R. Clemens
Introduction 363
Adenoviral Capsid Structure 364
Pathway of Infection 365
Adenoviral Vectors 368
Immunity Induced by Adenoviral Vectors 372
Targeting Adenoviral Vectors 375
Future Challenges 378
References 379

18. Retroviridae-Based Gene Transfer Vectors in Duchenne Muscular Dystrophy Therapy *391*
Michael L. Roberts, George Dickson, and Michael Themis
Molecular Biology of Retroviral Vectors and
  Their Application in DMD 391
Retroviral-Mediated Gene Delivery to Muscle Cells:
  In Vitro and Ex Vivo Approaches 396
Efficacy of Muscle-Directed Retroviral Delivery
  In Vivo 398
Cell-Based Strategies of Muscle-Directed Retroviral
  Delivery 399
Modern Approaches to Muscle-Directed Retroviral
  Delivery 402

The Development of Lentiviral Vectors for
   DMD Gene Therapy 405
Future Prospects 408
References 409

19. Gene Therapy of Muscular Dystrophy Using Adeno-Associated Viral Vectors: Promises and Limitations *413*
Michael J. Blankinship, Paul Gregorevic, and Jeffrey S. Chamberlain
Overview 413
AAV: The Genome and Capsid 413
AAV Serotypes 414
rAAV Cloning and Production 415
Safety of rAAV Vectors 417
Engineering of Microdystrophins 419
Dystrophin Replacement in Animal Models of
   DMD 422
rAAV Delivery of Nondystrophin Genes for the
   Treatment of DMD 424
Delivery of rAAV Vectors 426
Transduction of Myogenic Precursor Cells
   by rAAV Vectors 428
Conclusions 429
References 429

20. Regional and Systemic Gene Delivery Using Viral Vectors *439*
Leonard T. Su and Hansell H. Stedman
Introduction 439
Direct Intramuscular Injection 440
Regional Delivery 440
Future Directions: Applications of the Current
   Technology 448
References 449

Index *453*

Contributors

Roula Al-Dahhak Department of Neurology, Division of Neuromuscular Disease, The Ohio State University, Columbus, Ohio, U.S.A.

E. Bakker Center for Human and Clinical Genetics, Leiden University Medical Center, Leiden, Zuid-Holland, The Netherlands

Joshua O. Benditt Division of Pulmonary and Critical Care Medicine, Department of Medicine, University of Washington School of Medicine, Seattle, Washington, U.S.A.

Carmen Bertoni Department of Neurology and Neurological Sciences, Stanford University School of Medicine, Stanford, California, and GRECC and Neurology Service, VA Palo Alto Health Care System, Palo Alto, California, U.S.A.

Michael J. Blankinship Department of Neurology, Senator Paul D. Wellstone Muscular Dystrophy Cooperative Research Center, University of Washington School of Medicine, Seattle, Washington, U.S.A.

Karima Brimah Muscle Cell Biology Group, MRC Clinical Sciences Centre, Imperial College, London, U.K.

Gregory T. Carter Department of Rehabilitation Medicine, University of Washington School of Medicine, Seattle, Washington, U.S.A.

Jeffrey S. Chamberlain Department of Neurology, Senator Paul D. Wellstone Muscular Dystrophy Cooperative Research Center, University of Washington School of Medicine, Seattle, Washington, U.S.A.

Paula R. Clemens   Department of Neurology, University of Pittsburgh, Pittsburgh, Pennsylvania, U.S.A.

C. A. Collins   Muscle Cell Biology Group, MRC Clinical Sciences Centre, Imperial College, London, U.K.

Sandra Cooper   Institute for Neuromuscular Research, Children's Hospital at Westmead, University of Sydney, Sydney, New South Wales, Australia

Kay E. Davies   MRC Functional Genetics Unit, Department of Human Anatomy and Genetics, University of Oxford, Oxford, U.K.

J. T. den Dunnen   Center for Human and Clinical Genetics, Leiden University Medical Center, Leiden, Zuid-Holland, The Netherlands

George Dickson   School of Biological Science, Royal Holloway–University of London, Egham, Surrey, U.K.

H. B. Ginjaar   Center for Human and Clinical Genetics, Leiden University Medical Center, Leiden, Zuid-Holland, The Netherlands

Laura Goldberg   Department of Neurology, University of Pittsburgh, Pittsburgh, Pennsylvania, U.S.A.

Paul Gregorevic   Department of Neurology, Senator Paul D. Wellstone Muscular Dystrophy Cooperative Research Center, University of Washington School of Medicine, Seattle, Washington, U.S.A.

Robert C. Griggs   Department of Neurology, University of Rochester Medical Center, Rochester, New York, U.S.A.

Jay J. Han   Department of Rehabilitation Medicine, University of Washington School of Medicine, Seattle, Washington, U.S.A.

Hans Herweijer   Mirus Bio Corporation, Madison, Wisconsin, U.S.A.

John D. Hsu   Rancho Los Amigos Medical Center, Downey, and Department of Orthopedics, University of Southern California, Los Angeles, California, U.S.A.

John T. Kissel   Department of Neurology, Division of Neuromuscular Disease, The Ohio State University, Columbus, Ohio, U.S.A.

Contributors

L. M. Kunkel Howard Hughes Medical Institute at the Children's Hospital, and Department of Pediatrics, Harvard Medical School, Boston, Massachusetts, U.S.A.

K. Liadaki Howard Hughes Medical Institute at the Children's Hospital, and Department of Pediatrics, Harvard Medical School, Boston, Massachusetts, U.S.A.

Craig M. McDonald Department of Physical Medicine and Rehabilitation, University of California School of Medicine, Davis, California, U.S.A.

F. Montanaro Howard Hughes Medical Institute at the Children's Hospital, and Department of Pediatrics, Harvard Medical School, Boston, Massachusetts, U.S.A.

J. E. Morgan Muscle Cell Biology Group, MRC Clinical Sciences Centre, Imperial College, London, U.K.

Richard T. Moxley III Department of Neurology, University of Rochester School of Medicine and Dentistry, Rochester, New York, U.S.A.

Kathryn North Institute for Neuromuscular Research, Children's Hospital at Westmead, University of Sydney, Sydney, New South Wales, Australia

Eijiro Ozawa National Institute of Neuroscience, NCNP, Tokyo, Japan

T. A. Partridge Muscle Cell Biology Group, MRC Clinical Sciences Centre, Imperial College, London, U.K.

Kelly J. Perkins Department of Physiology and Pennsylvania Muscle Institute, University of Pennsylvania School of Medicine, Philadelphia, Pennsylvania, U.S.A.

Thomas W. Prior Division of Molecular Pathology, Department of Pathology, The Ohio State University, Columbus, Ohio, U.S.A.

Thomas A. Rando Department of Neurology and Neurological Sciences, Stanford University School of Medicine, Stanford, California, and GRECC and Neurology Service, VA Palo Alto Health Care System, Palo Alto, California, U.S.A.

Michael L. Roberts School of Biological Science, Royal Holloway–University of London, Egham, Surrey, U.K.

Irwin M. Siegel Departments of Orthopedic Surgery, Neurosciences, and PM&R, Rush University Medical Center, Chicago, Illinois, U.S.A.

Gayle Smythe School of Community Health, Charles Sturt University, Albury, New South Wales, Australia

Hansell H. Stedman Department of Surgery, University of Pennsylvania, Philadelphia, Pennsylvania, U.S.A.

Leonard T. Su Department of Surgery, University of Pennsylvania, Philadelphia, Pennsylvania, U.S.A.

Michael Themis Division of Biomedical Sciences, Imperial College of Science, Technology and Medicine, London, U.K.

G. J. B. van Ommen Center for Human and Clinical Genetics, Leiden University Medical Center, Leiden, Zuid-Holland, The Netherlands

Shannon L. Venance Department of Clinical Neurological Sciences, University of Western Ontario, London, Ontario, Canada

Dominic J. Wells Gene Targeting Group, Department of Cellular and Molecular Neuroscience, Division of Neuroscience and Mental Health, Imperial College, Charing Cross Hospital, London, U.K.

Steven J. Winder Department of Biomedical Science, Center for Developmental and Biomedical Genetics, University of Sheffield, Western Bank, Sheffield, U.K.

Jon A. Wolff Departments of Pediatrics and Medical Genetics, Waisman Center, University of Wisconsin–Madison, Madison, Wisconsin, U.S.A.

Introduction

Alan E. H. Emery
Green College, University of Oxford, Oxford, U.K.

EARLY CLINICAL STUDIES

The study of Duchenne muscular dystrophy (DMD) has a history going back to the mid-19th century—a history that in many ways mirrors the developments in medical science. Its clinical features were most clearly defined by Meryon in 1852, and a few years later by Duchenne (1,2). Meryon also showed at this time that the disease was familial with a predilection for males and that the spinal cord was not involved (and therefore the disease was myogenic and not neurogenic). His microscopic studies led him to suggest that the basic defect was a breakdown of the sarcolemma—some 135 years before this was proved. What is interesting is that these studies of DMD were carried out at a time when the overwhelming concern of most physicians was about infectious disease for which the causes were unknown and there was no effective treatment. Furthermore the detailed histological studies of Meryon, Duchenne and others at the time were only possible because they had access to the newly developed microscopes with achromatic lenses by Joseph Jackson Lister, father of the famous surgeon. Other improvements around the same time included the use of clearing agents that rendered tissues transparent, very thin coverslips, and mounting in Canada balsam. As so often happens in medical science, advances in our knowledge frequently depend on developments in unrelated fields. And this is very clearly evident in our understanding and knowledge of DMD (3).

After these early studies, there followed a period whereby the clinical features became increasingly refined. However, these studies that were conducted later revealed that cases of 'muscular paralysis' were clinically heterogeneous. Among these early investigators was Erb, who coined the term 'Dystrophia muscularis progressiva' or progressive muscular dystrophy (4), and who was the first to attempt to classify this group of diseases (5).

THE MECHANISM OF INHERITANCE

The next step in the history of this disease was the need to understand the mechanism of its inheritance. This had to await the emergence of Mendelism and in particular the interpretation of 'sex-linked inheritance'. This only became clear after the work on *Drosophila* by Thomas Hunt Morgan and colleagues in the early 1900s (6). That the gene was on the X-chromosome explained the pattern of inheritance that many had observed. The report of an affected young girl in a family with the disease who also had Turner's syndrome, and proved to be XO, confirmed the localization of the gene to the X-chromosome (7).

The next important step was the demonstration by Japanese scientists that the serum creatine kinase (SCK) level was significantly elevated in affected boys. Most importantly, SCK levels were also found to be raised in a proportion of carrier females, which proved extremely important in genetic counselling (8). The use of SCK levels in potential carriers was aided by the application of Bayesian statistics introduced by Tony Murphy in the United States (9). Bayesian methodology now finds wide application in various other branches of medicine and related subjects, but its first application was in DMD families.

There then followed a period of over 10 years when, in retrospect, much of the research contributed very little to our understanding of DMD except for the fact that raised serum enzyme levels pointed to a possible defect in the muscle membrane. An entirely new approach was needed.

GENE LOCATION AND FUNCTION

This came with the discovery of common restriction fragment length polymorphisms (RFLPs) and that these could be used as genetic markers to locate gene loci (10). The importance of this idea and the associated technology cannot be over-emphasized and led to the location of the DMD gene in 1982 (11). This and subsequent studies confirmed the gene location to be Xp21. The use of RFLP markers in this way to locate the DMD gene was yet another first. It provided a model for the localization of other disease genes.

The next step was to isolate, clone, and characterize the DMD gene. This was brilliantly achieved in 1985 by Louis Kunkel and colleagues in

Introduction xix

the United States (12) and Ronald Worton and colleagues in Canada (13). The gene turned out to be the largest identified to date in any organism. It is now known to be some 2,500 Kb in length and consists of at least 86 exons. It includes 7 promoters with 3 full-length isoforms (M, muscle; B, brain; and P, cerebellar Purkinje neurons), and 4 truncated isoforms (DP 280; DP 140; DP 116; and DP 71) generated by separate promoters within the gene. Reflecting the size of the gene, its product *dystrophin*, identified by Eric Hoffman and colleagues in 1987 (14), was large (427 kDa consisting of 3685 amino acids). The details and functions of these isoforms and their products are detailed in Chapters 2 and 3.

These various developments generated considerable interest in the field that involved international collaboration on a scale not previously witnessed in the biomedical sciences. One paper for example had no less than 77 coauthors, from all over the world (15).

The practical outcome was that by using gene specific probes, genetic counselling became more reliable and prenatal diagnosis became possible. Furthermore, it also became possible to predict more reliably the clinical course in an individual case.

Finally, dystrophin was localized at the sarcolemma in normal muscle, and within just two years after the gene product had first been identified, Campbell and Kahl showed that it was intimately associated with glycoprotein, forming a dystrophin-associated-glycoprotein (DAG) complex of the muscle membrane (16). The absence of dystrophin in Duchenne, and to a lesser extent in Becker dystrophy, added credence to the widely held belief that the muscle membrane was defective in these diseases.

All these exciting developments occurred over a period of less than ten years. But a detailed analysis of pathogenesis is still very much a matter of debate, and is proving to be more complex than was originally believed (17). However, one area of importance that has largely been neglected in this regard relates to the possible role of environmental factors.

ROLE OF ENVIRONMENTAL FACTORS

Several muscle proteins defective in certain dystrophies have now been shown to be targets for microorganisms. The enteroviral protease 2A of Coxsackie B3 specifically cleaves cardiac muscle dystrophin (18,19). Could such an infection in an individual with reduced dystrophin precipitate or exacerbate any possible cardiomyopathy in Duchenne or Becker muscular dystrophy? Furthermore it is known that nitric oxide inhibits dystrophin proteolysis by Coxsackie virus (20). Could the known reduction in nNOS in DMD (21) thereby predispose these children to cardiomyopathy if they should become infected with this virus? In normal children the spectrum of disease associated with Coxsackievirus infection varies considerably depending on the serotype, but most commonly is relatively benign and self-limited.

Certain bacteria and viruses bind to α-dystroglycan with a resultant up-regulation of matrix metalloproteinase (MMP) which cleaves β-dystroglycan. This may be a natural defense mechanism preventing an infectious agent gaining entry into the host cell. MMP is also activated in skeletal muscles in certain dystrophies (22). Laminin α2 (merosin) is significantly reduced in certain congenital dystrophies. It binds to α-dystroglycan, so if following an infection β-dystroglycan is cleaved, could the resultant reduction of α-dystroglycan, and therefore any bound laminin α2, accentuate any laminin associated dystrophy? In fact severe myocarditis has recently been reported in two sibs with merosin-deficient congenital muscular dystrophy following parvovirus B19 infection (23). This virus can of course be involved in a cardiomyopathy of adulthood (24).

The relationship between infections and the muscular dystrophies, affecting perhaps their onset, progression and severity, is almost an unexplored field. It presents a future challenge to both epidemiologists and molecular biologists.

TREATMENT

Over the years considerable progress has been made in the management of DMD. An effective treatment however still remains elusive. No fewer than 32 different drugs have been tried (17). Only steroids (e.g., prednisone, prednisolone, deflazacort) appear to slow the disease process. Currently there are several international studies designed to determine which particular steroid and dosage regime may be the most effective (see Chapter 11).

Investigators have naturally turned to some form of molecular therapy as holding out a better hope of perhaps finding a cure. A variety of approaches are currently being researched: DNA gene transfer directly or by viral vector, suppression of a stop codon, up-regulation of a possible compensatory protein such as utrophin or even suppression of myostatin, circumventing a mutation (exon skipping) with antisense oligonucleotides, and even perhaps some form of stem cell therapy. These various approaches are dealt with in Section IV of this book.

CONCLUSIONS

In this very brief review of a rapidly expanding field, certain points have been emphasized. Though DMD has been recognized as a distinct clinical entity for 150 years, progress in understanding its cause and possible treatment has only emerged in the last 20 years. Many advances have mirrored contemporary developments in medical science, and the history of the disease actually demonstrates many 'firsts'. It was the first X-linked disease for example to be reported in XO Turner's syndrome in 1957 (thus confirming location of the gene locus on the X chromosome). Bayesian statistics

Introduction

were used in medical genetics for the very first time in 1966 for risk calculations in DMD. Later the gene locus was shown to be linked to a restriction fragment length polymorphism (RFLP) in 1982; and the gene finally isolated in 1985 and its protein product (dystrophin) identified in 1987. This was all achieved by molecular genetic techniques when there was no prior knowledge as to the cause of the disease. Comparable techniques have been employed ever since to locate, identify, and characterize other disease genes.

Now we are entering the final stage in the story: the search for an effective treatment through a variety of molecular techniques.

There is currently an understandable euphoria among those working on the disease. There is little doubt, as Bertolt Brecht, the German playwright and poet put it so elegantly:

Beauty in nature is a quality which gives the human senses a chance to be skillful.

Hopefully such skills will soon benefit patients and their families.

REFERENCES

1. Meryon E. On granular and fatty degeneration of the voluntary muscles. Medico-Chirurgical Transactions 1852; 35:73–84.
2. Duchenne GBA. Recherches sur la paralysie musculaire pseudo-hypertrophique ou paralysie myo-sclérosique. Archives Générales de Médecine 1868; 11:5–25, 179–209, 305–321, 421–443, 552–588.
3. Emery AEH, Emery MLH. The History of a Genetic Disease. London: Royal Society of Medicine Press, 1995.
4. Erb WH. Über die 'juvenile Form' der progressiven Muskelatrophie und ihre Beziehungen zur sogenannten Pseudohypertrophie der Muskeln. Deutsches Archiv für Klinische Medizin 1884; 34:467–519.
5. Erb WH. Dystrophia muscularis progressiva–Klinische und pathologisch-anatomische Studien. Deutsche Zeitschrift für Nervenheilkunde 1891; 1:13–261.
6. Morgan TH, Sturtevant AH, Muller HJ, Bridges CB. The Mechanism of Mendelian Heredity. New York: Henry Holt & Co., 1915.
7. Walton JN. The inheritance of muscular dystrophy. Acta Genetica 1957; 7: 318–320.
8. Okinaka S, Sugita H, Momoi H, Toyokura Y, Kumagai H, Ebashi S, Fujie Y. Serum creatine phosphokinase and aldolase activity in neuromuscular disorders. Transactions of the American Neurological Association 1959; 84:62–64 (84th Annual Meeting, Atlantic City).
9. Murphy EA, Mutalik GS, Eldridge R. The application of Bayesian methods in genetic counselling. Proceedings of the 3rd International Congress of Human Genetics, Chicago, 1966:70.
10. Botstein D, White RL, Skolnick M, Davis RW. Construction of a genetic linkage map in man using restriction fragment length polymorphisms. American Journal of Human Genetics 1980; 32:314–331.

11. Murray JM, Davies KE, Harper PS, Meredith L, Mueller CR, Williamson R. Linkage relationship of a cloned DNA sequence on the short arm of the X chromosome to Duchenne muscular dystrophy. Nature 1982; 300:69–71.
12. Kunkel LM, Monaco AP, Middlesworth W, Ochs HD, Latt SA. Specific cloning of DNA fragments absent from the DNA of a male patient with an X chromosome deletion. Proceedings of the National Academy of Sciences USA 1985; 82:4778–4782.
13. Ray PN, Belfall B, Duff C, et al. Cloning of the breakpoint of an X:21 translocation associated with Duchenne muscular dystrophy. Nature 1985; 318: 672–675.
14. Hoffman EP, Brown RH, Kunkel LM. Dystrophin: the protein product of the Duchenne muscular dystrophy locus. Cell 1987; 51:919–928.
15. Kunkel LM, et al. Analysis of deletions in DNA from patients with Becker and Duchenne muscular dystrophy. Nature 1986; 322:73–77.
16. Campbell KP, Kahl SD. Association of dystrophin and an integral membrane glycoprotein. Nature 1989; 338:259–262.
17. Emery AEH, Muntoni F. Duchenne Muscular Dystrophy. 3rd. Oxford: Oxford University Press, 2003.
18. Badorff C, Lee G, Lamphear BJ, Martone ME, et al. Enteroviral protease 2A cleaves dystrophin; evidence of cytoskeletal disruption in an acquired cardiomyopathy. Nature Medicine 1999; 5:320–326.
19. Lee G-H, Badorff C, Knowlton KU. Dissociation of sarcoglycans and the dystrophin carboxyl terminus from the sarcolemma in enteroviral cardiomyopathy. Circulation Research 2000; 887:489–495.
20. Badorff C, Fichtlscherer B, Rhoads RE, Zeiher AM, Muelsch A, Dimmeler S, Knowlton KU. Nitric oxide inhibits dystrophin proteolysis by Coxsackie viral protease 2A through S-nitrosylation: a protective mechanism against enteroviral cardiomyopathy. Circulation 2000; 102:2276–2281.
21. Sander M, Chavoshan B, Harris SA, et al. Functional muscle ischaemia in neuronal nitric oxide synthase-deficient skeletal muscle of children with Duchenne muscular dystrophy. Proceedings of the National Academy of Sciences, USA 2000; 97:13818–13823.
22. Yamada H, Saito F, Fukuta-Ohi H, et al. Processing of β-dystroglycan by matrix metalloproteinase disrupts the link between the extracellular matrix and cell membrane via the dystroglycan complex. Human Molecular Genetics 2001; 10:1563–1569.
23. Beghetti M, Gervaix A, Haenggeli CA, Berner M, Rimensberger PC. Myocarditis associated with parvovirus B19 infection in two siblings with merosin-deficient congenital muscular dystrophy. European Journal of Pediatrics 2000; 159:135–136.
24. Kuhl U, Pauschinger M, Noutsias M, Seeberg B, Bock T, Lassner D, Poller W, Kandolf R, Schultheiss HP. High prevalence of viral genomes and multiple viral infections in the myocardium of adults with "idiopathic" left ventricular dysfunction. Circulation 2005; 111:887–893.

SECTION I: DUCHENNE MUSCULAR DYSTROPHY BACKGROUND

1

Clinical Overview of Duchenne Muscular Dystrophy

Richard T. Moxley III

Department of Neurology, University of Rochester School of Medicine and Dentistry, Rochester, New York, U.S.A.

HISTORICAL BACKGROUND

Clinical descriptions of Duchenne muscular dystrophy (DMD) have occurred since the mid-1800s. The clinical picture is one of a slowly progressive muscle-wasting disease marked by symptoms that develop before five years of age. Early in its course, DMD affects the proximal hip and shoulder girdle muscles as well as the anterior neck and abdominal muscles (1–4). The progression of weakness is relentless and becomes more disabling in late childhood. Patients receiving only supportive care typically become limited to a wheelchair in late childhood or early teens, and usually die of complications of respiratory insufficiency and/or cardiomyopathy in their late teens or early twenties (3–5).

The first clinical description of this disorder was not actually made by Duchenne. Meryon and Little (4) described the illness several years before Duchenne published his report in 1861. In 1852, Meryon described four brothers who were affected by this disease. He also observed pathologic alterations such as disrupted sarcolemma and oil globules on microscopic examination of skeletal muscle obtained at autopsy. To characterize the clinical course, Meryon described one of the affected brothers' condition. He noted that in infancy, the child was dead weight, and that throughout early childhood, he never jumped. At eight years of age, he had trouble climbing the stairs. At 11 years he could not stand, and by 14, his upper extremities had become extremely weak. At 16, he died. In 1853, Little (4) described two brothers with a typical pattern of weakness. They had hypertrophy of the calf muscles and were unable to walk by 11 years of age. Muscle pathology revealed adipose degeneration (4). In 1861, Duchenne (4) described boys who had hypertrophic paraplegia, which he initially thought was due to a cerebral cause. Later in 1868, he recognized that the disease had its origin in muscle. In 1886, Gowers described a number of boys with DMD and observed the classical sign named after him (Gowers' sign). He drew sketches depicting the way in which patients "walk up their legs" by using their hands to push up from the floor, then push on their knees/thighs to arise to a standing position (3,4) (Fig. 1). In 1891, Erb reported on 89 patients with progressive muscular dystrophy, 29 of whom appeared to have DMD (3). Erb described the clinical features and studied muscle specimens taken from these patients. He identified virtually all the light microscopic alterations that typify DMD, including abnormal variation in fiber size, fiber splitting, proliferation of fibrous and connective tissue, and increased numbers of nuclei in the muscle fibers (3).

In the first half of the twentieth century, clinicians extended our knowledge of the clinical and laboratory findings of inherited muscle disease. From the 1930s to the 1970s, there was increasing interest in muscle biochemistry. Reports described elevation of the serum level of the muscle enzymes, including creatine kinase, in patients with DMD and in the female carriers (6). In 1953, Becker and Kiener described a milder form of X-linked muscular dystrophy, and two years later, Walton described patients with this same milder form of X-linked muscular dystrophy (4). This milder form of dystrophy had similarities to DMD, such as hip girdle weakness and calf muscle hypertrophy, but had delayed onset of symptoms. Patients remained ambulatory into their teens and beyond. This disorder has come to be known as Becker muscular dystrophy. The cause for the muscle wasting and weakness in Duchenne and Becker muscular dystrophies remained a puzzle.

Throughout the 1950s, 1960s, and 1970s, different theories of the pathophysiology of DMD emerged. These theories proposed that the weakness and wasting might result from faulty function of the muscle membrane, neurogenic mechanisms, and vascular pathology (7). A specific focus was on the pathophysiology in the late 1980s with the discovery of the gene responsible for DMD.

DMD results from a mutation in the dystrophin gene which resides in the Xp21 region of the X-chromosome and is associated with the loss of dystrophin, a large cytoskeletal protein (3–5,8–12). Dystrophin attaches to the inner surface of the muscle fiber membrane as a part of a complex of glycoproteins (3–5,8–12). Other chapters in this book discuss the pathogenesis of the mutation and the effects of the mutation in detail. In brief, an alteration in one or more of the functions of dystrophin leads to the characteristic

Clinical Overview of Duchenne Muscular Dystrophy

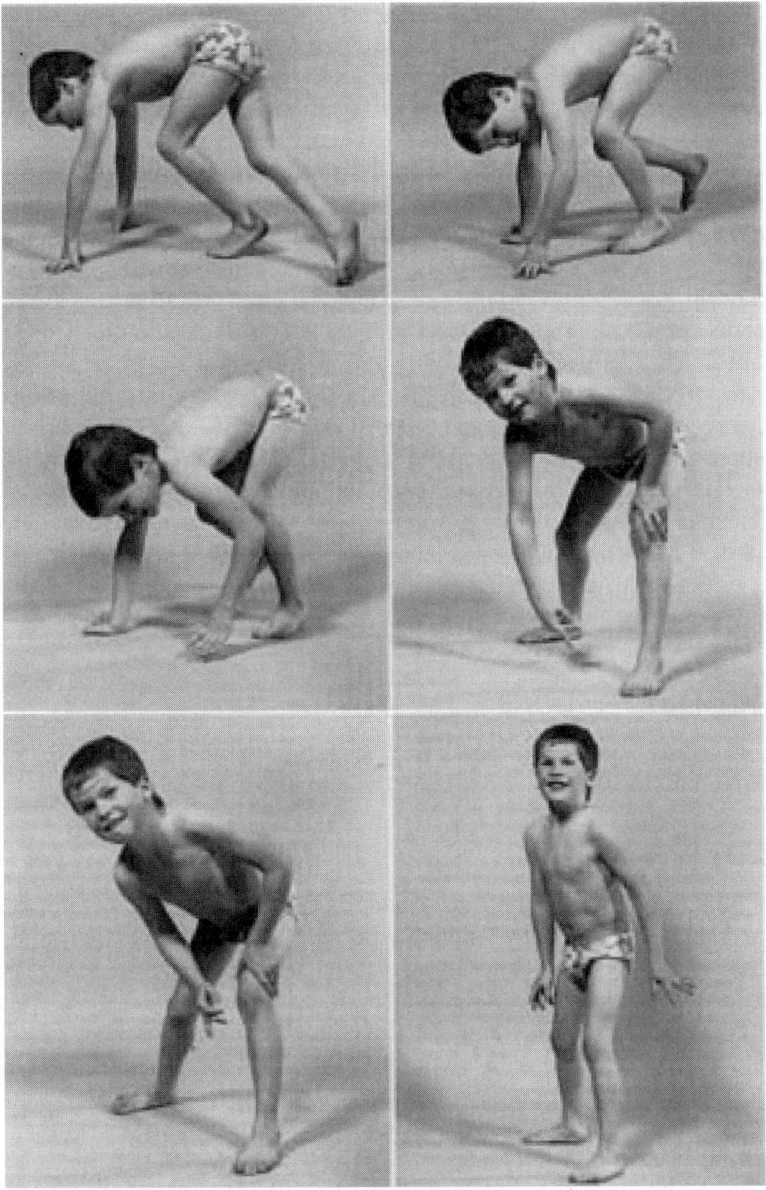

Figure 1 Photographs of Gowers' sign in a boy with DMD. He demonstrates the sequence of maneuvers that constitutes Gowers' sign. The child pushes off the floor with all four extremities, then prepares to push up by moving his hands along the floor close to the feet, and finally placing the hands on the thighs and pushing up to the erect position. The maneuver is necessary primarily because of marked weakness of hip extensor muscles.

pattern of muscle wasting and weakness, and causes damage to other tissues in which dystrophin is expressed, including the heart, respiratory muscles, gastrointestinal smooth muscle, and the brain (3–5,8–12).

A few of the key discoveries in the search for the gene mutation are noted below. In 1983, Dr. Kay Davies, (13) while working in the laboratory of Professor Bob Williamson in London, England, found a link between the polymorphic DNA marker (RC8) and the DMD gene. The marker mapped the DMD locus to the middle of the short arm of the X-chromosome, the Xp21 region. Becker muscular dystrophy also mapped to this region, indicating that this form of muscular dystrophy had a close link to or was allelic to the locus for DMD. In 1986 Louis Kunkel (14) isolated the Duchenne/Becker muscular dystrophy gene, and in 1987 Hoffman et al. (15) identified the protein product of that gene, dystrophin. The discovery that mutations in the dystrophin gene were responsible for DMD led to the development of diagnostic testing and new ideas about its pathomechanism and treatment. Whereas later chapters discuss details of diagnostic principles, mutation detection, and dystrophin protein analysis, this chapter gives an overview of the clinical picture and current management of DMD. This chapter also includes questions to consider as we address the challenges and the opportunities to develop better treatments.

CLINICAL MANIFESTATIONS

DMD progresses through three clinical stages: an ambulatory stage, an early nonambulatory stage, and a late nonambulatory stage.

Ambulatory Stage

In the ambulatory stage, symptoms usually become apparent between two and four years of age. Parents notice weakness of forward head flexion, and a limited ability to sit up persists beyond infancy. This weakness is accompanied by slowed motor development. Patients have difficulty keeping up with their peers, physically and sometimes cognitively. A selective deficit in verbal working memory skills is common (4). Early in this stage patients usually can play with their peers in most activities, but by the first or second grade some adaptation of physical education requirements becomes necessary. Special classes in school may also be necessary to assist patients in keeping up to grade level. Heel cord and elbow flexion contractures may become evident as patients have more difficulty walking. Respiratory, gastrointestinal, and significant cardiac problems are uncommon at this stage. Occasionally obstructive sleep apnea develops, or problems with fecal soiling occur. The typical cardiac findings are asymptomatic electrocardiographic alterations: Q waves in the lateral precordial leads and tall R and deep S waves in the early precordial leads (3,4).

Often by nine years of age, ambulatory patients not receiving treatment with glucocorticoids (see Chapter 7) lose their ability to rise from supine to standing position and to climb stairs (1,2). Patients often lose their ability to arise from a chair before they lose their ability to climb stairs (1). Eventually, patients are able to ambulate only with the help of braces, and the duration of this type of ambulation is relatively short. The average time between assisted ambulation with braces and being confined to a wheelchair is three years, with a range of one to six years (2). Once patients become unable to ambulate in braces, they can use the braces to permit standing and weight bearing.

Early Nonambulatory Stage

The natural history of DMD reveals that a patient will become wheelchair-dependent between 10 and 12 years of age (1,2). In the early nonambulatory stage of DMD, flexion contractures at the ankles and elbows become more apparent (see Chapter 9). Physical activity, such as standing in braces and aquatic therapy, may slow the rate of their progression (see Chapter 8). Patients who are able to stand in braces are often able to ambulate in water during aquatic therapy. Standing a few hours each day with the help of braces as well as weight bearing during aquatic therapy may also delay curvature of the spine, but after a few years of wheelchair dependency, patients typically develop significant scoliosis requiring orthopedic consultation and radiological evaluation (see Chapters 8 and 9).

Figures 2, 3, and 4 depict important features of the natural history of weakness in DMD in individuals between 3 and 16 years of age and provide a helpful overview of the clinical course during both the ambulatory and the early nonambulatory stages of the disease. The data were obtained from a study of 114 boys with the clinical diagnosis of DMD, none of whom had received corticosteroid therapy prior to or at the time of these evaluations (1). The DMD was diagnosed before the discovery of the gene for dystrophin, and subsequent analysis of DNA and muscle biopsies in this group has revealed that the "outliers" mentioned in the reports (1,2) (who had relatively preserved muscle strength and function) had Becker muscular dystrophy. Figure 2 shows a linear decline in average muscle strength from 3 to 16 years of age (1). This linear decline in average muscle score has served as a reproducible measure of treatment efficacy in subsequent therapeutic trials in DMD (see Chapters 7 and 11) (16,17). From three to eight years of age, patients typically have an average strength score that is well above the antigravity level; however, by nine years of age average strength declines, being only barely above the level required to move against gravity. At this point, the patient often struggles to continue walking. Figure 3 presents the same average strength score data as in Figure 2 as percentiles, with the centerline representing the 50th percentile for average

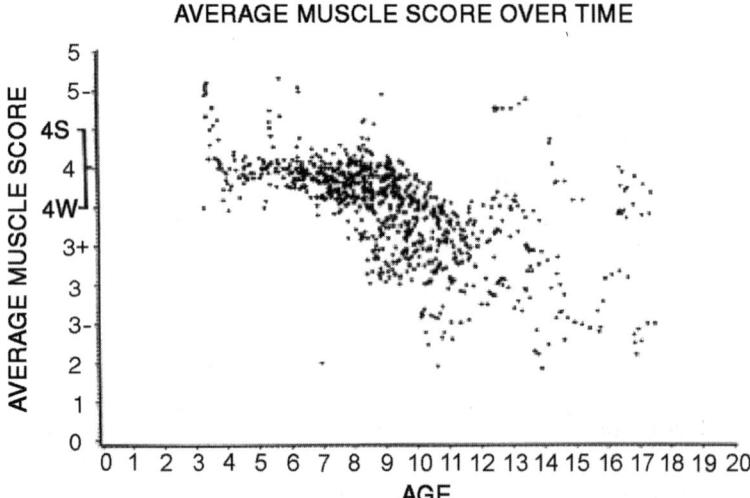

Figure 2 Scatter plot of average muscle score versus the age of the patient at the time the observation was made ($R = 0.47$; $P < 0.0001$). The average muscle score indicates the numerical average of a standard set of 34 muscles. Scores were from 114 patients with the clinical diagnosis of DMD ranging in age from 3 to 16 years and were determined from examinations performed serially: at baseline, 2, 3, 6, 9, and 12 years. Each patient took placebo pills daily. None had taken corticosteroids. These values demonstrate a linear decline in strength as the patients become older. The average value for the slopes of the serial muscle scores per year is 0.49 ± 0.86 units per year (mean $\pm$ standard deviation). *Source*: From Ref. 1.

strength score. Figure 4 presents the 50th percentile data for individual muscles and reveals the pattern of weakness that contributes to the loss of ambulation (1). Careful review of Figure 4 indicates that from early childhood until 16 years of age, the plantar flexor and foot invertor muscles remain close to normal in strength, and that the wrist flexor and extensor, ankle dorsiflexor, and neck extensor muscles also remain well above antigravity in power over the same age range. Knee flexor, shoulder abductor, elbow flexor, and extensor muscles show somewhat greater weakness throughout childhood and early teens. More prominent weakness occurs in the knee extensor, shoulder rotator, and hip flexor muscles. Taken together, these specific muscles go from being able to overcome gravity between three to eight years of age to becoming less than antigravity in power between nine to twelve years of age. However, the greatest muscle weakness in DMD occurs in the neck flexor, external rotators of the shoulder, hip extensor, and hip abductor muscles. The neck flexors remain less than antigravity in power throughout the clinical course of DMD in patients not treated with corticosteroids. The hip extensors and abductors typically become less than

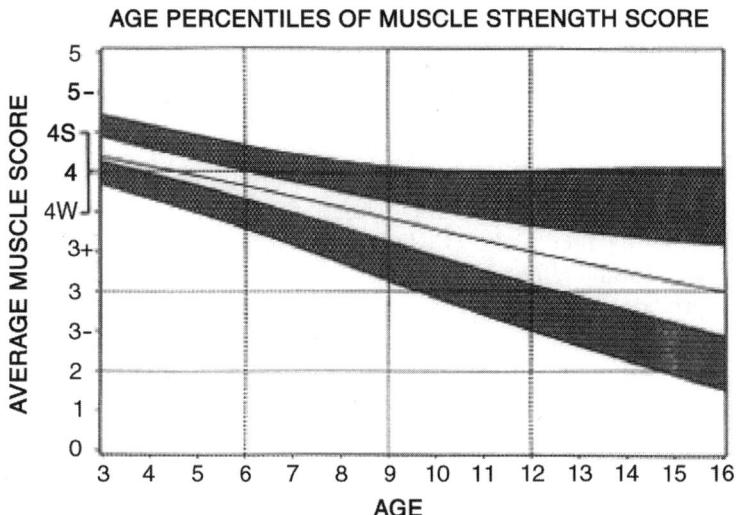

Figure 3 Same data as in Figure 2 plotted as percentiles of the population. The line in the center represents the 50th percentile; the shaded areas span from 5th to 25th percentile and 75th to 95th percentile.

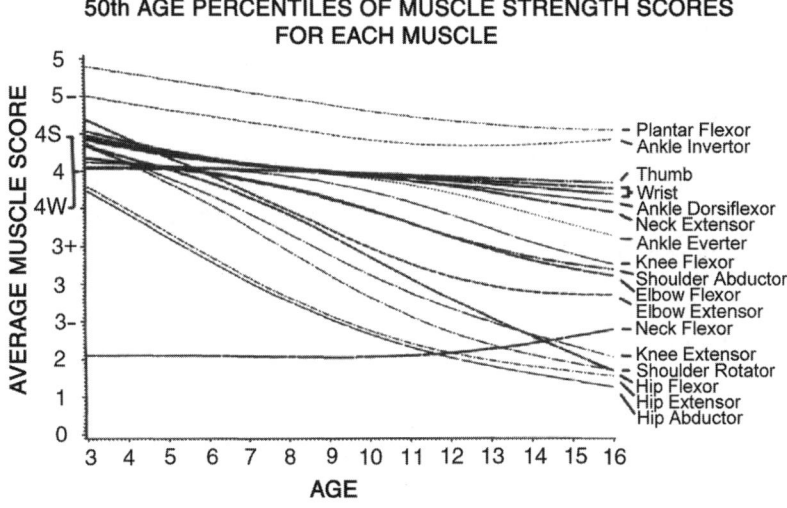

Figure 4 The strength data of individual muscles from the same patients in Figure 2 represented as the 50th percentile of muscle strength plotted against age.

antigravity in strength by eight years of age. One note of correction is necessary regarding the apparent improvement in neck flexor strength that appears in Figure 4 after 11 years of age. This is an artifact caused by the small group of outliers with Becker muscular dystrophy who participated in the study. They had greater than antigravity strength in their neck flexor muscles and exerted a disproportionate effect on the 50th percentile curve in the older age range. For a complete discussion of the natural history of muscle manifestations in patients with DMD (not receiving glucocorticoid treatment), the reader should refer to the two papers by Brooke et al. (1,2). These manuscripts provide an excellent description and commentary on the natural history of DMD.

Late Nonambulatory Stage

Transition of the patient from the early nonambulatory stage of DMD into the late nonambulatory stage is less easily described than the movement from the ambulatory to the early nonambulatory stage. Patients who have progressed into the late nonambulatory stage of the disease not only have a wheelchair-to-bed lifestyle, but also struggle with many of the serious long-term complications of DMD. These include respiratory insufficiency/ failure, cardiac problems, and gastrointestinal dysfunction (3–5). They also have more orthopedic problems related to the progressive joint contractures and scoliosis, which typically worsen in the late nonambulatory stage of illness.

Respiratory Insufficiency

The natural history of DMD in patients not receiving corticosteroid therapy indicates that between the ages of 11 and 20, the forced vital capacity will decline to less than 60% to 70% of normal (on average less than 2.0 L) (2). This reduction in forced vital capacity correlates with a decreased power of coughing and an increased occurrence of pneumonia. Decreased effective night-time ventilation during sleep occurs prior to frank respiratory failure (18,19), but more study of the natural history of diaphragm and other respiratory muscle weakness is needed (19). When the forced vital capacity falls to less than 1.0 L and/or the partial pressure of carbon dioxide ($PaCO_2$) is greater than 45 mm Hg, patients have a poor three to five year survival (18–20).

Cardiomyopathy

As noted above, electrocardiographic abnormalities occur even in the ambulatory stage (increased R/S amplitude in lead V1 and deep Q waves in V5, V6) (3,4). Atrial arrhythmias of varying types occur commonly in the late stage of DMD, and ventricular arrhythmias occur less frequently (3,4,21,22). Echocardiography reveals that the primary alteration develops in left ventricular function in the late stages of disease (23,24). Resting tachycardia is common throughout each stage of DMD and may be caused by autonomic dysfunction that is separate from dysfunction of the left ventricle (25,26). More study is necessary to determine the role of autonomic regulation of heart rhythm in the pathophysiology of DMD. Pathological study confirms the echocardiographic findings and demonstrates that the major damage occurs in the ventricles, especially in the posterobasilar area of the left ventricle (27,28).

Gastrointestinal Dysfunction

The esophageal and gastrointestinal complaints involve both voluntary and smooth muscles. This fits with the fact that there is a deficiency of dystrophin in voluntary and smooth muscles (3,4,28,29).

Bulbar weakness (both in the upper voluntary skeletal muscle portion of the pharyngeal–esophageal tract and in the lower involuntary smooth muscle portion) occurs, and there is frequent clearing of the throat and coughing (especially at the time of meals), in the late stage of DMD (30). Delayed gastric emptying may also become a problem (29). Acute gastric dilatation can occur occasionally and increase the risk of respiratory insufficiency due to pressure upward on the diaphragm (31). Chronic intestinal dysfunction with constipation, distention, hypomotility, and impaction is common in the late stages of DMD. Hypokalemia and insufficient intake of fluid, primarily water, aggravate the slowed intestinal motility and the difficulty in maintaining regular bowel movements. Chronic intestinal dysfunction can also hamper ventilation and diaphragmatic movement during sleep. There is a suspicion that chronic gastrointestinal distention may predispose patients to pelvic and lower extremity venous thrombosis, but this clinical impression has not been examined with controlled studies.

DIAGNOSIS

Diagnosis hinges on careful history taking and physical examination, as well as on laboratory testing (i.e., serum creatine kinase levels and leucocyte DNA testing for the DMD mutation), and in situations in which DNA testing is not informative, on obtaining a muscle biopsy. Creatine kinase levels are markedly elevated in the early ambulatory stage of DMD, being well above 10 times higher than normal (1,3,4). Figure 5 provides an algorithm to follow for the workup of a child with an elevation of creatine kinase and signs suggestive of DMD. Table 1 provides clinical and laboratory diagnostic criteria for DMD and contrasts that information with the diagnostic criteria for Becker muscular dystrophy. Other chapters (see Chapters 4 and 5) cover this information in detail. In the past few years, major advances have occurred in genetic screening for mutations in DMD. Now there are

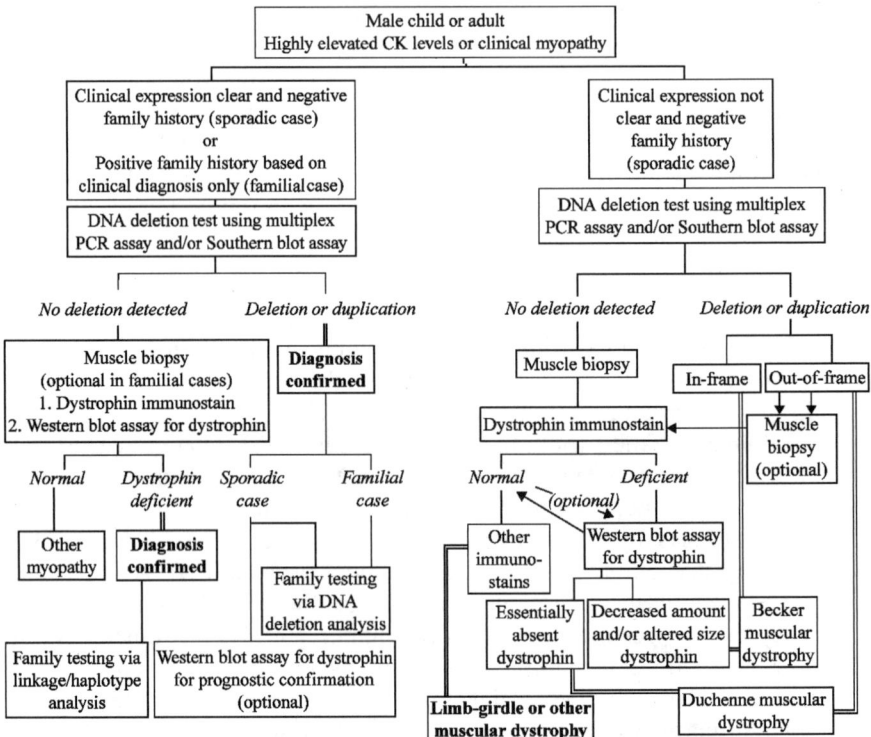

Figure 5 Workup for child who is suspected to have DMD. This figure is an algorithm for the laboratory diagnosis of sporadic and familial cases of Duchenne and Becker muscular dystrophy and for family testing (carrier detection and prenatal or presymptomatic diagnosis). *Abbreviations*: CK, creatine kinase; DMD, Duchenne muscular dystrophy; PCR, polymerase chain reaction. *Source*: From Ref. 4.

economical methods available to detect duplications of one or more exons (32) and to identify point mutations (33). Previously point mutations and duplications required lengthy procedures to be performed, and as a result the only feasible testing was to look for large deletions in the gene.

More unpleasant diagnostic testing for the patient, such as electrodiagnosis and muscle biopsy, are often not carried out. Electromyography and nerve conduction testing are rarely necessary. In sporadic cases of DMD, a muscle biopsy helps to distinguish many of the recently described autosomal dominant and autosomal recessive forms of limb-girdle muscular dystrophy (LGMD) (34–36). Certain forms of LGMD have a close clinical similarity to DMD, and without a clear abnormality on DNA testing to establish the diagnosis of DMD, muscle biopsy with appropriate membrane associated protein immunostaining is necessary along with Western blot analysis. Table 2 summarizes the major features of the dominant and

Table 1 Clinical and Laboratory Diagnostic Criteria for Duchenne Muscular Dystrophy and for Becker Muscular Dystrophy

	Duchenne dystrophy	Becker dystrophy
Onset	Before age 5; typically between 2 and 4 years of age	After age 5; can begin in adult life
Initial symptoms	Cannot run or keep up with peers; climbs only one step at a time	Fatigue or marked thigh weakness; trouble climbing steps; occasional calf or thigh cramps; patient can ambulate beyond the age of 15 years
Serum creatine kinase	At least 10 times above normal	At least 5 times above normal
Leukocyte DNA testing	Perform DNA testing as the initial diagnostic procedure (Fig. 5)	Same as Duchenne dystrophy
Muscle biopsy	Active myopathy, absence of dystrophin, severe reduction in dystrophin–associated proteins	Moderately active myopathy, absence or deficiency of dystrophin, reduction in dystrophin–associated proteins
Electrodiagnostic testing	Normal nerve conduction; myopathic EMG; electrodiagnostic testing usually not necessary	Normal nerve conduction; mildly myopathic EMG

Abbreviation: EMG, electromyography.

recessive forms of LGMD. Other myopathies, such as the congenital muscular dystrophies, congenital myopathies, childhood myotonic dystrophy (DM1), and facioscapulohumeral muscular dystrophy, can be distinguished by clinical evaluation and history taking.

It is mainly certain forms of LGMD and the occasional Becker muscular dystrophy presented by a patient before five years of age that pose a challenge in the differential diagnosis of DMD. The usual criterion to distinguish Becker dystrophy from DMD is that the patient with Becker dystrophy remains ambulatory after 15 years of age. This occurs without treatment with prednisone. In a patient with Becker dystrophy who is seen before 15 years of age and who has symptoms before five years of age, the diagnosis becomes very difficult. Greater reliance is placed upon the use of Western blot analysis of dystrophin and on immunostaining of the muscle biopsy for dystrophin. Even with Western blot data, there may be a limitation in predicting the clinical course in a particular patient.

Table 2 Distinguishing Features for Diagnosis of the Limb-Girdle Muscular Dystrophies

Disease	Age at onset, years	Dinstinctive feature	CK level	Linkage	Protein product	Diagnostic modalities
Autosomal dominant						
LGMD1A	20–40	Dysarthria	NL–10X	5q22.3–31.3	Myotilin	DNA only
LGMD1B	<10	Contractures	NL–20X	1q11–21	Lamin A/C	DNA only
LGMD1C	<10	Mounding/rippling	2–25X	3p25	Caveolin-3	IS, WB
LGMD1D	15–50	Cardiomyopathy	NL–4X	6q23	Unknown	
LGMD1E	30–50	No	NL–10X	7q	Unknown	
Autosomal recessive						
LGMD2A	5–40	Adductor weakness	NL–50X	15q15.1	Calpain-3	WB
LGMD2B	10–30	Distal leg weakness	10–150X	2p13	Dysferlin	IS, WB
LGMD2C-F	3–20	No	5–120X	13q, 17q, 4q, 5q	γ–, α–, β–, δ–sarcoglycan	IS, WB
LGMD2G	2–15	Brazilian	2–30X	17q11-q12	Telethonin	IS, WB
LGMD2H	5–30	Hutterite	NL–20X	9q31-q34	TRIM32	DNA only
LGMD2I	1–40	Respiratory dysfunction	5–40X	19q13.3	Fukutin related protein	DNA only
LGMD2J	5–20	Finns	NL–2X	2q31	Titin	DNA only

Abbreviations: CK, creatine kinase; IS, immunostaining; NL, normal; WB, western blotting; X, times above upper limit of normal.
Source: Ref. 37.

TREATMENT

Supportive Treatment

The overall goals in managing patients who have DMD are to maintain ambulation for as long as possible, to optimize the development of the patient's cognitive abilities, and to anticipate the occurrence of complications such as excessive weight gain, joint contractures (especially of the Achilles tendons), respiratory insufficiency, scoliosis, gastrointestinal hypomotility, and cardiomyopathy (3–5). Table 3 summarizes the principal problems and treatment options.

The patient/family need to work closely with the physicians, schoolteachers, physical educators, and physical and occupational therapists to develop an individualized care plan for each stage of DMD. Often, lightweight long-leg bracing is helpful in the final months of the ambulatory stage to prolong weight bearing and ambulation, both of which delay the development of joint contractures and scoliosis. Contractures develop primarily during the early and late nonambulatory stages of the disease after the patient becomes wheelchair bound. They do not appear at a specific age but depend largely on the functional ability of the patient. Once contractures begin to develop, usually at the ankles and elbows (flexion and pronation), it is important to obtain physical therapy and occupational therapy consultations. Other chapters (see Chapters 8 and 9) give a detailed description of treatment.

Scoliosis develops in the early nonambulatory stage (wheel-chair dependent) and often accelerates in the late nonambulatory stage (respiratory insufficiency) of DMD. Orthopedic consultation and serial follow-up to monitor contractures and degree of spinal curvature are part of the optimal care (see Chapter 9). Most spine surgeons recommend preventive stabilization surgery in DMD once the patient is nonambulatory and the major curve exceeds 20 degrees (see Chapter 9). Prior to spinal stabilization surgery and any major surgery in patients with DMD, it is necessary for the neurologist and primary care physician to obtain consultations with specialists in pulmonary medicine and cardiology.

An involved primary care physician is essential in the early, middle, and late stages of DMD treatment. Minor medical problems can provoke major complications. In the later stages, a mild cold may lead to atelectatic pneumonitis and acute respiratory insufficiency. Even chronic constipation can produce respiratory compromise in the later stages of DMD, due to abdominal distention and upward pressure on the diaphragm. Respiratory insufficiency is common in the late stages of DMD. Forced vital capacity declines, usually into the range of 600 to 1000 mL (2). Recent reports describe the management options, which include nasal ventilation rather than positive pressure ventilation via tracheostomy (18–20).

Periodic consultations by a pulmonologist are important once patients are wheelchair bound. Pulmonary consultation prior to and after general

Table 3 Complications and Treatment for Duchenne and Becker Muscular Dystrophy

	Duchenne dystrophy	Becker dystrophy
Muscle weakness	Treatment with prednisone 0.75 mg/kg/day or deflazacort 0.9 mg/kg/day slows or stabilizes muscle strength; lightweight long leg bracing maintains ambulation in later stages	No controlled studies of prednisone treatment; bracing is helpful in late stages
Respiratory problems	Forced vital capacity is monitored (in later stages, atelectatic pneumonitis is common); colds are treated aggressively; if signs of respiratory failure develop, nasal/oral ventilation should be considered	Uncommon until late stages; management then is as with Duchenne dystrophy
Cardiac problems	Occasionally cardiomyopathy leads to congestive heart failure—afterload reducing therapy often helps, though the role of digoxin is uncertain; patients should be monitored for intracardiac clots	Occasionally severe cardiomyopathy develops; treatment is the same as for Duchenne dystrophy
Orthopedic problems	Achilles tendon contractures respond to stretching in early stages; contractures at the hips, knees, elbows, and wrists usually develop after the patient becomes wheelchair bound; scoliosis often develops when patients stop ambulating, and spinal stabilization surgery helps maintain use of the arms and preserves pulmonary reserve	Uncommon; contractures are much less common than in Duchenne dystrophy; mainly occur in Achilles tendon
Nervous system symptoms	Increased incidence of cognitive and behavioral problems; some patients improve with small doses of methylphenidate	Uncommon
Gastrointestinal dysfunction	Hypomotility with constipation is common, especially late in the disease; careful dietary	Uncommon

(*Continued*)

Table 3 Complications and Treatment for Duchenne and Becker Muscular Dystrophy (*Continued*)

	Duchenne dystrophy	Becker dystrophy
	monitoring, stool softeners, and good water intake (urine specific gravities 1.007–1.010) usually are effective; occasionally acute gastric dilation occurs; it resolves over 2–3 days with NG tube decompression of the stomach and intravenous hydration	

Abbreviation: NG tube, nasogastric tube.

anesthesia is an integral part of elective surgery in DMD. The preoperative consultation often includes training of the patient/care providers in the use of assisted coughing techniques and in the use of nasal bilevel positive airway pressure (BIPAP). Using nasal BIPAP and assisted coughing techniques speeds up recovery after general anesthesia. These treatments lessen the likelihood of postoperative pneumonia, and in outpatients they help to prevent the development of pneumonia with troublesome upper respiratory infections (19).

In the later stages of DMD, considerable discussion about significant pulmonary problems is necessary to educate the patients and their families, and to guide them in choosing treatment they believe is most appropriate for the patients. Often neuromuscular physicians and nurses are the individuals who educate the family, and the roles of the pediatric pulmonologist, other specialists, and the primary care physician have to be tailored to each medical care setting.

Acute gastric dilation is an infrequent complication in the late stages of DMD (29,31). This typically occurs in association with an idiopathic metabolic acidosis and responds rapidly to nasogastric tube decompression of the stomach and intravenous hydration. Caution must be used with intravenous repletion of potassium because in the late stages of the disease, the muscle mass of the patient is considerably diminished and is not available to buffer an acute rise in extracellular potassium. The cause of the gastric dilation is unknown, but this problem, as well as the chronic intestinal hypomotility (constipation), probably results from the deficiency of dystrophin in the smooth muscle of the gastrointestinal (GI) tract (27–29). Good hydration, a balanced dietary intake, and regular bowel habits are the mainstays of treatment for these problems.

Symptomatic cardiomyopathy gradually develops in a significant number of patients in the late stages of DMD (3,4,21–27). A chest roentgenogram typically reveals cardiomegaly, and the cardiac ejection fraction falls to 10%

to 20% of normal. Heart failure is often exacerbated by coexisting respiratory insufficiency. In all these cases, simultaneous ventilatory support must be considered provided the patient/family have decided to pursue a vigorous course of treatment for illness. Heart failure in its advanced stage is difficult to manage, and early treatment with afterload reduction therapy is often more effective than digoxin. Typically, initial treatment is with an angiotensin converting enzyme inhibitor, and titrating the diastolic blood pressure to 60 to 70 mm of Hg. If left ventricular dysfunction persists or worsens, beta-blocker therapy is necessary with the goal of keeping heart rate between 55 and 70 beats per minute. Cardiology consultation needs to guide the care plan. Occasionally ventricular and/or atrial clots are present, and long-term anticoagulant therapy is necessary.

Corticosteroid Therapy (Prednisone, Deflazacort)

The only effective treatment for DMD is corticosteroid (glucocorticoid) therapy with prednisone, prednisolone, or deflazacort (16,17,38), a topic which is considered in detail in Ref. 38 and in Chapters 7 and 11. Patients treated with prednisone preferably should be monitored by or coordinated by technicians in specialized neuromuscular centers. The protocol for monitoring side effects and for assessing muscle strength and function have been published previously (16). To monitor the development of side effects, patients are seen every three months, and weight, blood pressure, pulse, forced vital capacity, urinalysis, and neuromuscular function are checked. At each visit, patients undergo timed function testing (time needed to travel 30 feet, to arise from supine to standing position, and to climb four standard steps). Patients undergo an evaluation of muscle strength (shoulder abductors, elbow flexors and extensors, knee extensors, and hip flexors and extensors). These measures of vital signs and neuromuscular status help guide the physician in adjusting the dosage of corticosteroid treatment. The blood count and serum electrolyte levels are measured at six month intervals. With close follow-up, patients have been kept stable or showed only very mild progression of muscle weakness for periods exceeding five years (16,17). Even in the late stages, corticosteroid therapy appears to maintain respiratory muscle power and has slowed the development of respiratory failure (16,17).

QUESTIONS AND OPPORTUNITIES RELATED TO FUTURE TREATMENT FOR DMD

Major challenges exist for patients, clinicians, and researchers as they join efforts to develop effective treatment for DMD. But, realistic hope for the identification of better treatment arises not only from the major advances in gene therapy and the breakthroughs in molecular biology, but also from the results of clinical trials. The success of corticosteroid therapy in DMD has led to a number of questions that when answered may lead to significant improvements in treatment. A number of questions are given below that need consideration.

What are the cellular mechanisms that underlie the beneficial effects of corticosteroids in DMD? What is the best approach to treatment (dosage and frequency) to optimize these beneficial effects and minimize side effects? Are corticosteroids more effective, even in lower dosages, if administration was started in very young patients? What is the most appropriate way to define the natural history of DMD in very young patients so that a reliable assessment of early treatment with corticosteroid therapy can occur? What are the limitations to establishing the diagnosis in the very young (birth to four years of age)? Are there other medications that can amplify, or "synergize," the beneficial effects? Does prednisone exert a beneficial effect on tissues other than skeletal muscle, such as heart, brain, and smooth muscle? How can better methods be developed and studies performed to assess the quality of life in patients with DMD from infancy to adulthood? How can those methods be used to examine the influence of long-term corticosteroid therapy on the quality of life in DMD patients?

There are questions related to the bone and joint manifestations in DMD. What changes occur in bone density and joint range of motion with long-term treatment with prednisone? What is the natural history of changes in bone density in DMD in the absence of corticosteroid treatment, and how is it used to compare the changes observed in other childhood neuromuscular diseases, such as spinal muscular atrophy, early onset congenital myopathies, various forms of limb girdle muscular dystrophy, and congenital muscular dystrophies? What effect does aquatic therapy have on joint range of motion and force vital capacity (FVC) in nonambulatory DMD patients with and without corticosteroid treatment?

Questions about the pulmonary and cardiac complications of DMD need to be explored. What are the most reliable early indications of respiratory insufficiency and cardiac failure in DMD? Would "preemptive treatment" with cardiac medications or corticosteroids improve the level of function and quality of life? What studies can be designed to document the natural history of the late stages of DMD and what investigations can be initiated to determine the efficacy of corticosteroid therapy when initiated late in the course of DMD (e.g., after 15 years of age)?

With all these questions, there are many opportunities for translational research in DMD. What have we learned about the role of dystrophin? What do animal models tell us, and do they provide a means of screening a potential treatment? How do we utilize the advances in gene transfer to treat DMD? How can we use the support of patients and be prepared to evaluate potential therapies? What are some strategies we can pursue to optimize therapy with prednisone?

REFERENCES

1. Brooke MH, Fenichel GM, Griggs RC, et al. Clinical investigation in Duchenne dystrophy: 2. Determination of the "power" of therapeutic trials based on the natural history. Muscle Nerve 1983; 6(2):91–103.
2. Brooke MH, Fenichel GM, Griggs RC, et al. Duchenne muscular dystrophy: patterns of clinical progression and effects of supportive therapy. Neurology 1989; 39(4):475–481.
3. Engel A, Yamamoto M, Fischbeck K. Dystrophinopathies. In: Engel A, Franzini-Armstrong C, eds. Myology: Basic and Clinical. New York: McGraw-Hill, Inc, 1994:1133–1187.
4. Darras BT, Menache CC, Kunkel LM. Dystrophinopathies. In: Jones HR, DeVivo DC, Darras BT, eds. Neuromuscular Disorders of Infancy, Childhood, and Adolescence—A Clinician's Approach. Amsterdam: Butterworth Heinemann, 2003:649–700.
5. Hoffman EP. Dystrophinopathies. In: Karpati G, Hilton-Jones D, Griggs RC, eds. Disorders of Voluntary Muscle. Cambridge: Cambridge University Press, 2001:385–482.
6. Pennington R. Serum enzymes. In: Rowland L, ed. Pathogenesis of Human Muscular Dystrophies. Amsterdam: Excerpta Medica, 1977:341–349.
7. Rowland LP. Pathogenesis of muscular dystrophies. Arch Neurol 1976; 33(5): 315–321.
8. Rando TA. The dystrophin-glycoprotein complex, cellular signaling, and the regulation of cell survival in the muscular dystrophies. Muscle Nerve 2001; 24(12):1575–1594.
9. Nobile C, Marchi J, Nigro V, Roberts RG, Danieli GA. Exon-intron organization of the human dystrophin gene. Genomics 1997; 45(2):421–424.
10. Ozawa E, Noguchi S, Mizuno Y, Hagiwara Y, Yoshida M. From dystrophinopathy to sarcoglycanopathy: evolution of a concept of muscular dystrophy. Muscle Nerve 1998; 21(4):421–438.
11. Ahn AH, Kunkel LM. The structural and functional diversity of dystrophin. Nat Genet 1993; 3(4):283–291.
12. Muntoni F, Gobbi P, Sewry C, et al. Deletions in the 5' region of dystrophin and resulting phenotypes. J Med Genet 1994; 31(11):843–847.
13. Davies KE, Pearson PL, Harper PS, et al. Linkage analysis of two cloned DNA sequences flanking the Duchenne muscular dystrophy locus on the short arm of the human X chromosome. Nucleic Acids Res 1983; 11(8):2303–2312.
14. Kunkel LM. Analysis of deletions in DNA from patients with Becker and Duchenne muscular dystrophy. Nature 1986; 322(6074):73–77.
15. Hoffman EP, Brown RH Jr, Kunkel LM. Dystrophin: the protein product of the Duchenne muscular dystrophy locus. Cell 1987; 51(6):919–928.
16. Moxley RT. Corticosteroid and anabolic hormone treatment of Duchenne's muscular dystrophy. In: Jones HR, DeVivo DC, Darras BT, eds. Neuromuscular Disorders of Infancy, Childhood, and Adolescence—A Clinician's Approach. Amsterdam: Butterworth Heinemann, 2003:1209–1225.
17. Manzur AY, Kuntzer T, Pike M, Swan A. Glucocorticoid corticosteroids for Duchenne muscular dystrophy. Cochrane Review 2004; (2):1–61.

18. Vianello A, Bevilacqua M, Salvador V, Cardaioli C, Vincenti E. Long-term nasal intermittent positive pressure ventilation in advanced Duchenne's muscular dystrophy. Chest 1994; 105(2):445–448.
19. Finder JCCP. Respiratory care of the patient with Duchenne muscular dystrophy: an official ATS consensus statement. Am J Respir Crit Care Med 2004; 170(4):456–465.
20. Phillips MF, Quinlivan RC, Edwards RH, Calverley PM. Changes in spirometry over time as a prognostic marker in patients with Duchenne muscular dystrophy. Am J Respir Crit Care Med 2001; 164:2191–2194.
21. Yanagisawa A, Miyagawa M, Yotsukura M, et al. The prevalence and prognostic significance of arrhythmias in Duchenne type muscular dystrophy. Am Heart J 1992; 124(5):1244–1250.
22. Chenard AA, Becane HM, Tertrain F, de Kermadec JM, Weiss YA. Ventricular arrhythmia in Duchenne muscular dystrophy: prevalence, significance and prognosis. Neuromuscul Disord 1993; 3(3):201–206.
23. de Kermadec JM, Becane HM, Chenard A, Tertrain F, Weiss Y. Prevalence of left ventricular systolic dysfunction in Duchenne muscular dystrophy: an echocardiographic study. Am Heart J 1994; 127(3):618–623.
24. Takenaka A, Yokota M, Iwase M, Miyaguchi K, Hayashi H, Saito H. Discrepancy between systolic and diastolic dysfunction of the left ventricle in patients with Duchenne muscular dystrophy. Eur Heart J 1993; 14(5):669–676.
25. Yotsukura M, Fujii K, Katayama A, et al. Nine-year follow-up study of heart rate variability in patients with Duchenne-type progressive muscular dystrophy. Am Heart J 1998; 136(2):289–296.
26. Lanza GA, Dello RA, Giglio V, et al. Impairment of cardiac autonomic function in patients with Duchenne muscular dystrophy: relationship to myocardial and respiratory function. Am Heart J 2001; 141(5):808–812.
27. Moriuchi T, Kagawa N, Mukoyama M, Hizawa K. Autopsy analyses of the muscular dystrophies. Tokushima J Exp Med 1993; 40(1–2):83–93.
28. Boland BJ, Silbert PL, Groover RV, Wollan PC, Silverstein MD. Skeletal, cardiac, and smooth muscle failure in Duchenne muscular dystrophy. Pediatr Neurol 1996; 14(1):7–12.
29. Barohn RJ, Levine EJ, Olson JO, Mendell JR. Gastric hypomotility in Duchenne's muscular dystrophy. N Engl J Med 1988; 319(1):15–18.
30. Jaffe KM, McDonald CM, Ingman E, Haas J. Symptoms of upper gastrointestinal dysfunction in Duchenne muscular dystrophy: case-control study. Arch Phys Med Rehabil 1990; 71(10):742–744.
31. Bensen ES, Jaffe KM, Tarr PI. Acute gastric dilatation in Duchenne muscular dystrophy: a case report and review of the literature. Arch Phys Med Rehabil 1996; 77(5):512–514.
32. White S, Kalf M, Liu Q, et al. Comprehensive detection of genomic duplications and deletions in the DMD gene, by use of multiplex amplifiable probe hybridization. Am J Hum Genet 2002; 71(2):365–374.
33. Flanigan KM, von Niederhausern A, Dunn DM, Alder J, Mendell JR, Weiss RB. Rapid direct sequence analysis of the dystrophin gene. Am J Hum Genet 2003; 72(4):931–939.

34. Laval SH, Bushby KM. Limb-girdle muscular dystrophies—from genetics to molecular pathology. Neuropathol Appl Neurobiol 2004; 30(2):91–105.
35. Bushby KM, Beckmann JS. The 105th ENMC sponsored workshop: pathogenesis in the non-sarcoglycan limb-girdle muscular dystrophies, Naarden, April 12–14, 2002. Neuromuscul Disord 2003; 13(1):80–90.
36. Mathews KD, Moore SA. Limb-girdle muscular dystrophy. Curr Neurol Neurosci Rep 2003; 3(1):78–85.
37. Wicklund MP, Hilton-Jones D. The limb-girdle muscular dystrophics: genetics phenotypic definition of a disrupted entity. Neurology 2003; 60:1230–1231.
38. Moxley RT III, Ashwal S, Pandya S, et al. Practice parameter: corticosteroid treatment of Duchenne dystrophy: report of the Quality Standards Subcommittee of the American Academy of Neurology and the practice commitee of the Child Neurology of Society. Neurology 2005; 64(1):13–20.

2

The Functional Biology of Dystrophin: Structural Components and the Pathogenesis of Duchenne Muscular Dystrophy

Eijiro Ozawa
*National Institute of Neuroscience, NCNP,
Tokyo, Japan*

KEYNOTES ON THE PATHOGENESIS OF DUCHENNE MUSCULAR DYSTROPHY

At least two keys from clinical and pathological observations are important in understanding the pathogenesis of Duchenne muscular dystrophy (DMD) at the molecular and the cellular levels. This chapter begins with a discussion of these keys.

The First Key: DMD Displays a Chronic Progressive Course

DMD is a chronic, debilitating disease resulting from progressive degeneration and necrosis of skeletal and cardiac muscles, though degenerated muscle fibers are efficiently regenerated with myogenic stem cells at the early stages of the disease. The primary cause of DMD is a mutation in the dystrophin gene, which is inherited in an X-linked recessive manner. DMD gene mutations result in the absence of the dystrophin protein that is normally present in the subsarcolemmal cytoskeletal network (1,2). Clinical symptoms are first observed at the age of three to five years. As the affected boys grow, the disease progresses in proportion to the increases in physical movement. Atrophy begins in muscles of the limb–girdle region, including the proximal portion of the extremities (3). However, the calf muscles appear hypertrophic in the early stages. As the disease advances, atrophy spreads and calf hypertrophy disappears. By the early teens, patients lose the ability to walk without assistance and require the use of a wheelchair. Unbalanced power because of differential muscle damage leads to bone deformities, such as the spine lordosis and scoliosis, which sometimes require surgery (see Chapter 9). The problem of power imbalance may become crucial in future gene therapy applications, as this imbalance could be maintained or exacerbated among the treated muscles. Eventually, patients become confined to bed and lose most of their ability to move. This course is always progressive and eventually respiratory or cardiac failure occurs, which generally leads to death. It was previously described in many textbooks that death occurs by the age of 20 years. However, with recently improved respiratory management, the patient's lifespan has been appreciably prolonged. In Japan, DMD patients usually live until their thirties in hospitals specialized in treating muscular dystrophy, and some pass 40 years of age.

The *mdx* mouse is a widely used animal model of human DMD that has a nonsense mutation in the dystrophin gene; dystrophin is not expressed at the cell membrane (4). However, the course of disease is not entirely similar to that in humans. In *mdx* mice, a surge of degenerative and necrotic changes appears in skeletal muscles approximately between three and eight weeks after birth, accompanied by marked infiltration of mononuclear cells in degenerating areas. The grade of cell infiltration is much more severe than that found in DMD muscles. Many of these cells are macrophages that scavenge the degenerated materials. At later ages, the degeneration process slows considerably and extensive regeneration is better able to compensate for the ongoing myofiber necrosis. Therefore, this surge of degeneration in mice is neither chronic nor progressive. The cycles of degeneration and regeneration continue throughout life, and ultimately, the regenerating muscles grow larger than normal muscles. In contrast to *mdx* mice, degeneration–regeneration surge has not been observed in human DMD. The molecular mechanisms of degeneration in *mdx* muscles therefore may not be completely the same as that in human DMD. Finally, it is worth noting that *mdx* mice live about 80% as long as normal mice (Chamberlain, personal communication). There are other animal models such as the *cxmd* dogs, but their pathogenesis at the molecular and the cellular levels has not been thoroughly investigated.

The Second Key: Muscle Contraction Is Linked to the Pathogenesis of DMD

The most essential function of muscle fibers is to contract, generating strong tension and heat. This function is different from that of most other types of cells. Here, the characteristics of human DMD muscles are summarized in terms of the relationship between the progression of disease and mechanical force.

1. The signs and symptoms of DMD are first noted after patients begin to stand and walk. Atrophy first appears in the limb–girdle muscles (3). These muscles support the upright posture and body weight and are used for movements such as walking, running, and climbing stairs; these muscles therefore support sustained contraction or generate explosive force. When patients grow, they become more mobile and, e.g., begin running. These functions become increasingly impaired because of atrophy of the related muscles. Clinically, it is difficult to determine whether muscle contraction causes atrophy or whether atrophy results in the impairment of muscle function. Typically, only the second possibility is assumed. However, the first possibility should also be considered during the following discussion.
2. The extrafusal muscle fibers that actively contract are strongly affected, whereas the structure of intrafusal muscle fibers that scarcely contract are preserved until the late stages of DMD (5). The intrafusal fibers arise from early muscle precursor cells and are located inside a membranous sheath surrounded by a mass of extrafusal muscle fibers. Similarly, in the human heart, the cells of the stimulus-conducting system are far less susceptible than the contracting cardiac cells. In these less contractile cells, dystrophin is normally expressed on the cell membrane (6), and myofibrils are formed in the cytoplasm, albeit they remain sparse.
3. Serum creatine kinase (CK) levels remain elevated throughout a patient's life, although the levels decrease with time because of reduced muscle mass. CK levels can fluctuate on an hourly basis, as the half-life of CK in serum is approximately two days in normal individuals (7). Serum CK levels apparently increase after movements and decrease following rest (8).

    Acute changes in CK levels may reflect the severity of injury resulting from muscle contractions. In addition to CK, aldolase, pyruvate kinase, aspartate aminotransferase, alanine aminotransferase, glucose phosphatase, lactic hydrogenase, carbonic anhydrase III, and enolase levels are also increased in DMD serum. Myoglobinemia is also observed (3). Reciprocally, serum albumin bound to Evans blue dye has been shown to freely enter degenerating muscle fibers from the serum (9). These observations indicate that hydrophilic macromolecules are released from muscles into the extracellular space and influxed from the space into the fiber, passing through the cell membrane. As the cell membrane is composed of a hydrophobic lipid bilayer, it does not normally allow such hydrophilic macromolecules to freely enter. Clearly, specific alterations in DMD muscles cause CK release during the contraction–relaxation cycle.

4. The degenerative changes in DMD are limited to the skeletal and cardiac muscles. Other non- or less-contractile cells of DMD patients do not show degenerative changes. Although smooth muscles that contract slowly also express dystrophin, pathological changes related to smooth muscles have rarely been observed in DMD patients. A low dystrophin expression level is observed in some neurons (10). Dystrophin loss is ascribed as the cause of mental retardation that is sometimes observed among DMD patients, although it is not known how this occurs.

5. Dystrophic changes begin after myotubes have acquired contractility during development and dystrophin is expressed on the cell membrane simultaneously with myotube maturation (11). Myoblasts and immature myotubes, which do not contract, do not degenerate in DMD.

Considering the above findings, it is evident that the progression of DMD is strongly related to muscle fiber contraction. Thus, the following discussions are restricted to extrafusal muscle fibers that vigorously contract. Regardless of these relations, an exceedingly sedentary life is not good for patients, as their muscles would quickly develop disuse atrophy.

SARCOLEMMAL AND CYTOSKELETAL ARCHITECTURES RELATED TO DMD

Dystrophin and Dystrophin-Associated Proteins

The proximate cause of DMD is the absence of dystrophin from the subsarcolemmal cytoskeletal network (Table 1). Dystrophin is encoded in a large gene composed of 79 exons that maps the Xp21 and occupies approximately 0.1% of the entire genome size, namely, 3 Mb (12). In muscle, the mRNA spans 14 kb, which is only 0.46% of the gene size. The dystrophin protein is composed of 3685 amino acid (AA) residues and has a molecular mass of 427 kDa (13). It is long and slender in shape, and is divided into the following four domains; the actin-binding (approximately exons 1–8), rod (approximately exons 9–62), cysteine-rich (approximately exons 63–69), and C-terminal (approximately exons 70–79) domains.

Utrophin, an autosomal homologue of dystrophin that is widely expressed in various cells, has a molecular mass of 395 kDa. Its molecular characteristics are similar to, if not the same as, those of dystrophin (14,15).

Table 1 Dystrophin-DAP and Their Related Proteins

Protein	Gene locus	Molecular mass (kDa)	Glycosyl chains	Transmembrane domains	Presence	Myopathy due to a mutation of the gene
Dystrophin	Xp21.2	427	−	−	Intracellular	DMD/BMD
Utrophin	6q24	395	−	−	Intracellular	Not known
α-Dystroglycan	3p21	156	+++	−	Extracellular	KO mice: lethal
β-Dystroglycan	3p21	43	+	+	Transmembranous	KO mice: lethal
α-Sarcoglycan	17q21	50	+	+	Transmembranous	α-Sarcoglycanopathy LGMD2D
β-Sarcoglycan	4q12	43	+	+	Transmembranous	β-Sarcoglycanopathy LGMD2E
γ-Sarcoglycan	13q12	35	+	+	Transmembranous	γ-Sarcoglycanopathy LGMD2C
δ-Sarcoglycan	5q33	35	+	+	Transmembranous	δ-Sarcoglycanopathy LGMD2F
Sarcospan	12q11.2	25	−	+++	Largely membrane Integrated	KO mice: normal
α-Dystrobrevin	18q12.1–2	90[a]		−	Intracellular	KO mice: dystrophic
α-Syntrophin	20q11.2	60	−	−	Intracellular	KO mice: normal
β1-Syntrophin	8q23–24	60	−	−	Intracellular	Not known
β2-Syntrophin	16q22–q23	60	−	−	Intracellular	Not known
nNOS	12q24.2	161	−	−	Intracellular	Not known
Caveolin-3	3p25	22–24	−	+	Partially membrane Integrated, mostly Intracellular	LGMD

(*Continued*)

Table 1 Dystrophin-DAP and Their Related Proteins (Continued)

Protein	Gene locus	Molecular mass (kDa)	Glycosyl chains	Transmembrane domains	Presence	Myopathy due to a mutation of the gene
Dysferlin	2p13	230	−	+	Transmembranous	LGMD and Miyoshi distal myopathy
Plectin	8q24.13-qter	466	−	−	Intracellular	Skin lesion and muscular dystrophy
Desmin	2q35	53	−	−	Intracellular	Desmin-related myopathy
Integrin α7	12q13	130	−	−	Intracellular	Congenital muscular dystrophy
Syncoilin	1p33–34	54	−	−	Intracellular	Not known
β-Synemin	15q26.3	160	−	−	Intracellular	Not known
Laminin α2	6q2	300	−	−	In the basal lamina	Congenital muscular dystrophy
Collagen VI	A1&A2:21q22 A3:2q37	A1&A2:140 A3:200–250	−	−	Outside of the basal lamina	Ullrich CMD and Bethlem myopathy

[a]Several isoforms are known due to alternative splicing.
Abbreviations: CMD, congenital muscular dystrophy; LGMD, limb-girdle muscular dystrophy.

In skeletal muscles, it is highly expressed at the neuromuscular and myotendinous junctions close to the site of dystrophin expression (see Chapter 12).

At least 10 types of proteins bind to dystrophin and are known collectively as dystrophin-associated proteins (DAP) (Fig. 1). Six of the DAPs are glycoproteins, and are termed dystrophin-associated glycoproteins (DAG) (16). DAGs can be divided into two subcomplexes: the dystroglycan (DG) and sarcoglycan (SG) complexes (17).

The DG complex is composed of two subunits: α- and β-DG (18). They are synthesized from a single mRNA as one polypeptide with 895 AA residues including the signal sequence at the N-terminus that is post-transcriptionally cleaved into two peptides of 626 (excluding the signal sequence) and 242 AAs that remain associated as a single protein subcomplex. The molecular mass of the core protein of α-DG is 74 kDa, whereas the molecular mass of glycosylated α-DG is estimated to be approximately 156 kDa. α-DG has O-linked sugar chains, composed mostly of four sugar residues (19) bound to various threonine or serine residues, which comprise 17% of the total α-DG AA sequence. α-DG also has long N-linked sugar chains bound to asparagine residues that comprise 2% of the total α-DG AA sequence. β-DG is a transmembranous glycoprotein. The molecular masses of the core and glycosylated β-DG protein are 27 and 43 kDa, respectively.

The SG complex is composed of four different transmembranous glycoproteins (α-, β-, γ-, and δ-SGs), each of which is encoded in different autosomal genes (20,21). The molecular masses of the core and glycosylated proteins are 40.2 and 50 kDa for α-SG, 34.8 and 43 kDa for β-SG, 32 and 35 kDa for γ-SG, and 32 and 35 kDa for δ-SG, respectively. Sarcospan, a 25 kDa protein, has four intramembranous sequences that occupy about 60% of the molecule, but has no glycosyl chain (22). In addition to these proteins, two intracellular proteins, α-dystrobrevin, and the syntrophins (α- and β- isoforms) form the DAP (Fig. 1).

Architecture of Dystrophin–DAP Complex

The architecture of the dystrophin–DAP complex together with other proteins superimposed on the sarcolemmal membrane is shown in Figure 1. Dystrophin binds to a γ-actin filament in the subsarcolemmal cytoskeleton by its N-terminal actin-binding domain (N-ABD) (23,24) and laterally by the basic residues present in rod repeats 11 to 17 (r-ABD) (25). As the intracellular domain of β-DG is small and the length of the rod domain is assumed to be approximately 125 nm (13), the actin filament must be present very close to the cell membrane. Thus, dystrophin does not bind to a myofibrillar α-actin filament, but binds to a subsarcolemmal cytoskeletal γ-actin filament. The dystroglycan-binding domain (DGBD) of dystrophin is located at the distal end of the rod and includes almost the entire cysteine-rich domain (26). β-DG, a transmembrane protein, extracellularly binds to α-DG, which

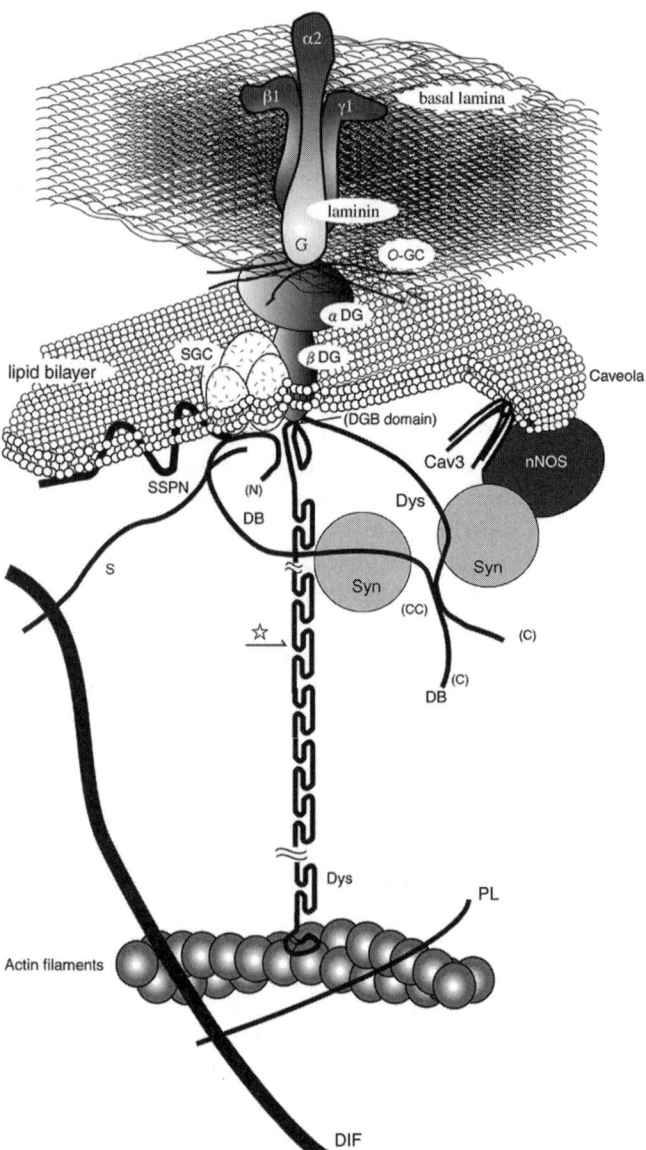

Figure 1 Molecular model of the dystrophin–DAP complex and other proteins superimposed on the sarcolemma and actin filaments. *Abbreviations*: cc, coiled-coil motif present on dystrophin (Dys) and dystrobrevin (DB); SSPN, sarcospan; Syn, syntrophin; Cav, caveolin-3; (N) and (C), N- and C-termini; O-GC, *O*-glycosyl chains; G, G-domain of laminin. The arrow with a star depicts the site of binding of actin filaments on the dystrophin rod (*Star*: r-ABD). *Source*: Redrawn from Ref. 28 with modifications.

in turn binds to laminin, one of the main components of the basal lamina. Thus, a structure (dystrophin-α-DG-β-DG), termed "dystrophin bolt," transmembranously connects the actin network and the basal lamina (Fig. 2) (27). Another structure (utrophin-α-DG-β-DG) observed in DMD muscles in place of the dystrophin bolt is termed "utrophin bolt."

The transmembranous SG complex binds to the DG complex at the cell membrane. Intracellularly, sarcospan and dystrobrevin (by its N-terminal) bind to the SG complex (28). At least three isoforms of α-dystrobrevin are expressed in muscles, the longest two of which bind dystrophin through homologous coiled-coil domains present in both dystrobrevin and dystrophin; the shortest dystrobrevin isoform in muscle, α-dystrobrevin-3, does not bind dystrophin. Dystrobrevin and the C-terminal domain of dystrophin each bind to various isoforms of syntrophin. The syntrophins bind to nNOS, which also binds caveolin-3.

The DG and SG complexes and sarcospan are synthesized in the endoplasmic reticulum (ER), where they remain as separate complexes (29). After translocation to the Golgi apparatus, a single large complex is assembled. Dystrophin is synthesized in polyribosomes and subsequently attaches to β-DG, which extrudes its intracellular domain from the Golgi membrane into the cytoplasm. Glycosylation of the DG and SG subunits occurs during transport from the ER to the cell membrane. The exact timing of when the dystrophin bolt is completed by binding with the actin networks is not known.

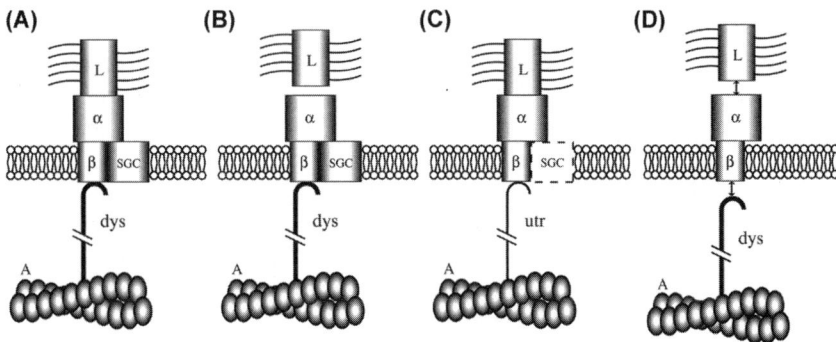

Figure 2 Structure of dystrophin or utrophin bolt. (A) The dystrophin bolt of normal muscle fibers. (B) Dystrophin bolt in various congenital muscular dystrophy muscle fibers. Note that the junction between laminin and α-dystroglycan is disrupted. (C) The utrophin bolt in DMD muscle fibers. Note that dystrophin is replaced by utrophin and SGC is almost absent or is greatly reduced. (D) The dystrophin bolt in sarcoglycanopathy muscle fibers. Note that the binding of dystrophin to β-dystroglycan, and that of β-dystroglycan to α-dystroglycan, is weak. This point is represented by double-headed arrows. *Abbreviations*: A, actin filament; dys, dystrophin; β, β-dystroglycan; α, α-dystroglycan; SGC, sarcoglycan complex; L, laminin.

Three Surface Layers of Muscle Fibers: Basal Lamina, Cell Membrane, and Actin Networks

The basal lamina is an extracellular mantle existing over the cell membrane (Fig. 1) and is composed of collagen IV, laminin, perlecan, and other components. It is a thick, mechanically strong structure composed of extendable networks that allow diffusion of water-soluble substances such as ions and proteins. Macrophages are even able to pass through the basal lamina in damaged muscle to scavenge necrotic materials.

The cell membrane is composed of a lipid bilayer containing various transmembrane proteins. The lipid bilayer prevents diffusion of hydrophilic substances through the cell membrane. When small hydrophilic substances are transported into or out of a cell, specific channels or pumps are used. Macromolecules such as various enzymes that are not synthesized in the ER or are not contained in endo- or exocytotic vesicles usually cannot diffuse across the cell membrane. It must be emphasized that one of the most important functions of the cell membrane is to act as a barrier that maintains the internal conditions of the cell within the normal physiologic range. Therefore, the cell membrane must always remain intact for cell viability.

The structure of the actin networks present immediately underneath the cell membrane is not well understood. It is complicated and includes both intermediate filaments and microfilaments. In normal muscle, dystrophin is found in this complicated structure (30).

Figuratively, a muscle fiber is similar to a long and slender bag filled with water; the cytosolic pressure generated upon contraction of the muscle fiber is evenly conducted to the cell membrane. If the cell membrane is not mechanically protected, it may be destroyed by high intracellular pressure or extracellular disturbances that occur during the contraction–relaxation cycle. The basal lamina serves as the outer defense layer and the actin networks as the inner defense layer of the cell membrane (16). The protective ability of the basal lamina is considered much stronger than that of the actin networks. This triple, or sandwich, structure is mechanically stronger than a naked cell membrane. Its defensive ability is reinforced when bound together by the dystrophin bolt in normal muscle fibers and, to some extent, by the utrophin bolt in DMD muscle fibers.

The Dystrophin Bolt

An understanding of the structure of the dystrophin bolt provides the theoretical basis of gene therapy for DMD (Fig. 2A). In DMD, dystrophin is absent while utrophin expression is upregulated. A small amount of β-DG is found bound to utrophin. A single utrophin bolt that is composed of one molecule each of utrophin and α- and β-DGs is structurally weaker than a single dystrophin bolt (26). Furthermore, the number of utrophin bolts present on the cell membrane of DMD muscle fibers is less than that of the dystrophin bolt present on the normal cell membrane. Consequently, the mechanical connection between the basal lamina and actin networks is weaker in DMD muscle fibers than in normal muscle fibers. The aim of conventional gene therapy for DMD is thus to reconstruct or replace the dystrophin bolt. Transduction of dystrophic muscle with a dystrophin expression cassette leads to reassembly of the DG complex to form new dystrophin bolts.

1. *Binding of the N-terminus of dystrophin to f-actin filaments*: Actin filaments are double helical threads composed of many g-(globular) actin monomers. G-actin is nearly spherical with a diameter of approximately 5 nm. Its molecular mass is about 42 kDa, similar to that of β-SG. The half turn of the double helix of f-actin is composed of 6.5 to 7 molecules of g-actin and spans 36 nm. This corresponds to about 30% of the length of the dystrophin rod domain. It is worth noting that the g-actin unit is typically drawn erroneously small compared with other proteins in most of the published schemes of the DAP complex. When the use of truncated dystrophins in DMD gene therapy is considered, the size of the actin molecule must also be considered, as mini-dystrophins bind to available actin filaments located very close to the cell membrane.

    Dystrophin binds to f-actin, but not to g-actin, at the N-ABD. However, the N-ABD binds to a single g-actin unit within an f-actin filament. The binding at N-ABD involves three actin-binding sites (ABSs) of dystrophin at AA 17 to 26 (in exon 1), 88 to 116 (in exons 4–5), and 128 to 156 (in exon 6). ABSs 1 and 3 bind to AA 83 to 117 and 350 to 373 located at the C-terminus of actin, respectively (16).

2. *Binding of the dystroglycan-binding domain (DGBD) of dystrophin to β-DG*: In vitro and in vivo experiments show that the DGBD of dystrophin spans AA 3026 to 3345 (26). This sequence includes a small part of the C-terminus of the rod, and most of the cysteine-rich domains. Deletions in this region interfere with dystrophin binding to β-DG. AA 3055 to 3088 is a WW domain, a motif that participates in a variety of protein–protein interactions (31,32). The dystrophin WW domain is exceptional in that it does not work alone, but requires the downstream cysteine-rich domain sequences for binding DG. X-ray analysis revealed that the molecular shape of the WW domain of dystrophin is slightly different from that of the WW domain present in other proteins (33,34). In an in vitro binding experiment, a polypeptide spanning AA 3026 to 3324 weakly bound to β-DG. However, a longer sequence was necessary for strong binding in vitro and also in vivo (26,35). The consensus AA sequence that binds to the WW domain is PPXY, and the C-terminus of β-DG includes a PPPY sequence.

3. Binding of β-DG to α-DG was described in an earlier section.
4. *Binding of α-DG to laminin*: This binding has only been studied in vitro and requires glycosylated α-DG and calcium ions in the micromolar range (18). The roles of the sugar chains are not well understood, although laminin does not bind to unglycosylated α-DG. This observation suggests that laminin directly binds to the sugar chains, or that the protein conformation of DG is changed in the presence of sugar chains, which forms a receptor site for laminin on the core α-DG protein. Whether the *O*- or *N*-glycosyl chains, or both, are required for binding has not been biochemically clarified. However, the *O*-glycosyl chain is known to be important for binding for two reasons. One, the *O*-glycosyl chains are much more abundant than *N*-glycosyl chain in α-DG, and two, an impairment of the synthesis of the *O*-glycosyl chains because of mutations in any of several genes encoding glycosylation enzymes or other related proteins results in various congenital muscular dystrophies (CMD). The major form of laminin in the muscle basal lamina is laminin 2, which is composed of α2-, β1-, and γ1-subunits. The *G*-domain present in the C-terminal region of the α2-subunit binds to α-DG (36).
5. *Binding of the SG complex to the dystrophin bolt*: The complex composed of the DG and SG complexes, as well as sarcospan, has been isolated directly from mammalian muscle (28). The SG subunits are classified into two groups. Group 1 includes the essential subunits, β- and δ-SG. These are universally used as the core of the SG complex. They directly and strongly bind to β-DG (37). Their messenger RNA (mRNA) are found in the myoblast stage, and their expression levels remain fairly constant during development when protein synthesis increases following myotube formation (38). Group 2 includes the variable subunits, α- and γ-SG. These are expressed in striated muscles and only weakly bind to β-DG. In addition, α-SG binds to α-DG and other SG subunits (37). The expression levels of their mRNAs increase before their protein synthesis (38). Ectopic expression of ε-SG was recently shown to functionally substitute for α-SG and lead to a phenotypic rescue of α-SG-mutant mice (39). Whether γ-SG is expressed in cardiac vascular smooth muscles or is replaced by ζ-SG is in dispute [reviewed in (21)].
6. Integrin bolt may be a functional unit that works independently of the dystrophin bolt, as the integrin system also connects laminin and actin networks. Integrin α is a laminin receptor that has sugar chains (40). However, laminin binds to the core protein but not to the sugar chains.

STRUCTURAL DEFECTS IN DMD

Defects of the Dystrophin–DAP Complex in DMD

Dystrophin

Large deletions in the dystrophin gene are found in about 60% of DMD patients. In out-of-frame deletions, a nonsense mutation is invariably encoded 3' side of the deletion resulting in markedly decreased mRNA levels via nonsense mediated decay (NMD) (41). Although some truncated dystrophin is likely synthesized, none has been detected. With in-frame mutations, which are mostly present in the rod domain, dystrophin with a short or elongated rod domain is produced depending on whether the mutation is a gene deletion or duplication. These mutations result in Becker muscular dystrophy (BMD), a mild form of DMD. In BMD, the amount of dystrophin expressed on the cell membrane is usually decreased, resulting in a pathologic phenotype. Accurately measuring the expression level of dystrophin mRNA has rarely been done because of technical challenges from the large size (14 kb) and the very low level (0.01–0.001% of total muscle mRNA) of the transcript in muscle (42).

Utrophin

In DMD, utrophin is upregulated and is fixed on the cell membrane where it partially replaces the dystrophin bolt to a certain extent (see Chapter 12) (43). Transgenic *mdx* mice expressing utrophin do not display a dystrophic phenotype (44), and dystrophin–utrophin double deficient mice show a more severe phenotype than dystrophin-deficient mice, even though utrophin deficient mice show an almost normal phenotype (45–47).

DG Complex

In DMD, β-DG expressed on the cell membrane is greatly decreased but is distinctly detectable (48), where it likely interacts with utrophin forming the utrophin bolt.

SG Complex

The expression of this complex on the cell membrane is greatly reduced or sometimes almost undetectable in DMD. It is not known to what extent the utrophin bolt is associated with the SG complex. This question needs to be addressed in more detail, because in the absence of the SG complex, the dystrophin bolt is mechanically weak (20,21).

Syntrophin, nNOS, Sarcospan, and Dystrobrevin

In DMD muscles, these proteins are absent or their expression levels on the cell membrane are greatly reduced (49–51). However, the knockout mutant mice for these proteins do not show dystrophic phenotypes, except the dystrobrevin mutants, which display a very mild phenotype (52–54). These proteins are recruited to the membrane by the expression of dystrophin (55).

Studies Using DNA Microarrays

In biopsies of DMD muscles, transcripts for numerous proteins show a wide variability, which can differ from one group of patients to another (56).

Structural Features of Dystrophin Critical for DMD Gene Therapy: Actin–Dystrophin and Dystrophin-β-DG Junctions and the Rod Domain

1. Actin-dystrophin and dystrophin-β-DG junctions in the following:
    a. Normal muscles (Fig. 3.1-a): The ligands of dystrophin, actin filaments, and β-DG are spanned by the full-length dystrophin.
    b. DMD muscles (Fig. 3.1-b): The actin filaments are not connected to β-DG by dystrophin but by utrophin (43). However, utrophin levels are low in DMD muscle fibers: utrophin binding to β-DG is weaker than that of dystrophin (26). Therefore, the connection between the actin networks and the basal lamina is likely weaker in DMD fibers than that in normal fibers.

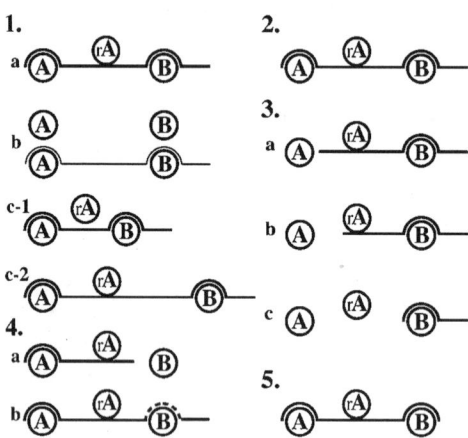

Figure 3 The N-terminal actin-binding domain (N-ABD), the rod actin-binding domain (r-ABD), and the dystroglycan-binding domain (DGBD) and dystrophin as affected by various mutations. (**A**) rA and (**B**) N-ABD, r-ABD, and DGBD, respectively. A bold line depicts dystrophin and a thin line utrophin (for details, see text).

c. BMD muscles: The actin filaments and β-DG are connected to truncated (Fig. 3.1-c1) or elongated (Fig. 3.1-c2) dystrophins. The amount of dystrophin is decreased in BMD muscle.
2. Artificial connection of actin filament–dystrophin and dystrophin–β-DG using exogenous transgenes. Exogenous full-length dystrophin in muscles of transgenic *mdx* mice has been shown to fully rescue the dystrophic phenotype and restore normal expression of the DAP complex (Fig. 3.2) (55).
3. Disruptions of dystrophin–actin filament interactions.
    a. In humans (Fig. 3.3-a), deletion of exons 3 to 7 (an out-of-frame mutation) has been observed to result in either DMD or BMD, although dystrophin is still detected on the sarcolemma using antibodies that bind epitopes in exons 10 to 13 (57). Dystrophin may have been produced by translational re-initiation at an AUG in exon 8. The deleted region corresponds to the N-ABD.

    Presumably, this truncated dystrophin binds actin via the r-ABD. The amounts of dystrophin detected in two patients with this mutation was 14% and 21% of normal, which results in DMD and BMD, respectively (57). This result is compatible with the observation that the severity of dystrophinopathy depends on the amount of dystrophin present (58).
    b. Transgenic *mdx* mice expressing the retinal isoform of dystrophin, Dp260, in skeletal muscle show a slow progression of the *mdx* phenotype. Dp260 includes r-ABD and the residual AA sequences up through the C-terminus (Fig. 3.3-b) (59).
    c. This shortest dystrophin isoform, Dp71, spans from the DGBD to the C-terminus. Dp71 expressed in transgenic *mdx* mouse muscles binds to β-DG and restores the DAP. However, dystrophy is not prevented (Fig. 3.3-c) (60,61). Similar results have been observed with transgenic expression of Dp116 in *mdx* muscles (Chamberlain, personal communication). These observations suggests that the mere presence of the DAP is not sufficient to prevent muscular dystrophy.
4. Disconnection of dystrophin and β-DG.
    a. In human DMD, dystrophin is usually completely absent except in the so-called revertant fibers. However, some exceptional cases are known which result from mutations that prevent expression of portions of the C-terminal rod domain through the cysteine-rich domain (Fig. 3.4-a). These truncated dystrophins localize to the cell membrane of DMD muscle fibers at a level similar to that of dystrophin in normal muscle fibers. These dystrophins contain both the N- and r-ABDs, but lack the DGBD (62–64).

b. Transgenic *mdx* mice expressing dystrophin constructs lacking small portions of the DGBD all display a fully dystrophic phenotype even though the transgenic dystrophin is expressed on the cell membrane (Fig. 3.4-b) (35).

   These observations reveal that the binding of dystrophin to actin filaments and β-DG is required to prevent severe muscular dystrophy. When dystrophin can bind to only one of them, the dystrophin bolt is broken (Fig. 3.3-c). When only the N- and r-ABDs are present, dystrophin might be fixed on the cell membrane but the muscles remain dystrophic (Fig. 3.4-a,b). However, when either of the N- or r-ABD and DGBD is present (Fig. 3.3-a,b) dystrophin is fixed and the dystrophic process is ameliorated although the severity of symptoms depends on the amount of dystrophin fixed. Therefore, at least either one of N- or r-ABD and DGBD are essential for dystrophin to be functional in terms of preventing muscular dystrophy.

   Other studies have addressed whether the entire rod domain is required to prevent severe muscular dystrophy. Clinical studies indicate that no specific portion of the rod domain encoded by exons 9 to 55 is necessary for a highly functional dystrophin, as in-frame deletions anywhere within this region lead to BMD (65–67). The rod domain is therefore considered to be a flexible and elastic spacer connecting the critical actin and DG binding domains.

5. *Absence of C-terminal domain*: Most of this domain is dispensable for the prevention of the dystrophic phenotype of DMD patients and *mdx* mice (68). Dystrophy was completely prevented by expression of a truncated dystrophin containing the N- and r-ABD, the rod domain and the DGBD, but lacking the C-terminal domain (Fig. 3.5) (see Chapter 16). Based on the above and related evidence, dystrophin function requires two essential structural features: (1) N- and r-ABDs and DGBD and (2) rod domain of sufficient length to join these domains (69,70). These features are the theoretical basis of minigene currently used in experimental gene therapy (71). Evidence supporting this concept has been confirmed in numerous subsequent publications (72–74).

Defects of the Dystrophin Bolt: Comparison of Pathomechanisms of Some Muscular Dystrophies Related to DMD

Replacement of the dystrophin bolt with a low amount of the mechanically weaker utrophin bolt causes DMD (26,43) while a defect of the extracellular junction, i.e., the connection of α-DG with laminin, results in CMD (Fig. 2).

CMDs are a group of muscular dystrophies whose primary symptoms appear soon after birth. The infants show only limited movements that continue for their entire lives and the clinical symptoms only gradually progress. Serum CK levels are high.

A defect of merosin, the α2 subunit of muscle-specific laminin 2, results in a CMD (merosinopathy) (75). Defect of sugar chain addition to α-DG resulting from impaired synthesis of glycosyl residues results in a decrease in the amount of sugar chains, which gives rise to several CMDs (76,77). Five responsible proteins including sugar transfer enzymes that function mainly in the Golgi complex have been identified or postulated to date (78). Because merosin and α-DG form a junction between the dystrophin bolt and the laminin, the strength of this junction is crucial for preventing CMDs. In addition, a defect of another junction between laminin and a transmembrane protein, integrin α7, also results in mild CMD (79). Therefore, when the attachments between the basal lamina, the "outer defense layer," and the cell membrane weaken, CMDs develop (80).

In developing human muscles, the basal lamina appears and develops by the 16th week of gestation together with the development of myotubes (81,82). The actin networks are present from the myoblast stage. In normal muscles, the utrophin bolt first appears to fix the membrane defense layers in myotubes and is then gradually replaced by the dystrophin bolt as myotubes mature into myofibers. Dystrophin begins to be expressed in muscle fibers at 11 to 12 weeks of gestation, and its expression levels increase with time (83). Utrophin expression becomes very low after birth and dystrophin is expressed on the sarcolemma thereafter (84–86).

In CMDs, since the laminin–α-DG junction is hereditarily defective, the connections between the basal lamina and actin network are disrupted from the beginning of the formation of the junction (Fig. 2B). The basal lamina covers the cell membrane: it is a thick, rather compact, and strong mat containing collagen fibers (81), whereas the actin-networks are coarse meshworks (30) that may be stretched. Thus, the protective ability of the basal lamina may be much higher than that of the actin networks in terms of structure and location. Because the basal lamina is not well fixed in CMD and is sometimes dissociated, the cell membrane may be easily injured by small movements of the fetus in utero. Such injuries may inhibit the normal differentiation and growth of muscle fibers. This may result in developmental arrest with reduced motility of the children. In support of this, CMD muscle fibers remain immature in terms of their morphological appearance and their protein isoform expression profiles (Toda T, personal communication). These may be related to the reduced movement of CMD patients.

In contrast to CMDs, in DMD the basal lamina is well developed (87), even though expression of the DG complex is low (88). In DMD muscle development, the utrophin bolt is initially formed, but is not replaced by the dystrophin bolt (Fig. 2C). However, it is not sufficiently strong to maintain the muscle in a healthy state. After birth when movements increase, DMD muscle fibers gradually degenerate because their cell membrane defense system remains immature, whereas the contractile system develops almost normally. This disproportional relationship causes DMD. Thus, with the increase in movement, muscle degeneration progresses and serum levels of CK increase (8). Therefore, the aim of gene or cell therapy of DMD is to form a mature defense system by constructing a functionally strong dystrophin or utrophin bolt.

In sarcoglycanopathy (SGP, autosomal recessive Duchenne-like muscular dystrophy), one of four SG subunit genes is mutated, and the entire SG complex is lost (20) or greatly reduced. Thus, the link between dystrophin and β-DG and between β-DG and α-DG is weakened (Fig. 2D). In SGP muscles, the dystrophin bolt is present at normal amounts, but it is weak (21).

In summary, these muscular dystrophies are grouped into diseases that result from defects of the dystrophin bolt. In CMDs, the number of dystrophin bolts may not be changed; however, the junction between laminin and its receptor, α-DG, is disrupted. In DMD, the dystrophin bolt is replaced by a small number of utrophin bolts. In SGP, the number of dystrophin bolts may not change, but it is structurally impaired and functionally weak.

TRANSVERSE FIXATION SYSTEM: THE STRUCTURAL BASIS FOR A MECHANICAL HYPOTHESIS OF DMD PATHOGENESIS

Myofibrils in normal skeletal muscle are regularly arranged in rows at the level of the Z-disc to form cross striations. Each myofibril is encircled and bound at the Z-disc by desmin intermediate filaments (DIF) that bind the neighboring myofibrils in register and that also radiate to the costamere on the cell membrane where the dystrophin bolts are present (89–92). The costameres are located along a circle on the cell membrane corresponding to the Z-disc.

DIFs are fixed to the Z-disc by plectin, syncoilin, and β-synemin [formerly called desmuslin (93)]. Because DIFs are connected to the subsarcolemmal actin networks via plectin and to dystrobrevin via syncoilin and β-synemin at the cell membrane (Fig. 4.2) (94,95) and since the actin networks and dystrobrevin bind to dystrophin, the dystrophin bolt may serve as the DIF tether on the cell membrane. Therefore, the DIFs ultimately connect the basal lamina via the dystrophin bolt. This connective structure is termed the transverse fixation system (TFS) (16). We note that the length of the DIF always remains constant, probably to prevent the tubular or T-systems that conduct excitation of the cell membrane to the sarcoplasmic reticulum from overstretching during strong contractions.

During contraction, the diameter of the muscle fiber increases. However, the diameter is not constant throughout the vertical axis of the muscle fiber like a cylinder, as the muscle fiber is constricted at each Z-disc. During contraction, the distance between the cell membrane and the center of the

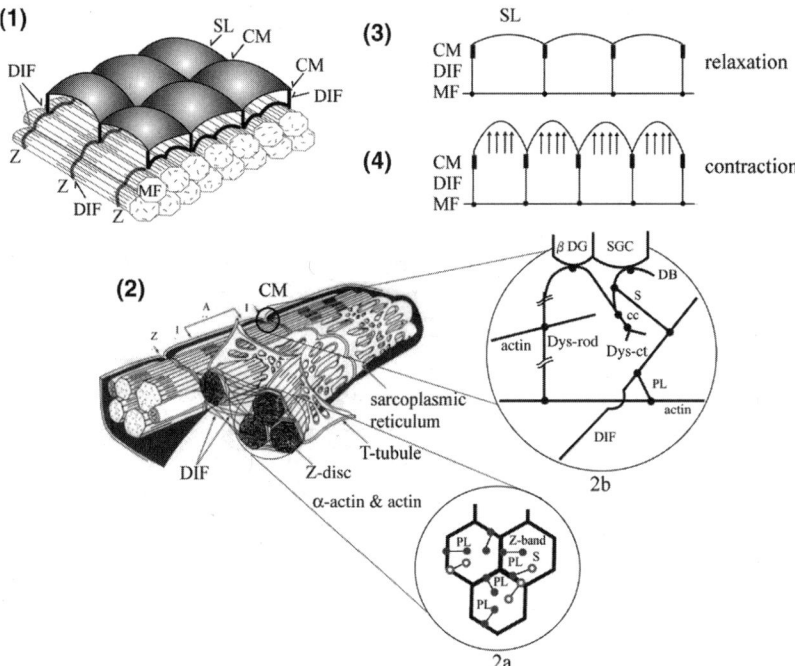

Figure 4 Transverse fixation system and the sarcolemma. (**1**) Myofibrils (MF) and sarcolemma (SL) connected to desmin intermediate filaments (DIF). Z: Z-disc, CM: costamere. (**2**) The DIFs tether MFs at Z discs and connect to CMs, where the DIF is associated with the dystrophin–DAP complex via various cytoskeletal proteins: (2a) Details of Z discs; (2b) Connection of the DAP complex and other components of the costameres. (**3, 4**) Longitudinal section of a muscle fiber containing DIFs and showing festooning. *Abbreviations*: S, syncoilin and/or β-synemin; DB, dystrobrevin; cc, coiled-coil motifs. *Source*: The central part of this figure is redrawn from Ref. 89 with modifications.

muscle fiber is maintained unchanged by the TFS at each costamere, whereas the extracostameric cell membrane is pushed outwards (Fig. 4.2, 4.3). Thus, the cell membrane appears as if it were pulled inward at the costamere (Fig. 4). The sarcolemma balloons similar to a parachute where the TFS corresponds to the strings and the general cell membrane to the canopy. In support of this, the sarcolemma was found to form continuous, multiple semicircles in the longitudinal section of the muscle fiber in which the costameres form depressions, and this is called "festooning" (96). This process becomes very distinct when the fiber undergoes strong shortening.

Let us consider the dynamics of this cell membrane extrusion. Tetanus power of mammalian muscle fibers reaches its plateau within several hundred milliseconds, when the fibers are frequently stimulated (97).

This reflects the movement in the living body. At the start of contraction, the cell membrane must be pushed not by hydrostatic pressure but by hydrodynamic pressure by strong and quick stream of cytosol to the membrane. Therefore, the cell membrane has to endure strong pressure.

In normal muscle fibers, dystrophin bolt is also distributed on the extracostameric cell membrane (98), the cell membrane can be protected. In DMD fibers, utrophin is upregulated to some extent in place of dystrophin (26). However, protection of cell membrane in DMD muscle is weaker than in normal muscle. Thus, the DMD cell membrane may be ruptured at its delicate loci when the fibers contract. Small clefts of cell membrane can be spontaneously resealed on relaxation (99). This scenario is supported by the finding that the leakage of various nonspecific water-soluble cytosolic proteins such as CK into serum is promoted by DMD muscle contraction (8,100).

The TFS is composed of many molecules responsible for various muscle diseases (Fig. 5). These proteins are arranged on the TFS from the outside to the center of the muscle fibers as follows: the proteins on the sarcolemma are laminin and the proteins required for normal glycosylation of α-DG that are responsible for CMDs, four proteins for SGP (20,21) and dystrophin for

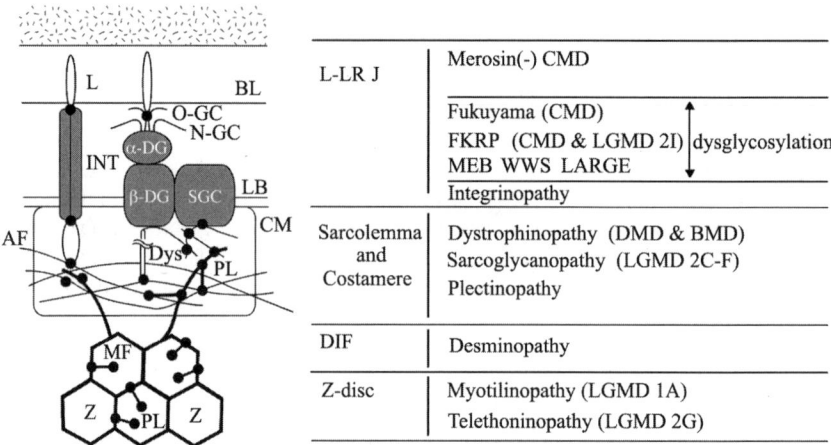

Figure 5 The array of proteins responsible for muscular dystrophy–myopathy present on the transverse fixation system. Figure and Table depict the relative position of dystrophin among various proteins responsible for different muscular dystrophies–myopathies. Note that dystrophin and α- and β-DGs form the dystrophin bolt. *Left column* of the table indicates site of defect and *right column* denotes name of disease. *Abbreviations*: AF, actin filament; BL, basal lamina; CM, costamere; Dys, dystrophin; FKRP, fukutin-related protein disorder; INT, integrin; L, laminin; LB, lipid bilayer; L-LR J, laminin–laminin receptor junction; MEB, muscle-eye-brain disease (CMD); MF, myofibril; N-GC, *N*-glycosyl chain; O-GC, *O*-glycosyl chain; PL, plectin; WWS, Walker-Warburg syndrome (CMD); Z, Z-disc.

DMD. There is also a plectin defect that results in muscular dystrophy associated with epidermolysis bullosa simplex (101). A mutation of desmin gene leads to a myopathy (102). Finally, myotilin and telethonin localize to the Z-disc and are responsible for limb–girdle muscular dystrophies (LGMD) 1A and 2G (103,104). In conclusion, the TFS serves as a contradystrophic array, playing mechanical roles during contraction. The pathogenesis of diseases resulting from defects of TFS components is likely to be closely related to this mechanical process.

WHAT INDUCES THE DEGENERATIVE PROCESSES IN DMD?

DMD muscle fibers can survive for long periods while undergoing repeated cycles of segmental necrosis and regeneration. Some fibers may last longer, and others may become necrotic and disappear within a shorter period. Until birth, nearly normal numbers of muscle fibers are formed in utero, although the dystrophin bolt is not established. Most fibers can grow larger and contract strongly for the first few years or more after birth, although degenerative changes in the muscles progress. Some specific molecular mechanisms must induce degeneration of muscle fibers. However, to date, there is no clear answer as to what triggers individual degeneration events and what promotes and sustains the long lasting degenerative process.

The Calcium–Calpain Hypothesis and a Strategy to Test It

Calcium ions (Ca^{2+}) have long been widely assumed to be the initial inducer of muscle degeneration (3). Since the late 1960s, it has been hypothesized that calcium enters muscle fibers by an unknown mechanism and activates the serine neutral protease calpain (105). Activated calpain then digests protoplasmic proteins including myofibrils, resulting in the atrophy of the myofiber. This scenario has been accepted without serious discussion, while other possibilities are scarcely proposed. Some studies partially support the hypothesis, although many additional problems need to be addressed before this hypothesis can be accepted as fact.

Some consideration is warranted as to what would be a strict and valid research strategy with which to test the calcium–calpain hypothesis. Generally, to demonstrate that a substance is a regulator of an enzyme that can influence a cellular process, the following criteria must be fulfilled. (i) The enzyme must exist in the cell. (ii) It must be activated to a sufficient level by an activating substance for it to influence a cellular process. (iii) The activating substance must be available at appropriate concentrations at the time when the enzyme functions and the activation of systems other than the enzyme by the same substance should be compatible with cell viability. (iv) Evidence must be present that the enzymatic reaction occurs in the cell, i.e., the substrates must be present and the products must be detectable.

Finally, (v) the enzymatic process must be qualitatively and quantitatively relevant to cellular phenomena. Too little or too much activity is not physiologically relevant. These criteria were originally devised for an activator–enzyme system functioning in a rapid cell process (106,107). They are essentially a modification of Koch's postulates for determination of a microorganism as the cause of an infectious disease (108).

Inspection of the Ca^{2+}–Calpain Hypothesis

Increases in the total amount of Ca^{2+} have been found in DMD muscle fibers. However, most Ca^{2+} is present in a sequestered form, such as those bound to mitochondria, within the sarcoplasmic reticulum, or those complexed with troponin C. Therefore, most Ca^{2+} present in muscles is not available for activation of calpain. In adult living muscle fibers, the intracellular concentration of free Ca^{2+} remains less than 10^{-7} M during relaxation, whereas it increases to more than 10^{-5} M during the strongest contractions (Fig. 6) (109). In a contraction–relaxation cycle, cytosolic Ca^{2+} ion concentrations vary within this range. Phosphorylase kinase, which is involved in glycogenolysis, is also activated by these same concentrations of Ca^{2+} ions (107). Thus, the energy-consuming system and energy-producing system are simultaneously controlled by the same amount of Ca^{2+}. In addition, there may be some cellular systems delicately regulated by Ca^{2+}. Disturbance of these systems would induce severe damage to the cells, and such crucial damage would not be compatible with the fact that the DMD muscle fibers live for many years.

There are at least two types of calpain present in muscles that differ in the Ca^{2+} ion concentration required for activation, m- and µ-calpains (110).

1. m-Calpain is activated by Ca^{2+} at millimolar concentrations in vitro (Fig. 6) (111), raising questions as to whether the enzymatic activity of this enzyme can be biologically relevant in contracting muscle fibers. For example, what could be the source of activating Ca^{2+} ions at such concentrations? If all the Ca^{2+} sequestering systems suddenly released their calcium as Ca^{2+} ions, the cytosolic Ca^{2+} ion concentration could become sufficiently high to activate m-Calpain. However, this could not occur in a myofiber without leading to necrosis because of the devastating effects that such elevated levels would have on other muscle processes. Thus, the Ca^{2+} ion must be derived from the extracellular space.
    a. In cases where Ca^{2+} ions are quickly taken through the "membrane cleft" upon contraction (see section "Transverse Fixation System"), free Ca^{2+} ion concentrations in serum range from 1.1 to 1.4 m mol/l (112). If the free-Ca^{2+} ion concentration of the extracellular fluid was also within this range, about one-third of the intracellular fluid would need to be replaced

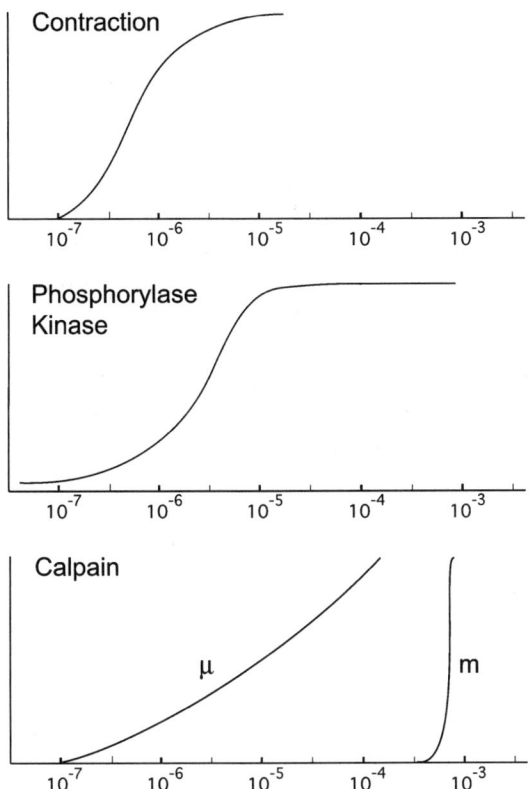

Figure 6 Relationship between the contractile or enzyme activity (ordinate, arbitrary units) and calcium ion concentration (expressed in molarity in the logarithmic scale, abscissa). (*Top*): Tension generated by isometric contraction of skinned fibers (calcium-receptor: troponin). (*Middle*): activity of phosphorylase kinase (calcium-receptor: calmodulin). (*Bottom*): activities of μ- and *m*-calpains, which are plotted against the calcium ion. Both enzymes contain their respective calcium-binding domains. *Source*: These curves are redrawn from Refs. 106, 108, and 115 with modifications.

by the same amount of extracellular fluid to activate *m*-calpain (Fig. 6). Ca^{2+} ions in the extracellular fluid would need to quickly enter the cytosol through the cleft during contraction, when the intracellular fluid pressure is higher than the extracellular fluid pressure. If the fluid exchange actually happens within a very short period, the cell would be disrupted chemically and physically, and could not remain viable.

b. In cases where Ca^{2+} ions gradually enter myofibers through Ca^{2+} channels (113) or by a long lasting repetition of gradual diffusion through the "membrane cleft," Ca^{2+} ion concentrations might gradually increase. Ca^{2+} ions would initially be sequestered but could gradually accumulate beyond the sequestering capacity. Ca^{2+} ions diffuse in the cytosol at a speed of approximately 1 mm/sec, so the entire fiber would be filled with Ca^{2+} ions at the same concentration within a short period.

If Ca^{2+} concentrations exceeded a threshold level of sequestering, both the contraction and glycogen-metabolic processes would be strongly activated (Fig. 6) (107,109), resulting in severe contracture of muscles as in rigor mortis. If the concentration was sustained at more than 10^{-5} M in multiple muscles of the body, the consequences would resemble those observed in malignant hyperthermia, a hereditary disorder caused by excessive Ca^{2+} release from the sarcoplasmic reticulum that is induced by drug administration (114). This increase in Ca^{2+} ions in the sarcoplasm induces strong contractions and high heat production, sometimes resulting in death. Although over-contraction has been observed in the middle stages of DMD (115), it does not reach the magnitude observed in malignant hyperthermia. Nonetheless, the elevated calcium concentrations associated with these strong contractures are insufficient to activate *m*-calpain. If Ca^{2+} ion concentrations were to continue increasing until *m*-calpain was activated, severe digestion of the cytoplasm would occur together with untreatable strong contractions and heat production. Considering that many degenerating muscle fibers survive many years through multiple rounds of regeneration, it seems unlikely that activation of *m*-calpain could be relevant to DMD muscle pathology, at least in the early and middle stages of the disease.

2. μ-Calpain: Ca^{2+} ions at the physiological concentration that reversibly induce muscle contraction and phosphorylase kinase activation can activate μ-calpain (Fig. 6) (116). In this case, protein degradation would be triggered during each contraction–relaxation cycle. If this process induces muscular dystrophy, every muscle fiber in a normal subject would be prone to degeneration. Nonetheless, there may be a few possible scenarios where μ-calpain could contribute to the development of the dystrophic pathology. One is that the enzyme level is very low in normal muscles but is increased in dystrophic muscles. The other is that changes in the concentration of phosphatidylinositol might enhance μ-calpain activity at a given concentration of Ca^{2+} ion (116). However, calpain activity must not be too high or muscle fibers would be

completely digested within a short period, and DMD does not follow such a chronic course.

Calpain digests some muscle proteins, including dystrophin, by producing partially degraded polypeptides (117,118). To explore a possible role for calpain in DMD muscle pathology, several calpain inhibitors such as E64 and leupeptin have been extensively studied. Such trials were, however, not successful. In contrast, calpastatin-transgenic *mdx* mice were reported to display a reduced surge of muscle necrosis (119). Calpastatin is an intrinsic calpain inhibitor. However, this degenerative surge occurs acutely in *mdx* mice, but is not observed in DMD patients. Different cellular pathways may well be involved in the acute degenerative process compared with those in the chronic degenerative processes. In addition, the protease content in skeletal muscles is fairly different among animal species, suggesting that pathways involved in muscle degeneration may be different depending on the species. In the case of human dystrophic muscle fibers at very late stages of the disease, contraction is severely impaired and minimal vestiges of the calcium-sequestration systems remain. In such fibers, calpain could very well be activated and might rapidly digest the remaining intracellular proteins, serving as a scavenger working together with enzymes from infiltrating macrophages. The digestive process at this stage of the disease could well be considerably faster than in the early and middle stages.

There are many difficult problems yet to be solved before the Ca^{2+}-calpain hypothesis can be accepted. In addition, there are some naïve questions. For example, could other enzymes participate in the degenerative process, such as cathepsin, whose expression increases several times more than does calpain 2, which is the *m*-calpain catalytic subunit in *mdx* muscles (120)?

Other Possibilities in Degeneration

It is important to always consider additional and alternate mechanisms that may contribute to degeneration, and that the primary mechanism contributing to degeneration might not be the same at all stages of the disease. For example, since the Ca^{2+}–calpain hypothesis implies that a decreased amount of protein leads to muscle necrosis, one should consider other mechanisms that can decrease protein concentrations in myofibers. One possibility is the leakage of cytoplasmic proteins such as creatine kinase. This leakage decreases the protein levels unless they are adequately replaced by new synthesis. In addition, long-term leakage of cytosolic contents could result in the disturbance of a variety of metabolic processes, since many of the components involved in these processes are enzymes. Furthermore, continuous loss of proteins from muscle fibers could contribute to malnutrition. Cytoplasmic proteins are normally degraded to AAs, which are then used for de novo synthesis of proteins (121). This AA recycling system could also be disturbed by the continuous release of the cytosolic contents into the extracellular milieu. Although an increased AA uptake may partially compensate, a prolonged loss of protein must be a heavy burden for muscle fiber, especially when continuous myofiber regeneration is occurring. Disturbances because of the leakage of smaller molecules, such as those functioning in signaling processes, coupled with the entrance of foreign substances from the extracellular fluid must be also considered as potentially contributing to myonecrosis.

In summary, our understanding of the mechanisms underlying the degenerative processes in dystrophic muscle fiber is still preliminary and requires consideration of multiple mechanisms and approaches to analysis. A clear strategy must be established for the study of chronic processes, although this is a very difficult task. Various processes occurring in normal and dystrophic muscle development have to be considered for a fuller understanding of how muscles degenerate.

EPILOGUE

In this chapter, DMD pathogenesis at the molecular and the cellular levels was explained based on the mechanical hypothesis. This hypothesis is based on the clinical observations of DMD patients and not only on laboratory experiments. Unfortunately, because numerous gaps remain in our knowledge of specific mechanisms, some parts of this explanation were constructed on circumstantial evidence, particularly the discussions in the previous two sections.

Disturbances in signaling systems secondarily induced by the lack of dystrophin are also important in DMD pathogenesis, and may modify the processes explained above (see Chapter 3). Even when detailed knowledge on signaling systems becomes available, the pathogenesis cannot be explained without considering the mechanical processes, because the principal function of muscle fibers is mechanical and the course of DMD is closely related to muscle contraction.

As an old Oriental saying goes, we cannot understand what the forest is, if we only gaze upon a single tree. It is very difficult to access the forest. Although we consider that a detailed investigation of a single tree is an important task, knowing how to apply these findings to understand the forest is crucial. Furthermore, we have to consider that the forest is not merely the sum of its trees. For a complete understanding of the pathogenesis of DMD, we must consider what is happening in a single entire muscle fiber in addition to various molecular phenomena. Furthermore, in the study of DMD therapies, the effects on the entire musculature have to be considered, because the problem of how to retain muscle functions in good balance in terms of the posture and movement of the living body will arise.

REFERENCES

1. Arahata K, Ishiura S, Ishiguro T, et al. Immunostaining of skeletal and cardiac muscle surface membrane with antibody against Duchenne muscular dystrophy peptide. Nature 1988; 333:861–863.
2. Watkins SC, Hoffman EP, Slayter HS, Kunkel LM. Immunoelectron microscopic localization of dystrophin in myofibres. Nature 1988; 333:863–866.
3. Engel A, Ozawa E. Dystrophinopathies. In: Engel A. Franzini-Armstrong C, ed. Myology. New York: McGraw-Hill, 2004:961–1025.
4. De Le Porte S, Morin S, Koenig J. Characteristics of skeletal muscle in mdx mutant mice. Int. Rev Cytol 1999; 191:99–148.
5. Batten FE. The muscle spindle under pathological conditions. Brain 1897; 20:138–179.
6. Tanaka H, Yoshida M, Ishiguro T, Eguchi C, Nonaka I, Ozawa E. Expression of dystrophin on the cell membrane of intrafusal fibers of human skeletal muscle. Protoplasma 1989; 152:109–111.
7. Noakes TD. Effect of exercise on serum enzyme activities in humans. Sports Med 1987; 4:245–267.
8. Florence JM, Fox PT, Planer GJ, Brooke MH. Activity, creatine kinase, and myoglobin in Duchenne muscular dystrophy: a clue to etiology? Neurology 1985; 35:758–761.
9. Matsuda R, Nishikawa A, Tanaka H. Visualization of dystrophic muscle fibers in mdx mouse by vital staining with Evans blue: evidence of apoptosis in dystrophin-deficient muscle. J Biochem (Tokyo) 1995; 118:959–964.
10. Lidov H, Byers TJ, Watkins SC, Kunkel LM. Localization of dystrophin to postsynaptic regions of central nervous system cortical neurons. Nature 1990; 348:725–728.
11. Hagiwara Y, Yoshida M, Nonaka I, Ozawa E. Developmental expression of dystrophin on the plasma membrane of rat muscle cells. Protoplasma 1989; 151:11–18.
12. Monaco AP, Kunkel LM. Cloning of the Duchenne/Becker muscular dystrophy locus. Adv Hum Genet 1988; 17:61–98.
13. Koenig M, Monaco AP, Kunkel LM. The complete sequence of dystrophin predicts a rod-shaped cytoskeletal protein. Cell 1988; 53:219–228.
14. Tinsley JM, Blake DJ, Zuelling RA, Davies KE. Increasing complexity of the dystrophin-associated protein complex. Proc Natl Acad Sci USA 1994; 91:8307–8313.
15. Blake DJ, Weir A, Sarah E Newey, Kay E Davies. Function and genetics of dystrophin and dystrophin-related proteins in muscle. Physiol Rev 2002; 82:291–329.
16. Ozawa E. The muscle fiber cytoskeleton: The dystrophin system. In: Engel A, Franzini-Armstrong C, eds. Myology. New York: McGraw-Hill, 2004:455–470.
17. Yoshida M, Suzuki A, Yamamoto, H, Noguchi S, Ozawa E. Dissociation of the complex of dystrophin and its associated proteins into several unique groups by n-octyl β-D-glucoside. Eur J Biochem 1994; 222:1055–1061.
18. Ibraghimov-Beskrovnaya O, Ervasti JM, Leveille CJ, Slaughter CA, Sernett SW, Campbell KP. Primary structure of dystrophin-associated glycoproteins linking dystrophin to the extracellular matrix. Nature 1992; 355:696–702.

19. Chiba A, Matsumura K, Yamada H, et al. Structures of sialylated O-linked oligosaccharides of bovine peripheral nerve alpha-dystroglycan. The role of a novel O-mannosyl-type oligosaccharide in the binding of alpha-dystroglycan with laminin. J Biol Chem 1997; 272:2156–2162.
20. Ozawa E, Noguchi S, Mizuno Y, Hagiwara Y, Yoshida M. From dystrophinopathy to sarcoglycanopathy: evolution of a concept of muscular dystrophy. Muscle Nerve 1998; 21:421–438.
21. Ozawa E, Mizuno Y, Hagiwara Y, Sasaoka T, Yoshida M. Molecular and cell biology of sarcoglycan complex. Muscle Nerve 2005; 32:563–576.
22. Crosbie RH, Heighway J, Venzke DP, Lee JC, Campbell KP. Sarcospan, the 25-kDa transmembrane component of the dystrophin–glycoprotein complex. J Biol Chem 1997; 272:31221–1224.
23. Winder SJ, Gibson TJ, Kendrick-Jones J. Dystrophin and utrophin: the missing links!. FEBS Lett 1995; 369:27–33.
24. Sutherland-Smith AJ, Moores CA, Norwood FL, et al. An atomic model for actin binding by the CH domains and spectrin-repeat modules of utrophin and dystrophin. J Mol Biol 2003; 329:15–33.
25. Rybakova I, Amann KJ, Ervasti JM. A new model for the interaction of dystrophin with F-actin. J Cell Biol 1996; 135:661–671.
26. Ishikawa-Sakurai M, Yoshida M, Imamura M, Davies K, Ozawa E. ZZ domain is essentially required for the physiological binding of dystrophin and utrophin to β-dystroglycan. Hum Mol Genet 2004; 13:693–702.
27. Ozawa E, Nishino I, Nonaka I. Sarcolemmopathy: muscular dystrophies with cell membrane defects. Brain Pathol 2001; 11:218–230.
28. Yoshida M, Hama H, Ishikawa-Sakurai M, et al. Biochemical evidence for association of dystrobrevin with the sarcoglycan–sarcospan complex as a basis for understanding sarcoglycanopathy. Hum Mol Genet 2000; 9:1033–1040.
29. Noguchi S, Wakabayashi E, Imamura M, Yoshida M, Ozawa E. Formation of sarcoglycan complex with differentiation in cultured myocytes. Eur J Biochem 2000; 267:640–648.
30. Wakayama Y, Shibuya S. Gold-labelled dystrophin molecule in muscle plasmalemma of mdx control mice as seen by electron microscopy of deep etching replica. Acta Neuropathol 1991; 82:178–184.
31. Andre B, Springer J-Y. WWWP, a new amino acid motif present in single or multiple copies in various proteins including dystrophin and SH3-binding Yes-associated protein YAP65. Biochem. Biophys Res Comm 1994; 205:1201–1205.
32. Bork P, Sudol M. The WW domain: a signaling site in dystrophin? TIBS 1994; 19:531–533.
33. Zarrinpar A, Lim WA. Converging on proline: the mechanism of WW domain peptide recognition. Nat Struct Biol 2000; 7:611–613.
34. Huang X, Poy F, Zhang R, Joakimiak A, Sudol M, Eck MJ. Structure of a WW domain containing fragment of dystrophin in complex with β-dystroglycan. Nat Struct Biol 2000; 7:634–638.
35. Rafael JA, Cox GA, Corrado K, Jung D, Campbell KP, Chamberlain JS. Forced expression of dystrophin deletion constructs reveals structure–function correlations. J Cell Biol 1996; 134:93–102.

36. Talts JF, Andac Z, Gohring W, Brancaccio A, Timpl R. Binding of the G domains of laminin α1 and α2 chains and perlecan to heparin, sulfatides, α-dystroglycan and several extracellular matrix proteins. EMBO J 1999; 18:863–870.
37. Sakamoto A, Ono K, Abe M, et al. Both hypertrophic and dilated cardiomyopathies are caused by mutation of the same gene, δ-sarcoglycan, in hamster: an animal model of disrupted dystrophin-associated glycoprotein complex. Proc Natl Acad Sci USA 1997; 94:13873–13878.
38. Noguchi S, Wakabayashi E, Imamura, Yoshida M, Ozawa E. Developmental expression of sarcoglycan gene products in cultured myocytes. Biochem Biophys Res Commun 1990; 262:88–93.
39. Imamura M, Mochizuki Y, Engvall E, Takeda S. ε-Sarcoglycan compensate for lack of α-sarcoglycan in a mouse model of limb–girdle muscular dystrophy. Hum Mol Genet 2005; 14:775–783.
40. Burkin DJ, Kaufman SJ. The α7β1 integrin in muscle developmemt and disease. Cell Tissue Res 1999; 296:183–190.
41. Kerr TP, Sewry CA, Robb SA, Roberts RG. Long mutant dystrophins and variable phenotypes: evasion of nonsense mediated decay? Human Genet 2001; 109:402–407.
42. Chelly J, Kaplan JC, Maire P, Gautron S, Kahn A. Transcription of the dystrophin gene in human muscle and non-muscle tissue. Nature 1988; 333:858–860.
43. Tanaka H, Ishiguro T, Eguchi C, Saito K, Ozawa E. Expression of a dystrophin-related protein associated with the skeletal muscle cell membrane. Histochemistry 1991; 96:1–5.
44. Squire S, Raymackers JM, Vandebrouck C, et al. Prevention of pathology in *mdx* mice by expression of utrophin: analysis using an inducible transgenic expression system. Hum Mol Genet 2002; 11:3333–3344.
45. Deckonick AE, Rafael JA, Skinner JA, et al. Utrophin-deficient mice as a model for Duchenne muscular dystrophy. Cell 1997; 90:717–727.
46. Grady RM, Teng H, Nichol MC, Cunningham JC, Wilkinson RS, Sanes JR. Skeletal and cardiac myopathies in mice lacking utrophin and dystrophin: a model for Duchenne muscular dystrophy. Cell 1997; 90:729–738.
47. Rafael JA, Tinsley, Potter AC, Deconinck AE, Davies KE. Skeletal muscle-specific expression of a utrophin transgene rescues utrophin–dystrophin deficient mice. Nat Genet 1998; 19:79–83.
48. Mizuno Y, Yoshida M, Nonaka I, Hirai S, Ozawa E. Expression of utrophin (dystrophin-related protein) and dystrophin-associated glycoproteins in muscles from patients with Duchenne muscular dystrophy. Muscle Nerve 1994; 17:206–216.
49. Ohlendieck K, Matsumura K, Ioanescu VV, et al. Duchenne muscular dystrophy: Deficiency of dystrophin associated proteins in the sarcolemma. Neurology 1993; 43:795–800.
50. Brenman JE, Chao DS, Xia H, Aldape K, Bredt DS. Nitric oxide synthase complexed with dystrophin and absent from skeletal muscle sarcolemma in Duchenne muscular dystrophy. Cell 1995; 82:743–752.
51. Metzinger L, Blake DJ, Squier MV, et al. Dystrobrevin deficiency at the sarcolemma of patients with muscular dystrophy. Hum Mol Genet 1997:1185–1191.

52. Kameya S, Miyagoe Y, Nonaka I, et al. α1-Syntrophin gene disruption results in the absence of neuronal-type nitric-oxide synthase at the sarcolemma but does not induce muscle degeneration. J Biol Chem 1999; 274:2193–2200.
53. Chao DS, Silvagno F, Bredt DS. Muscular dystrophy in *mdx* mice despite lack of neuronal nitric oxide synthase. J Neurochem 1998; 71:784–789.
54. Grady RM, Grange RW, Lau KS, et al. Role for α-dystrobrevin in the pathogenesis of dystrophin-dependent muscular dystrophies. Nat Cell Biol 1999; 1:215–220.
55. Cox GA, Cole NM, Matsumura K, et al. Overexpression of dystrophin in transgenic mdx mice eliminates dystrophic symptoms without toxicity. Nature 1993; 364:725–729.
56. Noguchi S, Tsukahara T, Fujita M, et al. cDNA microarray analysis of individual Duchenne muscular dystrophy patients. Hum Mol Genet 2003; 12: 595–600.
57. Winnard AV, Klein CJ, Coovert DD, et al. Characterization of translational frame exception patients in Duchenne/Becker muscular dystrophy. Hum Mol Genet 1993; 2:737–744.
58. Hoffman EP, Fischbeck KH, Brown RH, et al. Characterization of dystrophin in muscle-biopsy specimens from patients with Duchenne's or Becker's muscular dystrophy. N Engl J Med 1988; 26 (318):1363–1368.
59. Warner LE, DelloRusso C, Crawford RW, et al. Expression of Dp260 in muscle tethers the actin cytoskeleton to the dystrophin-glycoprotein complex and partially prevents dystrophy. Hum Mol Genet 2002; 11:1095–1105.
60. Cox GA, Sunada Y, Campbell KP, Chamberlain JS. Dp71 can restore the dystrophin-associated glycoprotein complex in muscle but fails to prevent dystrophy. Nat Genet 1994; 8:333–339.
61. Greenberg DS, Sunada Y, Campbell KP, Yaffe D, Nudel U. Exogenous Dp71 restores the levels of dystrophin associated proteins but does not alleviate muscle damage in *mdx* mice. Nat Genet 1994; 8:340–344.
62. Hoffman EP, Garcia CA, Chamberlain JS, Angelini C, Lupski JR, Fenwick R. Is the carboxyl-terminus of dystrophin required for membrane association? A novel, severe case of Duchenne muscular dystrophy. Ann Neurol 1991; 30:605–610.
63. Recan D, Chafey P, Leturcq F, et al. Are cysteine-rich and COOH-terminal domains of dystrophin critical for sarcolemmal localization? J Clin Invest 1992; 89:712–716.
64. Helliwell TR, Ellis JM, Mountford RC, Appleton RE, Morris GE. A truncated dystrophin lacking the C-terminal domains is localized at the muscle membrane. Am J Hum Genet. 1992; 50:508–514.
65. Koenig M, Beggs AH, Moyer M, et al. The molecular basis for Duchenne versus Becker muscular dystrophy: correlation of severity with type of deletion. Am J Hum Genet. 1989; 45:498–506.
66. Den Dunnen JT, Grootscholten PM, Bakker E, et al. Topography of the Duchenne muscular dystrophy (DMD) gene: FIGE and cDNA analysis of 194 cases reveals 115 deletions and 13 duplications. Am J Hum Genet 1989; 45:835–847.
67. Hodgson S, Hart K, Abbs S, et al. Correlation of clinical and deletion data in Duchenne and Becker muscular dystrophy. J Med Genet 1989; 26:682–693.

68. Crawford GE, Faulkner JA, Crosbie RH, Campbell KP, Froehner SC, Chamberlain JS. Assembly of the dystrophin-associated protein complex does not require the dystrophin COOH-terminal domain. J Cell Biol 2000; 150:1399–1410.
69. England SB, Nicholson LV, Johnson MA, et al. Very mild muscular dystrophy associated with the deletion of 46% of dystrophin. Nature 1990; 343:180–182.
70. Dunckley MG, Love DR, Davies KE, Walsh FS, Morris GE, Dickson G. Retroviral-mediated transfer of a dystrophin minigene into *mdx* mouse myoblasts in vitro. FEBS Lett 1992; 296:128–134.
71. Ozawa E, Yoshida M, Suzuki A, Mizuno Y, Hagiwara Y, Noguchi S. Dystrophin-associated proteins in muscular dystrophy. Hum Mol Genet 1995; 4:1711–1716.
72. Yuasa K, Miyagoe Y, Yamamoto K, Nabeshima Y, Dickson G, Takeda S. Effective restoration of dystrophin-associated proteins in vivo by adenovirus-mediated transfer of truncated dystrophin cDNAs. FEBS Lett 1998; 425:329–336.
73. Gregorevic P, Blankinship MJ, Allen JM, et al. Systemic delivery of genes to striated muscles using adeno-associated viral vectors. Nat Med 2004; 10:828–834.
74. Sakamoto M, Yuasa K, Yoshimura M, et al. Micro-dystrophin cDNA ameliorates dystrophic phenotypes when introduced into *mdx* mice as a transgene. Biochem Biophys Res Commun 2002; 293:1265–1272.
75. Tome FM, Evangelista T, Leclerc A, et al. Congenital muscular dystrophy with merosin deficiency. CR Acad Sci III 1994; 317:351–357.
76. Yoshida A, Kobayashi K, Manya H, et al. Muscular dystrophy and neuronal migration disorder caused by mutations in a glycosyltransferase, POMGnT1. Dev Cell 2001; 1:717–724.
77. Muntoni F, Voit T. The congenital muscular dystrophies in 2004: a century of exciting progress. Neuromuscul Disord 2004 ; 14:635–649.
78. Voit T, Tome FMS. The congenital muscular dystrophies. In: Engel A, Franzini-Armstrong C , eds. Myology. New York: McGraw-Hill, 2004:1203–1238.
79. Hayashi YK, Chou FL, Engvall E, et al. Mutations in the integrin alpha7 gene cause congenital myopathy. Nat Genet 1998; 19:94–97.
80. Osari S, Kobayashi O, Yamashita Y, et al. Basement membrane abnormality in merosin-negative congenital muscular dystrophy. Acta Neuropathol (Berl) 1996; 91:332–336.
81. Tomanek RJ, Colling-Saltin AS. Cytological differentiation of human fetal skeletal muscle. Am J Anat 1977; 149:227–245.
82. Chiu AY, Sanes JR. Development of basal lamina in synaptic and extrasynaptic portions of embryonic rat muscle. Dev Biol 1984; 103:456–467.
83. Clerk A, Strong PN, Sewry CA. Characterization of dystrophin during development of human skeletal muscle. Development 1992; 114:395–402.
84. Clerk A, Sewry CA, Dubowitz V, Strong PN. Characterization of dystrophin in fetuses at risk for Duchenne muscular dystrophy. J Neurol Sci 1992; 111:82–91.
85. Clerk A, Morris GE, Dubowitz V, Davies KE, Sewry CA. Dystrophin-related protein, utrophin, in normal and dystrophic human fetal skeletal muscle. Histochem J 1993; 25:554–561.
86. Tome FM, Matsumura K, Chevallay M, Campbell KP, Fardeau M. Expression of dystrophin-associated glycoproteins during human fetal muscle

development: a preliminary immunocytochemical study. Neuromuscul Disord 1994; 4:343–348.
87. Carpenter S, Karpati G. Duchenne muscular dystrophy: plasma membrane loss initiates muscle cell necrosis unless it is repaired. Brain 1979; 102:147–161.
88. Henry MD, Campbell KP. A role for dystroglycan in basement membrane assembly. Cell 1998; 95:859–870.
89. Lazarides E. Intermediate filaments as mechanical integrators of cellular space. Nature 1980; 283:249–256.
90. Pardo JV, Siliciano JD, Craig SW. A vinculin-containing cortical lattice in skeletal muscle: transverse lattice elements ("costameres") mark sites of attachment between myofibrils and sarcolemma. Proc Natl Acad Sci USA 1983; 80:1008–1012.
91. Danowski BA, Imanaka-Yoshida K, Sanger JM, Sanger JW. Costameres are sites of force transmission to the substratum in adult rat cardiomyocytes. J Cell Biol 1992; 118:1411–1420.
92. Hijikata T, Fujimaki N, Osawa H, Ishikawa H. The direct visualization of structural array from laminin to dystrophin in sarcolemmal vesicles prepared from rat skeletal muscles. Biol Cell 1998; 90:629–639.
93. Mizuno Y, Thompson TG, Guyon JR, et al. Desmuslin, an intermediate filament protein that interact with α-dystrobrevin and desmin. Proc Natl Acad Sci USA 2001; 98:6156–6161.
94. Hijikata T, Murakami T, Ishikawa H, Yorifuji H. Plectin tethers desmin intermediate filaments onto subsarcolemmal dense plaques containing dystrophin and vinculin. Histochem Cell Biol 2003; 119:109–123.
95. Blake DJ, Weir A, Newey SE, Davies KE. Function and genetics of dystrophin and dystrophin-related proteins in muscle. Physiol Rev 2001; 82:291–329.
96. Pardo JV, Siliciano JD, Craig SW. Vinculin is a component of an extensive network of myofibril-sarcolemma attachment regions in cardiac muscle fibers. J Cell Biol 1983; 97:1081–1088.
97. Dowben RM. Contractility. In: Mountcastle VB, ed. Medical Physiology. St Louis: C.V. Mosby Company, 1980:82–119.
98. Masuda T, Fujimaki N, Ozawa E, Ishikawa H. Confocal laser microscopy of dystrophin localization in guinea pig skeletal muscle fibers. J Cell Biol 1992; 119:543–548.
99. McNeil PL, Terasaki M. Coping with the inevitable: how cells repair a torn surface membrane. Nat Cell Biol 2001; 3:E124–129.
100. Ozawa E, Hagiwara Y, Yoshida M. Creatine kinase, cell membrane and Duchenne muscular dystrophy. Mol Cell Biochem 1999; 190:143–151.
101. Smith FJS, Eady RA, Leigh IM, et al. Plectin deficiency results in muscular dystrophy with epidermolysis bullosa. Nat Genet 1996; 13:450–457.
102. Dalakas MC, Park KY, Semino-Mora C, Lee HS, Sivakumar K, Goldfarb LG. Desmin myopathy, a skeletal myopathy with cardiomyopathy caused by mutations in the desmin gene. N Engl J Med 2000; 342:770–780.
103. Hauser MA, Horrigan SK, Salmikangas P, et al. Myotilin is mutated in limb girdle muscular dystrophy 1A. Hum Mol Genet 2000; 9:2141–2147.

104. Moreira ES, Wiltshire TJ, Faulkner G, et al. Limb-girdle muscular dystrophy type 2G is caused by mutations in the gene encoding the sarcomeric protein telethonin. Nat Genet 2000; 24:163–116.
105. Sorimachi H, Ishiura S, Suzuki K. Structure and physiological function of calpains. Biochem J 1997; 328:721–732.
106. Ozawa E, Hosoi S, Ebashi S. Reversible stimulation of muscle phosphorylase b kinase by low concentration of Ca ions. J Biochem (Tokyo) 1967; 61:531–533.
107. Ozawa E. Activation of muscular phosphprylase b kinase by a minute amount of Ca ion. J Biochem (Tokyo) 1972; 71:321–331.
108. Koch R. Die Aetiologie der Tuberklose. Addressed at the Berlin Physiological Society 1882. In: Porter R (Summarized). In: The Greatest Benefit to Mankind. New York: W W Norton Co, 1997:436–437.
109. Ebashi S, Endo M. Calcium ion and muscle contraction. Prog Biophys Mol Biol. 1968; 18:123–183.
110. Sorimachi H, Imajoh-Ohmi S, Emori Y, et al. Molecular cloning of a novel mammalian calcium-dependent protease distinct from both m- and mu-types. Specific expression of the mRNA in skeletal muscle. J Biol Chem 1989; 264:20106–20111.
111. Ishiura S, Tsuji S, Murofushi H, Suzuki K. Purification of an endogenous 68,000-dalton inhibitor of Ca^{2+}-activated neutral protease from chicken skeletal muscle. Biochim Biophys Acta 1982; 701:216–223.
112. Isselbacher KJ, et al., eds. Harrison's Principles of Internal Medicine. 13th edn. New York: McGraw Hill, Inc., 1994:2490.
113. Iwata Y, Katanosaka Y, Arai Y, Komamura K, Miyatake K, Shigekawa M. A novel mechanism of myocyte degeneration involving the Ca^{2+}-permeable growth factor-regulated channel. J Cell Biol 2003; 161:957–967.
114. Endo M, Yagi S, Ishizuka T, Horiuti K, Koga Y, Amaha K. Changes in the Ca-induced Ca release mechanism in the sarcoplasmic reticulum of the muscle from a patient with malignant hyperthermia. Biomed Res 1983; 4:83–92.
115. Cullen MJ, Fulthorpe JJ. Stages in fibre breakdown in Duchenne muscular dystrophy. An electron-microscopic study. J Neurol Sci 1975; 24:179–200.
116. Suzuki K, Saido TC, Hirai S. Modulation of cellular signals by calpain. Ann NY Acad Sci. 1992; 674:218–227.
117. Croall DE, DeMartino GN. Calcium-activated neutral protease (calpain) system: structure, function, and regulation. Physiol Rev 1991; 71:813–847.
118. Suzuki A, Yoshida M, Yamamoto H, Ozawa E. Glycoprotein-binding site of dystrophin is confined to the cysteine-rich domain and the first half of the carboxy-terminal domain. FEBS Lett 1992; 308:154–160.
119. Spencer MJ, Mellgren RL. Overexpression of a calpastatin transgene in *mdx* muscle reduces dystrophic pathology. Hum Mol Genet 2002; 11:2645–2655.
120. Porter JD, Khanna S, Kaminski HJ, et al. A chronic inflammatory response dominates the skeletal muscle molecular signature in dystrophic-deficient *mdx* mice. Human Mol Genet 2002; 11:263–272.
121. Zak R, Martin AF, Blough R. Assessment of protein turnover by use of radioisotopic tracers. Physiol Rev 1979; 59:407–447.

3

The Functional Biology of Dystrophin: Associated Signaling Pathways and Potential Targets for Therapeutic Intervention

Gayle Smythe
School of Community Health, Charles Sturt University, Albury, New South Wales, Australia

Steven J. Winder
Department of Biomedical Science, Center for Developmental and Biomedical Genetics, University of Sheffield, Western Bank, Sheffield, U.K.

Thomas A. Rando
Department of Neurology and Neurological Sciences, Stanford University School of Medicine, Stanford, California, and GRECC and Neurology Service, VA Palo Alto Health Care System, Palo Alto, California, U.S.A.

INTRODUCTION

The obstacles to gene therapy approaches in the treatment of Duchenne muscular dystrophy (DMD), as outlined in several chapters in this book (see Chapters 17–19), have led to many investigations to seek alternative therapeutic strategies. One of the hurdles to non-genetic therapy for DMD is the absence of a well-defined pathogenetic process leading from dystrophin deficiency to the pathological manifestations of DMD. The "function" of dystrophin is deduced primarily by what is observed in its absence, but this is complicated by the fact that the histological phenotype of dystrophin-deficiency can vary widely. Dystrophin-deficient muscle displays normal or nearly normal histology in very young dystrophin-deficient (*mdx*) mice and in certain muscle groups in both DMD patients and animal models (1–3). It appears predominantly hypertrophic in the feline model (4), it displays mild degenerative changes in specific cases in humans (5), and it displays severe degenerative changes in human limb and trunk muscles in typical DMD patients (6). Understanding the function of dystrophin by the examination of dystrophin-deficient muscle is further complicated by the fact that dystrophin is part of a multicomponent protein complex, generally referred to as the dystrophin-associated protein complex (DAPC) or more narrowly as the dystrophin–glycoprotein complex (7–9). This complex includes, at its core, the transmembrane dystroglycan complex (a heterodimer composed of a transmembrane β-subunit and an extracellular α-subunit) that binds dystrophin intracellularly and laminin extracellularly (10). The sarcoglycan complex likewise is a transmembrane protein complex tightly associated with the dystroglycan complex (11). Intracellularly, dystrophin and β-dystroglycan bind to numerous other proteins including, directly or indirectly, actin, dystrobrevins, and syntrophins (7–9). Dystrophin deficiency results in secondary deficiency or mislocalization of virtually every component of the DAPC. Ultimately, it will be critical to distinguish which aspects of DMD are caused by these secondary deficiencies. By considering the various domains of the dystrophin protein, specific biochemical deficits and physiological perturbations associated with deletions of those regions and the effects of restoring regions of the protein in transgenic *mdx* mice, it is possible to begin to develop a functional biology of dystrophin that may reveal multiple therapeutic targets.

Fundamentally, the issue is whether functional deficits that result from dystrophin deficiency can be prevented pharmacologically. This approach requires an understanding of the functional units of the DAPC. In that regard, the question is whether the functional units can be understood in terms of known signal transduction or metabolic pathways in the cell, and in terms of basic cell biological properties that relate to cell survival or cell death. This conceptual approach is supported by the increasing number of "booster genes" that, when overexpressed, can compensate for the absence of dystrophin (12). Although these have all been proof-of-principle demonstrations involving genetic manipulation, each one also reflects distinct biochemical pathways that may be amenable to pharmacological manipulation.

The previous chapter (Chapter 2) focuses on the biophysical aspects of dystrophin, its interactions with cytoskeletal elements, and the role of dystrophin in contractile functions. This chapter will focus on the functional biology of dystrophin as it relates to disrupted cellular functions in the setting of dystrophin mutations and dystrophin deficiency, and the potential that some of those functional deficits may present novel therapeutic targets. The first section deals with the different domains of the dystrophin protein and its specific cellular functions. The second section reviews various signaling cascades and their associated cellular processes that are disrupted in the setting of dystrophin deficiency.

DYSTROPHIN DOMAINS AND PROTEIN INTERACTIONS

Dystrophin is a large protein with several identified domains, including the N-terminal, rod, cysteine-rich, and C-terminal domains (Fig. 1). Within those domains, specific "functions" have been identified, that is, protein–protein interactions. The importance of these interactions is demonstrated by the consequences of their disruption. This section focuses on the four major domains of the dystrophin protein, highlights the known protein–protein interactions mediated by each domain, and serves as a prelude to the following section in which the physiologic processes mediated by an intact DAPC are considered.

N-Terminal Domain

The N-terminal domain of dystrophin has been identified, primarily, as a site of interaction with F-actin (13–15). By analogy, therefore, this domain is likened to other actin-binding proteins that link the structure and dynamics of cytoskeletal actin with transmembrane signaling proteins (16). Becker muscular dystrophy (BMD) patients with deletions in this region tend to have fairly mild disease, although a DMD patient with a missense mutation in this region has been reported (Fig. 1) (17,18).

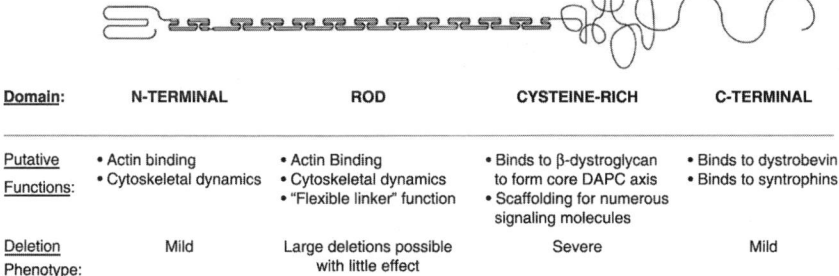

Figure 1 Dystrophin domain structure, function, and deletion phenotype. Dystrophin is presented schematically to illustrate its four major domains, to summarize the functional biology of each domain, and to categorize generally the severity of the muscular dystrophy associated with in-frame deletions within each domain.

Transgenic *mdx* strains that express dystrophin with a deletion in the actin-binding domain in this region have a mild phenotype (19). This might suggest that the binding to actin is not crucial to the function of the complex but the rod domain also has actin-binding sites (see below). Therefore, this may be a somewhat redundant property within the dystrophin protein. In fact, transgenic *mdx* strains expressing just the cysteine-rich and C-terminal domains of the protein have a severe phenotype despite the restoration of the DAPC, whereas expression of a transgene containing these regions and a portion of the rod domain containing the actin-binding sites produces a much milder dystrophy (20–22). Thus, the binding of actin either within the N-terminal or within the rod domain may be necessary for full functional capabilities. It remains to be determined whether the binding of actin to dystrophin is strictly a scaffolding function or if dystrophin participates in the regulation of cytoskeletal dynamics.

Rod Domain

The rod domain of dystrophin is notable for its homology to spectrin (23) and has been shown to have actin-binding properties (24). Much emphasis had been placed on a role for the rod domain as a flexible linker (25,26); however, more recently new roles have emerged, and the production of fully functional dystrophins with very little rod domain have reduced the emphasis on a flexible linker function. What is perhaps most notable about the rod domain is how much of it can be eliminated without profound consequences. In humans, there are well documented cases of BMD arising from deletion of massive regions of the rod domain (27,28). Based on these observations, truncated dystrophin transgenes ("mini-dystrophins" and "micro-dystrophins") that lack large portions of the rod domain have been developed for gene therapy approaches (29–31). Virtually all of the functional aspects of full-length dystrophin, at least in mice, have been restored by the expression of these shortened forms of dystrophin lacking very large portions of the rod domain, including the actin-binding domain. Again, this suggests that this functional aspect of the rod domain is not strictly essential, though these constructs all possessed a fully functional amino-terminal actin-binding domain. This is highlighted by the fact that overexpression of utrophin, which is very homologous to dystrophin but lacks the high affinity actin-binding property in its rod domain, prevents degeneration of dystrophin-deficient muscle (32,33). However, more recent studies have suggested that the utrophin rod domain may also contain actin-binding sites distinct from those of dystrophin (34). Furthermore, the rod domain can be reduced only so much before the functionality of the protein is lost in terms of preventing degeneration (31). It is not known whether these remaining regions are essential for actin binding, proper folding, spacing, or molecular dynamics of the protein itself or are involved in the other as yet undiscovered protein–protein interactions.

Cysteine-Rich and C-Terminal Domains

Many key protein–protein interaction domains are present in the cysteine-rich and C-terminal domains of dystrophin (35). The WW domain found at the N-terminal end of the cysteine-rich domain is essential for binding β-dystroglycan with the cysteine-rich region as a whole, whereas the coiled-coil motif of the C-terminus forms the binding site for dystrobrevin and syntrophins (35,36). In addition, it is via the increasing number of signaling proteins that bind to these domains that the scaffolding function of dystrophin is most dramatically revealed (Table 1). Also, with the exception of half of the WW domain being absent in the DP71 isoform, these domains are conserved throughout all of the dystrophin isoforms that are expressed in nonmuscle tissue (37). Thus variations of the muscle DAPC are found in tissues throughout the body, and these protein complexes presumably regulate many of the same cellular functions in those tissues as the DAPC does in muscle (38).

There are no examples of BMD with deletions in the cysteine-rich region; predicted in-frame deletions in this region all lead to the severe DMD phenotype (17,39). Even missense mutations in this region can lead to DMD because of the disruption of key cysteines involved in protein–protein interactions (36,40,41). However, deletions of the C-terminal domain can lead to a mild BMD phenotype, and deletions of proteins that bind specifically to the C-terminal domain, such as dystrobrevin, produce either a very mild myopathy or no pathology at all (42,43). This same pattern holds true in transgenic *mdx* mice. Even though deletion of the final C-terminal domain does not significantly affect the ability of the protein to protect against degenerative changes, deletions within the cysteine-rich domain are generally catastrophic (44). In fact, expression of transgenes containing only the cysteine-rich and C-terminal domains in *mdx* mice appears to worsen the dystrophy, perhaps by competing with utrophin for binding to dystroglycan and thus eliminating any protective effect being conferred by that dystrophin homolog (20,21). This is further suggested by the fact that overexpression of this isoform in wild-type mice leads to a muscular dystrophy (45). Thus, the full functional properties of dystrophin depend heavily on an intact cysteine-rich domain, almost certainly related to the binding to β-dystroglycan in this region and attesting to the central role of the laminin–dystroglycan–dystrophin axis in DAPC structure and function. It is likely that all of the sarcoglycan deficiencies also produce severe muscular dystrophies by interfering with the normal function of this axis and the cellular functions mediated by the DAPC.

Table 1 Interaction of DAPC Proteins with Signaling Proteins at the Muscle Sarcolemma

DAPC protein	Associated signaling proteins	DAPC protein function		Reference
		Scaffold	Substrate	
Dystrophin	Calmodulin	+	+	(103,104,130)
	CaM kinase		+	(106,122)
	ERK		+	(123,130,131)
	Casein kinase		+	(122,123,130)
	p34^{cdc2}		+	(130)
	Calcineurin		+	(130)
	PKA		+	(123)
	PKC		+	(122,123)
	PKG		+	(122)
β-Dystroglycan	Grb2	+		(66–68)
	MEK2, ERK	+		(132)
	Ezrin	+		(133)
	Src	+		(134)
	Fyn	+	+	(134)
	FAK	+		(67,134)
	Shc, Nck, Csk	+		(134)
Syntrophins	Grb2			(65)
	Calmodulin	+		(135)
	nNOS	+		(89,136)
	DGKζ	+		(124,125)
	SAPK-3	+	+	(62)
	Phosphatidylinositol 4, 5-bisphosphate	+		(88,137)
	CaM kinase		+	(106)
	Aquaporin	+		(87,138)
	MAST	+		(139)
Sarcoglycans	Src		+	(140)
Dystrobrevins	DAMAGE	+		(141)
Caveolin-3	nNOS	+		(88,142,143,144)
	H-Ras	+		(145)
	Src	+		(88,146,147)
	PKCα	+		(148)
	Phosphofructokinase-M	+		(146,149,150)
	cG-proteins	+		(151)
	β-Dystroglycan	+		(134)

DAPC proteins to which direct binding of a signaling protein or adaptor signaling protein have been identified or which have been demonstrated to be a substrate for an enzyme in a signaling pathway, are presented. Although caveolin-3 is not an integral DAPC protein, it is included here owing to its known association with the DAPC (152,153) and altered expression in DMD (142,154). The associations presented in this table are those that relate to the DAPC at the sarcolemma. There are numerous other signaling molecules that have been found to be associated with DAPC proteins at the neuromuscular junction and in other tissues. At the neuromuscular junction and in other tissues, other isoforms of dystrophin or utrophin would substitute for full-length dystrophin in the complex. In the latter case, the appropriate designation would be "UAPC" (utrophin associated protein complex) rather than DAPC.

Abbreviations: DAPC, dystrophin-associated protein complex; DMD, Duchenne muscular dystrophy; PKA, protein kinase A.

CELLULAR SIGNALING PATHWAYS ASSOCIATED WITH THE DAPC

In this section, we will segue from the domains of dystrophin and their interactions with specific proteins to the cellular functions and biochemical pathways that may relate to those interactions. The main focus of this section is to review those processes that may be regulated by an intact DAPC, are altered when the DAPC is disrupted, may account for aspects of DMD, and therefore may be targets for therapeutic intervention. Among the cardinal features of muscular dystrophies is the death of myofibers. Although necrotic cell death is one of the hallmarks of the pathology, it is clear that apoptotic death contributes to and may precede the necrotic phase of the disease (46–48). Not only have apoptotic myonuclei been detected in dystrophic muscle, but also changes in specific cell death pathways have been found. A number of pro-apoptotic proteins are upregulated in DMD muscle, including Bax and several caspase isoforms (48,49). In particular, caspase-3 expression is strongly correlated with apoptosis in DMD, being upregulated in 100% of muscle biopsies analyzed from DMD patients (48).

An intact DAPC protects muscle cells from the processes that lead to these forms of cell death. The protective function of the complex depends critically on the adhesive aspects of dystroglycan with the extracellular matrix. It is well established that cellular interactions with the extracellular matrix are key to the maintenance of cell survival and integrity and that disruption of these interactions leads to apoptotic cell death (50–52). The importance of the adhesion properties of the dystrophin complex in maintaining cell survival is demonstrated by recent reports showing that enhancing cellular adhesion can protect dystrophin-deficient muscle from degeneration. Transgenic overexpression of the $\alpha7\beta1$ integrin, which, like the DAPC, is expressed on myofiber membranes and binds to laminin, can ameliorate the dystrophic phenotype in mice that lack both dystrophin and utrophin (53). In addition, although overexpression of dystroglycan alone does not ameliorate the dystrophic phenotype, hyperglycosylation of this DAPC protein does significantly protect dystrophic muscle from degeneration, presumably by enhancing the adhesion/signaling properties of the complex through utrophin (54,55). Furthermore, overexpression of the glycosyltransferase LARGE can similarly overcome the molecular defect in a range of muscular dystrophies including Fukuyama congenital muscular dystrophy and muscle–eye–brain disease, by restoring glycosylation of dystroglycan (56). Therefore, understanding the signaling pathways by which interactions between the extracellular matrix and the DAPC regulate cell survival may reveal novel therapeutic targets for promoting cell survival in dystrophin-deficient muscle.

Clearly, the dystrophin complex interacts with numerous signaling proteins, as detailed in Table 1. Each of these regulates cellular defense mechanisms that may play a role in muscle cell survival. These defense mechanisms include anti-apoptotic pathways, stress response pathways, antioxidant defense pathways, and anti-inflammatory pathways, all of which have been implicated in the pathogenesis of DMD (57). In the following sections we have focused on the major pathways that have known interactions with the DAPC, that have been shown to be dysregulated in dystrophin-deficient muscle, and that have been implicated in disease pathogenesis.

Mitogen-Activated Protein Kinase

Mitogen-activated protein kinases (MAPKs), including extracellular signal–regulated protein kinases (ERKs), p38 MAPK, and c-Jun N-terminal kinases (JNKs), are components of signaling cascades that regulate cell survival and cell stress responses. They are rapidly emerging as targets for therapeutic intervention in several diseases (58,59). While ERK activation is usually associated with growth factor–mediated signaling and the promotion of cell survival, p38 and JNKs are usually activated in response to stressful stimuli and are therefore often referred to as stress-activated protein kinases (SAPKs) (58,59). The regulation of pro-apoptotic proteins including those of the Bcl family involves certain MAPK pathways. Phosphorylation and inactivation of the pro-apoptotic protein, Bad, can be regulated by ERKs, and Bcl-2 and Bcl-XL can both be similarly inhibited by JNK signaling (60,61).

There is evidence that multiple components of MAPK signaling pathways are associated with DAPC proteins, and that these pathways are disrupted in DMD. Skeletal muscle α1-syntrophin is a substrate for p38γ, and syntrophins bind the p46 JNK isoform (62,63). These interactions are likely mediated by the ubiquitous SH2/SH3 domain–containing adaptor protein, Grb2, which is commonly involved in signaling pathways initiated at receptor tyrosine kinases (64). Grb2 has been shown to bind at least two DAPC proteins. Grb2 binding to α1-syntrophin results in the formation of a Rac1–Grb2–SOS complex that recruits p46 JNK and promotes muscle cell survival (63,65), whereas Grb2 binding to β-dystroglycan appears to be involved in promoting cell adhesion (66–68).

Several modifications in MAPK signaling have been reported in DMD muscle that may reflect changes in myofiber responses to their extracellular environment. Persistent activation of SAPK signaling pathways has been reported in cardiac muscle from mice that are deficient in both dystrophin and utrophin, and to some extent in *mdx* hearts (69,70). In addition, p38 MAPK activation is significantly reduced in *mdx* diaphragm, which exhibits a severe dystrophic phenotype, compared with mildly affected limb muscles from the same mice in which p38 MAPK activation was normal (71). The same study reported comparable levels of ERK1/2 activation in *mdx* diaphragm and limb muscles, which were elevated compared with normal muscles. Increased phosphorylation of the p54 JNK isoform has been reported in *mdx* skeletal muscle, and expression of constitutively active p54 JNK causes compromised integrity and cell death in cultured myotubes (72). Treatment with p54 JNK inhibitors ameliorates the dystrophic phenotype (72). Interestingly, this JNK isoform is activated when the interaction between α-dystroglycan and laminin is disrupted, a process that results in apoptosis, in contrast to the p46 isoform that is phosphorylated in response to normal laminin binding (63).

Nuclear factor κB (NF-κB), a transcription factor that regulates expression of genes involved in cell survival and proliferation in response to stress, is a downstream target of JNKs and p38 MAPK (73,74). NF-κB activation precedes the onset of muscle degeneration in *mdx* mice, and applying mechanical stress to *mdx* myofibers results in further activation of this transcription factor (75). Furthermore, NF-κB is upregulated in human DMD muscle (76). However, as discussed below, NF-κB can be activated by multiple signaling pathways, including those mediated by phosphatidylinositol-3-kinase [PI(3)K]/AKT and calpains. Therefore, careful dissection of the upstream regulators of this transcription factor is required, and the effects of its upregulation in dystrophic muscle be determined, whether must be beneficial or detrimental.

PI(3)K/AKT

It is well established that signaling through the PI(3)K/AKT cascade promotes cell survival via canonical anti-apoptotic pathways. Thus, enhancing the activation of this pathway may skew the balance toward cell survival (77). Active AKT inhibits cell death by phosphorylating and inactivating Bad and by inactivating caspase-9 (78,79). Activated AKT also phosphorylates and inactivates proteins, such as YAP, GSK-3β, and members of the Forkhead family of transcription factors, all of which may be involved in the cell survival properties of AKT (79). In some cells, survival is directly promoted through activation of the NF-κB transcription factor downstream of AKT (79,80).

Like the MAPK pathways, the PI(3)K/AKT pathway can interact with the DAPC via the adaptor protein, Grb2 (81). The apoptotic cell death that occurs in muscle cells when the binding of the DAPC to laminin is disrupted is due to an inhibition of PI(3)K/AKT activity (51). This is consistent with the finding that apoptotic cell death is associated with decreased PI(3)K/AKT activity following loss of cell adhesion to the extracellular matrix (52). Furthermore, the beneficial effects of insulin-like growth factors (IGFs) in *mdx* mice may result from the ability of these factors to activate AKT in muscle cells (82–85). Taken together these studies suggest a crucial role for reduced PI(3)K/AKT signaling in the dystrophic process. While further analysis of the involvement of this pathway in altered muscle cell survival in

DMD is required, upregulating PI(3)K/AKT has strong potential as a therapeutic target for alleviating the dystrophic phenotype.

Neuronal Nitric Oxide Synthase

One of the most widely studied signaling proteins in DMD is neuronal nitric oxide synthase (nNOS), which catalyzes the production of nitric oxide. In normal skeletal muscle fibers, nNOS localizes to the sarcolemma and is preferentially expressed in fast (type I) fibers (86). nNOS binds the DAPC via the PDZ domain of α1-syntrophin, and it also binds directly to the scaffolding domain of the DAPC-associated protein, caveolin-3 (87,88). In *mdx* muscle, nNOS expression is significantly reduced, and it is mislocalized from the sarcolemma to the cytosol where it retains some enzymatic activity (89,90). There are conflicting arguments about the contribution of altered nNOS expression and activity to the dystrophic phenotype. While some suggest that aberrant localization and activation of nNOS promotes the dystrophic phenotype via increased free radical production, others hypothesize that an overall decrease in nNOS expression results in an increased susceptibility to inflammation (89,90). These conflicting hypotheses may be because of the complex properties of nNOS, which can be either anti- or pro-inflammatory, depending on multiple factors (86,91). Changes in nitric oxide production do not significantly affect the redox state of *mdx* muscle cells (92). Furthermore, it was recently reported that nNOS overexpression has anti-inflammatory properties and can protect skeletal muscle from exercise-induced injury (93). A complete absence of nNOS from *mdx* muscle neither promotes nor alleviates the dystrophy, while nNOS overexpression improves muscle histology primarily by reducing inflammatory parameters (94,95). Taken together these studies indicate that reduced total expression and activation of nNOS is a contributing factor to disease progression in DMD. Although it is clear that nNOS deficiency alone is insufficient to produce a dystrophic phenotype (96), in the presence of additional metabolic stressors, it is likely to be a major contributing factor.

Calcium Activated Signaling Pathways

The notion of dystrophin deficiency leading to alterations in cellular calcium level as a primary pathogenetic mechanism is an old one (97). Aside from the clear increase in cellular calcium that would accompany membrane breakdown at the early stages of necrotic cell death, evidence from pre-necrotic *mdx* mouse muscle indicates that steady-state increases in intracellular calcium levels may predispose the cells to either apoptotic or necrotic cell death (98). Two proteins that provide direct links between calcium regulatory pathways and the DAPC are calmodulin and calpain (99,100). Disrupted signaling via each of these in dystrophin-deficient muscle suggests possible therapeutic targets for intervening in pathogenetic mechanisms.

Calmodulin is a major calcium-sensing protein, and its interaction with calcium can regulate multiple signaling pathways. Among the downstream targets of calmodulin are calmodulin-dependent kinases (CaM-kinases) and phosphatases (calcineurin) (101). Both calmodulin and CaM-kinase II bind to DAPC proteins (Table 1) (102–106). Elevated cytosolic levels of calmodulin have been reported in human DMD muscles, suggesting that in the absence of an intact DAPC, calmodulin is mislocalized from the sarcolemma to the cytosol (107). Calcineurin is a calmodulin-dependent serine/threonine phosphatase with a catalytic subunit (calcineurin-A/protein phosphatase 2B) and a regulatory subunit (calcineurin-B). Calcineurin activity is elevated in *mdx* and utrophin/dystrophin-deficient mice, perhaps as part of an endogenous compensatory mechanism (69,70). Treatment of *mdx* mice with the immunosuppressant cyclosporin, a calcineurin inhibitor, exacerbates the dystrophic phenotype (108). Similarly, expression of constitutively active calcineurin results in reduced myofiber degeneration, upregulation of sarcolemmal expression of utrophin, and restoration of normal levels and localization of β-dystroglycan, syntrophin, and nNOS (109). The latter study suggested that upregulation of calcineurin restores DAPC expression at the sarcolemma by promoting sarcolemmal expression of utrophin, which is normally restricted to the neuromuscular junction. These findings may relate to reports that transplant recipients on long-term cyclosporin treatment experience muscle fiber atrophy and necrosis, myalgia, cramps, and elevated serum creatine kinase which, in most cases, were reversible side effects that disappeared after cyclosporin withdrawal (110). Taken together these studies indicate that calcineurin is an important calmodulin-dependent regulator of skeletal muscle growth and differentiation, and that altered intracellular calcium homeostasis in DMD could promote muscle fiber necrosis by indirectly disrupting calcineurin signaling. Furthermore, in vivo evidence strongly suggests that exogenous activation of calcineurin is a potential therapeutic target in DMD (108,109).

Calpains are a family of calcium-dependent, calmodulin-independent proteases, of which three isoforms [calpain-1 (μ-calpain), calpain-2 (m-calpain), and calpain-3] are expressed in skeletal muscle. Although calpains have not been shown to directly associate with the DAPC, calpain-1 is hyperactivated and calpain-2 overexpressed in DMD muscle (111). Furthermore, calpain inhibition by treatment with leupeptin or by inducing overexpression of the endogenous calpain inhibitor, calpastatin, significantly reduces the dystrophic phenotype in *mdx* mice. Calpains have multiple substrates, including protein kinase C (PKC), G-protein α-subunits, and Rac1, although no studies to date have examined a functional relationship between altered function of these signaling proteins and elevated calpain activity in DMD (112–114). Elevated calpain activity may also indirectly contribute to muscle degeneration by degrading the calpain-sensitive enzyme, nNOS (115). Calpains have also been reported to regulate NF-κB pathways, and a calpain-3 deficiency in skeletal muscle is known to disrupt NF-κB signaling and cause muscle cell apoptosis

(116–118). In contrast, calpains have been reported to cleave caspase-9, inhibiting cleavage of caspase-3 and, subsequently, inhibiting apoptosis (119). Thus, the role of calpains in controlling apoptotic mechanisms appears to be extremely complex and may be cell-type specific (119). Further characterizing the role of these proteases in skeletal muscle, and specifically in DMD, is likely to provide new opportunities for therapeutic development. However, while calpain inhibitors have strong potential for treating DMD, a calpain-3 deficiency is associated with a limb-girdle–type muscular dystrophy in humans (120), and calpains are involved in normal muscle regeneration and in normal sarcomere formation (111,113,121). Therefore, the use of isoform-specific calpain inhibitors, such as calpastatin, which inhibits calpain-1 and calpain-2, but not calpain-3, are likely to be the most suitable candidates for alleviating the dystrophic phenotype in DMD (113).

Other Cell Survival Regulatory Pathways

Although PKC expression and activation have not been shown to be regulated by aspects of the dystrophin complex, PKC may interact with and phosphorylate dystrophin (122,123). Expression of diacylglycerol kinase-ζ (DGK-ζ), an enzyme essential in the activation of certain PKC isoforms, is reduced at the sarcolemma of skeletal muscle from *mdx* mice (124). This protein binds syntrophins, an interaction that appears to have a role in regulating actin assembly and organization (124,125). Phosphorylation of DGK-ζ is required for normal actin assembly, and this appears to occur downstream of ERK (124). Furthermore, the DGK-ζ interaction with syntrophin may be important for regulating its subcellular localization (124). Therefore, decreased expression, and possibly mislocalization, of DGK-ζ in DMD muscle may contribute to disrupted assembly and organization of the actin cytoskeleton. Further studies on the signaling pathways both up- and downstream of this enzyme in skeletal muscle will clarify its potential as a therapeutic target.

In the *mdx* mouse diaphragm, where the onset of the dystrophic phenotype is early and progresses rapidly, phosphorylation of p70 S6 kinase was significantly elevated compared with limb muscles in which the dystrophy is less obvious (71). p70 S6 kinase participates in a range of signaling pathways, typically those downstream of receptor tyrosine kinase activation. In skeletal muscle cells p70 S6 kinase is activated in response to IGF-1 treatment, indicating that upregulation of this protein reflects the ongoing regeneration process in dystrophic muscle (126). Further studies are required to establish the exact signaling pathways that utilize this protein in dystrophic skeletal muscle and to determine if it is a suitable therapeutic candidate.

Another anti-apoptotic protein, apoptosis repressor with caspase recruitment domain (ARC), is highly expressed in skeletal muscle and protects myofibers from cell death primarily by interacting with caspases (127,128). However, despite an abnormal subcellular localization pattern of ARC in *mdx* skeletal muscle, overexpression of this protein does not significantly alter the dystrophic phenotype (129). Therefore, subcellular localization of ARC may be extremely important to its ability to exert anti-apoptotic effects in skeletal muscle. Further studies into the upstream regulators and downstream targets of this protein are warranted.

CONCLUSIONS

It is becoming increasingly clear that DMD is a complex disease that results from multiple contributing factors. Although replacement of the full-length dystrophin gene by viral- or nonviral mediated gene transfer represents an appealingly simple therapeutic approach in concept, gene therapy remains an extremely challenging practical option as outlined in other chapters. Furthermore, because gene transfer is increasingly focusing on truncated forms of dystrophin, the studies reviewed here clearly demonstrate the importance of identifying key dystrophin domains required for localization, phosphorylation, and binding to other DAPC proteins and associated signaling proteins in transgene design. Importantly, there are still multiple hurdles that must be overcome once appropriate transgenes and vectors are designed, including widespread delivery to muscle, transgene incorporation into appropriate genomic sites, and safety issues.

Beyond the value of understanding dystrophin functional domains for transgene design, the studies reviewed here also suggest potential alternate therapeutic approaches that do not involve gene transfer. In this chapter, we have focused on disrupted signal transduction pathways as one aspect of the dystrophic phenotype in DMD. The identification of contributing factors to the dystrophic process, such as individual signaling pathways that are perturbed, provides potential targets for non-genetic therapy approaches to modify the disease process. Although the sarcolemmal localization of associated signaling proteins probably cannot be restored in the absence of an intact DAPC, exogenous regulation of their downstream targets may promote muscle cell integrity and survival. Pharmacological modulation of any one signaling pathway may enhance muscle structure and function, but it may be that a "cocktail" of agents to simultaneously regulate multiple disrupted signaling pathways will potentially have more considerable beneficial effects.

ACKNOWLEDGMENTS

This work was supported by grants from the Medical Research Council to SJW and from the National Institutes of Health and the Muscular Dystrophy Association to TAR.

REFERENCES

1. Khurana TS, Prendergast RA, Alameddine HS, et al. Absence of extraocular muscle pathology in Duchenne's muscular dystrophy: role for calcium homeostasis in extraocular muscle sparing. J Exp Med 1995; 182:467–475.
2. Porter JD. Extraocular muscle sparing in muscular dystrophy: a critical evaluation of potential protective mechanisms. Neuromuscul Disord 1998; 8:198–203.
3. Dowling P, Culligan K, Ohlendieck K. Distal mdx muscle groups exhibiting up-regulation of utrophin and rescue of dystrophin-associated glycoproteins exemplify a protected phenotype in muscular dystrophy. Naturwissenschaften 2002; 89:75–78.
4. Gaschen FP, Hoffman EP, Gorospe JR, et al. Dystrophin deficiency causes lethal muscle hypertrophy in cats. J Neurol Sci 1992; 110:149–159.
5. Zatz M, Betti RT, Levy JA. Benign Duchenne muscular dystrophy in a patient with growth hormone deficiency. Am J Med Genet 1981; 10:301–304.
6. Emery AEH. Duchenne Muscular Dystrophy. 2d ed. New York: Oxford University Press, 1993.
7. Rando TA. The dystrophin–glycoprotein complex, cellular signaling, and the regulation of cell survival in the muscular dystrophies. Muscle Nerve 2001; 24:1575–1594.
8. Ehmsen J, Poon E, Davies K. The dystrophin-associated protein complex. J Cell Sci 2002; 115:2801–2803.
9. Spence HJ, Chen YJ, Winder SJ. Muscular dystrophies, the cytoskeleton and cell adhesion. Bioessays 2002; 24:542–552.
10. Henry MD, Campbell KP. Dystroglycan inside and out. Curr Opin Cell Biol 1999; 11:602–607.
11. Betto R, Biral D, Sandona D. Functional roles of dystrophin and of associated proteins. New insights for the sarcoglycans. Ital J Neurol Sci 1999; 20:371–379.
12. Engvall E, Wewer UM. The new frontier in muscular dystrophy research: booster genes. FASEB J 2003; 17:1579–1584.
13. Way M, Pope B, Cross RA, Kendrick-Jones J, Weeds AG. Expression of the N-terminal domain of dystrophin in *E. coli* and demonstration of binding to F-actin. FEBS Lett 1992; 301:243–245.
14. Hemmings L, Kuhlman PA, Critchley DR. Analysis of the actin-binding domain of alpha-actinin by mutagenesis and demonstration that dystrophin contains a functionally homologous domain. J Cell Biol 1992; 116:1369–1380.
15. Fabbrizio E, Bonet-Kerrache A, Leger JJ, Mornet D. Actin–dystrophin interface. Biochemistry 1993; 32:10457–10463.
16. Pavalko FM, Otey CA. Role of adhesion molecule cytoplasmic domains in mediating interactions with the cytoskeleton. Proc Soc Exp Biol Med 1994; 205:282–293.
17. Beggs AH, Hoffman EP, Snyder JR, et al. Exploring the molecular basis for variability among patients with Becker muscular dystrophy: dystrophin gene and protein studies. Am J Hum Genet 1991; 49:54–67.
18. Prior TW, Papp AC, Snyder PJ, et al. A missense mutation in the dystrophin gene in a Duchenne muscular dystrophy patient. Nat Genet 1993; 4:357–360.

19. Corrado K, Rafael JA, Mills PL, Cole NM, Faulkner JA, Wang K, Chamberlain JS. Transgenic *mdx* mice expressing dystrophin with a deletion in the actin-binding domain display a "mild Becker" phenotype. J Cell Biol 1996; 134:873–884.
20. Cox GA, Sunada Y, Campbell KP, Chamberlain JS. Dp71 can restore the dystrophin-associated glycoprotein complex in muscle but fails to prevent dystrophy. Nat Genet 1994; 8:333–339.
21. Greenberg DS, Sunada Y, Campbell KP, Yaffe D, Nudel U. Exogenous Dp71 restores the levels of dystrophin associated proteins but does not alleviate muscle damage in mdx mice. Nat Genet 1994; 8:340–344.
22. Warner LE, DelloRusso C, Crawford RW, et al. Expression of Dp260 in muscle tethers the actin cytoskeleton to the dystrophin–glycoprotein complex and partially prevents dystrophy. Hum Mol Genet 2002; 11:1095–1105.
23. Hoffman EP, Brown RH Jr, Kunkel LM. Dystrophin: the protein product of the Duchenne muscular dystrophy locus. Cell 1987; 51:919–928.
24. Rybakova IN, Amann KJ, Ervasti JM. A new model for the interaction of dystrophin with F-actin. J Cell Biol 1996; 135:661–672.
25. Winder SJ, Gibson TJ, Kendrick-Jones J. Dystrophin and utrophin: the missing links!. FEBS Lett 1995; 369:27–33.
26. Winder SJ. The membrane-cytoskeleton interface: the role of dystrophin and utrophin. J Muscle Res Cell Motil 1997; 18:617–629.
27. England SB, Nicholson LV, Johnson MA, et al. Very mild muscular dystrophy associated with the deletion of 46% of dystrophin. Nature 1990; 343:180–182.
28. Matsumura K, Burghes AH, Mora M, et al. Immunohistochemical analysis of dystrophin-associated proteins in Becker/Duchenne muscular dystrophy with huge in-frame deletions in the NH2-terminal and rod domains of dystrophin. J Clin Invest 1994; 93:99–105.
29. Phelps SF, Hauser MA, Cole NM, et al. Expression of full-length and truncated dystrophin mini-genes in transgenic *mdx* mice. Hum Mol Genet 1995; 4:1251–1258.
30. Wells DJ, Wells KE, Asante EA, et al. Expression of human full-length and minidystrophin in transgenic mdx mice: implications for gene therapy of Duchenne muscular dystrophy. Hum Mol Genet 1995; 4:1245–1250.
31. Harper SQ, Hauser MA, DelloRusso C, et al. Modular flexibility of dystrophin: implications for gene therapy of Duchenne muscular dystrophy. Nat Med 2002; 8:253–261.
32. Amann KJ, Guo AW, Ervasti JM. Utrophin lacks the rod domain actin binding activity of dystrophin. J Biol Chem 1999; 274:35375–35380.
33. Tinsley JM, Potter AC, Phelps SR, Fisher R, Trickett JI, Davies KE. Amelioration of the dystrophic phenotype of mdx mice using a truncated utrophin transgene. Nature 1996; 384:349–353.
34. Rybakova IN, Patel JR, Davies KE, Yurchenco PD, Ervasti JM. Utrophin binds laterally along actin filaments and can couple costameric actin with sarcolemma when overexpressed in dystrophin-deficient muscle. Mol Biol Cell 2002; 13:1512–1521.
35. Blake DJ, Weir A, Newey SE, Davies KE. Function and genetics of dystrophin and dystrophin-related proteins in muscle. Physiol Rev 2002; 82:291–329.

36. Ishikawa-Sakurai M, Yoshida M, Imamura M, Davies KE, Ozawa E. ZZ domain is essentially required for the physiological binding of dystrophin and utrophin to beta-dystroglycan. Hum Mol Genet 2004; 13:693–702.
37. Love DR, Byth BC, Tinsley JM, Blake DJ, Davies KE. Dystrophin and dystrophin-related proteins: a review of protein and RNA studies. Neuromuscul Disord 1993; 3:5–21.
38. Kramarcy NR, Vidal A, Froehner SC, Sealock R. Association of utrophin and multiple dystrophin short forms with the mammalian M_r 58,000 dystrophin-associated protein (syntrophin). J Biol Chem 1994; 269:2870–2876.
39. Koenig M, Beggs AH, Moyer M, et al. The molecular basis for Duchenne versus Becker muscular dystrophy: correlation of severity with type of deletion. Am J Hum Genet 1989; 45:498–506.
40. Lenk U, Oexle K, Voit T, et al. A cysteine 3340 substitution in the dystroglycan-binding domain of dystrophin associated with Duchenne muscular dystrophy, mental retardation and absence of the ERG b-wave. Hum Mol Genet 1996; 5:973–975.
41. Goldberg LR, Hausmanowa-Petrusewicz I, Fidzianska A, Duggan DJ, Steinberg LS, Hoffman EP. A dystrophin missense mutation showing persistence of dystrophin and dystrophin-associated proteins yet a severe phenotype. Ann Neurol 1998; 44:971–976.
42. McCabe ER, Towbin J, Chamberlain J, et al. Complementary DNA probes for the Duchenne muscular dystrophy locus demonstrate a previously undetectable deletion in a patient with dystrophic myopathy, glycerol kinase deficiency, and congenital adrenal hypoplasia. J Clin Invest 1989; 83:95–99.
43. Grady RM, Grange RW, Lau KS, et al. Role for α-dystrobrevin in the pathogenesis of dystrophin-dependent muscular dystrophies. Nat Cell Biol 1999; 1:215–220.
44. Rafael JA, Cox GA, Corrado K, Jung D, Campbell KP, Chamberlain JS. Forced expression of dystrophin deletion constructs reveals structure–function correlations. J Cell Biol 1996; 134:93–102.
45. Leibovitz S, Meshorer A, Fridman Y, et al. Exogenous Dp71 is a dominant negative competitor of dystrophin in skeletal muscle. Neuromuscul Disord 2002; 12:836–844.
46. Tidball JG, Albrecht DE, Lokensgard BE, Spencer MJ. Apoptosis precedes necrosis of dystrophin-deficient muscle. J Cell Sci 1995; 108:2197–2204.
47. Tews DS, Goebel HH. DNA-fragmentation and expression of apoptosis-related proteins in muscular dystrophies. Neuropathol Appl Neurobiol 1997; 23:331–338.
48. Sandri M, Minetti C, Pedemonte M, Carraro U. Apoptotic myonuclei in human Duchenne muscular dystrophy. Lab Invest 1998; 78:1005–1016.
49. Tews DS. Apoptosis and muscle fibre loss in neuromuscular disorders. Neuromuscul Disord 2002; 12:613–622.
50. Montanaro F, Lindenbaum M, Carbonetto S. α-Dystroglycan is a laminin receptor involved in extracellular matrix assembly on myotubes and muscle cell viability. J Cell Biol 1999; 145:1325–1340.
51. Langenbach KJ, Rando TA. Inhibition of dystroglycan binding to laminin disrupts the PI3K/AKT pathway and survival signaling in muscle cells. Muscle Nerve 2002; 26:644–653.

52. Zhan M, Zhao H, Han ZC. Signalling mechanisms of anoikis. Histol Histopathol 2004; 19:973–983.
53. Burkin DJ, Wallace GQ, Nicol KJ, Kaufman DJ, Kaufman SJ. Enhanced expression of the alpha 7 beta 1 integrin reduces muscular dystrophy and restores viability in dystrophic mice. J Cell Biol 2001; 152:1207–1218.
54. Hoyte K, Jayasinha V, Xia B, Martin PT. Transgenic overexpression of dystroglycan does not inhibit muscular dystrophy in mdx mice. Am J Pathol 2004; 164:711–718.
55. Nguyen HH, Jayasinha V, Xia B, Hoyte K, Martin PT. Overexpression of the cytotoxic T cell GalNAc transferase in skeletal muscle inhibits muscular dystrophy in mdx mice. Proc Natl Acad Sci USA 2002; 99:5616–5621.
56. Barresi R, Michele DE, Kanagawa M, et al. LARGE can functionally bypass alpha-dystroglycan glycosylation defects in distinct congenital muscular dystrophies. Nat Med 2004; 10:696–703.
57. Petrof BJ. Molecular pathophysiology of myofiber injury in deficiencies of the dystrophin-glycoprotein complex. Am J Phys Med Rehabil 2002; 81:S162–S174.
58. Kyriakis JM, Avruch J. Mammalian mitogen-activated protein kinase signal transduction pathways activated by stress and inflammation. Physiol Rev 2001; 81:807–869.
59. Johnson GL, Lapadat R. Mitogen-activated protein kinase pathways mediated by ERK, JNK, and p38 protein kinases. Science 2002; 298:1911–1912.
60. Scheid MP, Schubert KM, Duronio V. Regulation of bad phosphorylation and association with Bcl-x(L) by the MAPK/Erk kinase. J Biol Chem 1999; 274:31108–31113.
61. Lin A. Activation of the JNK signaling pathway: breaking the brake on apoptosis. Bioessays 2003; 25:17–24.
62. Hasegawa M, Cuenda A, Spillantini MG, et al. Stress-activated protein kinase-3 interacts with the PDZ domain of α1-syntrophin. A mechanism for specific substrate recognition. J Biol Chem 1999; 274:12626–12631.
63. Oak SA, Zhou YW, Jarrett HW. Skeletal muscle signaling pathway through the dystrophin glycoprotein complex and Rac1. J Biol Chem 2003; 278:39287–39295.
64. Chardin P, Cussac D, Maignan S, Ducruix A. The Grb2 adaptor. FEBS Lett 1995; 369:47–51.
65. Oak SA, Russo K, Petrucci TC, Jarrett HW. Mouse alpha1-syntrophin binding to Grb2: further evidence of a role for syntrophin in cell signaling. Biochemistry 2001; 40:11270–11278.
66. Yang B, Jung D, Motto D, Meyer J, Koretzky G, Campbell KP. SH3 domain-mediated interaction of dystroglycan and Grb2. J Biol Chem 1995; 270:11711–11714.
67. Cavaldesi M, Macchia G, Barca S, Defilippi P, Tarone G, Petrucci TC. Association of the dystroglycan complex isolated from bovine brain synaptosomes with proteins involved in signal transduction. J Neurochem 1999; 72:1648–1655.
68. Russo K, Di Stasio E, Macchia G, Rosa G, Brancaccio A, Petrucci TC. Characterization of the β-dystroglycan-growth factor receptor 2 (Grb2) interaction. Biochem Biophys Res Commun 2000; 274:93–98.
69. Nakamura A, Harrod GV, Davies KE. Activation of calcineurin and stress activated protein kinase/p38-mitogen activated protein kinase in hearts of utrophin-dystrophin knockout mice. Neuromuscul Disord 2001; 11:251–259.

70. Nakamura A, Yoshida K, Takeda S, Dohi N, Ikeda S. Progression of dystrophic features and activation of mitogen-activated protein kinases and calcineurin by physical exercise, in hearts of mdx mice. FEBS Lett 2002; 520:18–24.
71. Lang JM, Esser KA, Dupont-Versteegden EE. Altered activity of signaling pathways in diaphragm and tibialis anterior muscle of dystrophic mice. Exp Biol Med 2004; 229:503–511.
72. Kolodziejczyk SM, Walsh GS, Balazsi K, et al. Activation of JNK1 contributes to dystrophic muscle pathogenesis. Curr Biol 2001; 11:1278–1282.
73. Hagemann C, Blank JL. The ups and downs of MEK kinase interactions. Cell Signal 2001; 13:863–875.
74. Panwalkar A, Verstovsek S, Giles F. Nuclear factor-kappaB modulation as a therapeutic approach in hematologic malignancies. Cancer 2004; 100:1578–1589.
75. Kumar A, Boriek AM. Mechanical stress activates the nuclear factor-kappaB pathway in skeletal muscle fibers: a possible role in Duchenne muscular dystrophy. FASEB J 2003; 17:386–396.
76. Monici MC, Aguennouz M, Mazzeo A, Messina C, Vita G. Activation of nuclear factor-kappaB in inflammatory myopathies and Duchenne muscular dystrophy. Neurology 2003; 60:993–997.
77. Wu W, Lee WL, Wu YY, et al. Expression of constitutively active phosphatidylinositol 3-kinase inhibits activation of caspase 3 and apoptosis of cardiac muscle cells. J Biol Chem 2000; 275:40113–40119.
78. Datta SR, Brunet A, Greenberg ME. Cellular survival: a play in three Akts. Genes Dev 1999; 13:2905–2927.
79. Downward J. PI 3-kinase, Akt and cell survival. Semin Cell Dev Biol 2004; 15:177–182.
80. Hanada M, Feng J, Hemmings BA. Structure, regulation and function of PKB/AKT–a major therapeutic target. Biochim Biophys Acta 2004; 1697:3–16.
81. Leshem Y, Gitelman I, Ponzetto C, Halevy O. Preferential binding of Grb2 or phosphatidylinositol 3-kinase to the met receptor has opposite effects on HGF-induced myoblast proliferation. Exp Cell Res 2002; 274:288–298.
82. Smith J, Goldsmith C, Ward A, LeDieu R. IGF-II ameliorates the dystrophic phenotype and coordinately down-regulates programmed cell death. Cell Death Differ 2000; 7:1109–1118.
83. Gregorevic P, Plant DR, Leeding KS, Bach LA, Lynch GS. Improved contractile function of the mdx dystrophic mouse diaphragm muscle after insulin-like growth factor-I administration. Am J Pathol 2002; 161:2263–2272.
84. Lawlor MA, Rotwein P. Insulin-like growth factor-mediated muscle cell survival: central roles for Akt and cyclin-dependent kinase inhibitor p21. Mol Cell Biol 2000; 20:8983–8995.
85. Rommel C, Bodine SC, Clarke BA, et al. Mediation of IGF-1-induced skeletal myotube hypertrophy by PI(3)K/Akt/mTOR and PI(3)K/Akt/GSK3 pathways. Nat Cell Biol 2001; 3:1009–1013.
86. Stamler JS, Meissner G. Physiology of nitric oxide in skeletal muscle. Physiol Rev 2001; 81:209–237.

87. Adams ME, Mueller HA, Froehner SC. In vivo requirement of the alpha-syntrophin PDZ domain for the sarcolemmal localization of nNOS and aquaporin-4. J Cell Biol 2001; 155:113–122.
88. Venema VJ, Ju H, Zou R, Venema RC. Interaction of neuronal nitric-oxide synthase with caveolin-3 in skeletal muscle. Identification of a novel caveolin scaffolding/inhibitory domain. J Biol Chem 1997; 272:28187–28190.
89. Chang WJ, Iannaccone ST, Lau KS, et al. Neuronal nitric oxide synthase and dystrophin-deficient muscular dystrophy. USA: Proc Natl Acad Sci 1996; 93:9142–9147.
90. Brenman JE, Chao DS, Xia H, Aldape K, Bredt DS. Nitric oxide synthase complexed with dystrophin and absent from skeletal muscle sarcolemma in Duchenne muscular dystrophy. Cell 1995; 82:743–752.
91. Rando TA. Role of nitric oxide in the pathogenesis of muscular dystrophies: a "two hit" hypothesis of the cause of muscle necrosis. Microsc Res Tech 2001; 55:223–235.
92. Zhuang W, Eby JC, Cheong M, et al. The susceptibility of muscle cells to oxidative stress is independent of nitric oxide synthase expression. Muscle Nerve 2001; 24:502–511.
93. Nguyen HX, Tidball JG. Expression of a muscle-specific, nitric oxide synthase transgene prevents muscle membrane injury and reduces muscle inflammation during modified muscle use in mice. J Physiol 2003; 550:347–356.
94. Crosbie RH, Straub V, Yun HY, et al. *mdx* muscle pathology is independent of nNOS perturbation. Hum Mol Genet 1998; 7:823–829.
95. Wehling M, Spencer MJ, Tidball JG. A nitric oxide synthase transgene ameliorates muscular dystrophy in mdx mice. J Cell Biol 2001; 155:123–131.
96. Chao DS, Silvagno F, Bredt DS. Muscular dystrophy in *mdx* mice despite lack of neuronal nitric oxide synthase. J Neurochem 1998; 71:784–789.
97. Bodensteiner JB, Engel AG. Intracellular calcium accumulation in Duchenne dystrophy and other myopathies: a study of 567,000 muscle fibers in 114 biopsies. Neurology 1978; 28:439–446.
98. Dunn JF, Radda GK. Total ion content of skeletal and cardiac muscle in the mdx mouse dystrophy: Ca2+ is elevated at all ages. J Neurol Sci 1991; 103:226–231.
99. Madhavan R, Jarrett HW. Calmodulin-activated phosphorylation of dystrophin. Biochemistry 1994; 33:5797–5804.
100. Berchtold MW, Brinkmeier H, Muntener M. Calcium ion in skeletal muscle: its crucial role for muscle function, plasticity, and disease. Physiol Rev 2000; 80:1215–1265.
101. Berridge MJ, Bootman MD, Roderick HL. Calcium signalling: dynamics, homeostasis and remodelling. Nat Rev Mol Cell Biol 2003; 4:517–529.
102. Madhavan R, Massom LR, Jarrett HW. Calmodulin specifically binds three proteins of the dystrophin-glycoprotein complex. Biochem Biophys Res Commun 1992; 185:753–759.
103. Jarrett HW, Foster JL. Alternate binding of actin and calmodulin to multiple sites on dystrophin. J Biol Chem 1995; 270:5578–5586.
104. Anderson JT, Rogers RP, Jarrett HW. Ca^{2+}-calmodulin binds to the carboxyl-terminal domain of dystrophin. J Biol Chem 1996; 271:6605–6610.

105. Newbell BJ, Anderson JT, Jarrett HW. Ca^{2+}-calmodulin binding to mouse α1 syntrophin: syntrophin is also a Ca^{2+}-binding protein. Biochemistry 1997; 36:1295–1305.
106. Madhavan R, Jarrett HW. Phosphorylation of dystrophin and α-syntrophin by Ca^{2+}-calmodulin dependent protein kinase II. Biochim Biophys Acta 1999; 1434:260–274.
107. Niebroj-Dobosz I, Kornguth S, Schutta HS, Siegel FL. Elevated calmodulin levels and reduced calmodulin-stimulated calcium-ATPase in Duchenne progressive muscular dystrophy. Neurology 1989; 39:1610–1614.
108. Stupka N, Gregorevic P, Plant DR, Lynch GS. The calcineurin signal transduction pathway is essential for successful muscle regeneration in mdx dystrophic mice. Acta Neuropathol 2004; 107:299–310.
109. Chakkalakal JV, Harrison MA, Carbonetto S, Chin E, Michel RN, Jasmin BJ. Stimulation of calcineurin signaling attenuates the dystrophic pathology in mdx mice. Hum Mol Genet 2004; 13:379–388.
110. Breil M, Chariot P. Muscle disorders associated with cyclosporine treatment. Muscle Nerve 1999; 22:1631–1636.
111. Spencer MJ, Croall DE, Tidball JG. Calpains are activated in necrotic fibers from mdx dystrophic mice. J Biol Chem 1995; 270:10909–10914.
112. Badalamente MA, Stracher A. Delay of muscle degeneration and necrosis in mdx mice by calpain inhibition. Muscle Nerve 2000; 23:106–111.
113. Spencer MJ, Mellgren RL. Overexpression of a calpastatin transgene in mdx muscle reduces dystrophic pathology. Hum Mol Genet 2002; 11:2645–2655.
114. Sato K, Kawashima S. Calpain function in the modulation of signal transduction molecules. Biol Chem 2001; 382:743–751.
115. Laine R, de Montellano PR. Neuronal nitric oxide synthase isoforms alpha and mu are closely related calpain-sensitive proteins. Mol Pharmacol 1998; 54:305–312.
116. Baghdiguian S, Martin M, Richard I, et al. Calpain 3 deficiency is associated with myonuclear apoptosis and profound perturbation of the IkappaB alpha/NF-kappaB pathway in limb-girdle muscular dystrophy type 2A. Nat Med 1999; 5:503–511.
117. Richard I, Roudaut C, Marchand S, et al. Loss of calpain 3 proteolytic activity leads to muscular dystrophy and to apoptosis-associated IkappaBalpha/nuclear factor kappaB pathway perturbation in mice. J Cell Biol 2000; 151:1583–1590.
118. Baghdiguian S, Richard I, Martin M, et al. Pathophysiology of limb girdle muscular dystrophy type 2A: hypothesis and new insights into the IkappaBalpha/NF-kappaB survival pathway in skeletal muscle. J Mol Med 2001; 79:254–261.
119. Chua BT, Guo K, Li P. Direct cleavage by the calcium-activated protease calpain can lead to inactivation of caspases. J Biol Chem 2000; 275:5131–5135.
120. Richard I, Broux O, Allamand V, et al. Mutations in the proteolytic enzyme calpain 3 cause limb-girdle muscular dystrophy type 2A. Cell 1995; 81:27–40.
121. Kramerova I, Kudryashova E, Tidball JG, Spencer MJ. Null mutation of calpain 3 (p94) in mice causes abnormal sarcomere formation in vivo and in vitro. Hum Mol Genet 2004; 13:1373–1388.
122. Luise M, Presotto C, Senter L, et al. Dystrophin is phosphorylated by endogenous protein kinases. Biochem J 1993; 293:243–247.

123. Senter L, Ceoldo S, Petrusa MM, Salviati G. Phosphorylation of dystrophin: effects on actin binding. Biochem Biophys Res Commun 1995; 206:57–63.
124. Abramovici H, Hogan AB, Obagi C, Topham MK, Gee SH. Diacylglycerol kinase-zeta localization in skeletal muscle is regulated by phosphorylation and interaction with syntrophins. Mol Biol Cell 2003; 14:4499–4511.
125. Hogan A, Shepherd L, Chabot J, Quenneville S, Prescott SM, Topham MK, Gee SH. Interaction of gamma 1-syntrophin with diacylglycerol kinase-zeta. Regulation of nuclear localization by PDZ interactions. J Biol Chem 2001; 276:26526–26533.
126. Li M, Li C, Parkhouse WS. Differential effects of des IGF-1 on Erks, AKT-1 and P70 S6K activation in mouse skeletal and cardiac muscle. Mol Cell Biochem 2002; 236:115–122.
127. Koseki T, Inohara N, Chen S, Nunez G. ARC, an inhibitor of apoptosis expressed in skeletal muscle and heart that interacts selectively with caspases. Proc Natl Acad Sci USA 1998; 95:5156–5160.
128. Ekhterae D, Lin Z, Lundberg MS, Crow MT, Brosius FC III, Nunez G. ARC inhibits cytochrome c release from mitochondria and protects against hypoxia-induced apoptosis in heart-derived H9c2 cells. Circ Res 1999; 85:e70–e77.
129. Abmayr S, Crawford RW, Chamberlain JS. Characterization of ARC, apoptosis repressor interacting with CARD, in normal and dystrophin-deficient skeletal muscle. Hum Mol Genet 2004; 13:213–221.
130. Michalak M, Fu SY, Milner RE, Busaan JL, Hance JE. Phosphorylation of the carboxyl-terminal region of dystrophin. Biochem Cell Biol 1996; 74:431–437.
131. Shemanko CS, Sanghera JS, Milner RE, Pelech S, Michalak M. Phosphorylation of the carboxyl terminal region of dystrophin by mitogen-activated protein (MAP) kinase. Mol Cell Biochem 1995; 152:63–70.
132. Spence HJ, Dhillon AS, James M, Winder SJ. Dystroglycan, a scaffold for the ERK-MAP kinase cascade. EMBO Rep 2004; 5:484–489.
133. Spence HJ, Chen YJ, Batchelor CL, et al. Ezrin-dependent regulation of the actin cytoskeleton by {beta}-dystroglycan. Hum Mol Genet 2004; 13:1657–1668.
134. Sotgia F, Lee H, Bedford MT, Petrucci T, Sudol M, Lisanti MP. Tyrosine phosphorylation of beta-dystroglycan at its WW domain binding motif, PPxY, recruits SH2 domain containing proteins. Biochemistry 2001; 40:14585–14592.
135. Iwata Y, Pan Y, Yoshida T, Hanada H, Shigekawa M, calmodulin. α1-syntrophin has distinct binding sites for actin and calmodulin. FEBS Lett 1998; 423:173–177.
136. Brenman JE, Chao DS, Gee SH, et al. Interaction of nitric oxide synthase with the postsynaptic density protein PSD-95 and α1-syntrophin mediated by PDZ domains. Cell 1996; 84:757–767.
137. Chockalingam PS, Gee SH, Jarrett HW. Pleckstrin homology domain 1 of mouse α1-syntrophin binds phosphatidylinositol 4,5-bisphosphate. Biochemistry 1999; 38:5596–5602.
138. Neely JD, Amiry-Moghaddam M, Ottersen OP, Froehner SC, Agre P, Adams ME. Syntrophin-dependent expression and localization of Aquaporin-4 water channel protein. Proc Natl Acad Sci USA 2001; 98:14108–14113.
139. Lumeng C, Phelps S, Crawford GE, Walden PD, Barald K, Chamberlain JS. Interactions between β2-syntrophin and a family of microtubule-associated serine/threonine kinases. Nat Neurosci 1999; 2:611–617.

140. Yoshida T, Pan Y, Hanada H, Iwata Y, Shigekawa M. Bidirectional signaling between sarcoglycans and the integrin adhesion system in cultured L6 myocytes. J Biol Chem 1998; 273:1583–1590.
141. Albrecht DE, Froehner SC. DAMAGE, a novel alpha-dystrobrevin-associated MAGE protein in dystrophin complexes. J Biol Chem 2004; 279:7014–7023.
142. Vaghy PL, Fang J, Wu W, Vaghy LP. Increased caveolin-3 levels in *mdx* mouse muscles. FEBS Lett 1998; 431:125–127.
143. Garcia-Cardena G, Martasek P, Masters BS, et al. Dissecting the interaction between nitric oxide synthase (NOS) and caveolin. Functional significance of the nos caveolin binding domain in vivo. J Biol Chem 1997; 272:25437–25440.
144. Gath I, Ebert J, Godtel-Armbrust U, Ross R, Reske-Kunz AB, Forstermann U. NO synthase II in mouse skeletal muscle is associated with caveolin 3. Biochem J 1999; 340:723–728.
145. Carozzi AJ, Roy S, Morrow IC, et al. Inhibition of lipid raft-dependent signaling by a dystrophy-associated mutant of caveolin-3. J Biol Chem 2002; 277:17944–17949.
146. Song KS, Li S, Okamoto T, Quilliam LA, Sargiacomo M, Lisanti MP. Co-purification and direct interaction of Ras with caveolin, an integral membrane protein of caveolae microdomains Detergent-free purification of caveolae microdomains. J Biol Chem 1996; 271:9690–9697.
147. Smythe GM, Eby JC, Disatnik MH, Rando TA. A caveolin-3 mutant that causes limb girdle muscular dystrophy type 1C disrupts Src localization and activity and induces apoptosis in skeletal myotubes. J Cell Sci 2003; 116:4739–4749.
148. Rybin VO, Xu X, Steinberg SF. Activated protein kinase C isoforms target to cardiomyocyte caveolae: stimulation of local protein phosphorylation. Circ Res 1999; 84:980–988.
149. Scherer PE, Lisanti MP. Association of phosphofructokinase-M with caveolin-3 in differentiated skeletal myotubes Dynamic regulation by extracellular glucose and intracellular metabolites. J Biol Chem 1997; 272:20698–20705.
150. Sotgia F, Bonuccelli G, Minetti C, et al. Phosphofructokinase muscle-specific isoform requires caveolin-3 expression for plasma membrane recruitment and caveolar targeting: implications for the pathogenesis of caveolin-related muscle diseases. Am J Pathol 2003; 163:2619–2634.
151. Murthy KS, Makhlouf GM. Heterologous desensitization mediated by G protein-specific binding to caveolin. J Biol Chem 2000; 275:30211–30219.
152. Song KS, Scherer PE, Tang Z, et al. Expression of caveolin-3 in skeletal, cardiac, and smooth muscle cells. Caveolin-3 is a component of the sarcolemma and co-fractionates with dystrophin and dystrophin-associated glycoproteins. J Biol Chem 1996; 271:15160–15165.
153. Sotgia F, Lee JK, Das K, et al. Caveolin-3 directly interacts with the C-terminal tail of β-dystroglycan. Identification of a central WW-like domain within caveolin family members. J Biol Chem 2000; 275:38048–38058.
154. Repetto S, Bado M, Broda P, et al. Increased number of caveolae and caveolin-3 overexpression in Duchenne muscular dystrophy. Biochem Biophys Res Commun 1999; 261:547–550.

SECTION II: DIAGNOSTIC CONSIDERATIONS

4

Duchenne Muscular Dystrophy and Becker Muscular Dystrophy: Diagnostic Principles

H. B. Ginjaar, J. T. den Dunnen, E. Bakker, and G. J. B. van Ommen

Center for Human and Clinical Genetics, Leiden University Medical Center, Leiden, Zuid-Holland, The Netherlands

INTRODUCTION

Duchenne muscular dystrophy (DMD) and the milder phenotype, Becker muscular dystrophy (BMD), are allelic X-linked disorders characterized by progressive, degenerative myopathy (1). About 95% of the DMD patients are diagnosed before the age of six, whereas BMD patients may show variable phenotypes with symptoms ranging from less severe DMD-like to very mild in patients who remain ambulant throughout their lives. The first diagnostic test used in patients suspected of DMD is the measurement of serum creatine kinase (CK) levels. Markedly elevated serum CK activities are observed in both DMD and BMD patients (1). Muscle biopsies of these patients will then be examined (immuno)histochemically. In parallel with, or before immunological muscle analysis, genetic studies are used to confirm the clinical diagnosis in the index patient and to further investigate their families for carrier status, and in prenatal diagnosis. In the majority of patients, one or more exons are deleted (60%) or duplicated (6%) (2–5). These rearrangements are patient-specific and unevenly distributed. In most of the remaining DMD patients, nonsense, frameshift, and frameshifting splice site mutations are found to be the causative mutations. For the detection of these small mutations, various DNA-based techniques and RNA-based methods, such as the protein truncation test (PTT), which uses mRNA isolated from lymphocytes, frozen muscle sections (preferably), or MyoD-differentiated fibroblasts, are available (6,7). Additional reverse transcription–polymerase chain reaction (RT–PCR) studies are also performed in case novel mutations are revealed and are predicted to affect splicing. The large size (approximately 2.4 Mb) of the dystrophin gene and the high number of exons, 79, make a complete genetic analysis an arduous task.

CONFIRMATION DIAGNOSIS OF DMD/BMD

DMD is a severe X-linked neuromuscular disorder, whereas BMD is the allelic milder form, showing a rather variable phenotype. Both DMD and BMD are characterized by progressive, symmetrical proximal muscle weakness. In DMD, the age at onset of symptoms is usually between three and five, and hypertrophy of some muscles is observed early in the course of the disease next to a positive Gowers' sign (1). Clinical criteria for differentiating a DMD or BMD diagnosis are linked to the age at which the patient will become wheelchair bound: for DMD before the age of 13 and BMD, if the patient is still ambulant, after the age of 16. Strong additional support for the diagnosis of either BMD or DMD can be the evidence of an X-linked recessive inheritance pattern. Findings of elevated CK levels, DNA studies and dystrophin analysis by means of immunological studies have been very helpful in the diagnosis of sporadic cases of DMD/BMD and in differentiating between the two.

Serum CK

CK levels in the blood samples of the patients are determined. Both in DMD and BMD patients, markedly elevated CK activities are observed, increased over ten- and fivefold, respectively, compared with unaffected individuals (1). Elevated CK levels may indicate not only X-linked dystrophinopathies, but also phenotypically overlapping autosomal recessive limb-girdle muscular dystrophies types 2A–I (8). Therefore, independent methods such as immunological studies of muscle tissue, in addition to molecular genetic analysis, are necessary for the confirmation of the clinical diagnosis.

Muscle Pathology

Muscle Histochemistry

Microscopic examination will show characteristic muscle pathology such as abnormal variation in fiber size (atrophic and hypertrophic muscle fibers), focal necrotic and regenerative fibers, extensive fibrosis (replacement of muscle fibers with fat and connective tissue), increased numbers of nuclei at different places, and large hyalinized fibers.

Immunohistochemistry and Immunobiochemistry

In most DMD cases, a frozen needle biopsy yields sufficient material for both histopathological and immunohistochemical examinations. Immunohistochemical dystrophin analysis of DMD muscle tissue shows dystrophin to be absent in most fibers, with the exception of some revertant positive fibers (less than 5%). Nicholson et al. (9) described variable amounts of revertant fibers in about half of their DMD patients; this phenomenon is explained as additional somatic recovery of the reading frame through alternative splicing or multiple exon skipping (10,11).

Because dystrophin is present in BMD patients, immunohistochemical analysis is not sufficient as a confirmative test. Because of the aberrant size and/or quality of dystrophin in BMD, Western blot analysis is usually performed (12,13). Western blot analysis may be very informative by detecting reduced amounts of dystrophin and/or aberrant dystrophin bands. In a recent study by Hofstra et al. (14), minor mutations in the dystrophin gene were identified in BMD patients previously shown to display aberrant dystrophin molecules by immunological muscle analysis. Moreover, multiplex Western blot analysis, by which, on the same blots various proteins involved in autosomal recessive limb-girdle muscular dystrophies (types 2A–D) are analyzed, may even indicate which of these phenotypically overlapping muscular dystrophies are disease causing (15). Dystrophin analysis using these techniques is often performed using several different antibodies, for example, one directed against the beginning (N-terminus), the central portion, and the end (C-terminus) of the dystrophin molecule. Sometimes these analyses uncover exceptional cases. For example, Ginjaar et al. (16) reported nonsense mutations in BMD patients after immunohistochemical analysis of their muscle tissue pinpointed the relevant epitope or detected somatic mosaicism (17).

Molecular Genetic Analysis

DNA Studies

Large rearrangements: The X-linked location and predominant deletion-prone nature of the DMD gene (60% of the mutations) have facilitated rapid, PCR-based detection of about 98% of all deletion cases using two sets of nine exon primer pairs (the Chamberlain and Beggs sets) (18,19). A minor proximal and a major central deletion hotspot have been identified comprising 30% and 60% of the deletions, respectively (3,20). Duplications predominantly occur in the same regions, although the skew toward the central region of the gene is not seen. A duplication of exon 2 is the single most frequently occurring duplication, whereas exon 45 is the most commonly deleted exon (21). In both cases, extreme intron size (greater than 100 kb) may be related, although the differences seen between deletions and duplications suggest that different mechanisms are involved.

Genetic studies in patients showed that the type of mutation and the size of the deletion/duplication did not directly correlate with the clinical severity of the affected individuals (3,22–26). Already in 1989, Monaco et al. (27) had postulated the reading-frame theory based on DNA studies in BMD/DMD patients, which holds for about 92% of the deletions/duplications (3,28). In most cases, mutations that stop or disrupt the reading frame cause DMD, and mutations that leave the reading frame intact lead to the milder BMD. Truncating mutations shift the reading frame and generate an incomplete dystrophin, which lacks the C-terminal end necessary to anchor it to the glycoprotein complex. This truncated dystrophin molecule is unstable and usually undetectable. Consequently, these mutations cause a severe DMD phenotype. However, mutations that somehow retain the reading frame will generate a largely functional protein, i.e., containing the C-terminal anchor site of abnormal size and/or amount, and generally cause the less severe BMD phenotype. Most exceptions to the reading-frame rule are cases where very large sections of the dystrophin molecule are deleted. Other "exceptions" occur when DNA data are used to deduce the effect of the change on RNA and protein level, without analyzing RNA (see DNA vs. RNA).

If no deletion is detected, further screening by dosage analysis using techniques such as Southern blotting (21), quantitative multiplex PCR (29), multiplex amplifiable probe hybridization (MAPH), or multiplex ligation-dependent probe amplification (MLPA) is performed to scan for duplications (8% of the mutations) or a deletion outside the deletion hotspots (2% of all deletions) as well as to determine the extent of the deletion/duplication (5,30,31). Deletions/duplications have been primarily detected by Southern blotting and quantitative PCR, although accurate, faster, and cheaper techniques such as MAPH and MLPA have been recently developed, of which the latter is currently being implemented in genetic diagnosis (32). For quantitative Southern blotting, at least two different restriction enzymes are used, which generate fragments containing all 79 exons that can be identified through five to seven independent hybridizations using different DMD cDNA probes. Not only can the extent of a deletion/duplication be defined, but also junction fragments, caused by deletions/duplications beginning or ending within these fragments, can be visualized. Junction fragments are excellent tools for family studies because they can reveal a mutant dystrophin gene in female carriers, who have a second, normal copy of the gene unequivocally. Taken together, Southern blotting covers all exons of the DMD gene, but requires about six blots to do so, and is time consuming and needs skilled technicians for correct interpretation of the data. Quicker screening methods for detection of deletions/duplications of all 79 exons simultaneously are the MAPH and MLPA. In MLPA, multiple pairs of oligonucleotides (probes) are first ligated and then simultaneously amplified (31).

The probes contain terminal universal primer sequences for amplification, a stuffer sequence of variable length to allow separation, and two genomic target sequences that hybridize at adjacent positions. The number of ligated oligonucleotide fragments is proportional to the amount of original target DNA, and PCR products can thus be quantified. MAPH is a similar technique but more difficult to perform in a diagnostic setting (30). In case of a single exon deletion, one should always confirm the result by another technique such as sequencing to exclude polymorphisms around the ligation site, preventing ligation and thus amplification, and thereby mimicking a deletion.

Minor mutations: The remaining cases of DMD/BMD are presumed to be caused by minor mutations such as substitutions, deletions, or insertions of one or several nucleotides leading to direct stops (nonsense mutations), truncating frameshifts, amino acid substitutions (missense and neutral mutations), or changes affecting splicing. Minor mutations do not cluster in hotspots (21), a result of which is that the complete gene has to be screened, which is time consuming and expensive. RNA-based techniques (see section on RNA Studies) are very efficient if muscle tissue is available. However, muscle RNA is not always easy to obtain; DMD mRNA levels in peripheral blood lymphocytes are very low and in a diagnostic setting RNA is more laborious to work with. Minor mutations can be identified using genomic DNA and prescreening techniques such as denaturing high-performance liquid chromatography (DHPLC), denaturing gradient gel electrophoresis (DGGE), detection of virtually all mutations (DOVAM), or by direct sequence analysis (14,33–35). DGGE is one of the most sensitive prescreening techniques with a detection rate of nearly 100%, whereas the sensitivity of DHPLC is slightly less because 3% to 9% of point mutations are missed (36,37). Direct sequence analysis of genomic DNA for all exons and their flanking sequences detects virtually all point mutations, but sequencing is rather expensive and deep intronic mutations would be missed (38). Analysis of single-nucleotide mutations did not reveal a common mechanism for certain subsets of mutations (39).

In 2% to 5% of cases, no mutation could be found. This result could be because of the inversions within the DMD gene, or mutations deep within introns that affect splicing (38). So far, more than 1000 unique changes have been listed in the DMD/BMD mutation database (21).

RNA Studies

RNA isolated from lymphocytes, muscle tissue, or MyoD-differentiated fibroblasts is used as starting material for the PTT (6), a technique developed to screen for translation terminating mutations. The PTT is based on in vitro transcription and subsequent translation of RT–PCR products. After RNA isolation, RT–PCR is performed, followed by PTT, and the protein products are analyzed on gel. Once a truncated protein band is detected, subsequent sequence analysis of the corresponding PCR product and genomic DNA will be performed to reveal the underlying mutation in the gene (40). For patients suspected of BMD/DMD without large deletions/duplications, RNA studies are performed only when immunological analysis of their muscle tissue confirms the clinical diagnosis.

DNA vs. RNA

It should be noted that one cannot predict the phenotypic consequences of a duplication/deletion based on a diagnosis at the DNA level only. To be sure, it is essential to perform an RNA analysis. Although a deletion at the DNA level mostly equals that at the RNA level, exceptions occur in 5% to 10% of cases. Most of these deletions are clustered in a region at the 5'-end of the gene and are identified as frameshifting deletions of exons 3 to 7 leading to DMD, BMD, or an intermediate phenotype (3,28,41). Chelly et al. (42,43) performed RNA–PCR studies to investigate some exceptions to this rule in various parts of the gene, and explained them as splicing abnormalities. In 1995, Winnard et al. (44) suggested an alternative mechanism in BMD patients with out-of-frame 3–7 deletions based on RNA studies. They suggested a translational reinitiation in exon 8 because splicing abnormalities (and hence exon skipping) have not been identified. In these cases, muscle tissue should be analyzed immunohistochemically to investigate dystrophin expression. Similarly, nonsense mutations have been found in BMD patients where RNA studies showed that splicing was altered, simply by skipping the exon containing the mutation (3–7,16).

Carrier Status

Initially, DMD/BMD carrier prediction was based on segregation analysis only, applied as a "Bayesian" statistical method, later combined with the results of serum CK measurements. This technique allows positive identification of the carrier status if the CK is repeatedly elevated in female relatives of DMD patients. However, one out of every three definite carriers cannot be detected on the basis of elevated CK levels because of an overlap with the normal range (45–47). In familial cases, the mother of the patient is generally an obligate carrier, and dosage analysis (21) or linkage methods using polymorphic dinucleotide (CA) repeat markers can be used to determine carrier status in the family (48,49). Linkage analysis can still be very effective in incriminating or excluding a dystrophin gene haplotype. However, in sporadic cases, the mothers might be carriers or there may be a new mutation.

If a mutation in the index patient is revealed, then reliable-carrier detection becomes straightforward. At present, molecular genetic tests are routinely applied for carrier detection with an accuracy exceeding 99% in the majority of the cases (50). In sporadic cases without deletions/duplications, where a de novo mutation is expected based on the haplotypes found, further analysis to detect a minor mutation in the dystrophin gene is required. However, very sophisticated approaches, often only available in highly specialized research centers, might be needed to identify a specific mutation in the DMD gene in some exceptional cases (7).

Germ Line Mosaicism

About one-third of the DMD cases arise from new mutations, while two-third of the cases are transmitted by carrier mothers (1,51). The latter cases also include those transmitted by "noncarrier" mothers who turned out to be germinal mosaics for de novo mutations (52). Genetic studies in DMD families unraveled the phenomenon of germ line mosaicism, associated with the appearance of new mutations. Noncarrier mothers of DMD patients with an apparent de novo mutation were nonetheless found to transmit the deletion for a second time (approximately 7%). Empirical data from haplotype analysis in these DMD families revealed recurrence risks of about 14% in future pregnancies involving a male fetus, associated with transmission of the "at risk" X chromosome (53). This result indicates that the mutations in the majority of cases do not occur at meiosis, but at an early stage of mitotic germ line proliferation, leading to an unknown percentage of mutated germ cells. Detailed analysis has resulted in further splitting into a 30% recurrence risk for the less frequent proximal deletions and a 4% recurrence risk for more frequently occurring distal deletions (54). These data suggest that, for yet unexplained reasons, proximal deletions occur earlier in germ line proliferation than distal ones.

PRENATAL DIAGNOSIS

Preferably, the family should be analyzed before a prenatal diagnostic test is performed, so that either the disease causing mutation or the "at risk" haplotype is known. A chorionic villus biopsy is usually taken at the 11th week of gestation. Twenty milligrams of chorionic villi are sufficient to perform all tests. The sex of the fetus is determined cytogenetically or by means of a Y chromosome–specific PCR test. Only in the case of a male fetus are further molecular genetic tests performed. (Quantitative) Multiplex PCR or MAPH/MLPA, to detect a deletion/duplication, or sequence analysis, to reveal a minor mutation, is then performed. Simultaneously, a PCR of CA-repeat loci within the DMD gene is carried out to exclude maternal contamination and as a check on the haplotype. In some cases, Southern blot analysis is performed either to detect a deletion/duplication or to visualize a junction band, which is extremely helpful for accurate diagnosis.

The results of the prenatal test are available within one to two weeks. In a minority of cases (less than 5%), an elevated risk cannot be excluded, either because the mutation is unknown and recombinations hamper haplotype analysis or because the mother is likely to be a germ line mosaic (risk 14%, see section on Germ Line Mosaicism). In those cases, the MyoD technique (7,55) might provide the ultimate tool. This technique uses viral delivery of the MyoD gene to the cells, either amniocytes or chorionic villus cells, to transform these into muscle-like cells. Expression of the introduced MyoD gene induces differentiation of the cells into myogenic cells, which within a few days start to express early muscle proteins like desmin. Through serum deprivation, the cells further differentiate and fuse into multinucleated myotubules. For diagnosis of DMD, the MyoD-differentiated cell cultures are screened for the absence/presence of dystrophin immunohistochemically. Subsequent RNA analysis by PTT can then be performed to reveal the actual mutation. The whole procedure generally requires three to four weeks for completion (56).

CONCLUDING REMARKS

For the diagnosis of patients suspected of DMD/BMD, various tests are available. Because each test may not be sufficient by itself for confirmation of the clinical diagnosis, the following flowchart (Fig. 1) is recommended. First, serum CK activity is measured, and then histochemical/immunological analysis of muscle tissue is carried out in parallel with DNA- and/or

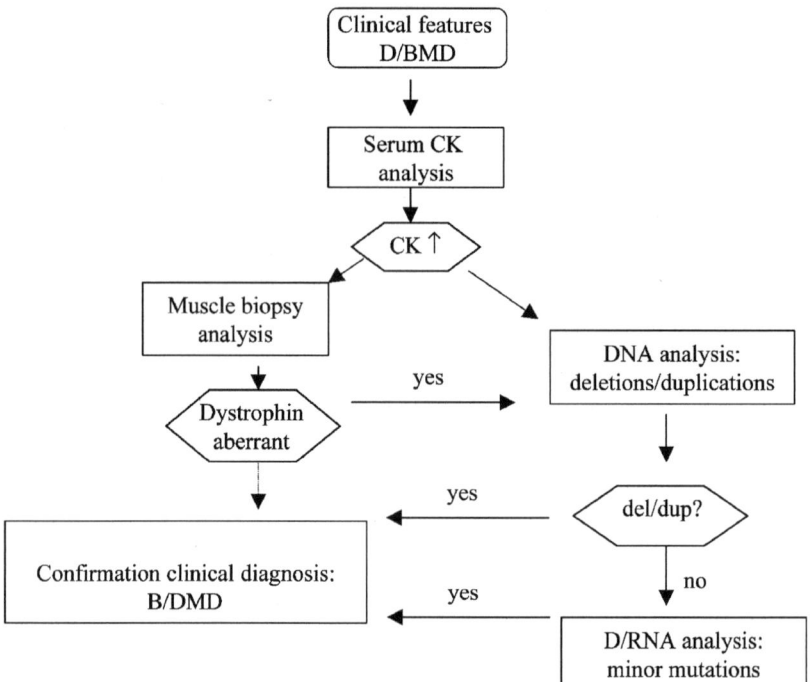

Figure 1 Diagnostic flowchart.

RNA-based genetic studies. For future familial studies such as carrier detection and prenatal diagnosis, prior molecular genetic analysis of the index patient's DNA is highly recommended. Moreover, in the light of future therapies such as antisense-induced exon skipping, gene therapy, or aminoglycoside treatment of patients, it will be required to identify the mutation (57).

Immunological studies may be informative for the diagnosis in those cases where initial DNA analysis did not reveal deletions/duplications, and before starting the search for minor mutations in the dystrophin gene. Due to the big clinical overlap between the X-linked dystrophinopathies and, in particular, the autosomal recessive limb-girdle muscular dystrophies, immunological studies of patient's muscle tissue, in particular, a multiplex Western blot, can reveal which of the dystrophin-associated glycoprotein complex (DGC) components, other structural muscle proteins, or muscle enzymes are aberrant (15). This result then identifies the genes encoding these proteins, on which subsequent genetic studies should be focused.

When material from patients is lacking, two approaches have been successfully applied for carrier detection. First, the MyoD technique has been implemented using fibroblast cell samples from patients to reveal mutations (see section on Prenatal Diagnosis) (7). Second, in a number of DMD families with deceased sporadic patients, for whom no DNA or muscle tissue was available, and when the relatives wanted to know their carrier status, unusual "archival" materials have been used. For example, milk teeth of six deceased patients have been employed for genetic analysis. Using DNA isolated from these teeth, a mutation was detected in half the number of patients. In three other DMD families, haplotype analyses have been performed for carrier detection (Ginjaar et al., unpublished results). In carrier studies, and in prenatal diagnosis in cases such as these, one should be especially aware of the possibility of germ line mosaicism.

RNA studies to establish the actual mutation may be needed in patients in whom the initial DNA studies confirmed the clinical diagnosis, but in whom clinical development is different than expected.

In case minor mutations have been detected in introns or exons, which may affect splicing, these observations should be verified by RNA studies.

Some techniques, such as the MyoD-induced in vitro differentiation, are highly specialized and are performed in only a few expert centers. In general, these centers are willing to help others when exceptional cases require special tools. Another issue is quality control and the introduction of international standards "best practice guidelines" for diagnostic analysis. In this respect, initiatives have been launched by organizing various national and international external quality assessment schemes in which diagnostic laboratories can participate to test and hence improve their individual performances. It is therefore strongly recommended that exceptional cases be referred to the molecular diagnostic centers working under high quality standards which are subjected yearly to external quality assessment.

REFERENCES

1. Emery AEH. Duchenne Muscular Dystrophy. 2d ed. Oxford University Press, 1993.
2. Koenig M, Hoffman EP, Bertelson CJ, Monaco AP, Feener C, Kunkel LM. Complete cloning of the Duchenne Muscular Dystrophy (DMD) cDNA and preliminary genomic organization of the DMD gene in normal and affected individuals. Cell 1987; 50:509–517.
3. den Dunnen JT, Grootscholten PM, Bakker E, et al. Topography of the DMD gene: fige- and cDNA analysis of 194 cases reveals 115 deletions and 13 duplications. Am J Hum Genet 1989; 45:835–847.
4. Hu X, Burghes AH, Bulman D, Ray PN, Worton RG. Partial gene duplications in Duchenne and Becker muscular dystrophies. J Med Genet 1988; 25:369–376.
5. White S, Kalf M, Liu Q, et al. Comprehensive detection of genomic duplications and deletions in the DMD gene, by use of multiplex amplifiable probe hybridization. Am J Hum Genet 2002; 71(2):365–374.
6. Roest PAM, Roberts RG, van der Tuijn AC, Sugine S, van Ommen GJB, den Dunnen JT. Protein truncation test (PTT) for rapid detection of translation terminating mutations. Hum Mol Genet 1993; 2:1719–1721.
7. Roest PAM, van der Tuyn AC, Ginjaar HB, et al. Application of in vitro myo-differentiation of nonmuscle cells to enhance gene expression and facilitate analysis of muscle proteins. Neuromuscul Disord 1996; 6:195–202.
8. Zatz M, de Paula F, Starling A, Vainzhof M. The 10 autosomal recessive limb-girdle muscular dystrophies. Neuromuscul Disord 2003; 13:532–544.
9. Nicholson LV, Johnson MA, Gardner-Medwin D, Bhattacharya S, Harris JB. Heterogeneity of dystrophin expression in patients with Duchenne and Becker muscular dystrophy. Acta Neuropathol (Berl) 1990; 80(3):239–250.
10. Nicholson LVB. The "rescue" of dystrophin synthesis in boys with Duchenne muscular dystrophy. Neuromuscul Disord 1993; 3:525–532.
11. Lu QL, Morris GE, Wilton SD, et al. Massive idiosyncratic exon skipping corrects the nonsense mutation in the dystrophic mouse muscle and produces functional revertant fibers by clonal expension. J Cell Biol 2000; 148:985–996.
12. Hoffman EP, Fischbeck KH, Brown RH, et al. Characterization of dystrophin in muscle-biopsy specimens from patients with Duchenne's or Becker's Muscular Dystrophy. New Engl J Med 1988; 318:1363–1368.
13. Arahata K, Ishiura S, Ishiguro T, et al. Immunostaining of skeletal and cardiac muscle surface membrane with antibody against Duchenne Muscular Dystrophy peptide. Nature 1989; 333:861–862.
14. Hofstra RMW, Mulder IM, Vossen R, et al. Whole gene DGGE-based mutation scanning of dystrophin gene in DMD/BMD patients. Human Mutat 2004; 23:57–66.
15. Anderson LVB. Multiplex Western Blot analysis of the muscular dystrophy proteins. In: Bushby KMD, Anderson LVB, eds. Muscular Dystrophy: Methods and Protocols. New Jersey: Humana Press, 2001.
16. Ginjaar IB, Kneppers ALJ, van der Meulen JDM, et al. Dystrophin nonsense mutation induces different levels of exon 29 skipping and leads to variable phenotypes within one BMD family. Eur J Hum Genet 2000; 8:793–796.

17. Helderman-van den Enden ATJM, Ginjaar HB, Kneppers ALJ, Bakker E, Breuning MH, de Visser M. Somatic mosaicism of a point mutation in the dystrophin gene in a patient presenting with an asymmetrical muscle weakness and contractures. Neuromuscul Disord 2003; 13:317–321.
18. Chamberlain JS, Gibbs RA, Ranier JE, Nguyen PN, Caskey CT. Deletion screening of the Duchenne muscular dystrophy locus via multiplex DNA amplification. Nucleic Acids Res 1988; 23:11141–11156.
19. Beggs AH, Koenig M, Boyce FM, Kunkel LM. Detection of 98% of DMD/BMD gene deletions by polymerase chain reaction. Hum Genet 1990; 86:45–48.
20. Forrest SM, Cross GS, Speer A, Gardner-Medwin D, Burn J, Davies K. Preferential deletion of exons in Duchenne and Becker muscular dystrophies. Nature 1987; 329:638–640.
21. http://www.DMD.nl.
22. Koenig M, Beggs AH, Moyer M. The molecular basis for Duchenne versus Becker muscular dystrophy: correlation of severity with type of deletion. Am J Hum Genet 1989; 45:498–506.
23. Roberts RG, Bentley DR, Bobrow M. Point mutations in the dystrophin. Proc Acad Natl Sci 1992; 89:52331–52335.
24. Roberts RG, Gardner RJ, Bentley DR. Searching for 1 in the 2,400,000: a review of dystrophin gene point mutations. Hum Mutat 1994; 4:1–11.
25. Lenk U, Hanke R, Thiele H, Speer A. Point mutations at the carboxy terminus of the human dystrophin gene: implications for association with mental retardation in DMD patients. Hum Mol Genet 1993; 2:1877–1881.
26. Prior TW, Papp AC, Snyder PJ, et al. Identification of two point mutations and a one base deletion in exon 19 of the dystrophin gene by heteroduplex formation. Hum Mol Genet 1993; 2:331–333.
27. Monaco AP, Bertelson CJ, Liechti-Gallati S, Moser H, Kunkel LM. An explanation for the phenotypic differences between patients bearing partial deletions of the DMD locus. Genomics 1988; 2:90–95.
28. Baumbach LL, Chamberlain JS, Ward PA, Farwell NJ, Caskey CT. Molecular and clinical correlation of deletion leading to Duchenne and Becker muscular dystrophies. Neurology 1989; 39:465–474.
29. www.lumc.nl/klingen.
30. Armour JA, Sismani C, Patsalis PC, Cross G. Measurement of locus copy number by hybridization with amplifiable probes. Nucleic Acids Res 2000; 28:605–609.
31. Schouten JP, McElgunn C, Waayer R, Zwijnenburg D, Diepvens F, Pals G. Relative quantification of 40 nucleic acid sequences by multiplex ligation-dependent probe amplification. Nucleic Acids Res 2002; 30:12–57.
32. Schwartz M, Duno M. Improved molecular diagnosis of dystrophin gene mutations using the multiplex ligation-dependent probe amplification method. Genet Test 2004; 8(4):361–367.
33. Bennett RR, den Dunnen J, O'Brien KF, Darras BT, Kunkel LM. Detection of mutations in the dystrophin gene via automated DHPLC screening and direct sequencing. BMC Genet 2001; 2(1):17.
34. Mendell JR, Buzin CH, Feng J, et al. Diagnosis of Duchenne dystrophy by enhanced detection of small mutations. Neurology 2001; 57:645–650.

35. Flanigan KM, von Niederhausern A, Dunn DM, Alder J, Mendell JR, Weiss RB. Rapid direct sequence analysis of the dystrophin gene. Am J Hum Genet 2003; 72(4):931–939.
36. Guldberg P, Henriksen KF, Guttler F. Molecular analysis of phenylketonuria in Denmark: 99% of the mutations detected by denaturing gradient gel electrophoresis. Genomics 1993; 17:141–146.
37. Xiao W, Oefner PJ. Denaturing high-performance liquid chromatography: a review. Hum Mutat 2001; 17:439–474.
38. Beroud C, Carrie A, Beldjord C, et al. Dystrophinopathy caused by mid-intronic substitutions activating cryptic exons in the DMD gene. Neuromuscul Disord 2004; 14(1):10–18.
39. Todorova A, Danieli GA. Large majority of single-nucleotide mutations along the dystrophin gene can be explained by more than one mechanism of mutagenesis. Hum Mutat 1997; 9:537–547.
40. Tuffery-Giraud S, Saquet C, Chambert S, et al. The role of muscle biopsy in analysis of the dystrophin gene in Duchenne muscular dystrophy: experience of a national referral centre. Neuromuscul Disord 2004; 14(10):650–658.
41. Malhotra SB, Hart KA, Klamut HJ, et al. Frame-shift deletions in patients with Duchenne and Becker muscular Dystrophy. Science 1988; 242:755–759.
42. Chelly J, Kaplan JC, Maire P, Gautron S, Kahn A. Transcription of the dystrophin gene in human muscle and nonmuscle tissues. Nature 1988; 333:858–860.
43. Chelly J, Gilgenkrantz H, Hugnot JP, et al. Illegitimate transcription: application to the analysis of truncated transcripts of the dystrophin gene in nonmuscle cultured cells from Duchenne and Becker patients. J Clin Invest 1989; 88:1161–1166.
44. Winnard AV, Mendell JR, Prior TW, Florence J, Burghes AH. Frameshift deletions of exons 3–7 and revertant fibers in Duchenne muscular dystrophy: mechanisms of dystrophin production. Am J Hum Genet 1995; 56(1):158–166.
45. Emery AEH. Carrier detection in sex linked muscular dystrophy. J Genet Hum 1965; 14:318–329.
46. Griggs RC, Mendell JR, Brooke MH. Clinical investigations in Duchenne dystrophy: V. Use of creatine kinase and pyruvate kinase in carrier detection. Muscle Nerve 1985; 8:60.
47. Hoogerwaard EM, Bakker E, Ippel PF, et al. Signs and symptoms of Duchenne muscular dystrophy and Becker muscular dystrophy among carriers in the Netherlands: a cohort study. Lancet 1999; 353:2116–2119.
48. Clemens PR, Fenwick RG, Chamberlain JS, et al. Carrier detection and prenatal diagnosis in Duchenne and Becker muscular dystrophy families, using dinucleotide repeat polymorphisms. Am J Hum Genet 1991; 49:951–960.
49. Schwartz LS, Tarleton J, Popovich B, Seltzer WK, Hoffman EP. Fluorescent multiplex linkage analysis and carrier detection for Duchenne/Becker muscular dystrophy. Am J Hum Genet 1992; 51(4):721–729.
50. van Essen AJ, Kneppers ALJ, Ginjaar HB, et al. The clinical and molecular genetic approach to Duchenne and Becker muscular dystrophy: an updated protocol. J Med Genet 1997; 34(10):805–812.
51. Zatz M, Lange M, Spence MA. Frequency of Duchenne muscular dystrophy carriers. Lancet 1977; 1:759.

52. Bakker E, Van Broeckhoven Ch, Bonten EJ, et al. Germ line mosaicism and Duchenne muscular dystrophy mutations. Nature 1987; 328:554–556.
53. Bakker E, Veenema H, den Dunnen JT, et al. Germinal mosaicism increases the recurrence risk for "new" Duchenne muscular dystrophy mutations. J Med Genet 1989; 26:553–559.
54. Passos-Bueno MR, Bakker E, Kneppers ALJ, et al. Different mosaicism frequencies for proximal and distal Duchenne muscular dystrophy (DMD) mutations indicate difference in etiology and recurrence risk. Am J Hum Genet 1992; 51:1150–1155.
55. Sancho S, Mongini T, Tanji K, et al. Analysis of dystrophin expression after activation of myogenesis in amniocytes, chorionic-villus cells, and fibroblasts. N Engl J Med 1993; 29:915–920.
56. Roest PA, Bakker E, Fallaux FJ, et al. New possibilities for prenatal diagnosis of muscular dystrophies: forced myogenesis with an adenoviral MyoD-vector. Lancet 1999; 353(9154):727–728.
57. van Deutekom JC, van Ommen GJ. Advances in Duchenne muscular dystrophy gene therapy. Nat Rev Genet 2003; 4(10):774–783.

5

Mutation Detection

Thomas W. Prior

*Division of Molecular Pathology, Department of Pathology,
The Ohio State University, Columbus, Ohio, U.S.A.*

GENE STUDIES

The Duchenne muscular dystrophy (DMD) gene is the largest human gene identified, spanning more than 2000 kb of genomic DNA, and is composed of 79 exons that encode a 14-kb transcript which is translated into a protein named dystrophin (1,2). It has been observed that approximately 60% to 65% of the mutations that cause DMD/BMD are large deletions in the dystrophin gene (3,4). The distribution of deletions within the *DMD* gene of DMD/BMD patients studied at The Ohio State University is shown in Figure 1. The deletions are nonrandomly distributed and occur primarily in the center (approximately 80%) and less frequently near the 5' end (approximately 20%) of the gene. The 200-kb region covering intron 44, exon 45, and intron 45 is the major deletion breakpoint region of the gene. The majority of the larger deletions are found to initiate at the 5' end of the gene. The distribution of deletions (Fig. 1) has been demonstrated in many populations and ethnic groups.

There is no apparent correlation between the size or location of the deletion and the severity and progression of the disorder. We identified one of the largest deletions encompassing exons 10–35, in a mild BMD patient. Furthermore, sequences deleted in DMD patients often overlap with those deleted in BMD patients. However, it was proposed that if a deletion disrupts the translational reading frame of the dystrophin mRNA

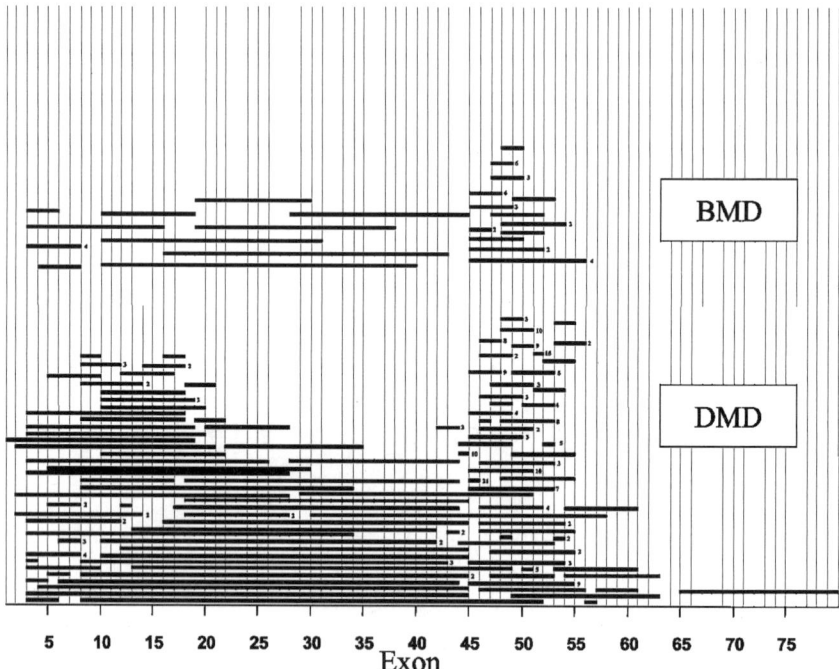

Figure 1 Distribution of deletions in the dystrophin gene in DMD and BMD patients. Each line above the gene exons represents a deletion observed in a patient. The number to the right of the deletion line indicates the number of independent patients sharing deletions of the same exons. *Abbreviations*: BMD, Becker muscular dystrophy; DMD, Duchenne muscular dystrophy.

triplet codons, then little or no dystrophin will be synthesized, resulting in the more severe DMD (5). In the milder BMD, the deletion maintains the translational reading frame, and a semifunctional protein is produced. The reading frame hypothesis explains the phenotypic differences observed in about 92% of the DMD/BMD cases. One major exception to the reading frame has been the identification of BMD patients with the out of frame exon three to seven deletion (6). It has been proposed that an alternate splicing mechanism or a new cryptic translational start site may account for the production of protein and the milder phenotype in these patients. A small number of DMD patients with in-frame deletions have also been identified. The more severe phenotype in these patients may be due to the overall effect of the deletion on the protein conformation or possibly may be the result of message instability. We have found some phenotypic variability in several of our patients who share identical gene deletions. The out of frame deletion of exon 45, one of the most commonly observed DMD deletions, has also been associated with BMD phenotypes (7). Some genetic variability may be due to modifier genes that affect splicing, or other molecules involved in destruction of damaged muscle fibers, in muscular regeneration, or in the cellular response to different hormones.

The large gene size, particularly the introns which average 35 kb, may account for part of the high deletion rate. However, in addition to target size, other factors must be involved. The observed nonrandom deletion pattern may reflect domain-associated variation in chromosomal stability. For instance, complications related to the maintenance of replication, correct transcription, and proper splicing of such a large gene may play an extremely important role.

Partial gene duplications have been revealed in about 5% to 10% of the patients (8). Unlike the deletion distribution, we have found about 80% of the duplications at the 5' end of the gene and only 20% in the central region (Fig. 2). The duplication distribution, like the deletion distribution, has also been demonstrated in different populations and ethnic groups. Out of frame duplications in DMD patients and in frame duplications have been observed in BMD patients, thus suggesting that the reading frame hypothesis also holds true for duplications (8).

There are now many reports of small mutations (point mutations and small deletions and duplications) detected in the dystrophin gene in the remaining DMD/BMD patients without deletions or duplications (9,10). The majority of these mutations have been unique to a single or a few patients and have resulted in truncated dystrophins lacking part or all of the C-terminus. The truncated proteins are presumably unstable, and little

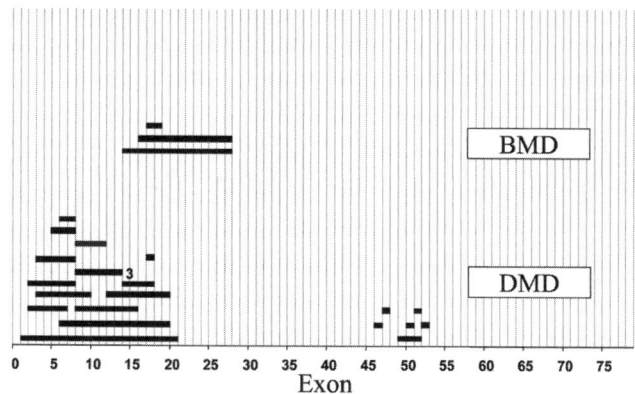

Figure 2 Distribution of duplications in the dystrophin gene in DMD and BMD patients. Each line above the gene exons represents a duplication observed in a patient. The number to the right of the duplication line indicates the number of independent patients sharing duplications of the same exons. *Abbreviations*: BMD, Becker muscular dystrophy; DMD, Duchenne muscular dystrophy.

or no dystrophin is produced. Therefore, these types of mutations provide little information on structural/functional relationships in the dystrophin protein. Missense mutations are rare in the dystrophin gene, even in the milder BMD patients. Although several base changes causing significant amino acid substitutions have been reported in the dystrophin gene, these are most likely polymorphic changes. The identification of mutations which do not cause protein truncation may provide us with further insight into the function of dystrophin as well as defining the essential regions and conformations necessary for dystrophin stability. DMD missense mutations, previously described in exons 3 and 16, have supported the important role of an intact actin-binding domain and of maintaining the proper conformation of the rod domain for dystrophin's function (10).

The small mutations have been shown to be more randomly distributed throughout the gene sequence. However, while less than 5% of the deletions are found in 3' of exon 55, we have found more than 40% of the small mutations to be located in this same region of the gene.

MOLECULAR DIAGNOSTICS

The analysis of gene mutations has greatly improved diagnosis, carrier detection, and genetic counseling. With the ability to identify deletions and duplications in approximately 70% of the affected patients, accurate direct DNA testing can be used for these cases. By using full-length dystrophin cDNA clones to probe Southern blots, it is possible to directly detect deletions and duplications. The cDNA probes detect the site of the mutation itself, so meiotic recombination events are irrelevant. Therefore, the chance of diagnostic error is greatly reduced. The digested and blotted DNA is sequentially hybridized with seven to nine cDNA probes, which cover the complete 14-kb transcript. Approximately 5 to 10 exons are scored for each cDNA hybridization. However, as shown in Figure 1, the deletions are primarily located in two hotspots, and therefore the majority of deletions can be identified by four cDNA probe hybridizations. The deletions are simply detected by examination of Southern blots for the presence or absence of each exon containing genomic restriction fragments which hybridize to the cDNA probe (Fig. 3). A duplication is revealed by an increased hybridization intensity of one or more DNA fragments when compared to the control (Fig. 4). Duplications should always be confirmed using a second different restriction enzyme digestion, and we routinely scan the autoradiogram by densitometry.

The most commonly used restriction enzyme for DMD analysis is *Hind*III, because the restriction pattern for all 79 exons is known, and the majority of exons are on single fragments. *Bgl*II and *Eco*RI are also commonly used enzymes. If a duplication or deletion starts or ends within the restriction enzyme exon fragment, an altered sized fragment will be detected

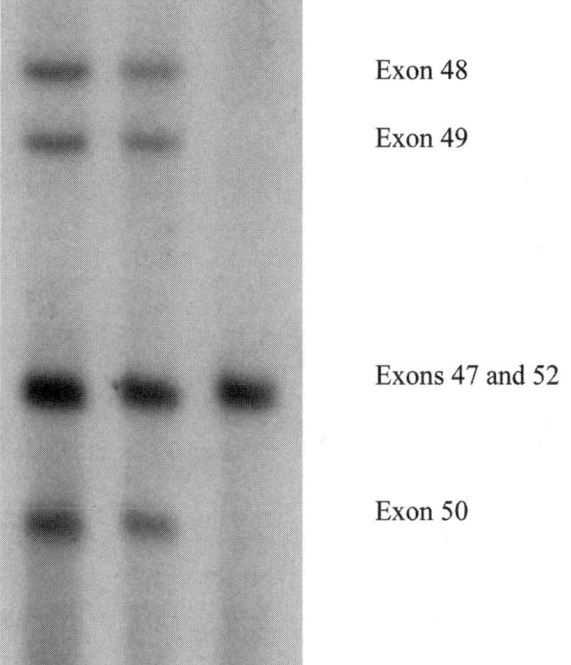

Figure 3 Southern hybridization, using dystrophin cDNA 8 (which hybridizes with exons 47–52), of DNA digested with BglII. The DNA sample analyzed in *lane 3* has a gene deletion of exons 48–50. *Abbreviation*: cDNA, complementary DNA.

(Fig. 5). The altered fragments are known as junction fragments, or J-bands, and are found in about 5% of the deletions. The J-bands can be helpful in determining the origin of the mutation and in carrier determinations; however normal restriction enzyme polymorphisms can also generate

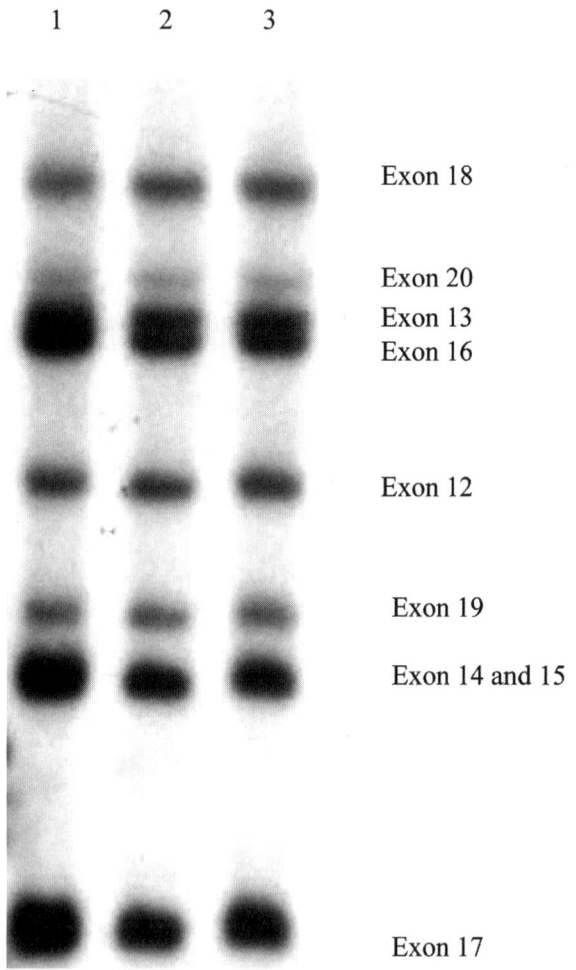

Figure 4 Southern hybridization, using dystrophin cDNA 2b-3 (which hybridizes with exons 12–20), of DNA digested with *Hind*III. The DNA sample analyzed in *lane 1* has a gene duplication of exons 13–17. *Abbreviation*: cDNA, complementary DNA.

new altered fragments. We have found several dystrophin gene *Hind*III polymorphisms in the African-American population, and care should be taken not to confuse these with deletions (11).

The Southern blotting technique requires isotope and high molecular weight DNA, is tedious, and is time consuming. Rapid and efficient deletion screening can be performed by the multiplex polymerase chain reaction (PCR) (12). The technique allows one to amplify specific deletion-prone exons within the *DMD* gene up to a millon-fold from nanogram amounts

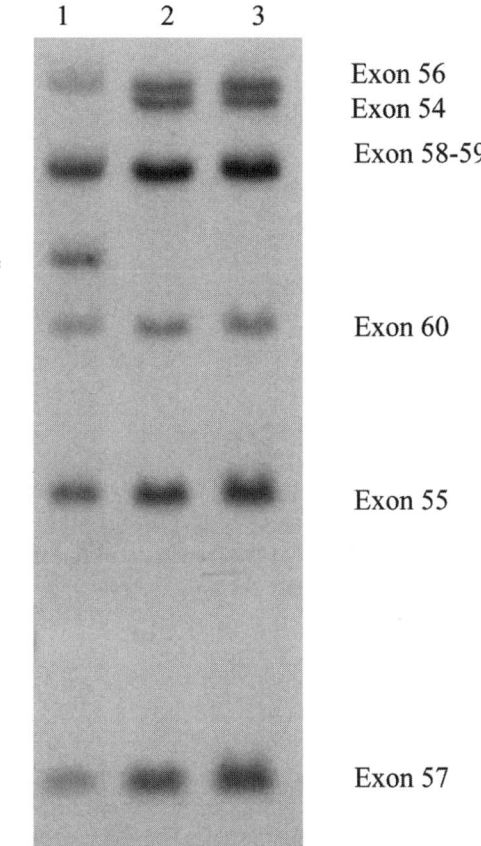

Figure 5 Southern hybridization, using dystrophin cDNA 9 (which hybridizes with exons 54–60), of DNA digested with *Hind*III. The DNA sample analyzed in *lane 1* is deleted for exons 45–53 and a junction fragment has resulted due to deletion terminating within the exon 54 *Hind*III restriction fragment. The normal exon 54 fragment has been displaced (*asterisk*). *Abbreviation*: cDNA, complementary DNA.

of genomic DNA. The exon products are discriminated from one another by size following gel electrophoresis. When any one of the coding sequences is deleted from a patient's sample, no ethidium bromide–stained amplification product, corresponding to the specific exon, is present on the gel (Fig. 6). Multiplex PCR, using primer sets for about 20 different exons, now detects approximately 98% of the deletions in the dystrophin gene (12,13). In contrast to Southern blotting, which may require several cDNA hybridizations and take several weeks to obtain results, the PCR can be completed in one day. This makes the technique ideal for prenatal diagnosis, when time is crucial.

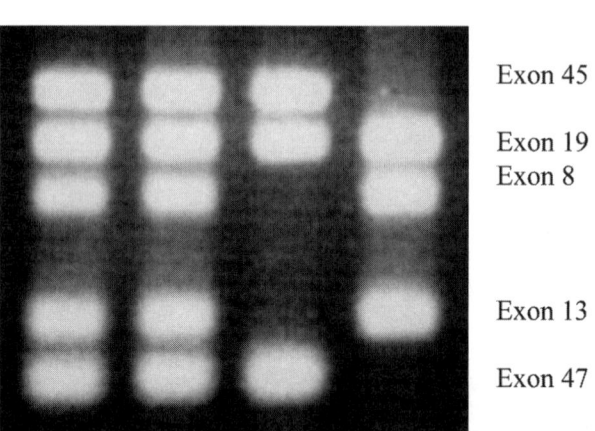

Figure 6 Multiplex PCR of DNA from DMD patients. *Lane 3* shows a DMD patient deleted for exons 8 and 13. *Lane 4* shows a DMD patient deleted for exons 45 and 47. *Abbreviations*: PCR, polymerase chain reaction DMD, Duchenne muscular dystrophy.

We have found that the two separate analyses, multiplex PCR and Southern blotting, complement each other, and therefore we test all of our patients using both methods. There are several reasons for our strategy. First, the identification of duplications by standard multiplex conditions and ethidium bromide–stained gels is technically difficult, for it is during the exponential phase that the amount of amplified products is proportional to the abundance of starting DNA. This occurs when the concentration of primers, nucleotides, and *Taq* polymerase are in a large excess over that of the template. In our experience, after the completion of an adequate number of cycles (about 25–30) to visualize the PCR products on an ethidium bromide–stained gel, the PCR is no longer in the exponential quantitative range, and the duplicated exons appear little or no brighter than the normal one copy exons. By using densitometry and multiple restriction digests, we have found the detection of duplications relatively straightforward by Southern blotting. However, the recent utilization of automated DNA fragment analysis using multiplex PCR with fluorescently labeled primers has allowed for more accurate detection of duplications. Secondly, Southern blotting allows for the determination of all deletion and duplication endpoints which is important in determining the effect of the mutation on the reading frame. Because the majority of labs tend to multiplex PCR about 20 deletion-prone exons, it is not possible to obtain all endpoints by PCR alone. Thirdly, the Southern blot technique allows for the detection of junction bands. Lastly, we have found it to be a good quality control practice to confirm all mutations by two separate analyses. A new technique was recently described for the detection of both dystrophin deletions and duplications, which combines both multiplex PCR and probe hybridization. The multiplex amplifiable probe hybridization is based on the quantitative recovery of probes after their hybridization to immobilized DNA (14). The probes are recovered by simultaneous PCR amplification, which produces different-sized products, and are analyzed on a 96-capillary sequencer. Therefore, changes in peak heights reflect either gene deletions or duplications. The technique was shown to be accurate and labor efficient.

The identification of a deletion in a DMD patient not only confirms the diagnosis but also allows one to perform accurate carrier detection in the affected family. Carrier status is determined by gene dosage, whereby one observes whether a female at risk exhibits no or 50% reduction in hybridization intensity in those bands that are deleted for the affected male (15,16). A 50% reduction (single-copy intensity) for the deleted band or bands on the autoradiograph indicates a deletion on one of her X chromosomes, and she would therefore be a carrier. Dosage determinations can be made from Southern blots or using a quantitative polymerase chain reaction.

A case study using quantitative PCR is shown in Figure 7. A DMD patient was found to have a molecular deletion for exon 19. This was an isolated case of the disease, and the mother and her daughters were tested for the deletion. To obtain quantitative results, one must measure PCR products during the exponential phase of the amplification process. This occurs when the concentration of primers, nucleotides, and *Taq* polymerase are in a large excess over that of the template. In our experience, after the completion of an adequate number of cycles (about 25–30) to visualize the PCR products on an ethidium bromide–stained gel, the PCR reaction is no longer in the quantitative range. Therefore exons 19 and 50 in the mother, daughters, proband, and a normal female control were amplified for 12 cycles, and hybridized with the corresponding cDNA probe; the resultant autoradiogram is shown in Figure 7. Exon 50 serves as an internal control, because this is an exon which is not deleted in the patient. Rather than directly comparing single bands, band ratios are calculated as a means of decreasing the error caused by differences in the amount of amplified product in each lane. The exon 19/50 ratio in the mother is approximately half the normal control ratio. These ratios were confirmed by densitometer. Therefore, the mother is a carrier of the exon 19 deletion, and the proband is not the result of a new sporadic mutation. Both daughters had normal exon 19/50 ratios and were therefore noncarriers.

Dosage determinations permit direct carrier analysis and eliminate the inherent problems of the restriction fragment length polymorphisms technique (recombinations, noninformative meioses, unavailability of family members, and spontaneous mutations). This is important because unlike the affected males, the heterozygous females are generally asymptomatic,

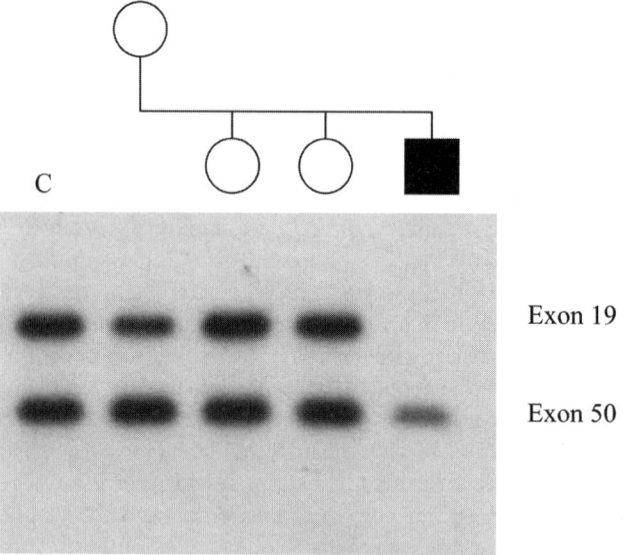

Figure 7 Carrier determination by gene dosage. The mother's DNA shows a 50% reduction of hybridization intensity for the exon 19/50 ratio. Exon 19 is deleted in the DNA from the proband and exon 50 is the endogenous standard, because the proband is not deleted for this exon. DNA from the daughters have normal exon 19/50 dosage ratios and are therefore noncarriers. "C" denotes noncarrier female control DNA.

and creatine kinase (CK) is only elevated in approximately 50% to 60% of known carriers.

Even when the dosage analysis indicates that the mother does not have a deletion, she still has an uncertain risk of carrier status, owing to the possibility of germline mosaicism (17). Cases of germline mosaicism in DMD have been reported, in which a deletion is transmitted to more than one offspring by a mother who shows no evidence of the mutation in her somatic cells. Cases of germline mosaicism have important counseling implications. The first and most obvious need is to perform carrier studies on all daughters of mothers with deletion cases. The sisters of DMD patients may possibly be carriers and should be investigated in a manner independent of the outcome of the mother. Furthermore, a negative deletion result in a mother does not rule out a recurrence risk for future pregnancies, and prenatal diagnosis should still be offered. Because it depends upon the frequency of the mutant germline cells in the mosaic mother, the exact recurrence risk in germline carriers is unknown. However, in these cases the risk is significantly increased relative to what had initially been perceived as a new mutation with a low recurrence risk. It has been estimated that mothers of apparently sporadic DMD cases have a 14% recurrence risk (17).

In the 35% of families with undefined mutations, carrier detection and prenatal diagnosis depend upon linkage analysis. The method relies on the co-inheritance of the disease gene with those DNA polymorphic variations known to be located very close to, or within, the disease gene. Thus, even when the responsible gene mutation remains unknown, the linkage technique allows one to trace the mutation through an affected family and make predictions about the inheritance of the disorder. Microsatellite sequences, which are short tandem repeats (di-, tri-, or tetranucleotides) and tend to be highly polymorphic in repeat number, have been found in several locations in the *DMD* gene and have significantly improved linkage analysis (18–20). The microsatellites vary in allele length and can easily be tested by PCR. Although the indirect approach can provide valuable information, it is limited by (i) the possibility of recombination between the microsatellite sequence and the unknown mutation, (ii) the presence of sporadic mutations, and (iii) the unavailability of family members. The intragenic recombination rate over the entire length of the *DMD* gene was estimated to be as high as 12% (21). The high recombinational error rate can be overcome by using markers at both ends of the gene. The results are still often extremely limited for extended family members of isolated cases of the disease, due to the possibility of the occurrence of a new mutation, for linkage indicates only whether the female at risk inherited the same X chromosome as the affected male, not whether she is a carrier of the defective gene. Furthermore, because the gene mutation remains unidentified, a correct diagnosis is essential. This is extremely important with patients presenting with the milder BMD, because this phenotype can overlap with other neuromuscular disorders. The diagnosis can usually be made clinically on the basis of symptoms and signs at presentation, increased CK levels, and myopathic findings. A family history in conjunction with the clinical findings would strongly suggest the diagnosis of DMD or BMD. However, if there is any question of the diagnosis, the Western blot assay of the dystrophin protein on a muscle biopsy specimen should be considered to confirm the diagnosis.

POINT MUTATION DETECTION IN THE DYSTROPHIN GENE

As previously described, using multiplex PCR and Southern blotting, large genomic deletions and duplications have been identified in approximately two-thirds of the DMD/BMD population. The other mutations are due to smaller types of mutations within the dystrophin gene, the detection of which would require some type of sequencing-based strategy. In most routine diagnostic services, these mutations have gone undetected because sequencing the entire gene is both expensive and labor intensive. However, the identification of these mutations is not only important for the confirmation of the diagnosis, but also for the determination of carrier studies. Due to the high mutation rate in the dystrophin gene, carrier testing based on indirect linkage results is often limited for extended family members of isolated cases of the disease. Knowledge of the exact causative mutation allows for the determination of the origin of mutation in families with simplex cases of the disease.

Using a variety of screening methods [single strand conformational polymorphism, denaturing high performance liquid chromatography, heteroduplex analysis, denaturing gradient gel electrophoresis, detection of virtually all mutations, protein truncation test (PTT)], several studies, performed primarily in research settings, have now identified smaller types of mutations in the dystrophin gene. Although some common mutations have been found, most mutations have been unique (private mutations) to single or few patients and are distributed throughout the gene, with no mutational hotspots. The majority of the mutations have been shown to affect only one or a few nucleotides and result in protein truncation, lacking part or all of the C-terminus. It is clear from numerous studies that the testing of the nondeletion/duplication patients, due to the large gene size and the lack of a point mutation hotspot, is laborious and expensive. Furthermore, the majority of methods described are DNA-based and will not detect the presence of mutations that may lie in regulatory regions or deep within introns. However, owing to the fact that the majority of mutations result in translational truncation, PTT has been successfully used by some investigators to detect point mutations in the *DMD* gene (22,23). Using de novo protein synthesis from RNA extracted from the patient, the coding region is screened for truncating types of mutations. The RNA is reverse transcribed, and the cDNA is then PCR-amplified with a primer which facilitates in vitro transcription by T7-RNA polymerase. A translation step then generates peptide fragments, which are analyzed on gels for the identification of shorter fragments indicative of a truncating mutation. The major limitation of the PTT is that it requires dystrophin RNA, which is most abundant in the muscle, and therefore muscle biopsies are the specimen of choice. Muscle biopsies are not always available from affected patients, and RNA extracted from lymphocytes is more difficult to utilize because its presence is very low.

Although a number of the current strategies have been shown to be fairly sensitive in detecting small types of alterations in the very large dystrophin gene, the majority of these methods cannot distinguish mutations from polymorphic variations. A final sequencing step is required to confirm the nature of all the positive screening tests. In order for the testing of the nondeletion/duplication patients to be performed routinely in a molecular diagnostic laboratory, more high throughput sequencing techniques are necessary. Recently, a single condition amplification/internal primer sequencing technique was described for point mutation detection in the dystrophin gene (24). The method relied on the amplification of dystrophin gene exons using a single set of PCR conditions, and sequencing was then performed using a second set of internal primers. The analysis was both automated and of high throughput, with all of the dystrophin exons being sequenced within three working days at a reasonable cost. The key features of this system, being sequence-based and automated, increase its desirability and potential for application in a routine molecular diagnostic laboratory.

CONCLUSIONS

As a result of the discovery of the dystrophin gene and elucidation of the mutational spectrum, clinical diagnostic testing for DMD and BMD has significantly improved. Until an effective treatment is found to cure or arrest the progression of the disease, prevention of new cases through accurate diagnosis and carrier and prenatal testing is of utmost importance. In the future, molecular therapies (such as antisense oligonucleotides, antibiotics, or chimeric RNA/DNA) that depend on the precise knowledge of the specific dystrophin mutation may be applied. This approach will require a complete mutation analysis and identification of all types of dystrophin mutations.

REFERENCES

1. Koenig M, Hoffman EP, Bertelson CJ, Monaco AP, Feener C, Kunkel LM. Complete cloning of the Duchenne muscular dystrophy (DMD) cDNA and preliminary genomic organization of the DMD gene in normal and affected individuals. Cell 1987; 50:509–517.
2. Hoffman EP, Brown RH, Kunkel LM. Dystrophin: the protein product of the Duchenne muscular dystrophy locus. Cell 1987; 51:919–928.
3. Forest S, Cross GS, Speer A, Gardner-Medwin D, Burner J, Davies K. Preferential deletion of exons in Duchenne and Becker muscular dystrophies. Nature 1987; 329:638–640.
4. Darras BT, Blattner P, Harper JF, Spiro AJ, Alter S, Franke U. Intragenic deletions in 21 Duchenne muscular dystrophy (DMD)/Becker muscular dystrophy (BMD) families studied with the dystrophin cDNA: location of breakpoints on *Hind*III and BglII exon-containing fragment maps, meiotic and mitotic origin of mutations. Am J Hum Genet 1988; 43:620–629.
5. Monaco AP, Bertelson CJ, Liechti-Gallati S, Moser H, Kunkel LM. An explanation for the phenotypic differences between patients bearing partial deletions of the DMD locus. Genomics 1988; 2:90–95.
6. Malhotra SB, Hart KA, Klamut HJ, et al. Frame-shift deletions in patients with Duchenne and Becker muscular dystrophy. Science 1988; 242:755–759.
7. Prior TW, Bartolo C, Papp AC, et al. Dystrophin expression in a Duchenne muscular dystrophy patient with a frameshift deletion. Neurology 1997; 48:486–488.
8. Hu X, Ray PN, Murphy E, Thompson MW, Worton RG. Duplicational mutation at the Duchenne muscular dystrophy locus: its frequency, distribution, origin and phenotype/genotype correlation. Am J Hum Genet 1990; 46:682–695.

9. Roberts RG, Gardner RJ, Bobrow M. Searching for the 1 in 2,400,000: a review of dystrophin gene point mutations. Hum Mutat 1994; 4:1–11.
10. Prior TW, Bartolo C, Pearl DK, et al. Spectrum of small mutations in the dystrophin coding region. Am J Hum Genet 1995; 57:22–33.
11. Prior TW, Papp AC, Snyder PJ, Burghes AHM, Wallace BH. A HindIII/BglII dystrophin gene polymorphism in the Black population. Hum Genet 1992; 89:687–688.
12. Chamberlain JS, Gibbs RA, Ranier JE, Nga Nguyen PN, Caskey CT. Deletion screening of the Duchenne muscular dystrophy locus via multiplex DNA amplification. Nucl Acids Res 1988; 16:11141–11156.
13. Beggs AH, Koenig M, Boyce FM, Kunkel LM. Detection of 98% of DMD/BMD gene deletions by PCR. Hum Genet 1990; 86:45–48.
14. White S, Kalf M, Liu Q, et al. Comprehensive detection of genomic duplications and deletions in the DMD gene, by use of multiplex amplifiable probe hybridization. Am J Hum Genet 2002; 71:365–374.
15. Darras BT, Koenig M, Kunkel LM, Francke U. Direct method for prenatal diagnosis and carrier detection in Duchenne/Becker muscular dystrophy using the entire dystrophin cDNA. Am J Med Genet 1988; 29:713–726.
16. Prior TW, Friedman KJ, Highsmith WE, Perry TR, Silverman LM. Molecular probe protocol for determining carrier status in Duchenne and Becker muscular dystrophies. Clin Chem 1990; 36:441–445.
17. Bakker E, Veenema H, den Dunnen JT, et al. Germinal mosaicism increases the recurrence risk for 'new' Duchenne muscular dystrophy mutations. J Med Genet 1989; 26:553–559.
18. Clemens PR, Fenwick RG, Chamberlain JS, et al. Carrier detection and prenatal diagnosis in Duchenne and Becker muscular dystrophy families, using dinucleotide repeat polymorphisms. Am J Hum Genet 1991; 49:951–960.
19. Oudet C, Helig R, Hanauer A, Mandel JL. Nonradioactive assay for new microsatellite polymorphisms at the 5' end of the dystrophin gene, and estimation of intragenic recombination. Am J Hum Genet 1991; 49:311–319.
20. King SC, Roche AL, Passos-Bueno MR, et al. Molecular characterization of further dystrophin gene microsatellites. Mol Cell Probes 1995; 9:361–370.
21. Abbs S, Roberts RG, Mathew CG, Bentley DR, Bobrow M. Accurate assessment of intragenic recombination frequency within the Duchenne muscular dystrophy gene. Genomics 1990; 7:602–606.
22. Roest PAM, Roberts RG, Sugino S, van Ommen GJB, den Dunnen JT. Protein truncation test (PTT) for rapid detection of translation-terminating mutations. Hum Mol Genet 1993; 2:1719–1721.
23. Gardner RJ, Bobrow M, Roberts RG. The identification of point mutations in Duchenne muscular dystrophy patients using reverse transcript PCR and the protein truncation test. Am J Hum Genet 1995; 57:311–320.
24. Flanigan KM, Niederhausern AV, Dunn DM, Alder J, Mendell JR, Weiss RB. Rapid direct sequence analysis of the dystrophin gene. Am J Hum Genet 2003; 72:931–939.

6

Protein Studies in Duchenne Muscular Dystrophy

Kathryn North and Sandra Cooper
Institute for Neuromuscular Research, Children's Hospital at Westmead, University of Sydney, Sydney, New South Wales, Australia

BACKGROUND

Indications for Protein Diagnosis in the Dystrophinopathies

A "dystrophic" pattern of findings on muscle biopsy (characterized by variation in fiber size, the presence of degenerating and regenerating muscle fibers, and an increase in fibrous connective tissue) is common to all forms of muscular dystrophy. While the clinical presentation or family history may suggest or confirm the diagnosis of Duchenne muscular dystrophy (DMD) or Becker muscular dystrophy (BMD), in some patients it is not possible to differentiate these conditions from other forms of limb girdle muscular dystrophy (LGMD) solely on the basis of clinical findings. This is particularly true for sporadic or isolated cases within a family, in whom the differential diagnosis of DMD from sarcoglycanopathy, or BMD from other classes of LGMD, may be impossible based on clinical examination alone. There are currently at least 19 identified disease candidates for the LGMD, and several more yet unidentified disease loci (1–3).

Dystrophin DNA analysis in current clinical practice can result in the molecular diagnosis of a dystrophinopathy in approximately two-thirds of

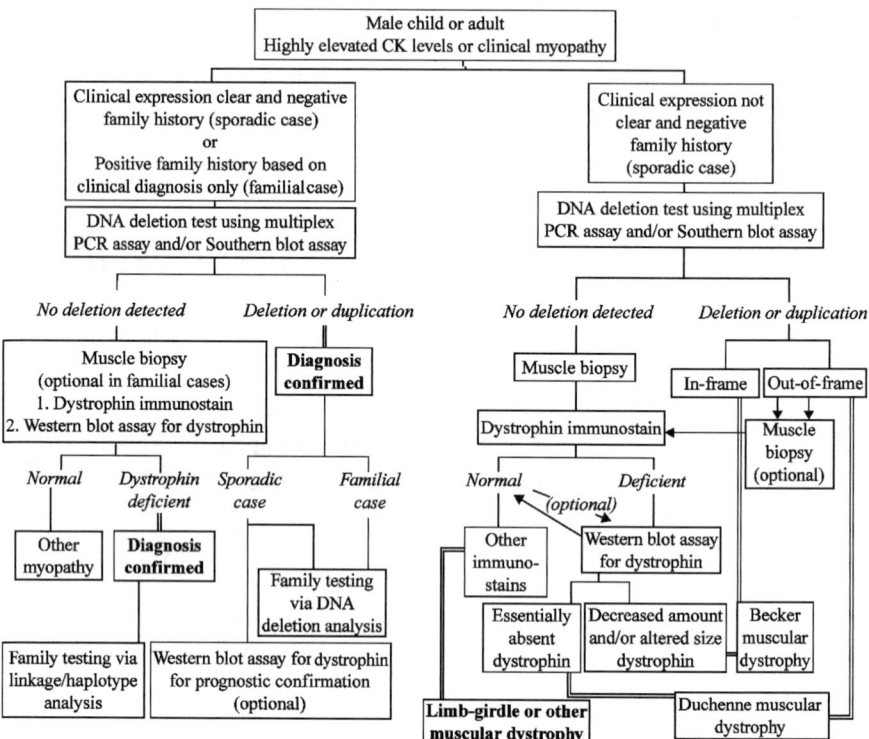

Figure 1 Algorithm for the laboratory diagnosis of sporadic and familial cases of DMD and BMD and for family testing (carrier detection and prenatal or presymptomatic diagnosis). *Abbreviations*: BMD, Becker muscular dystrophy; DMD, Duchenne muscular dystrophy. *Source*: From Ref. 4.

patients in whom dystrophin abnormalities are observed by protein studies (see Chapter 5). Thus, a muscle biopsy may not be necessary in many patients, particularly those with a classical clinical phenotype, a family history and/or an identified mutation in the dystrophin gene. The principle indications for a muscle biopsy (in a patient presenting with clinical findings suggestive of a muscular dystrophy) are to confirm diagnosis in dystrophin deletion–negative patients, to provide prognostic information from the quantitation of dystrophin in isolated cases (to distinguish between Duchenne and Becker subtypes—see below), or to explore the diagnosis of another specific muscular dystrophy subtype in patients with normal dystrophin. In these cases, the muscle biopsy is analyzed by immunohistochemistry (IHC), followed by quantitative analysis of proteins by Western blot. The algorithm in (Fig. 1) summarizes a diagnostic approach to the dystrophinopathies, utilizing clinical, genetic, and protein analysis in sequential steps (4). Early and definitive diagnosis of the various forms of muscular dystrophy is essential for provision of accurate prognostic information and genetic counseling to patients and their families.

Dystrophin Expression in the Muscular Dystrophies

The clinical utility of protein diagnosis in DMD and BMD was demonstrated soon after the identification of the dystrophin gene (5). Portions of the coding sequence were used to produce polyclonal antiserum to characterize dystrophin in normal muscle and in muscles of DMD and BMD patients (6). In normal muscle, dystrophin is a 427 kDa protein of low abundance (0.002% total muscle protein), localized to the inner surface of the plasma membrane of all myofibers (7). DMD is characterized by complete deficiency or significant reduction (less than 5% normal levels) in the levels of dystrophin expressed in the skeletal muscle of affected patients. BMD is characterized by reduced levels of dystrophin, and/or, an abnormally sized dystrophin protein product detected by immunoblot analysis (8,9). In BMD, dystrophin may have a reduction in apparent molecular weight due to intragenic deletions (about 80% of cases) or increased molecular weight due to duplication of exons within the dystrophin gene (approximately 5% of cases). Reduced levels of normal-sized dystrophin (due to small deletions or point mutations) are present in approximately 15% of BMD patients (10–13).

Early studies, which used immunoblotting of the dystrophin protein, also showed a correlation between the severity of the clinical phenotype and the quantity of dystrophin present in the muscle (9). Patients with 3% to 20% of the normal quantity of dystrophin, regardless of size, conformed to the severe Becker (intermediate) phenotype, and those with 20% to 50% had mild or moderate BMD. Most BMD patients with abnormal-sized dystrophin had higher levels of dystrophin protein (greater than 40% of normal levels, range 20–100%), compared with patients expressing normal-sized dystrophin. Subsequent quantitative studies have demonstrated a greater degree of overlap in the relative amount of dystrophin in severe, intermediate, and mild Becker phenotypes, suggesting that a prognosis based solely on dystrophin protein levels may be inaccurate (10). In one rare case, normal levels of dystrophin were detected by immunoblot analysis in biopsy samples from a patient exhibiting a DMD phenotype, who was later found to possess a single missense mutation and amino acid change within the cysteine-rich domain of dystrophin (G10211C, D3335H) (14). Immunohistochemical analysis of frozen muscle sections remains the most effective and rapid primary screen for dystrophin abnormalities. Successful immunohistochemical staining for dystrophin using formalin-fixed, paraffin-embedded sections has also been reported (15). Dystrophin immunostaining of muscle biopsy samples from patients with DMD, using

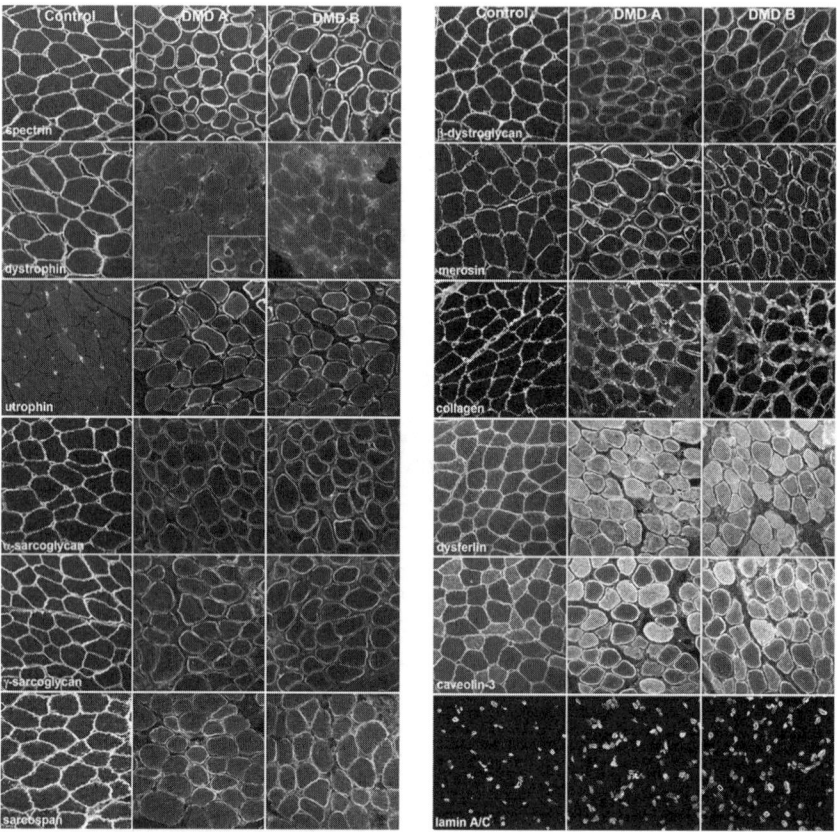

Figure 2 Immunohistochemical expression profiles of DAPC components and other muscular dystrophy disease candidates in DMD. (*Left column*): Control muscle, five years. (*Middle column*): DMD patient (Δ45–51), 5.5 years. *Dytrophin Insert*—demonstrates revertant fibers staining positively for Dys 1. (*Right column*): DMD patient (Δ45), four years. Biopsy samples (quadriceps) were stained with primary antibodies followed by CY3-conjugated secondary antibodies. Images were captured using a Leica SP2 scaning confocal microscope. For each antibody, control and patient samples were imaged under identical conditions to enable comparison of fluorescent intensities.

a panel of antidystrophin antibodies, results in negative staining of the sarcolemmal membrane, with perhaps occasional fibers that stain positively for dystrophin (Fig. 2). Occasional (less than 1%) dystrophin-positive fibers are detected in muscle sections from approximately 80% of DMD patients. These are often termed "revertant fibers" and are thought to result from alternative splicing, exon-skipping, or secondary somatic mutations within

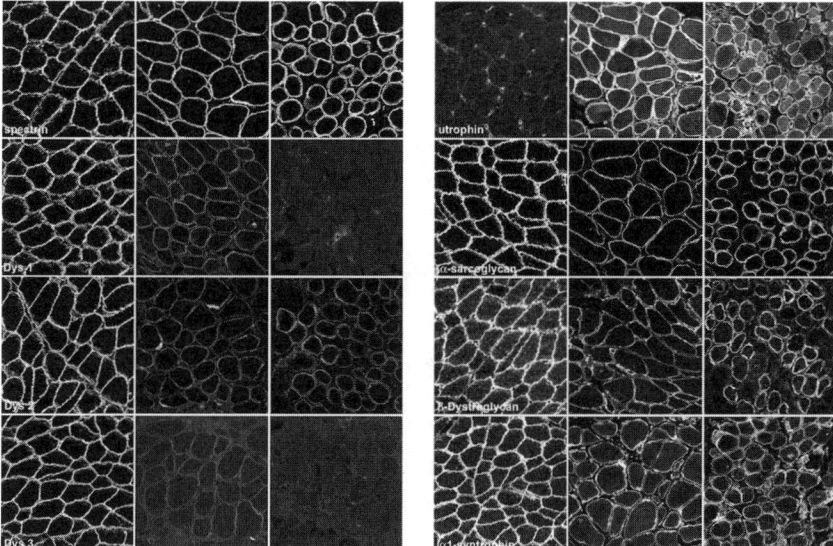

Figure 3 Immunohistochemical analysis of dystrophin and DAPC components in BMD. (*Left column*): Control muscle, five years. (*Middle column*): BMD patient (Δ3–6), nine years. (*Right column*): BMD patient (Δ3–34), 2.5 years. Biopsy samples (deltoid or quadriceps) were stained with primary antibodies followed by CY3-conjugated secondary antibodies. Images were captured using a Leica SP2 scaning confocal microscope. For each antibody, control and patient samples were imaged under identical conditions to enable comparison of fluorescent intensities.

myoblast clones, resulting in a dystrophin message with an "in-frame" coding sequence that may be successfully translated into a dystrophin protein product (16,17). For patients with BMD, dystrophin immunostaining may appear normal, or patchy and reduced, using different antidystrophin antibodies (Fig. 3). Patchy or discontinuous dystrophin immunostaining of the sarcolemmal membrane in BMD muscle sections may be more apparent when viewed at higher magnification, which is recommended for evaluation of stained slides. Female carriers of DMD usually exhibit a distinct mosaic pattern of dystrophin immunostaining that results from random X-inactivation within local nuclei of the muscle myofibers (Fig. 4). In some manifesting carriers of DMD, skewed X-inactivation may be apparent, represented by a greater number of negatively staining myofibers. However, many female carriers of DMD or BMD show no abnormalities in dystrophin immunostaining, either due to skewed X-inactivation in favor of the normal dystrophin allele, or due to even distribution of dystrophin protein products synthesized from "normal nuclei" to membrane regions surrounding "dystrophin-defective" nuclei.

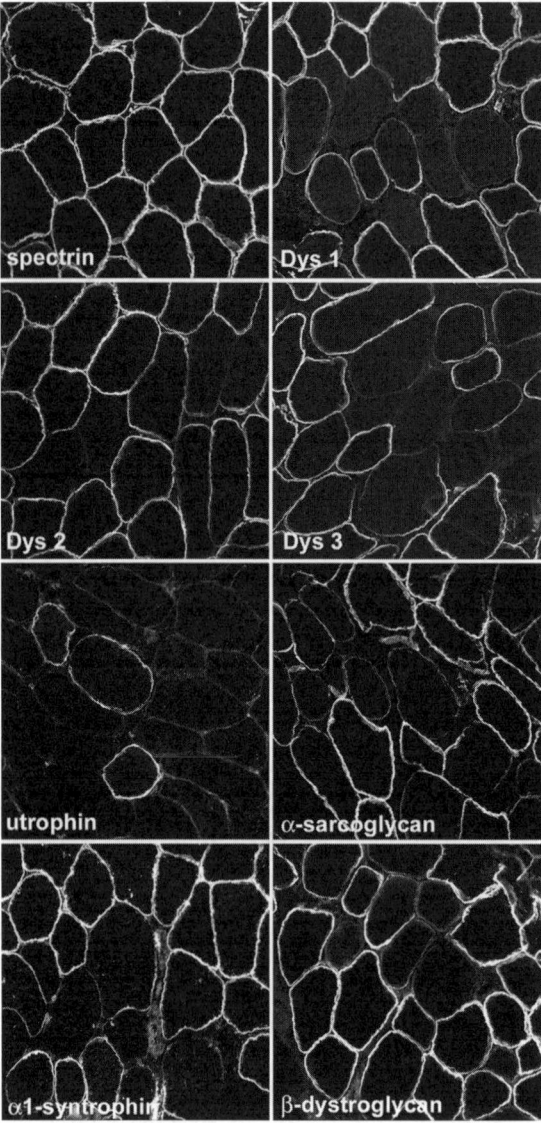

Figure 4 Immunohistochemical analysis of dystrophin and DAPC components in a manifesting carrier of DMD. Eight-micron biopsy cryosections were stained with primary antibodies followed by CY3-conjugated secondary antibodies. While spectrin uniformly stains the sarcolemma of all fibers, a mosaic staining pattern for dystrophin is observed, with negative and faintly stained fibers apparent. Utrophin appears upregulated, and there is concomitant downregulation of DAPC components in dystrophin-negative fibers.

Abnormal or deficient dystrophin expression may secondarily affect the expression levels and/or localization of other components of the dystrophin-associated protein complex, many of which can also cause muscular dystrophy disease. Typically, reduced levels and/or changes in the distribution of the sarcoglycans, dystroglycans, sarcospan, nNOS and AQP-4, syntrophin, and dystrobrevin may be observed in DMD (18–24). In contrast, levels of utrophin, caveolin-3, and α7β1 integrin may be elevated (Table 1) (25–27). Vice versa, muscle samples from patients with primary mutations in the sarcoglycans, for instance, may have abnormalities in dystrophin immunostaining (28). These findings highlight the necessity, in some cases, for qualitative and quantitative analysis of dystrophin by Western blot technique to distinguish between primary and secondary abnormalities observed by IHC techniques, for accurate diagnosis of a primary dystrophinopathy.

Skin biopsy and dystrophin immunostaining of smooth muscle under the skin (arrector pili muscle) has been studied as an alternate means for the

Table 1 Summary of IHC Expression Profiles for Components of the DAPC and Other Muscular Dystrophy Candidates in DMD (Fig. 1)

Spectrin	Normal, patchy in necrotic fibers
Laminin α2	Normal
Collagen 6	Highlights increased connective tissue
α-Sarcoglycan	Reduced/patchy
β-Sarcoglycan	Reduced/patchy
δ-Sarcoglycan	Reduced/patchy
γ-Sarcoglycan	Reduced/absent
Sarcospan	Reduced/patchy
β-Dystroglycan	Reduced
Dysferlin	Normal or elevated/cytoplasmic localization
Caveolin-3	Elevated
Myotilin	Normal or elevated
AQP4	Reduced, abnormal distribution, loss of fiber-type specificity
nNOS	Reduced, lost from the sarcolemma
α1-Syntrophin	Reduced, abnormal distribution
β1-Syntrophin	Elevated, abnormal distribution, loss of fiber-type specificity
β2-Syntrophin	Reduced, abnormal distribution, loss of fiber-type specificity
α-Dystrobrevin 1	Reduced, abnormal distribution
α-Dystrobrevin 2	Reduced, abnormal distribution

Abbreviations: DAPC, dystrophin-associated protein complex; DMD, Duchenne muscular dystrophy; IHC, immunohistochemistry.

diagnosis of dystrophinopathy (29,30). Dystrophin is known to be expressed in smooth muscle under the transcriptional control of the muscle promoter, although it is subject to alternate splicing compared with the skeletal muscle dystrophin isoform (31–33). Weakly positive dystrophin immunostaining was detected using a C-terminal dystrophin antibody in the six DMD patients studied, suggesting that this approach may not be sufficiently robust for accurate diagnosis of DMD (30).

METHODOLOGICAL APPROACH TO PROTEIN DIAGNOSIS OF DYSTROPHINOPATHIES

Immunohistochemistry

For patients fulfilling the clinical profile of DMD or BMD, initial screening employs immunohistochemical analysis of the muscle biopsy specimen using a panel of antibodies that recognize distinct regions of the large dystrophin protein, together with analysis of one or two of the sarcoglycans, merosin (laminin α2) to evaluate the integrity of the basal lamina, and β-spectrin for preservation of the plasma membrane within the sample. The proportion of regenerating fibers can be estimated through staining for fetal (NCL-devMHC, Novocastra) or developmental (NCL-neoMHC, Novocastra) myosin heavy chain isoforms. Analysis of an age-matched, unaffected control sample should always be performed in parallel, and comparison of results using known DMD and/or BMD samples may also be beneficial. Reduced expression of both β-spectrin and dystrophin may be observed in necrotic and regenerating fibers, resulting in a false-negative result. Therefore, interpretation of dystrophin immunostaining results requires careful comparison with results obtained using β-spectrin and fetal myosin.

Several commercial antidystrophin antibodies are available for use:

Dystrophin N-terminus	NCL-DYS3	Novocastra	Amino acids 67–713
Dystrophin rod domain	NCL-DYS1	Novocastra	Amino acids 1181–1388
	MANDYS8	Sigma	Amino acids 1431–1505
Dystrophin C-terminus	NCL-DYS2	Novocastra	Extreme C-terminus
	MANDRA1	Sigma	Amino acids 3200–3684

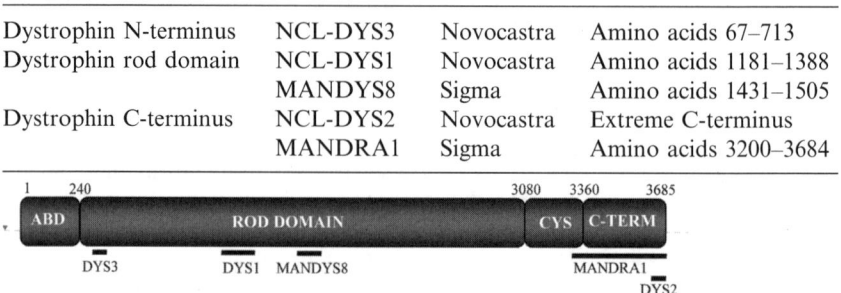

Weakly positive immunoreactivity to rod domain or N-terminal dystrophin antibodies has been reported in DMD, a phenomenon not observed

using C-terminal antibodies (10,34,35). Thus, staining the different regions of the dystrophin protein with multiple antibodies is essential for the accurate diagnosis of dystrophinopathies and to distinguish between BMD and DMD.

In BMD, immunostaining with a particular dystrophin antibody may be reduced uniformly in all fibers in a cryosection, or it may vary from fiber to fiber, or be patchy within single fibers. Furthermore, positive immunostaining of BMD muscle samples may be observed with one dystrophin antibody, whereas staining with another dystrophin antibody may be negative, due to deletion mutations that remove specific antibody recognition sites within the dystrophin protein (Fig. 3). Occasionally, dystrophin immunostaining may appear indistinguishable from controls, particularly when secondary antibodies, conjugated to horseradish peroxidase (HRP) or alkaline phosphatase, are used. Therefore, for accurate diagnosis of BMD, it is important to titrate dystrophin primary antibody concentrations up to an informative range. Use several dilutions of primary antibody to stain control muscle specimens, and employ a dilution that hovers at the point of saturation. These conditions should also be established for secondary antibodies, and be reconfirmed with each new antibody batch.

Several detection systems may be employed for dystrophin IHC. Historically, secondary antibodies conjugated to HRP or alkaline phosphatase are used for enzymatic conversion of diaminobenzamine (DAB), yielding a very stable brown product, and samples may be stored over many years at room temperature. Alternatively, secondary antibodies conjugated to fluorochromes may be used, and is our method of choice for detection. Indirect fluorescent microscopy provides high resolution against the contrast of a black background, permits dual-labeling of two antigens using species-specific secondary antibodies, and is nontoxic (DAB is carcinogenic). Improvements in photostable fluorochromes (i.e., Alexa, Cyanine, Rhodamine, and Texas red) and development of mounting reagents that prevent photobleaching have opened up the possibility of fluorescent-labeled slides being stable for several years even when stored in the dark. For either development system, results may be enhanced using a three-step detection sandwich, employing a biotinylated secondary antibody followed by streptavidin conjugated to your detection system of choice. Multiple streptavidin-conjugates may bind the biotinylated secondary antibody, increasing the emitted signal by several fold.

Detailed IHC Methodology Using Fluorescent Detection

Muscle biopsy specimens are cryosectioned (8 µm) and captured on poly-L-lysine–treated slides and allowed to dry at room temperature. An aqueous barrier may be formed around the specimen using a wax-pen. Muscle specimens are then incubated in primary antibody, diluted in blocking buffer [phosphate buffered saline (PBS) containing 10% fetal calf serum or 2% bovine serum albumin] for two hours at room temperature, in a humidified chamber. Approximately 50 μL of diluted primary antibody is applied to the sample as a droplet. Unbound primary antibody is removed by washing three times in PBS. The slides are carefully dried off using a Kim-wipe™ (Kimberly-Clark Corporation, Roswell, Georgia, U.S.A.), and taking care to avoid the circle of wax and muscle specimen. Samples are then incubated in fluorescent-labeled secondary antibody diluted in blocking buffer, for one to two hours at room temperature, in a humidified chamber. Excess secondary antibody is removed by washing three times in PBS. The slides are again dried using a Kim-wipe and then mounted with a glass coverslip using a suitable mounting reagent compatible with fluorescent microscopy.

Western Blotting

Western blot analysis is used for dystrophin quantitation and to assess the molecular weight of the residual dystrophin protein. As described above, immunoblot analysis can provide definitive diagnosis of DMD and BMD, as well as valuable prognostic information on the individual patient (9). However, immunoblot analysis of muscle biopsy specimens in patients has not been performed routinely as part of diagnostic screening for the muscular dystrophies. This is, in part, due to the fact that widely used protocols describing muscle immunoblot analysis recommend the solubilization of a comparatively large quantity of muscle tissue, i.e., 20 to 100 mg, in many cases requiring the remaining part of the specimen after biopsy (1,9). Recent progress using multiplex immunoblot analysis for simultaneous screening of a range of disease candidates has improved the diagnostic scope of Western blot analysis, but continues to require the use of a significant portion of a muscle biopsy specimen (20–30 mg) (36).

Ho Kim et al. (37) have demonstrated that effective and accurate analysis of dystrophin expression may be reliably performed using significantly less muscle tissue. We have shown that solubilization of muscle tissue according to traditional protocols (using 19 volumes w/v of lysis buffer) results in relatively inefficient solubilization of large and/or membrane-associated proteins including dystrophin, likely caused by lysis buffer saturation, due to the extremely high protein content of muscle. To this end, we have developed a methodological protocol for dystrophin immunoblot analysis that uses only one or two biopsy cryosections—"Single Section Western Blot" (Fig. 5) (38). We have defined "a single biopsy cryosection" as an eight micron section encompassing a surface area of 10 mm^2, and have shown that this provides sufficient tissue for multiplex analysis of dystrophin along with multiple muscular disease candidates (Fig. 6).

A myosin-loading gel is first used to ensure that equal amounts of "muscle protein" are loaded for both patient and control samples. Muscle lysates derived from severely dystrophic biopsy samples invariably contain less total protein than those derived from control muscle, due to less dense

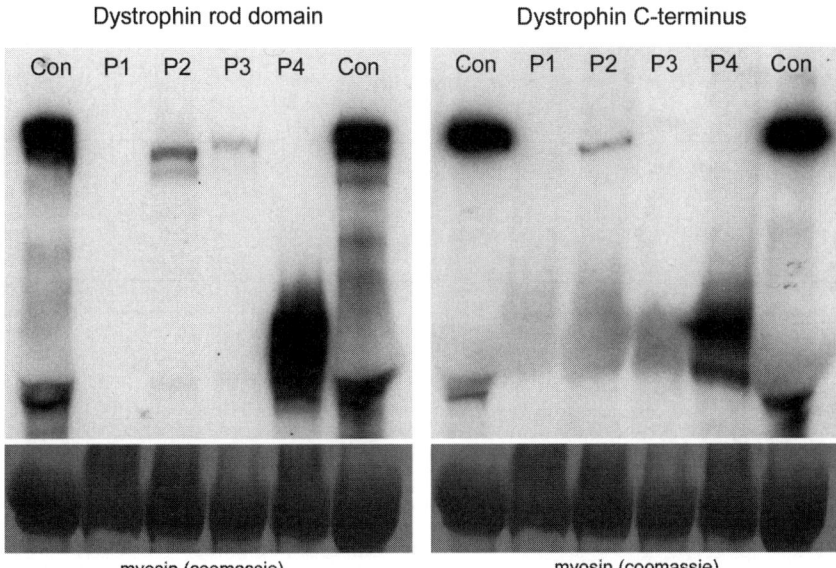

Figure 5 "Single Section Western Blot" for diagnosis of dystrophinopathies. Soluble muscle lysates were normalized for myosin content, separated on 2% to 9% polacrylamide gels and transferred to PVDF membranes. The blot was sectioned and the two halves probed with either rod domain or C-terminal antidystrophin antibodies. The gel is flanked by two samples from unaffected age-matched controls. Lane 1 contains muscle lysate from a patient with DMD (Δ 45–51). Lanes 2 to 4 contain muscle samples from BMD (P2—Δ exons 3–6; P3—unknown; P4—Δ exons 3–34). No detectable deletion was identified for the patient in lane 3, although our results suggest a small truncation of the C-terminus (based on observations of a slightly smaller dystrophin product and the absence of immunoreactivity to DYS2, a C-terminal antibody). *Abbreviations*: BMD, Becker muscular dystrophy; DMD, Duchenne muscular dystrophy; PVDF, poly(vinylidene difluoride).

myofibrillar packing of dystrophic muscle (soluble proteins levels are $\frac{1}{2}-\frac{1}{3}$ that of age-matched control muscle; our unpublished observations). Furthermore, muscle-specific proteins present in the lysate may be 'diluted' to some extent by protein components of fibrotic tissue. Therefore, for biopsy material, known by histological analysis to be severely dystrophic, we section and solubilize twice as much muscle tissue in the same volume of lysis buffer used for control muscle.

As with immunocytochemistry of muscle cryosections, multiple antibodies directed against different epitopes of dystrophin should be used in immunoblot analysis to make an accurate distinction between DMD and BMD. In DMD, dystrophin levels are typically 0% to 5% of normal control values. The majority of DMD mutations are "out-of-frame deletions,"

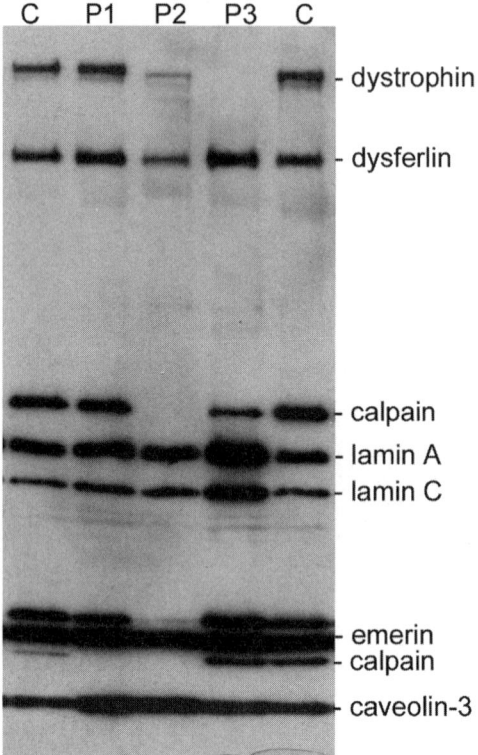

Figure 6 "Single Section Western Blot" for diagnostic screening of LGMD. Soluble lysates were separated by SDS-PAGE and transferred to PVDF membranes. Membranes were probed with an antibody cocktail containing antibodies recognizing dystrophin (Dys 1), dysferlin (Hamlet), calpain (2C4), lamin A/C, emerin, and caveolin (C38320), followed by an HRP-conjugated secondary antibody. The gel is flanked by control samples. Patient 1 appears normal for all proteins. Patient 2 has lower levels of dystrophin, suggestive of BMD, although also has reduced levels of dysferlin and absent calpain, perhaps indicating proteolytic degradation within the sample. Patient 3 appears a likely case of DMD, and also has increased levels of lamin, frequently observed in dystrophic muscle due to increased number of nuclei. *Abbreviations*: BMD, Becker muscular dystrophy; DMD, Duchenne muscular dystrophy; HRP, horseradish peroxidase; LGMD, limb girdle muscular dystrophy; PVDF, poly(vinylidene difluoride); SDS-PAGE, sodium dodecyl sulfate–polyacrylamide gel electrophoresis. *Source*: From Ref. 39.

introducing a premature stop codon that results either in degradation of mRNA by nonsense-mediated decay, or production of an unstable truncated dystrophin protein that is rapidly metabolized (40). In BMD, where deletions remove the epitope recognized by a specific antibody, dystrophin may be undetectable by Western blot analysis using that antibody. In addition, in patients with a deletion starting in exon 45 and extending to exons

47, 48, 49, or 54, a 210- to 230-kDa degradation fragment, likely due to proteolytic cleavage of dystrophin at the deletion junctions, may be detected using N-terminal and rod domain antibodies (but not C-terminal antibodies) (41). Therefore, we would recommend the use of multiple antibodies which recognize N-terminal, rod domain, and the C-terminal for Western blot analysis. While this approach results in a high level of diagnostic accuracy, results must always be interpreted in the context of the patient's clinical presentation.

Densitometric analysis of banding on autoradiographic film may be used for quantification of levels of dystrophin in BMD. Probing for β-spectrin provides a membrane-loading control, and results are best presented as a ratio of dystrophin and spectrin between controls and patients.

Detailed Western Blot Methodology

SDS-PAGE sample preparation: Biopsy samples are cryosectioned (8-μm sections) and transferred to an Eppendorf™ (Eppendorf AG, Hamburg, Germany), precooled on dry ice, using a sterile needle, also precooled on dry ice, and gently tapped to the bottom of the tube. Cross-sectional area of biopsy samples are estimated at the time of sectioning, using a ruler as a guide to approximate surface area. Typically, approximately 40 mm^2 (i.e., the equivalent of four, 10-mm^2 biopsy sections) for each patient is sectioned at one time, to enable repeat sodium dodecyl sulfate (SDS)–polyacrylamide gel electrophoresis (PAGE) and immunoblot analysis if required. Immediately transfer the Eppendorf containing the biopsy sections onto ice, and add an appropriate volume of lysis buffer (LB; 4% SDS, 125 mM Tris pH 8.8, 20% glycerol, 100 mM DTT, bromophenol blue, protease inhibitor cocktail). We recommend the use of 20 μL (mini-gel format) to 40 μL (large-gel format) of LB per 10-mm^2 biopsy cryosection. Vortex well and spin briefly to sediment the lysate (i.e., 1000 g, 20 seconds). Triturate the lysate to an even suspension using a Gilson pipette. Sonicate the samples to shear chromosomal DNA (reduce viscosity) and to aid solubilization, then heat inactivate at 94°C for four minutes in a water-filled well of a heating block. Following heat inactivation, the samples may be handled at room temperature. Prior to loading, spin the samples briefly (three minutes, 13,000 g) in a benchtop microfuge, to sediment particulate material.

SDS-PAGE and myosin loading gels for sample standardization: For each sample, separate 5 μL of the solublized lysate on a single phase 5% acrylamide minigel. Coomassie stain and destain the gel. Using the intensity of the myosin band from control samples as standard, normalize loading of patient samples and control samples for myosin content. Load samples onto SDS-PAGE gels and electrophorese until the dye-front runs off. For users not familiar with SDS-PAGE methodologies, the use of preprepared commercial gels may help with diagnostic reproducibility.

Electroblotting: A low concentration of SDS should be included in the transfer buffer, to assist the solubility and transfer of large proteins such as dystrophin. We typically use Towbin's transfer buffer (25 mM Tris, 192 mM glycine, pH 8.3) containing 0.075% SDS. Gels are electroblotted overnight at 35 V constant voltage (approximately 280–330 mA), with stirring, and with recirculating water cooled to 18°C. Under these conditions, myosin is barely detectable on the post-transfer gel, demonstrating very efficient protein transfer.

Antibody probing: Block free protein-binding sites on the poly(vinylidene difluoride) (PVDF) membranes using PBS or Tris buffered saline (TBS) (15 mM Tris, pH 8.0, 150 mM NaCl) containing 5% skim-milk powder plus 0.1% Tween-20 for at least one hour. Primary antibodies should be diluted in blocking buffer and incubated for two hours at room temperature, or overnight at 4°C. Wash the membranes thoroughly (four, 5-minute washes) with PBS/0.1% Tween-20 or TBS/0.1% Tween-20, reblock for 10 minutes, then incubate with appropriate HRP-conjugated secondary antibodies, also diluted in blocking solution, for two hours at room temperature. Wash membranes thoroughly and develop with chemiluminescent substrates, according to the manufacturer's instructions.

ACKNOWLEDGMENTS

We wish to thank Harriet Lo, Adam Maxwell, and Alison Compton for their assistance in the preparation of figures.

REFERENCES

1. Bushby KMD, Anderson LVB. Multiplex Western blot analysis of muscular dystrophy proteins. In: Bushby KMD, Anderson LVB, eds. Methods in Molecular Medicine: Muscular Dystrophy: Methods and Protocols. Vol. 43. Totowata, New Jersey: Humana, 2001:369–386.
2. Cohn RD, Campbell KP. Molecular basis of muscular dystrophies. Muscle Nerve 2000; 23(10):1456–1471.
3. Guglieri M, Magri F, Comi GP. Molecular etiopathogenesis of limb girdle muscular and congenital muscular dystrophies: boundaries and contiguities. Clinica Chimica Acta 2005; 361(1–2):54–79.
4. Darras BT, Jones HR Jr. Diagnosis of pediatric neuromuscular disorders in the era of DNA analysis. Pediatr Neurol 2000; 289–300.
5. Koenig M, Hoffman EP, Bertelson CJ, Monaco AP, Feener C, Kunkel LM. Complete cloning of the Duchenne muscular dystrophy (DMD) cDNA and preliminary organisation of the DMD gene in normal and affected individuals. Cell 1987; 50(3):509–517.
6. Hoffman EP, Brown RH Jr, Kunkel LM. Dystrophin: the protein product of Duchenne muscular dystrophy locus. Cell 1987; 51(6):919–928.

7. Arahata K, Ishiura S, Ishiguro T, et al. Immunostaining of skeletal and cardiac muscle surface membrane with antibody against Duchenne muscular dystrophy peptide. Nature 1988; 333(6176):861–863.
8. Arahata K, Hoffman EP, Kunkel LM, et al. Dystrophin diagnosis: comparison of dystrophin abnormalities by immunofluorescence and immunoblot analyses. Proc Natl Acad Sci USA 1989; 86(18):7154–7158.
9. Hoffman EP, Fischbeck KH, Brown RH, et al. Characterisation of dystrophin in muscle biopsy specimens from patients with Duchenne's and Becker's muscular dystrophy. N Engl J Med 1988; 318(21):1363–1368.
10. Bulman DE, Murphy EG, Zubrzycka-Gaarn EE, Worton RG, Ray PN. Differentiation of Duchenne and Becker muscular dystrophy phenotypes with amino- and carboxy-terminal antisera specific for dystrophin. Am J Hum Genet 1991; 48(2):295–304.
11. Hoffman EP, Kunkel LM. Dystrophin abnormalities in Duchenne/Becker muscular dystrophy. Neuron 1989; 2(1):1019–1029.
12. Nicholson LV, Johnson MA, Bushby KM, et al. Integrated study of 100 patients with Xp21 linked muscular dystrophy using clinical, genetic, immunochemical, and histopathological data. Part 1. Trends across the clinical groups. J Med Genet 1993; 30(9):728–756.
13. Nicholson LV, Johnson MA, Bushby KM, et al. Integrated study of 100 patients with Xp21 linked muscular dystrophy using clinical, genetic, immunochemical, and histopathological data. Part 2. Correlations within individual patients. J Med Genet 1993; 30(9):737–744.
14. Goldberg LR, Hausmanowa-Petrusewicz I, Fidzianska A, Duggan DJ, Steinberg LS, Hoffman EP. A dystrophin missense mutation showing persistence of dystrophin and dystrophin-associated proteins yet a severe phenotype. Ann Neurol 1998; 44(6):971–976.
15. Hoshino S, Ohkoshi N, Watanabe M, Shoji S. Immunohistochemical staining of dystrophin on formalin-fixed paraffin embedded sections in Duchenne/Becker muscular dystrophy and manifesting carriers of Duchenne muscular dystrophy. Neuromuscul Disord 2000; 10(6):425–429.
16. Watkins SC, Hoffman EP, Slayter HS, Kunkel LM. Dystrophin distribution in heterozygote mdx mice. Muscle Nerve 1989; 12(10):861–868.
17. Wallgren-Pettersson C, Jasani B, Rosser LG, Lazarov LP, Nicholson LV, Clarke A. Immunohistological evidence for second or somatic mutations as the underlying cause of dystrophin expression by isolated fibres in Xp21 muscular dystrophy of Duchenne type severity. J Neurol Sci 1993; 118(1):56–63.
18. Evasti JM, Ohlendieck K, Kahl SD, Gaver MG, Campbell KP. Deficiency of a glycoprotein component of the dystrophin complex in dystrophic muscle. Nature 1990; 345(6273):315–319.
19. Ibraghimov-Beskrovnaya O, Ervasti JM, Leveille CJ, Slaughter CA, Sernett SW, Campbell KP. Primary structure of dystrophin-associated glycoproteins linking dystrophin to the extracellular matrix. Nature 1992; 355(6362):696–702.
20. Crosbie RH, Heighway J, Venke DP, Lee JC, Campbell KP. Sarcospan, the 25 kDa transmembrane component of the dystrophin-glycoprotein complex. J Biol Chem 1997; 272(50):31221–31224.
21. Chang WJ, Iannaccone ST, Lau KS, et al. Neuronal nitric oxide synthase and dystrophin-deficient muscular dystrophy. Proc Natl Acad Sci USA 1996; 93(17):9142–9147.

22. Frigeri A, Niccha GP, Repetto S, Bado M, Minetti C, Svelto M. Altered aquaporin-4 expression in human muscular dystrophies: a common feature? FASEB J 2002; 16(9):1120–1121.
23. Tachi N, Ohya K, Chiba S, Matsuo M, Patria SY, Matsumara K. Deficiency of syntrophin, dystroglycan, and merosin in a female infant with a congenital muscular dystrophy phenotype lacking cysteine-rich and C-terminal domain of dystrophin. Neurology 1997; 49(2):579–583.
24. Metzinger L, Blake DJ, Squier MV, et al. Dystrobrevin deficiency at the sarcolemma of the patients with muscular dystrophy. Hum Mol Genet 1997; 6(7):1185–1191.
25. Nguyen TM, Ellis JM, Love DR, et al. Localization of the DMDL gene-encoded dystrophin-related protein using a panel of nineteen monoclonal antibodies: presence at the neuromuscular junctions, in the sarcolemma of dystrophic skeletal muscle, in vascular and other smooth muscles, and in proliferating brain cell lines. J Cell Biol 1991; 115(6):1695–1700.
26. Repetto S, Bado M, Broda P, et al. Increased number of caveolae and caveolin-3 over expression in Duchenne muscular dystrophin. Biochem Biopys Res Commun 1999; 261(3):547–550.
27. Hodges BL, Hayashi YK, Nonaka I, Wang W, Arahata K, Kaufman SJ. Altered expression of the alpha7beta1 integrin in human and murine muscular dystrophies. J Cell Sci 1997; 110(Pt 22):2873–2881.
28. Fanin M, Angelini C. Regeneration in sarcoglycanopathies: expression studies of sarcoglycans and other muscle proteins. J Neurol Sci 1999; 165(2):170–177.
29. Marbini A, Marcello N, Bellanova MF, Guidetti D, Gemignani F. Dystrophin expression in skin biopsy immunohistochemical localisation of striated muscle type dystrophin. J Neurol Sci 1995; 129(1):29–33.
30. Niiyama T, Higuchi I, Sakoda S, Matsumara T, Fukunaga H, Osame M. Diagnosis of dystrophinopathy by skin biopsy. Muscle Nerve 2002; 25(3):398–401.
31. Walsh FS, Pizzey JA, Dickson G. Tissue specific isoforms of dystrophin. Trends Neurosci 1989; 12(7):235–238.
32. Byers TJ, Kunkel LM, Watkins SC. The subcellular distribution of dystrophin in mouse skeletal, cardiac and smooth muscle. J Cell Biol 1991; 115(2):411–421.
33. Feener CA, Koenig M, Kunkel LM. Alternate splicing of human dystrophin mRNA generates isoforms at the carboxy terminus. Nature 1989; 338(6215):509–511.
34. Nicholson LV, Johnson MA, Gardner-Medwin D, Bhattacharya S, Harris JB. Heterogeneity of dystrophin expression in patients with Duchenne and Becker muscular dystrophy. Acta Neuropathol (Berl) 1990; 80(3):239–250.
35. Arahata K, Beggs AH, Honda H, et al. Preservation of the C terminus of dystrophin molecule in the skeletal muscle from Becker muscular dystrophy. J Neurol Sci 1991; 101(2):148–156.
36. Anderson LV, Davison K. Multiplex Western blotting system for the analysis of muscular dystrophy proteins. Am J Pathol 1999; 154(4):1017–1022.
37. Ho Kim MA, Bedard A, Vincent M, Rogers PA. Dystrophin: a sensitive and reliable immunohistochemical assay in tissue and cell culture homogenates. Biochem Biophys Res Commun 1991; 181(3):1164–1172.

38. Cooper ST, Lo HP, North KN. Single section Western blot: Improving the molecular diagnosis of the muscular dystrophies. Neurology 2003; 61(1):93–97.
39. Lo HP, Cooper St, Macarthur DG, Yang N, North KN. The role of dysferlin and calpain 3 in limb girdle muscular dystrophy. Xth International Congress on Neuromuscular Disorders, Vancouver, British Columbia, Jul 7–12, 2002.
40. Kerr TP, Sewry CA, Robb SA, Roberts RG. Long mutant dystrophins and variable phenotypes: evasion of nonsense-mediated decay?. Hum Genet 2001; 109(4):402–407.
41. Beggs AH, Hoffman EP, Kunkel LM. Additional dystrophin fragment in Becker muscular dystrophy may result from proteolytic cleavage at deletion junctions. Am J Med Genet 1992; 44(3):378–381.

SECTION III: CURRENT THERAPEUTICS

7

Medical Management of Duchenne Muscular Dystrophy

Roula Al-Dahhak and John T. Kissel

*Department of Neurology, Division of Neuromuscular Disease,
The Ohio State University, Columbus,
Ohio, U.S.A.*

INTRODUCTION

The identification of the genetic basis for Duchenne muscular dystrophy (DMD) in 1987 understandably raised hopes that meaningful therapy for this disorder was just around the corner (1,2). Aside from the excitement generated by the possibility of "gene therapy," there was cautious optimism that defining the molecular pathogenesis of the disease might lead to pharmacotherapies that could interrupt the inexorable muscle deterioration associated with this disorder. These hopes were raised even higher two years later when a prospective, randomized, placebo-controlled trial demonstrated that prednisone improved strength in DMD (3).

Unfortunately, these initial lofty expectations have slowly been replaced by a sobering reality. There is still no cure for DMD; although many agents have been evaluated in clinical trials, none, aside from the corticosteroids prednisone and deflazacort, have proved clinically useful (Table 1). Both prednisone and deflazacort have many side effects, and there is little agreement about when, how, and even if they should be used routinely in DMD. Further complicating the situation is the fact that the mechanism by which corticosteroids improve strength in DMD is uncertain, making it difficult to devise new pharmacologic strategies.

Table 1 Clinical Trials on Corticosteroids in Patients with DMD

Drug	Author	Year	Design	No. of patients	Age	Duration	Dosage	Primary outcome	Results[a]	Reference
Prednisone	Siegel	1974	DB-RCT	14	6–9	36 mos	5 mg/kg/qod	Ambulation	No effect	(4)
	Drachman	1974	Open-label	14	3–10	28 mos	2 mg/kg/day	Strength Function	Improved	(5)
	Mendell	1989	DB-RCT	103	5–15	6 mos	1.5 mg/kg/day vs. 0.75 mg/kg/day	MMT Function	Improved	(3)
	Fenichel	1991	DB-RCT	9	5–15	6 mos	2.5 mg/qod 1.25 mg/kg/qod 1 pred at 6 mos	MMT Function	Improved	(9)
	Griggs	1991	DB-RCT	99	5–15	6 mos	0.75 mg/kg/day 0.3 mg/kg/day	MMT	Improved	(11)
	Griggs	1993	DB-RCT	99	5–15	12 mos	0.3 mg/kg/1day + aza 0.75 mg/kg/day	MMT	Improved	(12)

Drug	Author	Year	Study	N	Age	Duration	Dose	Outcome measures	Result	Ref
	Sansome	1993	Open-label	32	6–14	18 mos	0.75 mg/kg/day first 10 days/mos	Strength	Improved	(18)
	Backman	1995	DB-RCT	41	4–19	6 mos	0.35 mg/kg/day	Strength	Improved	(14)
Deflazacort	Mesa	1991	DB-RCT	28	5–11	9 mos	1 mg/kg/day	Function	Improved	(28)
	Angelini	1994	DB-RCT	28	6–9	24 mos	2 mg/kg/qod	Function	Improved	(29)
	Brooke	1996	DB-RCT	196	>5	12 mos	0.75 mg/kg pred 0.9 mg/kg deflz 1.2 mg/kg deflz	MMT Weight	Improved Less weight gain with deflz	(36)
	Bonifati	2000	DB-RCT	25	5–14	12 mos	0.75 mg/kg pred 0.9 mg/kg deflz	Function	Improved	(34)
	Reiter	2000	DB-RCT	80	>5	24 mos	0.75 mg/kg pred 0.9 mg/kg deflz	MMT Function	Improved	(35)

[a]See text for details.

Abbreviations: DB-RCT, double-blind, randomized, controlled trial; DMD, Duchenne muscular dystrophy; MMT, manual muscle testing.

Despite these difficulties, the dream of effective pharmacotherapy for DMD persists. Several clinical trials either now underway or in the planning stages should provide invaluable information about how best to use corticosteroids in DMD. In addition, several exciting new trials are planned based on novel rationales which will hopefully generate a number of therapeutic possibilities while improving the clinical status of patients with this disease. This chapter will highlight the current status of medical management of DMD, and review the most important clinical trials related to this disorder. The information will be organized by the pharmacologic class of agents used in pertinent trials.

CORTICOSTEROIDS

Background and Rationale

The first clinical trials of prednisone in DMD were reported independently in 1974 by two groups of investigators (4,5). The rationale for both studies was based on earlier encouraging anecdotal reports and the fact that biopsies from DMD patients often contain inflammatory cells. Given the current opinion on the superiority of blinded, controlled trials, it is ironic that the study of Siegel et al., which was a blinded, placebo-controlled study comparing 5 mg/kg alternate day prednisone to placebo in 14 boys treated for one year, showed no benefit, while the study of Drachman et al., which was a six-month, open-label, uncontrolled trial of 2 mg/kg/day in 14 patients, reported a favorable effect on strength and function. Although these studies were provocative and controversial, it was 15 years before more definitive studies of prednisone in DMD were performed by the Collaborative Investigations in Duchenne Dystrophy (CIDD) group (3,6–12).

Subsequent Clinical Trials

The CIDD group was formed in the late 1970s specifically to conduct clinical trials in DMD (6,7). On the basis of the Drachman study, and a report that prednisone was beneficial in a form of chicken dystrophy, the group performed an open-label trial of prednisone in 33 boys with DMD, which demonstrated a clear benefit compared to natural history controls (8,13). This led to a larger, randomized, double-blind, placebo-controlled trial on 103 boys, which showed significant beneficial effects of two different doses of prednisone (0.75 mg/kg/day and 1.5 mg/kg/day) on multiple outcome measures including strength (assessed by manual muscle testing), timed functional tests (e.g., time to climb four stairs or walk 10 m), and pulmonary function tests (3). The effect could be documented within the first month of initiating treatment, peaked at three months, and was maintained through the six month study.

Despite these unequivocally positive results, the group was cautious in the interpretation of their findings, noting that "Despite the importance of this observation, we are by no means advocating prednisone administration as a specific treatment for this disorder." Despite this disclaimer, however, a remarkable series of subsequent studies by the same group answered many important questions raised by the initial study, and the CIDD prednisone regimen came to be accepted by many neuromuscular clinicians as standard therapy. In the first of these studies, patients in the original cohort were randomized to receive alternate day therapy at either 2.5 mg/kg or 1.25 mg/kg (9). The results of this study confirmed that daily dosing was superior to alternate day schedules in improving strength. In a second study, the group documented that improvement was sustained for at least three years (10). The improvement was also shown to be rapid, occurring within 10 days after initiation of therapy, and dose dependent, such that a lower dose of 0.3 mg/kg/day was less effective than 0.75 mg/kg/day (11). Subsequent studies have confirmed this important finding, but also confirmed that side effects were less at lower dosages (11,14). Finally, the group documented that another immunosuppressive agent, azathioprine, had no effect on strength in DMD, either alone or as a steroid-sparing agent (12).

Although only one additional randomized, controlled trial of prednisone monotherapy has been performed over the past decade, multiple open-label trials and subsequent analyses of the original cohorts have provided additional information about the effects of prednisone (14). Most importantly, several analyses have shown that prednisone prolongs ambulation compared to the natural history of DMD by two to four years, and that a positive effect can probably be detected for up to 15 years after initiation of therapy (Table 2) (15–17). Unfortunately, this benefit comes at a price, and long-term studies have documented significant side effects associated with long-term prednisone use. The most comprehensive of these studies followed 226 of the original CIDD patients, and found that after a mean of eight years of follow-up, 50% of patients had discontinued treatment, most often because of weight gain (85%) or mood changes (13%) (discussed further in this chapter) (16).

Table 2 Effects of Long-Term Steroid Therapy on Ambulation

Study	Year	Dose	No.	Duration	Effect on walking[a]
DeSilva	1987	2 mg/kg/day	16	11 yrs	+2 yrs
Pandya	2001	0.75 mg/kg/day	30	15 yrs	+4 yrs
Tunca	2001	0.75 mg/kg/day	66	5 yrs	+3 yrs

[a]Numbers represent years of walking beyond control or natural history cohorts.

In an attempt to limit the significant side effects of corticosteroids, two principal strategies have recently been formulated. The first involves alternative dosing strategies. One proposed regimen involves administering prednisone at a dose of 0.75 mg/kg/day in intermittent pulses of 10 days on and 10 days off (18,19). Kinali et al. (19) described their long-term experience in 37 patients with DMD on such a regimen. In this analysis, in which some patients were followed for up to 10 years, there was improved function noted within six months of treatment, with a slow decline by 24 months and loss of ambulation at a median age of 9.5 years. Additional support for this regimen came from a report describing two four-year old boys treated with this pulsed regimen over five years; both boys showed marked functional improvement and achieved complete clinical remissions (20). One boy remained in a complete remission, while the second boy had a sustained response for five years before a rapid decline that resulted in loss of ambulation by age 10.

Another proposed alternative steroid regimen involves administering 5 mg/kg of prednisone for two consecutive days each week. A preliminary uncontrolled report of this regimen in 20 boys (average age: 8.0) treated for up to 27 months described similar improvements in strength to that seen with standard dosing regimens, with less weight gain and mood changes (21).

Although the preliminary reports on both of these new regimens are provocative, there is not enough experience to recommend them for routine clinical use, especially because neither regimen has been compared to the standard prednisone regimen in a controlled trial. Fortunately, large, randomized, controlled trials that will compare both the new regimens to standard therapy are planned. The results of these trials may fundamentally alter how prednisone is administered in DMD, and are eagerly awaited.

Deflazacort

A second approach to limit the side effects of prednisone therapy is to find a similar agent with fewer side effects. Deflazacort is an oxazolone derivative of prednisolone synthesized in 1967 with anti-inflammatory and immunosuppressive effects comparable to prednisone (22,23). The rationale for its clinical use came from the fact that the oxazoline side chain at the carbon 17 position (Fig. 1) would reduce lipid solubility, so that noncirculating cells such as osteoclasts and osteoblasts might be less exposed to the drug than circulating lymphocytes and monocytes (23). In preliminary studies, deflazacort did have bone-sparing effects with less effect on calcium absorption, urinary calcium excretion, and vertebral bone loss than prednisone (23–27).

Several small, randomized, double-blind, placebo-controlled clinical trials showed that deflazacort improved strength and function in patients with DMD when administered daily for nine months or on alternate days for up to three years (28,29). Other retrospective reports showed prolonged ambulation, improved pulmonary function, and preserved cardiac function

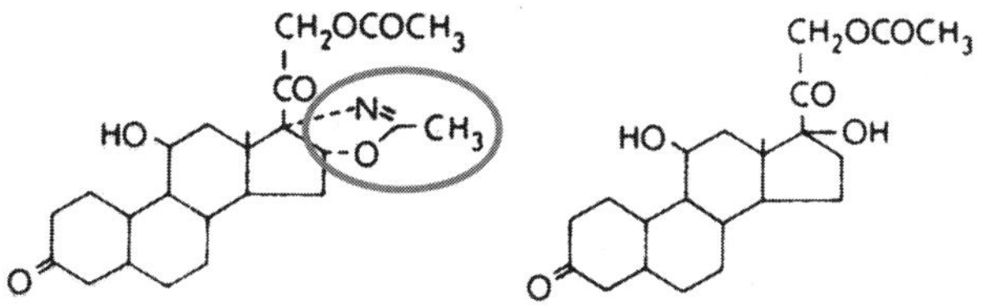

Figure 1 Chemical structure of deflazacort and prednisolone. The oxazoline side chain at the carbon 17 position is circled.

in patients treated with deflazacort for more than three years (30–33). More importantly, several large, double-blind, randomized trials comparing prednisone at 0.75 mg/kg with deflazacort at 0.9 mg/kg reported similar efficacy, with significantly less frequent and less severe weight gain with deflazacort (34–36). In these studies, however, it was observed that other side effects such as behavioral changes and growth retardation were similar for both drugs, while the incidence of cataracts was actually greater with deflazacort (31,35). In addition, measures of bone resorption were no different in some studies in the deflazacort compared to prednisone groups, suggesting that there may not be a benefit to deflazacort in terms of osteoporosis (37). For this and other reasons, the drug is not marketed in the United States and is unavailable for routine clinical use in DMD.

Mechanism of Action

The mechanism by which steroids produce benefits in DMD remains uncertain, although numerous possibilities have been proposed and tested (Table 3). Any plausible explanation must take into account the fact that

Table 3 Possible Mechanisms for the Beneficial Effect of Corticosteroids in DMD

Mechanism
Increased dystrophin expression
Increased expression of alternative cytoskeletal protein (e.g., utrophin)
Immunosuppression of inflammatory muscle damage
Stimulation of myoblast proliferation and differentiation
Growth inhibition
Stabilization of cellular membranes
Stabilization of lysosomal-bound proteases
Prevent loss of chloride conductance
Increased protease cathepsin D

positive effects on strength and function can be demonstrated within 10 days of the start of therapy, that the effects persist for years, and that the effect is associated with a decrease in muscle proteolysis and increase in muscle mass as measured by 24-hour urine creatinine and 3-methylhistidine assays (3,38). These anabolic effects are paradoxical to those seen in the muscle of normal individuals exposed to prolonged corticosteroids.

Although an intuitively appealing hypothesis is that steroids might act as a transcriptional modifier to augment dystrophin expression in muscle, immunohistochemical and western blot analyses on patients from the original CIDD cohorts showed that this was not the case (39). Alternatively, the expression of a different, functionally related cytoskeletal protein might be upregulated to compensate for the dystrophin deficiency (40). For example, the expression of utrophin, an autosomal homologue of dystrophin, has been shown to be upregulated in dexamethasone-treated *mdx* muscle cultures and methylprednisolone-treated *mdx* mice, as well as in corticosteroid-treated human myotube cultures from DMD patients (41,42).

Another possibility relates to the immunosuppressive qualities of prednisone and deflazacort. Support for this hypothesis came from quantitative immunohistochemical analyses of the mononuclear cellular infiltrates from muscle biopsies of 33 DMD patients from a CIDD cohort (43). This analysis demonstrated a statistically significant decrease in the number of mononuclear cells, total T cells, CD8+ cytotoxic cells, and muscle fibers focally invaded by lymphocytes in the prednisone-treated patients compared to those in placebo-treated controls. Further analyses, however, showed that azathioprine induced identical changes in muscle biopsies, despite having no clinical benefits (44). These findings indicated that changes in composition of the cellular infiltrates were not sufficient to explain the positive effects of prednisone in DMD, although other immunologic mechanisms could certainly be operative. Gene chip microarray analyses have indicated that human leukocyte antigen-related proteins are markedly upregulated in DMD, providing a possible template whereby corticosteroids might exert immunologic effects (45).

Corticosteroids also exert multiple metabolic and proliferative effects on muscle that might result in increased muscle mass (46–55). Steroids stimulate myoblast proliferation and differentiation, enhance muscle regeneration, and promote muscle repair and fiber growth in muscle cultures from *mdx* mice (46). They also inhibit muscle degeneration by stabilizing lysosomal-bound proteases and muscle cell membranes, limiting calcium influx into muscle cells, and preventing loss of membrane chloride conductance (48–50).

With long-term use of corticosteroids, another mechanism which may be operative in DMD relates to growth suppression. Boys with DMD and concurrent growth hormone deficiency have a milder phenotype than boys of normal stature, a finding so striking that it led to an unsuccessful clinical trial of growth hormone inhibitors in DMD (56–58). Because long-term steroid use in children invariably results in delayed bone maturation and growth inhibition, the resultant small stature may exert a protective effect on muscle degeneration. This mechanism, however, cannot be invoked to explain the onset of improvement within 10 days of starting therapy.

Given the genetic, biochemical, endocrinologic, and physiologic effects of corticosteroids on essentially every organ system and metabolic process in the body, it is unlikely that any one of the mechanisms accounts for all of the beneficial effects of these agents in DMD. More likely, the increase in muscle mass that occurs with these agents results from multiple effects on multiple processes involved in muscle differentiation and catabolism. Further investigations to define these effects and processes completely are needed so that other beneficial pharmacologic agents can be identified and developed.

Side Effects

Despite the unquestionable efficacy of the corticosteroids, controversy persists on whether they should be used routinely in DMD. This controversy stems in large part from the significant side effects associated with long-term steroid use (Table 4). The most common, noticeable, and troubling side effect that concerns patients and families is weight gain. The CIDD group reported weight gain greater than 10% baseline after six months in 80% of treated patients compared to 20% on placebo, with similar figures reported in subsequent studies (3,9–12). The weight gain is dose dependent, and increases with longer duration therapy (11). In patients followed for 12 months, weight gain greater than 20% baseline occurred in 75% of patients on a dose of 0.75 mg/kg/day, and in 68% of patients on 0.3 mg/kg/day (12). In long-term studies, weight gain is by far the most common reason

Table 4 Prednisone Side Effects in DMD Clinical Trials[a]

Side effect	Percent with effect	
	DMD	Placebo
Weight gain (>10%)	40–80	5–20
Increased appetite	60–70	30–40
Cushingoid appearance	40–70	17–35
Behavioral change	50–65	5–45
Abdominal distress	55–60	15–40
Hair growth	10–50	13–22
Acne	9–40	10–22
Cataracts	3–9	0

[a]Figures represent range of side effects reported in prospective, controlled trials of prednisone.
Source: From Refs. 3, 9–12, 14.

for discontinuing therapy (16). Multiple factors are involved in the weight gain seen with corticosteroids, including increased appetite, water and sodium retention, retention and redistribution of fat deposits, and the decreased activity inherent in DMD. Weight gain may be greater in wheelchair-dependent patients, even with lower dose therapy (14). Weight gain also decreases function and limits strength gains induced by the corticosteroid, and also promotes scoliosis, especially in wheelchair-dependent patients.

Other side effects of corticosteroids seen in DMD studies include cushingoid appearance (40–70%), behavioral changes (50–65%), abdominal distress (55–60%), hair growth (10–22%), and cataracts (3–9%). Although a discussion of each of these effects is beyond the scope of this review, it is worth noting that after weight gain, behavioral change is the most common side effect leading to discontinuation of therapy. Cataracts are seldom severe enough to limit vision. Growth delay can be profound, with most patients falling below the fifth percentile on growth charts, a factor that may contribute to the milder phenotype in these patients.

Unfortunately, the most serious and functionally limiting side effect of long-term corticosteroid use, namely osteoporosis, was not investigated in most DMD clinical trials because they were relatively brief in duration (less than one year). Osteoporosis results from the multiple metabolic effects of corticosteroids on bone and calcium metabolism (59–62). Among other effects, glucocorticoids decrease intestinal absorption of calcium, increase urinary calcium excretion, induce a mild hyperparathyroidism, and result in accelerated bone resorption (61). Osteoporosis occurs to some degree in 80% to 90% of patients treated with chronic corticosteroids, and affects mainly trabecular bone, which has an increased turnover rate and is therefore more susceptible to metabolic influences (60). The degree of osteoporosis depends on both the dose and duration of therapy, with approximately 15% of bone loss occurring within the first year of therapy. The frequency of osteoporosis-related fractures therefore increases after the first months of treatment, and is maintained throughout the treatment period (59–64). The bone loss can be demonstrated by both ultrasound and dual-energy X-ray absorptiometry (DEXA) (62,63). Alternate day steroid regimens have not been proved superior to daily therapy in preventing bone loss.

The impact of osteoporosis in DMD was highlighted by a recent retrospective analysis of 143 boys with a mean age of 15.5 years. In this cohort, 75 boys had been treated with steroids (prednisone, deflazacort, or both) for a mean duration of 8.7 years, while 68 boys had never received corticosteroids. In this analysis, the incidence of both long-bone fractures (51% vs. 20%) and vertebral compression fractures (32% vs. 0%) was significantly greater in the steroid-treated group ($p < 0.0001$ for both comparisons) (65). More aggressive management of osteoporosis and the other side effects of corticosteroids is therefore mandatory in patients on chronic steroid therapy (discussed later in the chapter).

Summary and Clinical Use

There is universal agreement that corticosteroids improve strength and function and prolong ambulation in boys with DMD. They also improve pulmonary status and "shift the curve" of progression to the right by three to four years and possibly more. Although deflazacort has fewer side effects than prednisone in regard to weight gain and cushingoid appearance, there are no convincing data that deflazacort is superior in terms of growth suppression or bone metabolism. Because deflazacort is not available in the United States, prednisone remains the only reasonable option for the majority of patients.

There is no consensus about when to initiate therapy, and the issue is controversial. Although some reports have suggested that there may be a benefit in very young patients (i.e., under five years), most clinicians are reluctant to prescribe steroids to patients under age 5. Typically, steroids are initiated at a time when a modest boost in strength may make a large functional difference, such as when the child starts falling or struggling to go up and down the steps. It is crucial that parents be counseled concerning realistic expectations for improvement in treatment. The optimal dosage of prednisone is 0.75 mg/kg/day (for deflazacort, 0.9 mg/kg/day). Although various intermittent dosing regimen are promising, they cannot be recommended at this time, because they have never been compared "head-to-head" with the standard regimen.

Any decision to initiate therapy with corticosteroids must be accompanied by a firm commitment to limit steroid-related side effects and to treat these when they develop. Weight gain must be scrupulously monitored, with parents and patients instructed in a low calorie, low sodium, low simple–sugar diet. Unacceptable weight gain can be addressed by a concerted approach, involving a team composed of the physician, physical therapist, dietician, and sometimes a psychologist to help insure satisfactory compliance. Blood pressure must be monitored closely, especially in the early phases of treatment, and ocular examinations with intraocular pressure checks should be performed every 6 to 12 months, with therapy initiated immediately for elevated intraocular pressures. Behavioral changes may respond to counseling, but antidepressants or other mood stabilizing agents are sometimes indicated. Bone density should be determined by DEXA on all patients before starting therapy and at least yearly as long as therapy continues. Patients should take supplemental calcium (1000–1500 mg/day), and most patients should also be started on vitamin D (800–1000 IU/day) or calcitriol (0.25–0.50 µg/day) (66). Bisphosphonates such as alendronate (5–10 mg/day or 50–70 mg once weekly) prevent and treat steroid-induced osteoporosis, and also reduce the incidence of corticosteroid-related vertebral fractures (67–73). They should be considered in most patients who develop osteoporosis, and should be continued as long as the patient is receiving corticosteroids. Referral to an endocrinologist with expertise in bone metabolism is appropriate for these patients, especially when reports link high-dose bisphosphonate use in children with osteopetrosis due to increased bone density and defective remodeling (74,75).

While on corticosteroids, patients should be seen at least every three to six months to monitor side effects and to determine the robustness of the clinical response and its impact on the patient's quality of life. This information is indispensable for making dosage adjustments and determining optimal duration of therapy. A common mistake occurs when the clinician "chases" the steroid-induced weight gain by rapidly and repeatedly increasing the prednisone dose to maintain the 0.75 mg/kg/day dose. This quickly leads to intolerable weight gain and cushingoid effects without an appreciable increase in benefit. A better approach is usually to maintain the appropriate initial dosing for at least one to two years, with subsequent dosing adjustments made to accommodate normal aging and growth, based on estimates of lean body mass.

When to discontinue treatment is another controversial area on which there is little agreement, because there have been few long-term studies on steroid-treated DMD patients. In general, it is best to continue therapy for as long as there is perceived benefit on quality of life. In most cases, older patients decide themselves if and when to withdraw therapy. Many elect to discontinue steroids when they lose the ability to ambulate and become wheelchair-dependent. For these individuals, whatever continued benefits the corticosteroids may be having are not worth the weight gain, dietary limitations, and other restrictions and risks imposed by these agents. For other patients, however, steroid withdrawal results in unacceptable deterioration in arm strength, pulmonary function, or both, so that they elect to continue medication. In either case, changes in prednisone dosing must be made slowly and in small increments, usually at a rate no faster than 5 mg every two to four weeks depending on treatment duration. Patients must be watched closely during this tapering off process for possible deterioration in strength and for signs of adrenal insufficiency.

Unresolved Issues

The effective clinical use of corticosteroids in DMD is complicated by the fact that there are multiple unresolved issues related to their use. Fundamental questions such as when to initiate therapy, whether alternative dosing regimens are superior to standard dosing, how long to continue therapy, and exactly how steroids work all need to be clarified. The long-term effects of corticosteroids on pulmonary and cardiac function, growth, cognition, immunologic status, and personality are particularly important issues that need to be addressed in prospective, controlled trials. Two closely related issues concern whether corticosteroids are beneficial in patients confined to a wheelchair, and whether strict prophylactic measures to limit weight gain, osteoporosis, behavioral changes, and the other dose-limiting side effects of prednisone can be effective in the DMD population. Finally, there have been no studies to determine whether combination therapy involving a corticosteroid and another agent (such as oxandrolone; see next section) might be more efficacious than prednisone monotherapy with acceptable side effects. Better information in these areas might fundamentally alter the use of corticosteroids in DMD, and lead to more effective therapeutic regimens.

OTHER AGENTS

In addition to the corticosteroids, several other drugs have been investigated through clinical trials in DMD (Table 5). Most of these agents have been clearly shown to be ineffective in well-designed trials. Although several agents have shown *some* positive results in at least one study, the benefits are either unconfirmed or too insufficient to recommend for routine clinical use.

Oxandrolone

Oxandrolone is an anabolic, androgenic steroid used to promote growth in children with Turner's syndrome and in boys with constitutional growth and pubertal delay (76,77). It increases total body protein content and fat-free body mass, and is safe, with no significant adverse effects recorded for periods up to one year (76–78). In a pilot study, 10 boys with DMD received 0.1 mg/kg/day of oxandrolone for three months. The mean change in average muscle score determined by manual muscle testing improved by 0.315 ± 0.097 in the group compared to the expected small deterioration of 0.1 in the natural history controls (79). This encouraging preliminary evidence led to a larger, six-month, randomized, placebo-controlled, double-blind clinical trial in 51 boys with DMD (80). Although there was no significant difference between the two groups in this study in the primary efficacy measure, which was the change in average manual muscle testing score from baseline to six months, there was a statistically significant improvement in the computerized quantitative muscle testing in the treated patients compared to those receiving placebo. The effects were small, however, and despite the fact that there were no side effects reported with oxandrolone, the drug has not been found to be of any practical benefit in boys with DMD. Whether the drug might have an additive effect if used in conjunction with a corticosteroid has not been determined. Because oxandrolone accelerates linear growth, its long-term use in DMD might be problematic on this basis alone.

Table 5 Noncorticosteroid Clinical Trials in DMD[a]

Drug	Author	Year	Design	No. of patients	Age	Duration	Dosage	Primary outcome	Results	Reference
Mazindol	Zatz	1986	DB-RCT	2	7.5	12 mos	2 mg/day	Function	Progression arrested	(58)
Oxandrolone	Fenichel	1997	Open	10	6–9	3 mos	0.1 mg/kg/day	MMT	Improved	(79)
	Fenichel	2001	DB-RCT	26	5–10	12 mos	0.1 mg/kg/day	MMT	No change	(80)
Creatine	Louis	2002	DB-RCT crossover	15	6–16	3 mos	3.0 gm/day	Strength PFTs	Improved	(87)
	Escolar	2003	DB-RCT	50	5–10	6 mos	5.0 gm/day	QMT MMT	Improved (young boys)	(88)
Cyclosporin	Sharma	1993	Open	15	5–10	2 mos	5.0 mg/kg/day	Strength	Improved	(91)
	Mendell	1995	DB-RCT	12	5–10	12 mos	5.0 mg/kg/day	QMT	No change	(92)

Drug	Author	Year	Type	n	Age	Duration	Dose	Outcome measures	Result	Ref
Flunarizine	Dick	1986	DB-RCT	27	5–14	12 mos	5 mg/qod 5 mg/day 5 mg/bid	Strength Function PFTs	No change	(102)
Nifidipine	Moxley	1987	DB-RCT	97	2–27	18 mos	0.75–1 mg/kg/day × 6 mos; then 1.5–2 mg/kg/day × 12 mos	MMT Function PFTs	No change	(103)
Verapamil	Bertorini	1988	DB-RCT	22	6–18	24–32 mos	8 mg/kg/day	Function	No change	(104)
Gentamicin	Wagner	2001	Open	4	6–18	2 wks	7.5 mg/kg/day	Dystrophin	No change	(110)
	Mendell	2001	Open	12	>5	2 wks	7.5 mg/kg/day	Function	No change	(111)
	Pollitano	2003	Open	4	>5	12 days	7.5 mg/kg/day	Dystrophin	Expression	(112)

^aSee Table 1 for corticosteroid trials.

Abbreviations: DB-RCT, double-blind, randomized, controlled trial; DMD, Duchenne muscular dystrophy; MMT, manual muscle testing; PFTs, pulmonary funtion tests; QMT, computerized quantitative muscle testing.

Creatine

Creatine monohydrate is a guanidine compound produced endogenously as a metabolite of glycine, arginine, and methionine. It plays a role in muscle energy metabolism, probably by increasing muscle stores of phosphocreatine and adenosine triphosphate synthesis (81–83). It has been used widely by athletes to improve performance and muscle strength, and has been shown to increase lean body mass, power output, and strength (84,85). Although the mechanism by which it might exert an anabolic effect is uncertain, it may reflect increased muscle energy production resulting from increased levels of intramuscular phosphocreatine and enhanced energy shuttling or stimulation of protein synthesis.

In reference to DMD, a single anecdotal report described a nine-year-old DMD boy whose strength improved after 155 days of creatine supplementation. An eight-week randomized, placebo-controlled, double-blind crossover trial in patients with several types of muscular dystrophy (including eight with DMD and 10 with Becker dystrophy) revealed a mild, but significant, improvement in muscle strength and daily life activities with 5 to 10 g/day of creatine and no significant adverse events (81,86). Louis et al. studied 15 boys who had DMD or Becker dystrophy. Eight of them received 3 g of creatine daily for three months, and the remaining boys received placebo. After two months of washout period, the treatment was switched for another three months. The authors reported improved strength and increased resistance to fatigue among the treated group that was not related to level of activity. There was also increased bone density by 3% in boys who were not using wheelchairs. There were no side effects (87).

These encouraging results have recently been further assessed through a prospective, randomized, double-blind, placebo-controlled trial in 50 DMD boys treated with either creatine (5 g/day), glutamine (0.6 g/kg/day) or placebo (88). In this study, boys less than seven years of age showed no response to creatine or glutamine. Older boys showed a tendency towards less deterioration in strength measured by computerized muscle testing than boys treated with either placebo or glutamine, although there was no effect on strength assessed by manual testing. Although these results suggest that there may be a modest effect of creatine on strength in DMD, they are not significant enough to indicate that creatine should be used routinely in DMD.

Cyclosporin

On the assumption that the beneficial effects of corticosteroids result from immunosuppressive actions, therapeutic trials of several alternative immunomodulatory agents have been performed in DMD. The unsuccessful trial of azathioprine has already been mentioned (12). Cyclosporin is a fungal cyclic peptide commonly used to prevent transplant rejection that acts principally by reducing the transcription of interleukin-2. It seemed a particularly appealing agent to try in DMD because, in addition to immunosuppressive qualities, it might also act to increase muscle mass, alter calcium metabolism, or act on vascular smooth muscle (89,90). In an open trial, 15 boys with DMD age 5 to 10 received cyclosporin at 5 mg/kg/day for eight weeks. Within two weeks of treatment, there was a significant improvement in tetanic force and maximum voluntary contraction in anterior tibial muscles (91). The improvement lasted until the drug was stopped; then a slow decline occurred. In contrast, there was a significant decline in the isometric force generation during four months of natural history and three months of drug washout. Although these results were encouraging, a subsequent analysis of cyclosporin in a DMD myoblast transfer study involving 12 patients showed no effect on strength (92). This study and the considerable side effects associated with cyclosporin have negated its use in DMD.

β2-Adrenergic Agonists

The β2-adrenergic agonists exert a number of effects on skeletal muscle. They induce satellite cell proliferation and muscle protein production and inhibit muscle proteolysis. These effects result in increased lean body mass and skeletal muscle protein content in normal animals and in multiple animal models of muscle injury, including the *mdx* mouse (93,94). The mechanical properties of muscle, including contractile strength, also improve with β2-agonists (95,96). Several studies in normal humans documented a positive effect of β2-agonists on muscle mass and strength (97,98). On the basis of this work and a prospective, double-blind, placebo-controlled trial showing a positive effect of the β2-agonist albuterol on muscle mass in facioscapulohumeral dystrophy, a prospective, randomized trial of albuterol in DMD is currently underway (99,100).

Calcium Channel Blockers

Before the discovery of dystrophin, a leading hypothesis for the pathogenesis of DMD involved increased membrane permeability to calcium, which might then activate neutral proteases and initiate a cascade of events that resulted in damage to the muscle cells. This hypothesis led to a series of clinical trials involving various calcium channel blockers, including flunarizine, nifedipine, verapamil, and diltiazem (101–104). Although the drugs were generally well tolerated in the DMD population, no clinically significant effects could be demonstrated that would justify their routine use.

Gentamicin

The use of gentamicin represents a novel approach to the pharmacotherapy of DMD. Approximately 15% of DMD cases result from point mutations resulting in premature stop codons (105–107). The aminoglycoside antibiotic gentamicin can suppress premature stop codons in cultured cells by causing misreading of the RNA code, allowing insertion of different amino acids at the site of the mutational stop codon. This effect has been demonstrated in cystic fibrosis, where gentamicin can suppress premature termination in the transmembrane conductance regulator gene in cultured cells, resulting in translation of a full-length functional protein (108). When given to *mdx* mice, gentamicin induced the reappearance of 10% to 20% of the normal amount of membrane-localized dystrophin, protection of muscle fibers from contraction-induced damage, and return of creatine kinase levels to normal (109). Also encouraging was the fact that the dystrophin–glycoprotein complex was partially restored in the gentamicin-treated mice.

On the basis of this work, three small trials of gentamicin in DMD patients have been conducted. In the first, no dystrophin was detected in post-treatment biopsies in four patients treated for two weeks with 7.5 mg/kg/day of gentamicin (110). In the second study, 12 DMD and sarcoglycan-deficient patients were treated for two weeks with 7.5 mg/kg/day of intravenous gentamicin. Although there was no improvement in strength, functional testing, or dystrophin expression compared to pretreatment levels, creatine kinase levels decreased significantly (111).

In the third study, four patients were given two six-day cycles of gentamicin spaced seven weeks apart; three of the four patients showed some evidence, either by western blot or immunocytochemistry, of dystrophin reexpression (112). The value of gentamicin therapy is currently being further assessed through a larger, 12-month, dose-escalated, blinded trial involving 12 DMD patients. In theory, however, gentamicin, or similar agents, could become an important means of treating DMD patients with point mutations resulting in premature stop codons, as well as other dystrophies resulting from stop mutations.

SUMMARY AND CONCLUSIONS

From the previous discussion, it is clear that in regard to DMD, the pharmacotherapy "glass" is either half empty or half full, depending on one's perspective. On the negative side, after 30 years of clinical trials, it seems increasingly unlikely that pharmacotherapy alone will ever prove curative in DMD. It is also humbling to consider that corticosteroids remain the only available medications shown to be unequivocally beneficial in well-designed, controlled trials, and the mechanism of these agents remains uncertain. On the positive side, corticosteroids have been shown to produce a clinically significant, sustained benefit that impacts positively on function and quality of life. Additional studies have suggested that other agents might also exert a nonspecific anabolic effect, raising the tantalizing possibility that combination therapy with "drug cocktails" might significantly prolong the clinical course of this steadily progressive disease. In addition, new approaches to medical management of DMD are currently being assessed in well-designed, controlled trials. Over the next 5 to 10 years, these studies should lead to better pharmacologic management of this disorder, while more definitive, gene-based therapies are being developed.

REFERENCES

1. Hoffman EP, Brown RHJ, Kunkel LM. Dystrophin: the protein product of the Duchenne muscular locus. Cell 1987; 51:919–928.
2. Hoffman EP, Fischbeck KH, Brown RH, et al. Characterization of dystrophin in muscle-biopsy specimens from patients with Duchenne's or Becker's muscular dystrophy. N Engl J Med 1988; 318:1363–1368.
3. Mendell JR, Moxley RT, Griggs RC, et al. Randomized, double-blind six-month trial of prednisone in Duchenne's muscular dystrophy. N Engl J Med 1989; 320:1592–1597.
4. Siegel IM, Miller JE, Ray RD. Failure of corticosteroid in the treatment of Duchenne (pseudo-hypertrophic) muscular dystrophy. Report of a clinically matched three year double-blind study. Ill Med J 1974; 145:32–33.
5. Drachman DB, Toyka KV, Myer E. Prednisone in Duchenne muscular dystrophy. Lancet 1974; 2:1409–1412.
6. Brooke MH, Griggs RC, Mendell JR, Fenichel GM, Shumate JB, Pellegrino RJ. Clinical trial in Duchenne dystrophy I. The design of the protocol. Muscle Nerve 1981; 4:186–197.
7. Brooke MH, Fenichel GM, Griggs RC, et al. Clinical investigation in Duchenne dystrophy: 2. Determination of the "power" of therapeutic trials based on the natural history. Muscle Nerve 1983; 6:91–103.
8. Brooke MH, Fenichel GM, Griggs RC, et al. Clinical investigation of Duchenne muscular dystrophy. Interesting results in a trial of prednisone. Arch Neurol 1987; 44:812–817.
9. Fenichel GM, Mendell JR, Moxley RT, et al. A comparison of daily and alternate-day prednisone therapy in the treatment of Duchenne muscular dystrophy. Arch Neurol 1991; 48:575–579.
10. Fenichel GM, Florence JM, Pestronk A, et al. Long-term benefit from prednisone therapy in Duchenne muscular dystrophy. Neurology 1991; 41:1874–1877.
11. Griggs RC, Moxley RT, Mendell JR, et al. Prednisone in Duchenne dystrophy. A randomized, controlled trial defining the time course and dose response. Clinical Investigation of Duchenne Dystrophy Group. Arch Neurol 1991; 48:383–388.
12. Griggs RC, Moxley RT, Mendell JR, et al. Duchenne dystrophy: randomized, controlled trial of prednisone (18 months) and azathioprine (12 months). Neurology 1993; 43:520–527.
13. Entrikin RK, Larson D, Dela Vega D, Abresch R. Therapeutic trials in muscular dystrophy of the chicken. Muscle Nerve 1986; 9(suppl):271.
14. Backman E, Henriksson KG. Low-dose prednisolone treatment in Duchenne and Becker muscular dystrophy. Neuromuscul Dis 1995; 5:233–241.

15. DeSilva S, Drachman DB, Mellits D, Kuncl RW. Prednisone treatment in Duchenne muscular dystrophy. Long-term benefit. Arch Neurol 1987; 44:818–822.
16. Pandya S, Moxley RT. Effect of daily prednisone on independent ambulation in patients with Duchenne muscular dystrophy treated up to 15 years (abstr). World Muscle Society Congress, Snowbird, Salt Lake City, Utah, Sep. 5–8, 2001.
17. Tunca O, Kabaskus N, Herguner O, et al. Alternate day prednisone therapy in Duchenne muscular dystrophy. Neuromuscul Dis 2001; 11:630.
18. Sansome A, Royston P, Dubowitz V. Steroids in Duchenne muscular dystrophy; pilot study of a new low-dosage schedule. Neuromuscul Dis 1993; 3: 567–569.
19. Kinali M, Mercuri E, Main M, Muntoni F, Dubowitz V. An effective, low-dosage, intermittent schedule of prednisolone in the long-term treatment of early cases of Duchenne dystrophy. Neuromuscul Dis 2002; 12(suppl 1): 169–174.
20. Dubowitz V, Kinali M, Main M, Mercuri E, Muntoni F. Remission of clinical signs in early Duchenne muscular dystrophy on intermittent low-dosage prednisolone therapy. Eur J Paed Neurol 2002; 6:153–159.
21. Connolly AM, Schierbecker J, Renna R, Florence J. High dose weekly oral prednisone improves strength in boys with Duchenne muscular dystrophy. Neuromuscul Dis 2002; 12:917–925.
22. Pagano G, Cavallo-Perin P, Cassader M, et al. An in vivo and in vitro study of the mechanism of prednisone-induced insulin resistance in healthy subjects. J Clin Invest 1983; 72:1814–1820.
23. Hahn BH, Pletscher LS, Muniain M. Immunosuppressive effects of deflazacort—a new glucocorticoid with bone-sparing and carbohydrate-sparing properties: comparison with prednisone. J Rheum 1981; 8:783–790.
24. Hahn TJ, Halstead LR, Strates B, Imbimbo B, Baran DT. Comparison of subacute effects of oxazacort and prednisone on mineral metabolism in man. Cal Tissue Int 1980; 31:109–115.
25. Lo Cascio V, Bonucci E, Imbimbo B, et al. Bone loss after glucocorticoid therapy. Cal Tissue Int 1984; 36:435–438.
26. Gennari C, Imbimbo B. Effects of prednisone and deflazacort on vertebral bone mass. Cal Tissue Int 1985; 37:592–593.
27. Caniggia A, Marchetti M, Gennari C, Vattimo A, Nicolis FB. Effects of a new glucocorticoid, oxazacort, on some variable connected with bone metabolism in man: a comparison with prednisone. Int J Clin Pharm Biopharm 1977; 15:126–134.
28. Mesa LE, Dubrovsky AL, Corderi J, Marco P, Flores D. Steroids in Duchenne muscular dystrophy–deflazacort trial. Neuromuscul Dis 1991; 1:261–266.
29. Angelini C, Pegoraro E, Turella E, Intino MT, Pini A, Costa C. Deflazacort in Duchenne dystrophy: study of long-term effect. Muscle Nerve 1994; 17: 386–391.
30. Dubrovsky AL, De Vito E, Suarez A, et al. Deflazacort treatment and respiratory function in DMD. Neurology 1999; 52(suppl 2):A544.
31. Schara U, Mortier W. Long-term steroid therapy in Duchenne muscular dystrophy; positive versus side effects. J Clin Neuromuscul Dis 2001; 2:179–183.
32. Biggar WD, Gingras M, Fehlings DL, Harris VA, Steele CA. Deflazacort treatment of Duchenne muscular dystrophy. J Ped 2001; 138:45–50.
33. Silversides CK, Webb GD, Harris VA, Biggar DW. Effects of deflazacort on left ventricular function in patients with Duchenne muscular dystrophy. Am J Cardio 2003; 91:769–772.

34. Bonifati MD, Ruzza G, Bonometto P, et al. A multicenter, double-blind, randomized trial of deflazacort versus prednisone in Duchenne muscular dystrophy. Muscle Nerve 2000; 23:1344–1347.
35. Anonymous. Workshop Report. 75th European Neuromuscular Centre International Workshop: 2nd Workshop on the Treatment of Muscular Dystrophy 10–12 December, 1999, Naarden, The Netherlands. Neuromuscul Dis 2000; 10:313–320.
36. Brooke MH. A randomized trial of deflazacort and prednisone in Duchenne muscular dystrophy: efficacy and toxicity. Neurology 1996; 46:A476.
37. Cacoub P, Chemlal K, Khalifa P, et al. Deflazacort versus prednisone in patients with giant cell arteritis: effects on bone mass loss. J Rheumatol 2001; 28:2474–2479.
38. Rifai Z, Welle S, Moxley RT, Lorenson M, Griggs RC. Effect of prednisone on protein metabolism in Duchenne dystrophy. Am J Physiol 1995; 268:67–74.
39. Burrow KL, Coovert DD, Klein CJ, Bulman DE, Kissel JT, Rammohan KW, Burghes AH, Mendell JR. Dystrophin expression and somatic reversion in prednisone-treated and untreated Duchenne dystrophy. CIDD Study Group. Neurology 1991; 41:661–666.
40. Ringold GM. Steroid hormone regulation of gene expression. Ann Rev Pharm Toxicol 1985; 25:529–566.
41. Burton EA, Tinsley JM, Holzfeind PJ, Rodrigues NR, Davies KE. A second promoter provides an alternative target for therapeutic up-regulation of utrophin in Duchenne muscular dystrophy. Proc Nat Acad Sci USA 1999; 96:14025–14030.
42. Courdier-Fruh I, Barman L, Briguet A, Meier T. Glucocorticoid-mediated regulation of utrophin levels in human muscle fibers. Neuromuscul Dis 2002; 12(suppl 1):95–104.
43. Kissel JT, Burrow KL, Rammohan KW, Mendell JR. Mononuclear cell analysis of muscle biopsies in prednisone-treated and untreated Duchenne muscular dystrophy. CIDD Study Group. Neurology 1991; 41:667–672.
44. Kissel JT, Lynn DJ, Rammohan KW, et al. Mononuclear cell analysis of muscle biopsies in prednisone- and azathioprine-treated Duchenne muscular dystrophy. Neurology 1993; 43:532–536.
45. Noguchi S, Tsukahara T, Fujita M, et al. cDNA microarray analysis of individual Duchenne muscular dystrophy patients. Hum Molecul Genet 2003; 12:595–600.
46. Guerriero VJ, Florini JR. Dexamethasone effects on myoblast proliferation and differentiation. Endocrinology 1980; 106:1198–1202.
47. Skrabek RQ, Anderson JE. Metabolic shifts and myocyte hypertrophy in deflazacort treatment of MDX mouse cardiomyopathy. Muscle Nerve 2001; 24:192–202.
48. Rabe A, Fromter E. Micromolar concentrations of steroids and of aldosterone antagonists inhibit the outwardly rectifying chloride channel with different kinetics. Pflugers Arch 2000; 439:559–566.
49. Sklar RM, Hudson A, Brown RHJ. Glucocorticoids increase myoblast proliferation rates by inhibiting death of cycling cells. In vitro cellular and developmental biology. J Tissue Cult Assoc 1991; 27A:433–434.

50. Ball EH, Sanwal BD. A synergistic effect of glucocorticoids and insulin on the differentiation of myoblasts. J Cell Physiol 1980; 102:27–36.
51. Seeman PM. Membrane stabilization by drugs: tranquilizers, steroids, and anesthetics. Int Rev Neurobiol 1966; 9:145–221.
52. Jacobs SC, Bootsma AL, Willems PW, Bar PR, Wokke JH. Prednisone can protect against exercise-induced muscle damage. J Neurol 1996; 243:410–416.
53. Dubowitz V. Special Centennial Workshop—101st ENMC International Workshop: Therapeutic Possibilities in Duchenne Muscular Dystrophy, 30th November–2nd December 2001, Naarden, The Netherlands. Neuromuscul Dis 2002; 12:421–431.
54. Whitaker JN, Bertorini TE, Mendell JR. Immunocytochemical studies of cathepsin D in human skeletal muscle. Ann Neurol 1983; 13:133–142.
55. Passaquin AC, Lhote P, Ruegg UT. Calcium influx inhibition by steroids and analogs in C2C12 skeletal muscle cells. Br J Pharmacol 1998; 124:751–759.
56. Zatz M, Betti RT, Levy JA. Benign Duchenne muscular dystrophy in a patient with growth hormone deficiency. Am J Med Gen 1981; 10:301–304.
57. Zatz M, Betti RT. Benign Duchenne muscular dystrophy in a patient with growth hormone deficiency: a five years follow-up. Am J Med Gen 1986; 24:567–572.
58. Zatz M, Betti RT, Frota-Pessoa O. Treatment of Duchenne muscular dystrophy with growth hormone inhibitors. Am J Med Gen 1986; 24:549–566.
59. Bothwell JE, Gordon KE, Dooley JM, MacSween J, Cummings EA, Salisbury S. Vertebral fractures in boys with Duchenne muscular dystrophy. Clin Ped 2003; 42:353–356.
60. Sambrook P, Birmingham J, Kempler S, et al. Corticosteroid effects on proximal femur bone loss. J Bone Miner Res 1990; 5:1211–1216.
61. Lukert BP, Raisz LG. Glucocorticoid-induced osteoporosis: pathogenesis and management. Ann Int Med 1990; 112:352–364.
62. van Staa TP, Leufkens HG, Abenhaim L, Zhang B, Cooper C. Oral corticosteroids and fracture risk: relationship to daily and cumulative doses. Rheumatology 2000; 39:1383–1389.
63. van Staa TP, Leufkens HG, Abenhaim L, Zhang B, Cooper C. Use of oral corticosteroids and risk of fractures. J Bone Miner Res 2000; 15:993–1000.
64. Larson CM, Henderson RC. Bone mineral density and fractures in boys with Duchenne muscular dystrophy. J Ped Orthoped 2000; 20:71–74.
65. King WK, Ruttencutter RE, Hoyle CJ, Hilling CJ, Mendell JR, Kissel JT. Orthopedic effects of steroid-treatment in Duchenne dystrophy. Neurology 2003; 60(suppl 1):A234.
66. Reid IR. Preventing glucocorticoid-induced osteoporosis. Zeit Rheum 2000; 59(suppl 2):II97–II102.
67. Saag KG, Emkey R, Schnitzer TJ, et al. Alendronate for the prevention and treatment of glucocorticoid-induced osteoporosis. Glucocorticoid-Induced Osteoporosis Intervention Study Group. N Engl J Med 1998; 339:292–299.
68. Brown JP, Chines AA, Myers WR, Eusebio RA, Ritter-Hrncirik C, Hayes CW. Improvement of pagetic bone lesions with risedronate treatment: a radiologic study. Bone 2000; 26:263–267.
69. Adachi JD, Bensen WG, Brown J, et al. Intermittent etidronate therapy to prevent corticosteroid-induced osteoporosis. N Engl J Med 1997; 337:382–387.

70. Cohen S, Levy RM, Keller M, et al. Risedronate therapy prevents corticosteroid-induced bone loss: a twelve-month, multicenter, randomized, double-blind, placebo-controlled, parallel-group study. Arthritis Rheum 1999; 42:2309–2318.
71. Roux C, Oriente P, Laan R, et al. Randomized trial of effect of cyclical etidronate in the prevention of corticosteroid-induced bone loss. Ciblos Study Group. J Clin Endocrinol Metab 1998; 83:1128–1133.
72. Wallach S, Cohen S, Reid DM, et al. Effects of risedronate treatment on bone density and vertebral fracture in patients on corticosteroid therapy. Calif Tissue Int 2000; 67:277–285.
73. Adachi JD, Saag KG, Delmas PD, et al. Two-year effects of alendronate on bone mineral density and vertebral fracture in patients receiving glucocorticoids: a randomized, double-blind, placebo-controlled extension trial. Arthritis Rheum 2001; 44:202–211.
74. Whyte MP, Wenkert D, Clements KL, McAlister WH, Mumm S. Bisphosphonate-induced osteopetrosis. N Engl J Med 2003; 349:457–463.
75. Marini JC. Do bisphosphonates make children's bones better or brittle? N Engl J Med 2003; 349:423–426.
76. Albanese A, Kewley GD, Long A, Pearl KN, Robins DG, Stanhope R. Oral treatment for constitutional delay of growth and puberty in boys: a randomised trial of an anabolic steroid or testosterone undecanoate. Arch Dis Child 1994; 71:315–317.
77. Wilson DM, McCauley E, Brown DR, Dudley R. Oxandrolone therapy in constitutionally delayed growth and puberty. Bio-Technology General Corporation Cooperative Study Group. Pediatrics 1995; 96:1095–1100.
78. Bhasin S, Storer TW, Berman N, et al. The effects of supra physiologic doses of testosterone on muscle size and strength in normal men. N Engl J Med 1996; 335:1–7.
79. Fenichel G, Pestronk A, Florence J, Robison V, Hemelt V. A beneficial effect of oxandrolone in the treatment of Duchenne muscular dystrophy: a pilot study. Neurology 1997; 48:1225–1226.
80. Fenichel GM, Griggs RC, Kissel J, et al. A randomized efficacy and safety trial of oxandrolone in the treatment of Duchenne dystrophy. Neurology 2001; 56:1075–1079.
81. Walter MC, Lochmuller H, Reilich P, et al. Creatine monohydrate in muscular dystrophies: a double-blind, placebo-controlled clinical study. Neurology 2000; 54:1848–1850.
82. Walter MC, Reilich P, Lochmuller H, et al. Creatine monohydrate in myotonic dystrophy: a double-blind, placebo-controlled clinical study. J Neurol 2002; 249:1717–1722.
83. Francaux M, Poortmans JR. Effects of training and creatine supplements on muscle strength and body mass. Eur J Appl Physiol Occup Physiol 1999; 80:165–168.
84. Terjung RL, Clarkson P, Eichner ER, et al. American College of Sports Medicine roundtable. The physiological and health effects of oral creatine supplementation. Med Sci Sports Exerc 2000; 32:706–717.
85. Vandenberghe K, Goris M, Van Hecke P, Van Leemputte M, Vangerven L, Hespel P. Long-term creatine intake is beneficial to muscle performance during resistance training. J Appl Physiol 1997; 83:2055–2063.

86. Felber S, Skladal D, Wyss M, Kremser C, Koller A, Sperl W. Oral creatine supplementation in Duchenne muscular dystrophy: a clinical and 31P magnetic resonance spectroscopy study. Neurol Res 2000; 22:145–150.
87. Louis M, Lebacq J, Poortmans JR, et al. Beneficial effects of creatine supplementation in dystrophic patients. Muscle Nerve 2003; 27:604–610.
88. Escolar DM, Buyse G, Henricson E, et al. CINRG investigators. Creatine and Glutamine therapeutic trial in Duchenne muscular dystrophy (DMD) by the Cooperative International Neuromuscular Research Group (CINRG). Work in Progress Abstract; American Neurological Association Meeting; San Francisco, 2003.
89. Meyer-Lehnert H, Schrier RW. Cyclosporine A enhances vasopressin-induced $Ca2+$ mobilization and contraction in mesangial cells. Kid Int 1988; 34:89–97.
90. Meyer-Lehnert H, Schrier RW. Potential mechanism of cyclosporine A-induced vascular smooth muscle contraction. Hypertension 1989; 13:352–360.
91. Sharma KR, Mynhier MA, Miller RG. Cyclosporine increases muscular force generation in Duchenne muscular dystrophy. Neurology 1993; 43:527–532.
92. Mendell JR, Kissel JT, Amato AA, et al. Myoblast transfer in the treatment of Duchenne's muscular dystrophy. N Engl J Med 1995; 333:832–838.
93. Zeman RJ, Peng H, Danon MJ, Etlinger JD. Clenbuterol reduces degeneration of exercised or aged dystrophic (mdx) muscle. Muscle Nerve 2000; 23:521–528.
94. Hayes A, Williams DA. Examining potential drug therapies for muscular dystrophy utilising the dy/dy mouse: I. Clenbuterol. J Neurol Sci 1998; 157:122–128.
95. Lynch GS, Hayes A, Campbell SP, Williams DA. Effects of beta 2-agonist administration and exercise on contractile activation of skeletal muscle fibers. J Appl Physiol 1996; 81:1610–1618.
96. Dodd SL, Powers SK, Vrabas IS, Criswell D, Stetson S, Hussain R. Effects of clenbuterol on contractile and biochemical properties of skeletal muscle. Med Sci Sport Exer 1996; 28:669–676.
97. Martineau L, Horan MA, Rothwell NJ, Little RA. Salbutamol, a beta 2-adrenoceptor agonist, increases skeletal muscle strength in young men. Clin Sci 1992; 83:615–621.
98. Maltin CA, Delday MI, Watson JS, et al. Clenbuterol, a beta-adrenoceptor agonist, increases relative muscle strength in orthopaedic patients. Clin Sci 1993; 84:651–654.
99. Kissel JT, McDermott MP, Natarajan R, et al. Pilot trial of albuterol in facioscapulohumeral muscular dystrophy. FSH-DY Group. Neurology 1998; 50:1402–1406.
100. Kissel JT, McDermott MP, Mendell JR, et al. FSH-DY Group. Randomized, double-blind, placebo-controlled trial of albuterol in facioscapulohumeral dystrophy. Neurology 2001; 57:1434–1440.
101. Emery AEH, Skinner R, Howden LC, Mathews MB. Verapamil in Duchenne muscular dystrophy. Lancet 1982; I:559.
102. Dick DJ, Gardner D, Gates PG, Gibson M, Simpson JM, Walls TJ. A trial of flunarizine in the treatment of Duchenne muscular dystrophy. Muscle Nerve 1986; 9:349–354.

103. Moxley RT, Brooke MH, Fenichel GM, et al. CIDD Group. Clinical investigation in Duchenne dystrophy. VI. Double-blind controlled trial of nifedipine. Muscle Nerve 1987; 10:22–33.
104. Bertorini TE, Palmieri GMA, Griffin JW, et al. Effect of chronic treatment with the calcium antagonist diltiazem in Duchenne muscular dystrophy. Neurology 1988; 38:609–613.
105. Prior TW, Bartolo C, Pearl DK, et al. Spectrum of small mutations in the dystrophin coding region. Am J Hum Genet 1995; 57:22–33.
106. Mendell JR, Buzin CH, Feng J, et al. Diagnosis of Duchenne dystrophy by enhanced detection of small mutations. Neurology 2001; 57:645–650.
107. Kapsa R, Kornberg AJ, Byrne E. Novel therapies for Duchenne muscular dystrophy. Lancet Neurol 2003; 2:299–310.
108. Howard M, Frizzell RA, Bedwell DM. Aminoglycoside antibiotics restore CFTR function by overcoming premature stop mutations. Nat Med 1996; 2:467–469.
109. Barton-Davis ER, Cordier L, Shoturma DI, Leland SE, Sweeney HL. Aminoglycoside antibiotics restore dystrophin function to skeletal muscles of mdx mice. J Clin Invest 1999; 104:375–381.
110. Wagner KR, Hamed S, Hadley DW, et al. Gentamicin treatment of Duchenne and Becker muscular dystrophy due to nonsense mutations. Ann Neurol 2001; 49:706–711.
111. Serrano C, Wall CA, Moore SA, et al. Gentamicin treatment for muscular dystrophy patients with stop codon mutations. Neurology 2001; 56:A79.
112. Pollitano L, Nigro G, Nibro V, et al. Gentamicin administration in Duchenne patients with premature stop codon. Preliminary results. Acta Myologica 2003; 22:15–21.

8

Rehabilitation Management of Duchenne Muscular Dystrophy

Craig M. McDonald
*Department of Physical Medicine and Rehabilitation,
University of California School of Medicine, Davis,
California, U.S.A.*

Gregory T. Carter and Jay J. Han
*Department of Rehabilitation Medicine,
University of Washington School of Medicine, Seattle,
Washington, U.S.A.*

Joshua O. Benditt
*Division of Pulmonary and Critical Care Medicine, Department of Medicine,
University of Washington School of Medicine, Seattle,
Washington, U.S.A.*

INTRODUCTION

The focus of this chapter will be on the rehabilitation management of Duchenne muscular dystrophy (DMD). The diagnostic evaluation, molecular genetic etiology, pathophysiology, and medical management of DMD are thoroughly covered in other chapters of this text. The orthopedic surgical management of DMD is also covered in a separate chapter, but will be discussed in this chapter only as it applies to specific rehabilitation modalities.

Briefly, DMD is an inherited, X-linked recessive disease characterized by the absence of the structural protein dystrophin, resulting in an unstable muscle cell membrane and impaired intracellular homeostasis (1,2).

The incidence of DMD has been estimated to be around 1:3500 male births (3). It is a progressive myopathy affecting skeletal muscle throughout the body including the diaphragm as well as myocardium. Death usually occurs due to respiratory or cardiac complications. Although potential curative treatments through genetic manipulation are on the horizon, current treatment regimens remain largely supportive. Thus, knowledge of the basic principles of rehabilitation management of DMD is essential for providing the appropriate care to this population and improving the quality of life. The following discussion will review general principles in the rehabilitation management of childhood neuromuscular disease as well as focus on specific rehabilitation treatments pertaining to the care of DMD patients. Several specific conditions encountered in the care of DMD patients will be highlighted to illustrate key concepts.

INITIAL REHABILITATION EVALUATION

Initial confirmation of the diagnosis is critical and is a primary responsibility of the consulting pediatric neurologist. A physician specializing in physical medicine and rehabilitation (physiatrist) or a pediatric neurologist with expertise in rehabilitation would be best suited to direct the rehabilitation team and oversee a comprehensive, goal-oriented treatment plan. Irrespective, a single primary physician who coordinates all rehabilitative care should be identified early in the process. In some centers, care coordination is also facilitated by a neuromuscular nurse practitioner.

A multidisciplinary approach is the best way to deliver effective care for DMD patients. The Muscular Dystrophy Association sponsors clinics designed specifically to care for patients with DMD and other neuromuscular disorders. Enrollment in a clinical trial, if available, should be encouraged and facilitated. It not only furthers science, but also provides some hope for the family and ensures frequent follow-up. A clinic that specializes in the care of patients with chronic neuromuscular diseases should have the necessary staff, including a pulmonologist with experience in DMD as well as physical and occupational therapists (PT/OT). Due to the learning disabilities experienced by some of the boys with DMD, a neurodevelopmental speech-language pathologist (SLP) can also be a valuable member of the team.

At initial evaluation the parents should be thoroughly educated about the expected outcome and what problems may be encountered. The family should be informed of the expected clinical problems that are likely to be encountered, including loss of functional muscle fiber leading to progressive weakness, decreased endurance, limb contractures, spine deformity, body composition changes, decrease in mobility, decreased pulmonary function, and occasionally cardiac impairment if the myocardium is affected. Dystrophin is expressed in the central nervous system, and subsequent structural protein alterations may lead to intellectual impairment (4). Rehabilitation approaches directed at mitigating impairment and/or resultant disability may substantially improve the quality of life and community integration of boys with DMD.

The initial rehabilitation evaluation will usually occur when the child is around five years old, shortly after the diagnosis has been confirmed. Table 1 outlines the major problems encountered in DMD and compares them to a less severe dystrophinopathy, Becker muscular dystrophy (BMD). While the history of hypotonia and delayed motor milestones is often reported in retrospect, the parents are often unaware of any abnormality until the child starts walking. There has been variability reported in the age of onset (4,5). In 74% to 80% of instances, the onset has been noted before the age of four (4–6). However, the vast majority of cases are identified by five to six years of age. The most frequent presenting symptoms have been abnormal gait, frequent falls, and difficulty in climbing steps. Pain in the muscles, especially the calves, is a common symptom. Parents frequently note toe walking, which is a compensatory adaptation to knee extensor weakness, and a lordotic lumbar spine, which is a compensatory change due to hip extensor weakness (Fig. 1). Difficulty in negotiating steps is an early feature as is a tendency to fall due to the child tripping or stumbling on a plantar-flexed ankle. Knee buckling or giving way due to knee extensor weakness also contributes to falling or stumbling. In addition, progressive difficulty in getting up from the floor or deep-seated position is noted.

General inspection of a boy with DMD at initial evaluation will reveal focal or diffuse muscle wasting or focal enlargement of muscles ("pseudohypertrophy"). The tongue is frequently enlarged. There is also commonly an associated wide arch to the mandible and maxilla with separation of the teeth, presumably secondary to the macroglossia. Enlargement of the calf muscles is commonly noted, and this increase in calf circumference is caused

Table 1 DMD vs. BMD

	DMD	BMD
Clinical onset	2–6 yr	4–12 yr (or later)
Age to wheelchair	7–13 yr (mean age 10 years)	>16 yr
Restrictive lung disease	Progresses to severe RLD (second decade)	Mild severity RLD
Cardiomyopathy	Severe (mid-to-late second decade)	Severe in third to fourth decade
Scoliosis	Severe in 80% to 90%	Rare
Life expectancy	17–25 (if patient does not opt for vent)	Fourth to sixth decade

Abbreviations: DMD, Duchenne muscular dystrophy; BMD, Becker muscular dystrophy, RLD, restrictive lung disease.

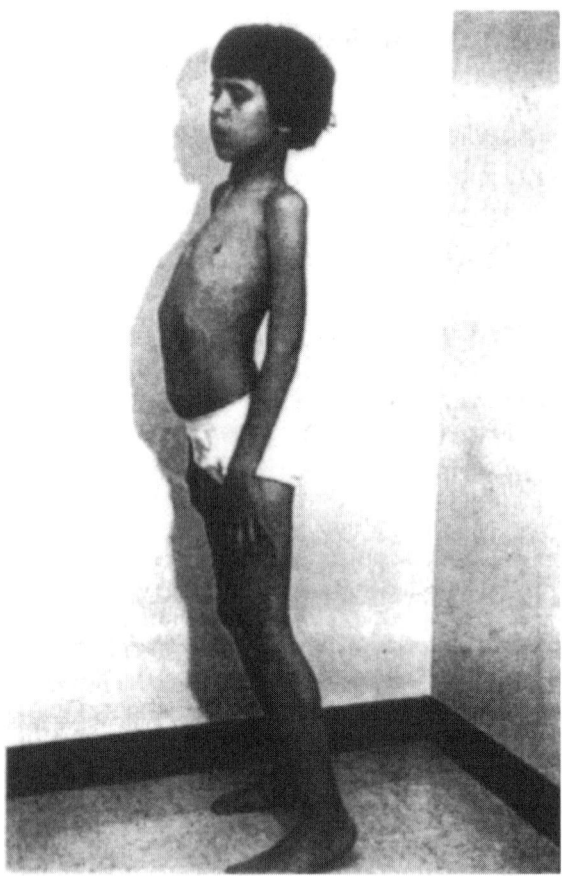

Figure 1 Photograph demonstrating hyperlorodotic positioning of the spine as well as heel cord tightness. The boy is leaning back on his Y ligaments to maintain his center of gravity.

by an increase in fibro fatty connective tissue deposition, not secondary to true muscle fiber hypertrophy of the gastrocnemius (7). Over time, a reduction in the muscle bulk is noted with more pronounced loss in the proximal musculature. This is presumably due to a more "active" dystrophic process with severe muscle fiber loss affecting the proximal muscles, which must move larger mass through space compared to the distally located muscles. Recently, children of age 8 to 11 years with DMD have been noted to exhibit an unusual clinical examination sign that results from selective hypertrophy and wasting in different muscles in the same region (8). When viewing these patients from behind with their arms abducted to 90° and elbows flexed to 90°, they demonstrate a linear or oval depression (due to wasting) of the posterior axillary fold with hypertrophied or preserved muscles on its two borders (i.e., infraspinatus inferomedially and deltoid superolaterally) as if there is a valley between two mountains.

Earliest weakness is seen in the neck flexors during preschool years. Weakness is generalized, but early in the disease course, proximal weakness is predominant and is therefore more noticeable. Pelvic girdle weakness predates shoulder girdle weakness by several years. Ankle dorsiflexors are weaker than ankle plantar flexors, ankle everters are weaker than ankle inverters, knee extensors are weaker than knee flexors, hip extensors are weaker than hip flexors, and hip abductors are weaker than hip adductors (4).

Because of proximal weakness involving the pelvic girdle muscles, boys with DMD may rise off the floor using the classic "Gowers' sign" where the patient usually assumes a four point stance on knees and hands, brings the knees into extension while leaning forward with the upper extremities, substitutes for hip extension weakness by pushing off the knees with the upper extremities, and sequentially moves the upper extremities up the thigh until an upright stance with full hip extension is achieved.

Patients with DMD often exhibit a classic myopathic gait pattern. Initially, weakness of the hip extensors produces anterior pelvic tilt and a tendency for the trunk to be positioned anterior to the hip joint. Boys with DMD compensate for this by maintaining lumbar lordosis which positions their center of gravity/weight line posterior to the hip joints, thus stabilizing the hip in extension on the anterior capsule and the ligamentous support of the hip joint. Subsequently, weakness of the knee extensors produces a tendency for patients to experience knee instability and knee buckling with falls. To gain more stability during the stance phase, the boys with DMD will compensate by positioning the ankle increasingly into more plantar flexion over time. This produces a knee extension moment at foot contact and the plantar flexion of the ankle during mid-to-late stance phase of gait, which helps position the weight line or center of gravity anterior to the knee joint, in effect producing a stabilizing knee extension moment. Again, patients with DMD progressively demonstrate toe walking with initial floor contact with the foot increasingly forward onto the mid-foot and finally onto the forefoot as they reach the transitional phase of ambulation before wheelchair reliance. Finally, weakness of the hip abductors produces a tendency toward lateral pelvic tilt and pelvic drop of the swing phase side. Bending or lurching the trunk laterally over the stance-phase hip joint compensates for proximal hip abduction weakness. This produces the so-called "gluteus medius lurch" or Trendelenburg gait pattern.

A thorough functional examination is essential in the diagnostic evaluation of a patient with suspected neuromuscular disease. This includes the evaluation of head control, bed/mat mobility, transitions from supine to sit, sit to stand, sitting ability without hand support, standing balance, gait, stair climbing, and overhead reach.

EVALUATING DISEASE PROGRESSION

Knowledge of the natural history of DMD helps in the ongoing rehabilitative management of progressive impairments, disabilities, and handicap. The weakness progresses steadily, but the rate may be variable during the disease course. Quantitative strength testing shows greater than 40% to 50% loss of strength by six years of age (4). With manual muscle testing, DMD subjects exhibit loss of strength in a fairly linear fashion from ages 5 to 13, and measurements obtained several years apart will show fairly steady disease progression. A variable course may be noted when analyzing individuals over a shorter time course (4,9). Previous investigators have noted a change in the rate of strength loss at ages approximately 14 to 15 (4,9). This change in the rate of progression did not appear to be associated with achievement of a particular score on the manual muscle test scale but rather consistently occurred in various muscle groups in the early second decade. Thus, the authors recommend that natural history control trials evaluating therapies in DMD should be cautious about including subjects transitioning to the teenage years because of the flattening of the MMT strength curve with increasing age (4,6). Quantitative strength measures have been shown to be more sensitive for demonstrating strength loss than manual muscle testing, particularly when strength is graded 4 to 5 on the 5-point Medical Research Council (MRC) scale (4).

Average age to wheelchair in an untreated DMD population has been 10 with a range of 7 to 13 years. Timed motor performance is useful for the prediction of time when ambulation will be lost without the aid of long-leg braces. One large natural history study showed that all DMD subjects who took nine seconds or longer to ambulate 30 feet lost ambulation within two years. All DMD subjects who took 12 seconds or longer to ambulate 30 feet lost ambulation within one year (4). Ambulation past the age of 14 should raise the suspicion of a milder form of muscular dystrophy such as BMD or limb girdle muscular dystrophy. Ambulation beyond 16 years was previously used as exclusionary criterion for DMD. Immobilization for any reason can lead to a marked and often precipitous decline in muscle power and ambulatory ability. A fall with resultant fracture leading to immobilization and loss of ambulatory ability is not an uncommon occurrence (10–12).

REHABILITATION MANAGEMENT

Joint Contractures

Contracture is defined as the lack of full active or passive range of motion (ROM) due to joint, muscle, or soft tissue limitation. Contractures may be arthrogenic, with the involvement of soft tissue, or myogenic in nature, and a combination of intrinsic structural changes of muscle and extrinsic factors leads to myogenic contractures in DMD. These factors include the following: (i) degree of fibrosis and fatty tissue infiltration, (ii) static positioning and lack of full active and passive ROM, (iii) imbalance of agonist and antagonist muscle strength across the joint, (iv) lack of upright weight bearing and static positioning in sitting, (v) compensatory postural changes used to biomechanically stabilize joints for upright standing, and (vi) functional anatomy of muscles and joints (multi-joint muscle groups in which the origins and insertions cross multiple joints). In general, dystrophic muscles have a high degree of fibrosis and fatty infiltration, placing these patients at higher risk for contractures, and significant joint contractures have been found in nearly all DMD children older than age 13 (4,5,13).

The most common contractures include ankle plantar flexion, knee flexion, hip flexion, iliotibial band involvement, elbow flexion, and wrist flexion contractures (4,13). Significant contractures are rare in DMD before age nine. There is no association between muscle imbalance around a specific joint (defined as grade 1 or greater difference in flexor and extensor strength) and the frequency or severity of contractures involving the hip, knee, ankle, wrist, and elbow in DMD (4,10). The presence of lower extremity contractures in DMD has been shown to be strongly related to onset of wheelchair use (4). Lower extremity contractures were rare while DMD subjects were still upright, but developed soon after they developed a sitting position in a wheelchair for most of the day. The occurrence of elbow flexion contractures also appears to be directly related to prolonged static positioning of the limb, and these contractures develop soon after wheelchair reliance. These are illustrated in Figure 2. Mild contractures of the iliotibial bands, hip flexor muscles, and heel cords occur in most DMD patients by six years of age (14). Limitations of knee, elbow, and wrist extension occur about two years later; however, these early observed contractures were relatively mild (15–17). The lack of lower extremity weight bearing likely contributes to the rapid acceleration in the severity of these contractures after transition to a wheelchair (16,17). Ankle plantar flexion contractures are not felt to be a significant cause of wheelchair reliance, as few subjects exhibit plantar flexion contractures of greater than or equal to 15° before their transition to a wheelchair (4,18,19). Natural history data suggest that weakness is the major cause of loss of ambulation in DMD, not contracture formation (4).

Prevention of fixed contractures requires early diagnosis and initiation of physical medicine approaches such as passive ROM and splinting while they are still mild. Advanced contractures become fixed and show little response to stretching programs. A major rationale for controlling contractures of the lower extremity is to minimize the adverse effect of contractures on independent ambulation. However, the major cause of wheelchair reliance in DMD is generally weakness, not contracture formation.

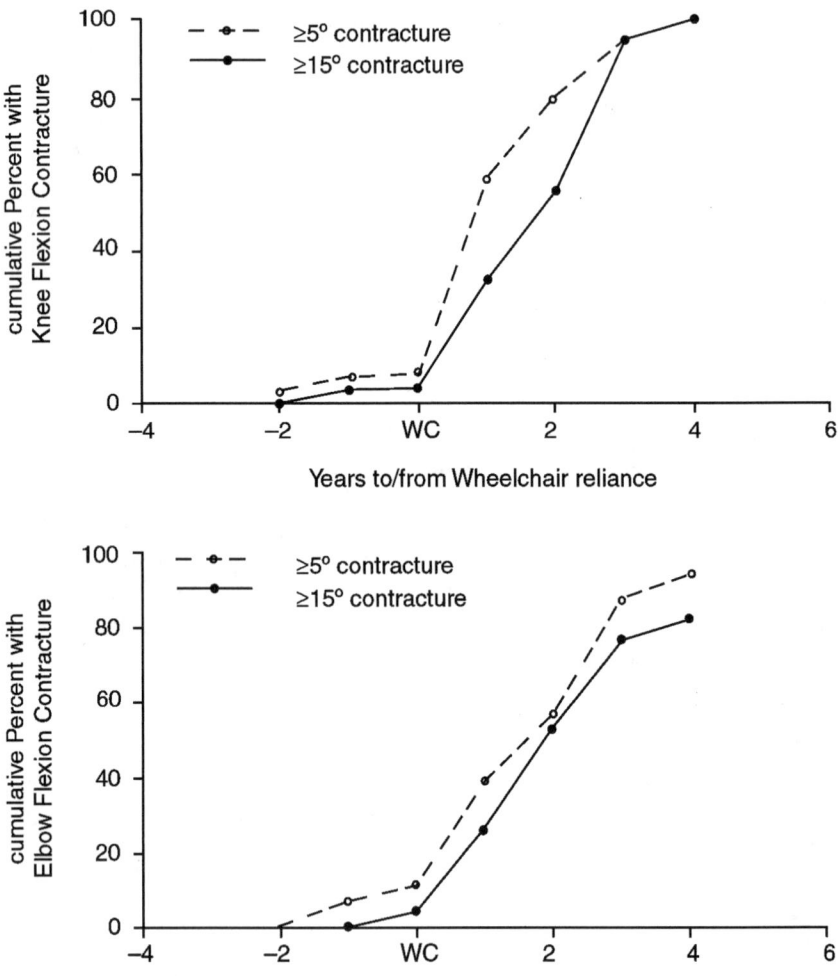

Figure 2 Graphic illustration of the relationship between wheelchair reliance versus elbow and knee contractures.

Principal therapy modalities must be regularly carried out to prevent or delay the development of lower extremity contractures for those at risk for musculoskeletal deformity. These include (i) regularly prescribed periods of daily standing and walking if the patient is functionally capable of being upright; (ii) passive stretching of muscles and joints with a daily home program; (iii) positioning of the leg to promote extension and oppose joint flexion when the patient is non-weight-bearing through the lower extremities; (iv) splinting, which is a useful measure for the prevention or delay of ankle contracture; and (v) reqular monitoring of joint ROM by

PT/OT using objective goniometric measurement. Upper extremity contractures may not negatively impact the function if they are mild. Elbow flexion contractures in DMD may occur soon after transition to the wheelchair, secondary to static positioning of the arms and elbow flexion on the armrests of the wheelchair (20,21). Passive stretching of the elbow flexors may be combined with passive stretching into forearm supination to help prevent contractures. Upper extremity orthoses should emphasize wrist and finger extension, but any splinting should not compromise sensation or function.

Bracing and surgical management of contractures may help prolong ambulation in DMD. The late phase of ambulation often is associated with more marked joint contractures involving the iliotibial bands and heel cords, because DMD patients spend more time sitting and less time standing (Fig. 3). Generally the release of contractures at both the heel cord and iliotibial band is necessary to obtain successful knee–ankle–foot orthosis (KAFO) bracing (18–20). Other authors have reported bracing of DMD patients without surgical release of the iliotibial bands (18,19). Hip and knee flexion contractures generally are not severe enough to interfere with bracing at the time of transition to wheelchair (4). The iliotibial band contractures may be released with a low Young fasciotomy and a high Ober fasciotomy (13,21).

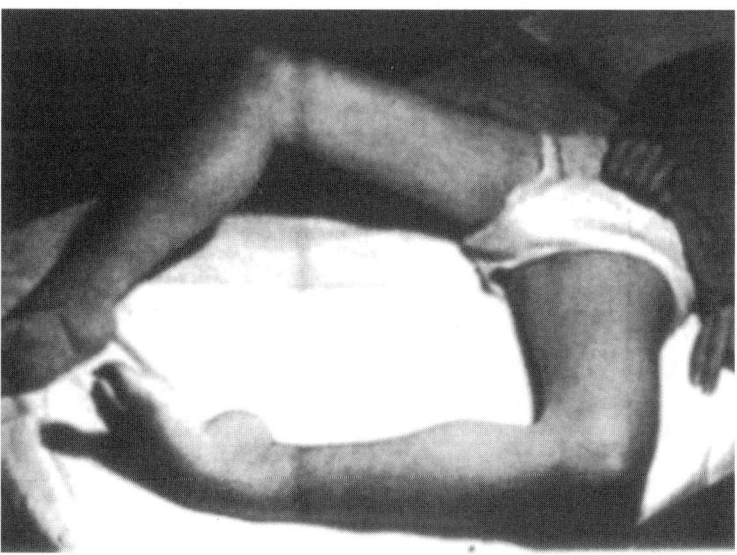

Figure 3 Thirteen-year-old boy with DMD and severe hip flexion, knee flexion, and ankle equinovarus contractures developed subsequent to wheelchair reliance. *Abbreviation*: DMD, Duchenne muscular dystrophy.

The ankle deformity may be corrected by either a tendo-achilles lengthening (TAL) or a TAL combined with a surgical transfer of the posterior tibialis muscle tendon to the dorsum of the foot (13,18). The posterior tibialis tendon transfer corrects the equinovarus deformity but prolongs the cast and recovery time, and it increases the risks of prolonged sitting (13,18).

Orthopedic surgical release of these contractures allows the DMD patient to be braced in lightweight polypropylene KAFOs with the sole and ankle set at 90°, drop-lock knee joints and ischial weight-bearing polypropylene upper thigh component (22). DMD patients who are braced may or may not require a walker for additional support (23).

While DMD subjects are still ambulating independently without orthotics, they often use their ankle equinus posturing from the gastrocnemius-soleus group to create a knee extension moment at foot contact, thus stabilizing the knee when the quadriceps muscle is weak. Several authors have cautioned against isolated heel cord tenotomies while DMD patients are still ambulating independently (4,24). Overcorrection of the heel cord contracture in a DMD patient may result in immediate loss of the ability to walk without bracing unless the quadriceps are grade 4 or better (24).

The duration of ambulation in DMD has been successfully prolonged by prompt surgery and bracing, immediately implemented following loss of independent ambulation. Generally, the gains in additional walking time have been variable, but generally reported between two and five years (25). Little evidence supports the efficacy of early prophylactic lower extremity surgery in DMD for independently producing prolonged ambulation (4,24,26).

Scoliosis

Reported ultimate prevalence of scoliosis in DMD varies from 33% to 100% (26). This marked variability is primarily because of retrospective selection for scoliosis, the inclusion or exclusion of functional curves, and dissimilar age groups. The prevalence of scoliosis is strongly related to age. Fifty percent of DMD patients acquire scoliosis between ages 12 and 15, corresponding to the adolescent growth spurt. Ten percent of older DMD subjects with no treatment of scoliosis show no clinical spinal deformity. This is consistent with Oda's report that 15% of older DMD patients show mild nonprogressive curves (usually 10° to 30°) (15). The rate of progression of the primary or single untreated lateral curve has been reported to range from 11° to 42° per year, depending on the age span studied. Johnson and Yarnell (27) reported an association between side of curvature, convexity, and hand dominance. Other studies showed no correlation between side of primary convexity and handedness (4,28). Oda et al. (15) reported that the likelihood of severe progressive spinal deformity could be predicted by type of curve and early pulmonary function measurements. Those without significant kyphosis or hyperlordosis and a peak obtained absolute forced vital capacity (FVC) greater than 2000 mL tended not to show severe progressive scoliosis (29).

No cause-and-effect relationship has been established between onset of wheelchair reliance and occurrence of scoliosis (4,27,28). Wheelchair reliance and scoliosis have been found to be age-related phenomena. The causal relationship between loss of ambulatory status and scoliosis is doubtful, given the substantial time interval between the two variables in most subjects (scoliosis usually develops after three to four years in a wheelchair).

Both wheelchair reliance and spinal deformity may be significantly related to other factors (e.g., age, adolescent growth spurt, increase in weakness of trunk musculature, and other unidentified factors) and thus represent coincidental signs of disease progression.

The surgical management of neuromuscular scoliosis will be covered in detail in another chapter. However, it is worth noting here that the severe spinal deformity often found in DMD may lead to multiple problems, including poor sitting balance, difficulty with upright seating and positioning, pain, difficulty in parental or attendant care, and potential exacerbation of underlying restrictive respiratory compromise. Severe scoliosis and pelvic obliquity can, in some instances, completely preclude upright sitting in a wheelchair (28,30).

Close clinical monitoring is essential for boys with DMD at risk for scoliosis. Curves may progress rapidly during the adolescent growth spurt, and children need to be monitored every three to four months during this time with clinical assessment and spine radiographs if indicated (28). In addition, patients who are likely to require surgical arthrodesis at some point should be monitored with pulmonary function tests every six months. A FVC falling below 30% to 40% of what has been predicted may contraindicate surgery, irrespective of scoliosis severity, because of increased perioperative morbidity (29). Nutrition is also critical as there is a high incidence of postoperative malnutrition (31). Thus, there is often a critical window of time where the spinal deformity is evident and likely to progress, and the restrictive lung disease (RLD) or nutritional issues are not of a severity which would contraindicate surgery.

The management of spinal deformity with orthotics is ineffective in DMD and does not change the natural course of the curve (4). Spinal orthoses are often reported to be uncomfortable and poorly tolerated by DMD patients, and may reduce vital capacity (4). Spinal fusion (arthrodesis) is the only effective treatment for scoliosis in DMD. For further details, see Chapter 9.

Respiratory Management

The medical management of cardiopulmonary symptoms in DMD is outlined in Table 2. Respiratory muscle weakness in DMD leads to decreases in RLD,

Table 2 Medical Management of Cardiopulmonary Symptoms in DMD

Respiratory muscle weakness and fatigue
   Signs of impending respiratory failure in DMD include FVC < 25 to 30% predicted, MIP < 25–30 cm H_2O, and $PaCO_2$ > 55
   Noninvasive ventilation with BiPAP

Cardiomyopathy in DMD
   Clinically significant cardiomyopathy rare before age 10
   Fibrosis posterior wall left ventricle
   Myocardium exhibits abnormal contractility
   Purkinje abnormalities lead to tachyarrhythmias
   Regular monitoring with ECG, Echo, Holter monitor
   Treatment with digitalis, afterload reduction, antiarrhythmics

Abbreviations: DMD, Duchenne muscular dystrophy; BiPAP, Bi-level positive airway pressure; ECG, electrocardiogram; FVC, forced vital capacity.

hypercarbia, and ultimately respiratory failure, if untreated. A linear decline in percent predicted FVC is apparent between 10 and 20 years of age in DMD (4). Rideau et al. (29) reported FVC to be predictive of the risk of rapid scoliosis progression. McDonald et al. (4) found that those patients with higher peak FVC (greater than 2500 mL) had a milder disease progression, losing 4% predicted FVC per year. Those with peak predicted FVC less than 1700 mL lost 9.6% predicted FVC per year (Fig. 4). Thus, the obtained peak absolute values of FVC usually occurring in the early part of the second decade are an important prognostic indicator for severity of spinal deformity as well as ultimate severity of restrictive pulmonary compromise due to muscular weakness.

In most cases of DMD, the respiratory insufficiency develops more insidiously unless an acute decompensation occurs from an event such as an aspiration episode. Signs and symptoms of significant respiratory difficulties may include subcostal retractions, accessory respiratory muscle recruitment, nasal flaring, exertional dyspnea or dyspnea at rest, orthopnea, generalized fatigue, and paradoxical breathing patterns. A history of nightmares, morning headaches, and daytime drowsiness may indicate nocturnal hypoventilation with sleep-disordered breathing. Pulmonary function tests have been used to help in the decision-making process regarding the institution of mechanical ventilation. In one study of 53 patients with proximal myopathy, hypercapnia occurred when the maximal inspiratory pressure was less than 30% of the predicted value and vital capacity was less than 55% of the predicted value (32). Other authors have noted lower values for vital capacity measurements in their patients with DMD at the time they require institution of mechanical ventilatory support (33,34). Hahn et al. (35) have reported the predicted value of maximal static airway pressures in predicting impending

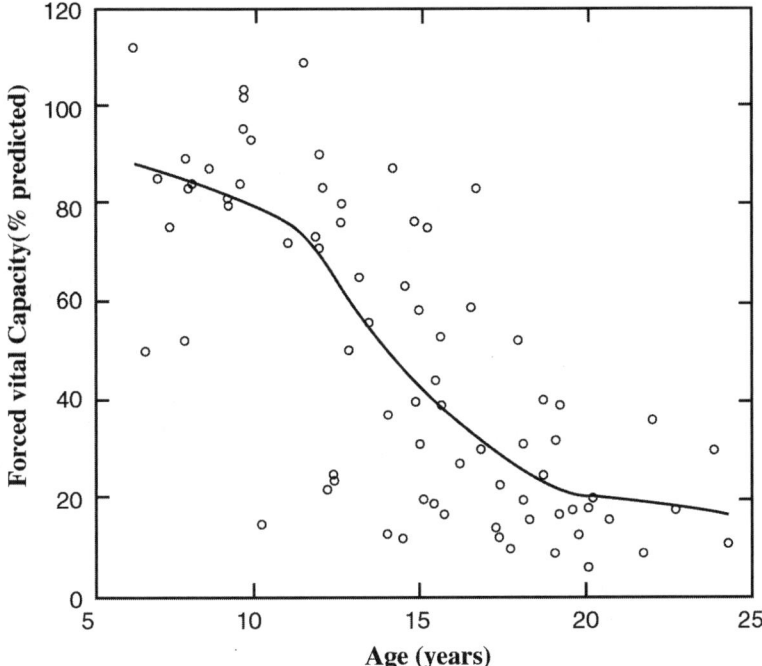

Figure 4 Lowess regression of percent predicted forced vital capacity for DMD subjects at initial evaluation vs. age. *Source*: From Ref. 4.

respiratory failure. Splaingard et al. (36) reviewed a series of 40 patients with a diverse group of neuromuscular disease conditions. They noted that all their patients who required mechanical ventilation had a vital capacity of less than or equal to 25% with at least one of the following associated findings: (i) $PaCO_2$ greater than 55 mmHg, (ii) recurrent atelectasis or pneumonia, (iii) moderate dyspnea at rest, or (iv) congestive heart failure.

Noninvasive forms of both positive- and negative-pressure ventilation are being increasingly applied to boys with DMD. These are outlined in Table 3. Initially, patients may require ventilatory support only for a part of the day. Noninvasive nocturnal ventilation has become a widely accepted clinical practice, providing ventilatory assistance for patients while sleeping and allowing them to breathe on their own during the day. The long-term use of noninvasive ventilation may be associated with fewer complications than ventilation via a tracheotomy (37–39). Ventilatory support has been shown to prolong survival and acceptable quality of life in DMD (34,38–41).

Improved pulmonary toilet and clearance of secretions can be achieved with assisted cough, deep breathing and set-up spirometry, and percussion and postural drainage, and in more severe cases, the additional

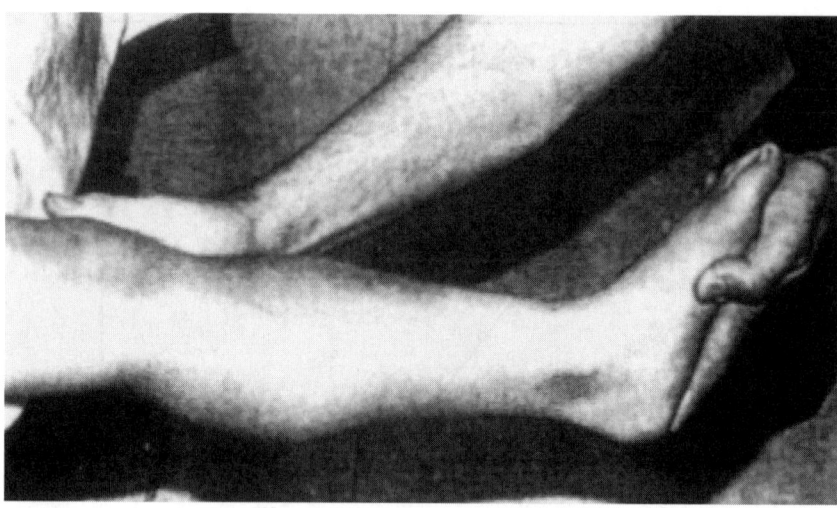

Figure 5 Eleven-year-old patient with DMD and severe ankle plantar flexion contractures one year after transition to the wheelchair. At time of transition to the wheelchair the ankle plantar flexion contracture measured less than 5.

use of intrapulmonary percussive ventilation, given 2 to 3 times daily. Respiratory muscle training may also have a modest beneficial effect (42,43). All patients with DMD should receive a pneumococcal vaccination and a yearly influenza vaccination. If FVC is less than 60% of the predicted value, patients should also avoid close contact with people who have upper respiratory tract infections. If the expiratory muscles are too weak to generate an adequate cough, patients can be helped by either manually assisted coughing or an in-exsufflator (Cough Assist manufactured by J.H. Emerson Co., Cambridge, Massachusetts, U.S.A.) (44). If the patient's vital capacity is less than 1.5 L, cough force can be improved by providing the patient with an insufflation using a manual resuscitator, an intermittent positive-pressure breathing machine, a portable ventilator, or the in-exsufflator. The in-exsufflator is a machine with a pneumatic motor that can be used to deliver a positive-pressure (insufflation) to fully inflate the lungs and provide vacuum and negative-pressure (exsufflation) to secretions of the suction from the lungs. Pressure is delivered via an anesthesia facemask; after exsufflation, secretions and mucous plugs are carried into the mouth and facemask from where they can be removed with the suction of the oral cavity. The in-exsufflator can generate a peak flow rate of 7 to 11 L/sec, which is better than that achieved with manually assisted coughing. The in-exsufflator can also be used in place of tracheal suctioning in patients who have tracheotomies. In addition, caregivers

Table 3 Devices Available for Mechanical Ventilation of Neuromuscular Disease Patients

Negative-pressure ventilators
    Fully boy ventilator (tank ventilator or iron lung)
    Raincoat ventilator ("poncho" or "pneumowrap")
    Cuirass ventilator (chest shelf)
    Pneumosuit ventilator with leggings
Positive-pressure ventilators
    Via tracheotomy
    Noninvasive
    Via full face mask (e.g., BiPAP)
    Via nasal mask (e.g., BiPAP)
    Via mouth piece with lip seal
    Via IPPB using mouth piece adapter
Ventilators resulting in passive movement of the diaphragm
    Pneumobelt
    Rocking bed

Abbreviation: IPPB, intermittent positive-pressure breathing.

can manually assist with the patient's cough by providing an abdominal thrust and anterior chest compression synchronized with the patient's attempts to cough. This technique can generate a peak flow of 5 to 7 L/sec (44).

Providing DMD patients with supplemental oxygen is not recommended as it may suppress respiratory drive, exacerbate alveolar hypoventilation, and ultimately lead to CO_2 narcosis and respiratory arrest (44).

Both negative- and positive-pressure devices can provide noninvasive ventilatory assistance, although positive-pressure methods are more commonly used. Noninvasive positive-pressure ventilation (NPPV) can be delivered through a variety of oral or nasal masks and interfaces using bi-level positive airway pressure (BiPAP) machines or portable volume-cycled ventilators. Either nasal interfaces or more traditional BiPAP masks can be used. Sometimes custom-molded devices may be required. Masks tend to be preferred by most patients for nocturnal ventilation. If air leakage from the mouth is excessive, a chinstrap can be used to hold the mouth closed. Oral interfaces include mouthpieces that must be held in place using a voluntary lip seal or those held in place by straps placed over the head when voluntary lip seal alone is inadequate. When an oral interface is used, blocking the nares with cotton pledgets can prevent air leaks from the nostrils. Combined oral and nasal interfaces are also available, but they tend to make patients feel claustrophobic. Some patients require the use of two or three interfaces be used on a rotating basis to prevent pressure-related skin breakdown over the bridge of the nose or other areas.

The BiPAP machine is essentially a pressure-cycled ventilator. With BiPAP, the tidal volume plateaus when a pressure of 15 cm H_2O is reached, so the lungs cannot be inflated as completely as it is done with a volume-cycled ventilator. Inspiratory and expiratory pressures can be set independently. For the most effective ventilation, the inspiratory pressure should be set at maximum and the expiratory pressure as low as possible unless the patient tends to have apneic episodes caused by hypopharyngeal collapse. BiPAP machines may not adequately ventilate patients with no vital capacity. In this case volume-cycled ventilators should be considered. Although BiPAP is the preferred method of assisted ventilation at night, many DMD patients like to use a "sip and puff," volume-cycled ventilator during the day. The ventilator may be mounted on the back of the wheelchair. A specific volume of air is delivered via a tube that the patient grasps with his mouth. By sucking on the tube the machine is triggered to deliver a breath (assist-control mode). The tidal volume is adjusted as needed to compensate for any air leakage. In general, tidal volumes are greater than those used for a patient with a tracheotomy, which is essentially a closed system. The goal of ventilatory support is to generate an intrapulmonary pressure of 20 cm H_2O, which is adequate for full lung inflation. If intermittent mandatory ventilation mode is used, the ventilator rate should be set to maintain $PaCO_2$ between 30 and 40 mmHg.

Guidelines as to when to initiate NPPV vary. Symptoms of respiratory distress or the presence of nocturnal hypoventilation are certainly indications for NPPV. We suggest NPPV be initiated when the supine FVC falls below 50% of the predicted value, depending on the clinical symptomatology. The rate of the patient's disease progression must also be considered in deciding when to initiate NPPV. Initially, NPPV is used only at night. As patients continue to show a decrease in vital capacity, the use of ventilator extends into the day for varying periods and eventually becomes continuous. It often takes several weeks for patients to become comfortable using the ventilator and to be able to sleep through the night with it. If NPPV is started before respiratory distress occurs, the patient can become slowly accustomed to the equipment and may gradually extend the daily period of use until overnight use is tolerated. The decision to undergo tracheotomy in a boy with DMD may be required if NPPV fails to provide adequate ventilation. However, this should only be done after all modalities of NPPV have been tried without success. Noninvasive ventilation is less costly than ventilation by tracheotomy because fewer expensive supplies are needed, and a less costly level of skilled home help can be used. Other advantages of noninvasive ventilation include more natural speech, a decreased risk of infection because the normal mucosal barriers are not bypassed, and sometimes, greater patient comfort. Boys or men with DMD and respiratory failure who have previously undergone tracheotomy may ultimately be able to be reverted to noninvasive ventilation, although there are no prospective studies documenting this.

Cardiac Management

The dystrophin protein is present in both the myocardium and the cardiac Purkinje fibers (45). Abnormalities of the heart may be detected by clinical examination, electrocardiogram (ECG), echocardiography, and Holter monitoring (46,47). Cardiac examination is notable for the point of maximal impulse palpable at the left sternal border due to the marked reduction in anteroposterior chest dimension common in DMD. A loud pulmonic component of the second heart sound suggests pulmonary hypertension in patients with restrictive pulmonary compromise (48). Nearly all patients over the age of 13 demonstrate abnormalities of the ECG (4,49,50). Q-waves in the lateral leads are the first abnormalities to appear, followed by elevated ST-segments and poor R-wave progression, increased R/S ratio, and finally resting tachycardia and conduction defects (4). ECG abnormalities have been demonstrated to be predictive of death from cardiomyopathy with the major determinants including R-wave in lead V1 less than 0.6 mV; R-wave in lead V5 less than 1.1 mV; R-wave in lead V6 less than 1.0 mV; abnormal T-waves in leads II, III, AVF, V5, and V6; cardiac conduction disturbances; premature ventricular contraction; and sinus tachycardia (51). Sinus tachycardia may be due to low stroke volume from the progressive cardiomyopathy or in some cases may be sudden in onset and labile, suggesting autonomic disturbance or direct involvement of the sinus node by the dystrophic process (52,53).

Autopsy studies and thallium 201 single photon emission computed tomography (SPECT) imaging have demonstrated left ventricular lateral and posterior wall defects that may explain the lateral Q-waves and the increased R/S ratio in V1 seen on ECG (54,55). Localized posterior wall fibrosis was found to be peculiar to DMD and was not found in other types of muscular dystrophy. Pulmonary hypertension leading to right ventricular enlargement also is known to affect prominent R-waves in V1 and has been demonstrated in patients with DMD (48).

Ventricular ectopy and sudden death are known complications of the cardiomyopathy in DMD, and this association likely explains observed cases of sudden death. Severe ventricular ectopy in DMD has been associated with left ventricular dysfunction and sudden death (47,56). Yanagisawa et al. (47) reported an age-related increase in the prevalence of cardiac arrhythmias detected by ambulatory 24-hour electrocardiographic recordings. They also noted an association between ventricular arrhythmias and sudden death in DMD. Clinically evident cardiomyopathy is usually first noted after age 10 and is apparent in nearly all patients over age 18 (47,49). Development of cardiomyopathy is a predictor of poor prognosis (57). Echocardiography has been used extensively to follow the development of cardiomyopathy and predict prognosis in patients with DMD. The onset of systolic dysfunction noted by echocardiography is associated with a poor short-term prognosis (57).

Themyocardial impairment remains clinically silent until late in the course of the disease, possibly caused by the absence of exertional dyspnea, secondary to lack of physical activity. Death has been attributed to congestive heart failure in as many as 40% to 50% of patients with DMD by some investigators (58,59). Regular cardiac evaluations with an ECG, echocardiography, and Holter monitor should be employed in teenagers with pre-clinical cardiomyopathy.

The management of cardiac complications in DMD often starts with low dose angiotensin converting enzyme inhibitors and is usually initiated when the measured ejection fraction falls below 35% (60). Digitalis has been demonstrated to be effective in decreasing morbidity from heart failure, but not mortality, and probably is also indicated for the treatment of heart failure observed in DMD patients with cardiomyopathy. Patients with known arrhythmias who are at risk for fatal tachyarrhythmias may benefit from antiarrhythmic medication, including beta-blockers.

Treatment with coenzyme Q10 remains controversial (60). Symptoms of cor pulmonale, confirmed on echocardiography, may improve with supplemental oxygen. DMD patients with mitral valve prolapse and mitral regurgitation should be given antibiotic prophylaxis for dental and surgical procedures in accordance with current guidelines.

Body Composition and Nutritional Management

Substantial anthropometric alterations have been described in DMD. Short stature and slow linear growth with onset shortly after birth have been reported (61,62). Accurate measurement of linear height is extremely difficult in this population. Arm span measurements are an alternative measure of linear growth although are inaccurate if elbow flexion contractures of greater than 30° are present. Forearm segment is an alternative linear measurement. Longitudinal weight measurements in DMD confirm significant rates of weight loss in subjects of ages 17 to 21 (4,63,64). This is likely caused by relative nutritional compromise during the later stages when boys with DMD have higher protein and energy intake requirements because of hyper-catabolic protein metabolism. Protein and calorie requirements may often be 160% of the predicted value for able-bodied populations during the later stages of DMD (65,66). RLD becomes more problematic during this time, and this may also influence caloric intake and requirements. Self-feeding often becomes impossible during this period because of biceps weakness. In addition, boys with DMD may develop signs and symptoms of upper gastrointestinal dysfunction (67).

DMD patients typically gain excessive weight between 9 and 13 years of age, subsequent to the onset of wheelchair reliance. This is likely due to a reduction in total daily energy expenditure with increased sedentary lifestyle. Edwards et al. (68) demonstrated that weight reduction through a medically supervised decrease in energy intake could be achieved successfully in DMD without compromising skeletal muscle mass. Protein and calorie needs in DMD may be approximately 160% of that required for able-bodied adolescents. Beneficial effects in weight gain, anthropometric measurements, and nitrogen balance were recently documented for DMD patients aged 10 to 20 years, subsequent to a three month nutritional supplementation which consisted of an additional 1000 kcal and 37.2 g of protein (69,70). The positive effects on metabolism observed in this study warrant further investigation. Stewart et al. (71) conducted a trial of branched-chain ketoacid supplementation. Leucine, valine, and isoleucine were administered orally as ornithine salts at a dosage of 0.45 g/kg body weight/day for four days in nine boys with DMD, aged five to nine years. An equivalent amount of protein was removed from the diet during this time. A small but significant reduction in muscle protein degradation was observed as a result of the treatment, and this warrants further investigation.

DMD patients have a high prevalence of dysphagia during the late stages of the disease (67). Swallowing is best evaluated with a fluoroscopic video dynamic swallowing evaluation. DMD patients may also develop acute gastric dilatation secondary to gastric paresis (72). Poor nutritional status, labored feeding, and/or symptoms of dysphagia are indications for initiation of supplemental enteral feedings via nasogastric tube or gastrostomy. Gastroesophageal reflux with risk of aspiration may be an indication for placement of a gastrojejunostomy tube.

Cognitive Impairment

A dystrophin isoform is present in the brain (73). Previous studies on intellectual function of children with DMD have generally revealed decreased IQ scores when these children are compared with both control and normative groups (4). A mean score, 1.0 to 1.5 SD below population norms, has been reported for the DMD population, with relative deficits in verbal IQ (74–76). On neuropsychological testing, a large proportion of DMD subjects fell within the "mildly impaired" or "impaired" range according to normative data (4). Identification of learning disability in a DMD patient necessitates an individual education plan with involvement of the school system and a school psychologist (and/or an SLP).

THE ROLE OF EXERCISE

Exercise prescriptions and recommendations in DMD need to consider the specific disease condition as well as the developmental and maturational status of the child. The inherent instability of the dystrophin-deficient sarcolemmal membrane predisposes to membrane injury due to mechanical loads. Eccentric or lengthening contractions produce more mechanical stress on muscle fiber than the concentric or shortening contractions do (77,78). Indeed, many of the muscle groups that show the greatest weakness early in the course of DMD, perform a great deal of eccentric activity such as the hip extensors, knee extensors, and ankle dorsiflexors. In addition, lower extremity muscles, in this population experience more mechanical loads than upper extremity muscles, and weakness in the lower extremities generally predates weakness in the upper extremities. Edwards et al. (79) proposed that routine eccentric contractions occurring during gait are a likely source of the pattern of weakness typically seen in myopathies. This was confirmed by studies in the *mdx* mouse showing significant increase in muscle injury with concentric exercise (78).

There may be increased weakness following strengthening exercise in DMD (80). There are other instances that have raised concerns regarding overwork weakness in dystrophic myopathies. The dominant upper limb has been found to be weaker in persons with FSH muscular dystrophy than the nondominant, providing circumstantial evidence for overwork weakness (81,82). Studies evaluating strengthening intervention in DMD subjects have shown maintenance of strength or even mild improvement in strength over the period of the investigation. However, these studies are limited by use of primarily nonquantitative measures, lack of a control group, and use of the opposite limb as a control without considering the effects of cross training (83–85). Animal work in both dystrophic mice and dogs has shown significant increases in creatine kinase values immediately following the exercise (77,78,86).

Thus far, no systematic studies of the DMD population have shown any definitive deleterious effects of resistance exercise. Based on the theoretic susceptibility of the dystrophin-deficient sarcolemmal membrane to mechanical injury and the relative paucity of investigations, it is prudent to recommend a submaximal-strengthening program in DMD and other rapidly progressive dystrophic disorders (87). Incorporation of the activity into recreational pursuits and aquatic-based therapy are probably the most reasonable approaches for the pre-adolescent child.

Recently, a moderate resistance home exercise program (using a less supervised approach) was devised that demonstrated strength gains in both neuromuscular disease patients and normal control subjects without evidence of overwork weakness (88). Based on this encouraging result, the home program was advanced to high-resistance training in similar subjects without apparent additive beneficial effects; in fact, eccentrically measured elbow flexor strength actually decreased significantly (89).

Based on the above investigations, we believe that there is adequate evidence to generally advocate a submaximal strengthening program for persons with slowly progressive neuromuscular disorders. There seems to be no additional benefit to high-resistance, low-repetition training sets, and the risk of actually increasing weakness becomes greater. Improvement in strength will hopefully translate to more functional issues such as improved endurance and mobility.

Aerobic exercise refers to rhythmic, prolonged activity of the level sufficient to provide a beneficial training stimulus to the cardiopulmonary and muscular systems but below the threshold where anaerobic metabolism of fuels is the primary source of energy. The response of normal skeletal muscle to this type of training includes increased capillary density in the muscle to improve substrate transfer, increased skeletal muscle mitochondrial size and density, higher concentrations of skeletal muscle oxidative enzymes, and improvement in utilization of fat as an energy source for muscular activity. Boys with DMD have been demonstrated to have low cardiovascular capacity and peripheral oxygen utilization with higher resting heart rate compared with controls (90). There is also emerging evidence that boys with DMD have a chronotropic insufficiency, i.e., they have decreased ability to raise their heart rate in response to exercise. Physical ability and exercise capacity are more likely to be limited by muscle strength than by deterioration of cardiorespiratory function. In a recent study using a home-based aerobic walking program, slowly progressive neuromuscular disease subjects showed modest improvement in aerobic capacity without evidence of overwork weakness or excessive fatigue (91). It is likely that alternative exercise approaches, such as aquatic-based therapy, will need to be utilized in boys with DMD who are nonambulatory and have less than antigravity muscle strength.

IMPROVING FUNCTIONAL MOBILITY

Generally, antigravity quadriceps are required for community ambulation. Some patients with more severe weakness may achieve short distance ambulation using KAFO bracing with or without a walker. Such orthotic intervention is often provided to boys with DMD. As the disease progresses it will be necessary for the boys to utilize power mobility devices for functional mobility. Generally, children can be taught to safely operate a power wheelchair when they are at the developmental age of approximately two years (92,93).

These boys will develop the need for a power recline system, and the chair should be able to accommodate such a recline or be retrofit. As the disability worsens, the power wheelchair electronics should be sufficiently sophisticated to incorporate alternative drive control systems, environmental control adaptations, and possibly communication systems in patients who are unable to vocalize. Indeed, with the advent of better, more portable mechanical ventilation systems, the life expectancy of men with DMD has markedly increased (94). Thus, the adequacy and performance of a powered mobility system are critical to maintaining their community integration and quality of life.

ACKNOWLEDGMENT

The National Institute on Disability and Rehabilitation Research, United States Department of Education through the Research and Training Center Grant H133B80016 supported this work.

REFERENCES

1. Roberts RG, Coffey AJ, Bobrow M, Bentley DR. Exon structure of the human dystrophin gene. Genomics 1993; 16:536–540.
2. Hoffman EP, Fischbeck KH, Brown RH, Johnson M, Medori R, Loike JD. Characterization of dystrophin in muscle biopsies from Duchenne and Becker muscular dystrophy patients. N Engl J Med 1988; 318:1363–1368.
3. Emery AH. Population frequencies of inherited neuromuscular diseases—a world survey. Neuromuscul Disord 1991; 1:19–24.
4. McDonald CM, Abresch RT, Carter GT, et al. Profiles of neuromuscular diseases: Duchenne muscular dystrophy. Am J Phys Med Rehabil 1995; 74: S70–S92.
5. Brooke MH, Fenichel GM, Griggs RC, Mendell JR, Moxley R, Florence J. Duchenne muscular dystrophy: patterns of clinical progression and effects of supportive therapy. Neurology 1989; 39:745–751.
6. Mendell JR, Province MA, Moxley RT, Griggs RC, Brooke MH. Clinical investigation of Duchenne muscular dystrophy: a methodology for therapeutic trials based on natural history controls. Arch Neurol 1987; 44:808–815.
7. Cros D, Harnden P, Pellisier JF, Serratrice G. Muscle hypertrophy in Duchenne muscular dystrophy: a pathological and morphometric study. J Neurol 1989; 236:43–49.
8. Pradhan S. New clinical sign in Duchenne muscular dystrophy. Pediatr Neurol 1994; 11:298–301.
9. Kilmer DMD, Abresch RT, Fowler WM Jr. Serial manual muscle testing in Duchenne muscular dystrophy. Arch Phys Med Rehabil 1993; 74:1168–1174.
10. Steffensen BF, Lyager S, Werge B, Rahbek J, Mattson E. Physical capacity in nonambulatory people with Duchenne muscular dystrophy or spinal muscular atrophy: a longitudinal study. Dev Med Child Neurol 2002; 44(9):623–632.
11. McDonald DG, Kinali M, Gallagher AC, et al. Fracture prevalence in Duchenne muscular dystrophy. Dev Med Child Neurol 2002; 44(10):695–698.
12. Bakker JP, De Groot IJ, Beelen A, Lankhorst GJ. Predictive factors of cessation of ambulation in patients with Duchenne muscular dystrophy. Am J Phys Med Rehabil 2002; 81(12):906–912.
13. Johnson ER, Fowler WM Jr, Lieberman JS. Contractures in neuromuscular disease. Arch Phys Med Rehabil 1992; 73:807–814.
14. Brooke MH, Fenichel GM, Griggs RC, Mendell JR, Moxley R, Miller JP, Province MA. Clinical investigation in Duchenne dystrophy II: determination of the "power" of therapeutic trials based on the natural history. Muscle Nerve 1983; 6:91–99.
15. Oda T, Shimizu N, Yonenobu K, Ono K, Nabeshima T, Kyoh S. Longitudinal study of spinal deformity in Duchenne muscular dystrophy. J Pediatr Orthop 1993; 13:478–486.

16. Scott OM, Hyde SA, Goddard C, Dubowitz V. Prevention of deformity in Duchenne muscular dystrophy: a prospective study of passive stretching and splintage. Physiotherapy 1981; 67:177–188.
17. Vignos PJ Jr, Archibald KC. Maintenance of ambulation in childhood muscular dystrophy. J Chron Dis 1960; 12:273–279.
18. Eyring EJ, Johnson EW, Burnett C. Surgery in muscular dystrophy. JAMA 1972; 222:1067–1071.
19. Siegel IM, Miller JE, Ray RD. Subcutaneous lower limb tenotomy in the treatment of pseudohypertrophic muscular dystrophy. J Bone Joint Surg 1986; 50-?A:1437–1444.
20. Spencer GE, Vignos PJ Jr. Bracing for ambulation in childhood progressive muscular dystrophy. J Bone Joint Surg 1962; 44-A:234–240.
21. Liu M, Mineo K, Hanayama K, Fujiwara T, Chino N. Practical problems and management of seating through the clinical stages of Duchenne muscular dystrophy. Arch Phys Med Rehabil 2003; 84(6):818–824.
22. Heckmatt JZ, Dubowitz V, Hyde SA, Florence J, Gabain AC, Thompson N. Prolongation of walking in Duchenne muscular dystrophy with lightweight orthoses: review of 57 cases. Dev Med Child Neurol 1985; 27:149–155.
23. McDonald C. Limb contractures in progressive neuromuscular disease and the role of stretching, orthotics, and surgery. Rehabil Neuro Disorders 1998; 9:187–194.
24. Vignos PJ Jr. Management of musculoskeletal complications in neuromuscular disease: limb contractures and the role of stretching, braces, and surgery. Phys Med Rehabil: State Art Rev 1988; 2:509–515.
25. Hart DA, McDonald CM. Spinal deformity in progressive neuromuscular disease: natural history and management. Phys Med Rehabil Clin N Am 1998; 9:213–220.
26. Manzur AY, Hyde SA, Rodillo E, Heckmatt JZ, Bentley G, Dubowitz V. A randomized controlled trial of early surgery in Duchenne muscular dystrophy. Neuromuscul Disord 1992; 2:379–386.
27. Johnson E, Yarnell S. Hand dominance and scoliosis in Duchenne muscular dystrophy. Arch Phys Med Rehabil 1976; 57:462–470.
28. Lord J, Behrman B, Varzos N, Cooper D, Lieberman JS, Fowler WM. Scoliosis associated with Duchenne muscular dystrophy. Arch Phys Med Rehabil 1990; 71:13–19.
29. Rideau Y, Jankowski L, Grellet J. Respiratory function in the muscular dystrophies. Muscle Nerve 1981; 4:155–162.
30. Rideau Y, Glorion B, Delaubier A, Tarle O, Bach J. The treatment of scoliosis in Duchenne muscular dystrophy. Muscle Nerve 1984; 7:281–285.
31. Iannaccone ST, Owens H, Scott J, Teitell B. Postoperative malnutrition in Duchenne muscular dystrophy. J Child Neurol 2003; 18(1):17–20.
32. Braun NMT, Aurora NS, Rochester DF. Respiratory muscle and pulmonary function in poliomyositis and other proximal myopathies. Thorax 1983; 38:316–321.
33. Curran FJ. Night ventilation by body respirators for patients in chronic respiratory failure due to late stage Duchenne muscular dystrophy. Arch Phys Med Rehabil 1981; 62:270–275.
34. Bach JR. Pulmonary rehabilitation. In: The obstructive and paralytic conditions. Philadelphia: Hanley & Belfus, 1995:303–315.

35. Hahn A, Bach JR, Delaubier A, Renardel-Irani A, Guillou C, Rideau Y. Clinical implications of maximal respiratory pressure determinations for individuals with Duchenne muscular dystrophy. Arch Phys Med Rehabil 1997; 78:1–12.
36. Splaingard ML, Frates RC Jr, Harrison GM, Carter RE, Jefferson LS. Home positive-pressure ventilation. Twenty years' experience. Chest 1983; 84(4):376–381.
37. Bach JR, Want TG. Noninvasive long-term ventilatory support for individuals with spinal muscular atrophy and functional bulbar musculature. Arch Phys Med Rehabil 1995; 76:213–217.
38. Bach JR, Campagnolo DI, Hoeman S. Life satisfaction of individuals with Duchenne muscular dystrophy using long-term mechanical ventilatory support. Am J Phys Med Rehabil 1991; 70:129–137.
39. Baydur A, Kanel G. Tracheobronchomalacia and tracheal hemorrhage in patients with Duchenne muscular dystrophy receiving long-term ventilation with uncuffed tracheostomies. Chest 2003; 123(4):1307–1311.
40. Gilgoff IS, Kahlstrom E, MacLaughlin E, Keens TG. Long-term ventilatory support in spinal muscular atrophy. J Pediatr 1989; 115:904–908.
41. Wang TG, Bach JR, Avila C, Alba AS, William Yang GF. Survival of individuals with spinal muscular atrophy on ventilatory support. Am J Phys Med Rehabil 1994; 73:207–215.
42. Topin N, Matecki S, Le Bris S, Rivier F, Echenne B, Prefaut C, Ramonatxo M. Dose-dependent effect of individualized respiratory muscle training in children with Duchenne muscular dystrophy. Neuromuscul Disord 2002; 12(6):576–583.
43. Eagle M. Report on the muscular dystrophy campaign workshop: exercise in neuromuscular diseases Newcastle, January 2002. Neuromuscul Disord 2002; 12(10):975–983.
44. Benditt JO. Management of pulmonary complications in neuromuscular disease. Phys Med Rehabil Clin N Am 1998:167–185.
45. Yamamoto S, Matsushima H, Suzuki A. A comparative study of thallium-201 single photon emission computed tomography and electrocardiography in Duchenne and other types of muscular dystrophy. Am J Cardiol 1988; 61:836–641.
46. Mori H, Utsunomiya T, Ishijima M. The relationship between 24-hour total heart beats or ventricular arrhythmias and cardiopulmonary function in patients with Duchenne muscular dystrophy. Japan Heart J 1990; 31(5):599–610.
47. Yanagisawa A, Miyagawa M, Yotsukura M. The prevalence and prognostic significance of arrhythmias in Duchenne type muscular dystrophy. Am Heart J 1992; 124:1244–1251.
48. Yotsukura M, Miyagawa M, Tsuya T. Pulmonary hypertension in progressive muscular dystrophy of the Duchenne type. Japan Circ J 1988; 52:321–326.
49. Nigro G, Comi LI, Politano L. The incidence and evolution of cardiomyopathy in Duchenne muscular dystrophy. Int J Cardiol 1990; 26(3):277–284.
50. Nigro G, Comi LI, Politano L, Limongelli FM, Nigro V, DeRimini ML. Evaluation of the cardiomyopathy in Becker muscular dystrophy. Muscle Nerve 1995; 18(3):283–289.
51. Akita H, Matsuoka S, Juroda Y. Predictive electrocardiographic score for evaluating prognosis in patients with Duchenne muscular dystrophy. Tokushima J Exp Med 1995; 40:55–61.

52. Miller G, D'Orsogna L, O'Shea JP. Autonomic function and the sinus tachycardia of Duchenne muscular dystrophy. Brain Dev 1989; 22:247–255.
53. Perloff JK. Cardiac rhythm and conduction in Duchenne muscular dystrophy. J Am Coll Cardiol 1984; 3:1263–1270.
54. Sanyal SK, Johnson WW, Thapar MK. An ultrastructural basis for the electrocardiographic alteration associated with Duchenne progressive muscular dystrophy. Circulation 1978; 57:1122–1130.
55. Takenaka A, Yokota M, Iwase M. Discrepancy between systolic and diastolic dysfunction of the left ventricle in patients with Duchenne muscular dystrophy. Eur Heart J 1993; 14(5):669–675.
56. Chenard AA, Becane HM, Tertrain F, Weiss YA. Systolic time intervals in Duchenne muscular dystrophy: evaluation of left ventricular performance. Clin Cardiol 1998; 11:407–411.
57. Nagai T. Prognostic evaluation of congestive heart failure in patients with Duchenne muscular dystrophy: a retrospective study using non-invasive cardiac function tests. Japan Circ J 1989; 53(5):406–412.
58. Gilroy J, Cahalan J, Berman R. Cardiac and pulmonary complications in Duchenne progressive muscular dystrophy. Circulation 1963; 27:484–488.
59. Leth A, Wulff K. Myocardiopathy in Duchenne progressive muscular dystrophy. Acta Paediatr Scand 1976; 65:28–35.
60. Lewis W, Yadlapalli S. Management of cardiac complications in neuromuscular disease. Phys Med Rehabil Clin N Am 1998; 9:145–156.
61. Rappaport D, Colleto GM, Vainzof M, Duaik MC, Zatz M. Short stature in Duchenne muscular dystrophy. Growth Regulation 1991; 1:11–21.
62. Eiholzer U, Boltshauser E, Frey D, Molinari L, Zachmann U. Short stature: a common feature in Duchenne muscular dystrophy. Eur J Pediatr 1988; 147:602–610.
63. Scott OM, Hyde SA, Goddard C, Dubowitz V. Quantitation of muscle function in children: a prospective study in Duchenne muscular dystrophy. Muscle Nerve 1982; 5:291–301.
64. Willig TN, Carlier L, Legrand M, Riviere H, Navarro J. Nutritional assessment in Duchenne muscular dystrophy. Dev Med Child Neurol 1993; 35:1074–1081.
65. Okada K, Manabe S, Sakamoto S, Ohnaka M, Niiyama Y. Protein and energy metabolism in patients with progressive muscular dystrophy. J Nutr Sci Vitaminol (Tokyo) 1992; 38:141–155.
66. Okada K, Manabe S, Sakamoto S, Ohnaka M, Niiyama Y. Predictions of energy intake and energy allowance of patients with Duchenne muscular dystrophy and their validity. J Nutr Sci Vitaminol (Tokyo) 1992; 38:155–161.
67. Jaffe KM, McDonald CM, Ingman E, Haas J. Symptoms of upper gastrointestinal dysfunction: case–control study. Arch Phys Med Rehabil 1990; 71:742–751.
68. Edwards RHT, Round JM, Jackson MJ. Weight reduction in boys with muscular dystrophy. Dev Med Child Neurol 1984; 26:384–390.
69. Goldstein M, Meyer S, Freund HR. Effects of overfeeding children with muscle dystrophies. J Parent Enteral Nutr 1989; 13:603–610.
70. McCrory M, Wright N, Kilmer D. Nutritional aspects of neuromuscular diseases. Phys Med Rehabil Clin N Am 1998; 9:127–136.

71. Stewart PM, Walser M, Drachman DB. Branched-chain ketoacids reduce muscle protein degradation in Duchenne muscular dystrophy. Muscle Nerve 1982; 5:197–215.
72. Benson ES, Jaffe KM, Tarr PI. Acute gastric dilatation in Duchenne muscular dystrophy: a case report and review of the literature. Arch Phys Med Rehabil 1996; 77:512–517.
73. Nudel L, Zuk D, Zeelan E. DMD gene product is not identical in muscle and brain. Nature 1989; 337:76–78.
74. Dorman C, Hurley AD, D'Avignon J. Language and learning disorders of older boys with Duchenne muscular dystrophy. Dev Med Child Neurol 1988; 30:316–321.
75. Marsh GG, Munsat TL. Evidence of early impairment of verbal intelligence in Duchenne muscular dystrophy. Arch Dis Child 1974; 49:118–125.
76. Sollee ND, Latham EE, Kinndlon DJ, Bresnan MJ. Neuropsychological impairment in Duchenne muscular dystrophy. J Clin Exp Neuropsychol 1985; 7:486–491.
77. Carter GT, Kikuchi N, Abresch RT, Walsh SA, Horasek S, Fowler WM. Effects of exhaustive concentric and eccentric exercise on murine skeletal muscle. Arch Phys Med Rehabil 1994; 75(5):555–559.
78. Carter GT, Wineinger MA, Walsh SA, Horasek SJ, Abresch RT, Fowler WM. Effect of voluntary wheel-running exercise on muscles of the mdx mouse. Neuromuscul Disord 1995; 5(4):323–331.
79. Edwards RHT, Newham DJ, Jones DA, Chapman SJ. Role of mechanical damage in pathogenesis of proximal myopathy in man. Lancet 1984; 8376:548–555.
80. Bonsett CA. Pseudohypertrophic muscular dystrophy: distribution of degenerative features as revealed by anatomical study. Neurology 1963; 13:728–733.
81. Johnson EW, Braddom R. Over-work weakness in facioscapulohumeral muscular dystrophy. Arch Phys Med Rehabil 1971; 52:333–338.
82. Kilmer DD, Abresch RT, McCrory MA, et al. Profiles of neuromuscular diseases: facioscapulohumeral muscular dystrophy. Am J Phys Med Rehabil 1995; 74:S131–S139..
83. Vignos PJ Jr, Watkins MP. Effect of exercise in muscular dystrophy. JAMA 1966; 197:843–850.
84. Scott OM, Hyde SA, Goddard C. Effect of exercise in Duchenne muscular dystrophy: controlled six-month feasibility study of effects of two different regimes of exercises in children with Duchenne dystrophy. Physiotherapy 1981; 67:174–180.
85. DeLateur BJ, Giaconi RM. Effect on maximal strength of submaximal exercise in Duchenne muscular dystrophy. Am J Phys Med 1979; 58:26–33.
86. Carter GT, Abresch RT, Fowler WM. Adaptations to exercise training and contraction-induced muscle injury in animal models of neuromuscular disease. Am J Phys Med Rehabil 2002; 81:S151–S161.
87. Vignos PJ Jr. Physical models of rehabilitation in neuromuscular disease. Muscle Nerve 1983; 6:323–325.
88. Aitkens SG, McCrory MA, Kilmer DD, Bernauer EM. Moderate resistance exercise program: its effect in slowly progressive neuromuscular disease. Arch Phys Med Rehabil 1993; 74:711–719.

89. Kilmer DD, McCrory MA, Wright NC, Aitkens SG, Bernauer EM. The effect of a high resistance exercise program in slowly progressive neuromuscular disease. Arch Phys Med Rehabil 1994; 75:560–565.
90. Sockolov R, Irwin B, Dressendorfer RH, Fowler WM. Exercise performance in 6 to 11 year old boys with Duchenne muscular dystrophy. Arch Phys Med Rehabil 1977; 58:195–201.
91. Wright NC, Kilmer DD, McCrory MA, Aitkens SG, Holcomb BJ, Bernauer EM. Aerobic walking in slowly progressive neuromuscular disease: effect of a 12-week program. Arch Phys Med Rehabil 1996; 77:64–70.
92. Butler C, Okamoto G, McKay T. Motorized wheelchair driving by disabled children. Arch Phys Med Rehabil 1984; 65:95–101.
93. Butler C, Okamoto G, McKay T. Powered mobility for very young disabled children. Dev Med Child Neurol 1983; 25:472–476.
94. Eagle M, Badouin SV, Chandler C, Giddings DR, Bullock R, Bushby K. Survival in Duchenne muscular dystrophy: improvement in life expectancy since 1967 and the impact of home nocturnal ventilation. Neuromuscul Disord 2002; 12(10):926–929.

9

Orthopedic Interventions in the Management of Duchenne Muscular Dystrophy
A Review of Current Practice and Clinical Outcomes

Irwin M. Siegel
Departments of Orthopedic Surgery, Neurosciences and PM&R, Rush University Medical Center, Chicago, Illinois, U.S.A.

John D. Hsu
Rancho Los Amigos Medical Center, Downey, and Department of Orthopedics, University of Southern California, Los Angeles, California, U.S.A.

INTRODUCTION

The principles of orthopedic rehabilitation in Duchenne muscular dystrophy (DMD) are based on an understanding of the natural evolution of patterns of weakness, contracture, and deformity, so that therapeutic measures can be staged appropriately to ensure full use of available strength (1).

BIOMECHANICS

Principal functional loss is noted in the limb girdle musculature; the most severe contractures occurring in muscles that span two joints, are involved in eccentric contractions, and exercise a postural function (2).

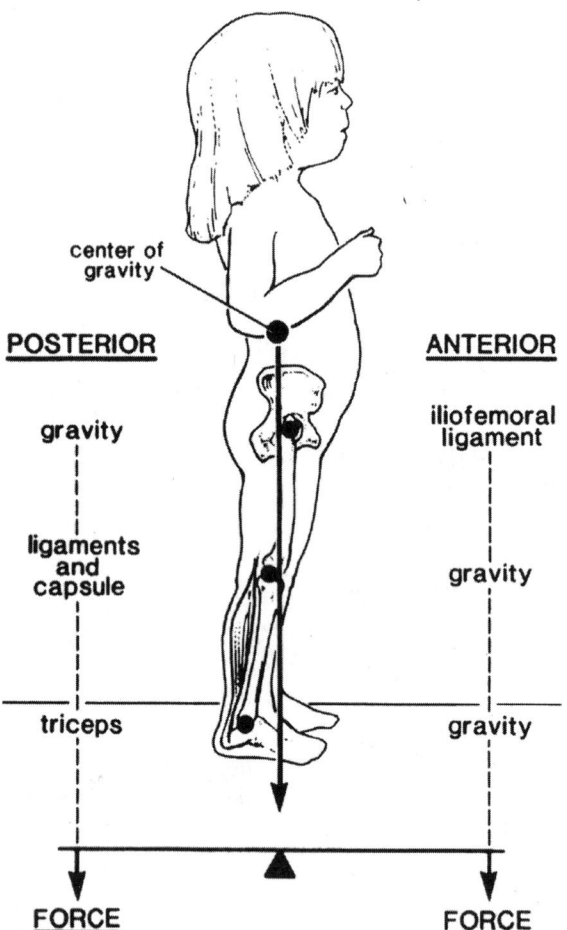

Figure 1 Placement of line of gravity.

The abiotrophic half-life of dystrophic muscle is about 4.8 years. Therefore, a child who is ambulatory at this age has lost approximately 50% of the voluntary musculature. As axial and proximal muscles weaken, the child finds it increasingly difficult to maintain torso-pelvic alignment by keeping the line of gravity behind the hips, anterior to the knees, and within the child's base of support (Fig. 1). With progression of quadriceps weakness, contracture advances in (i) the hip flexors, (ii) tensor fasciae latae, and (iii) gastrocsoleus (Fig. 2). Lumbar lordosis (concavity) increases; loss of strength in the shoulder depressors makes the torso balance awkwardly, as parascapular weakening draws the shoulders forward; abdominal and lumbar extensor weakness contribute to an unstable and effortful stance

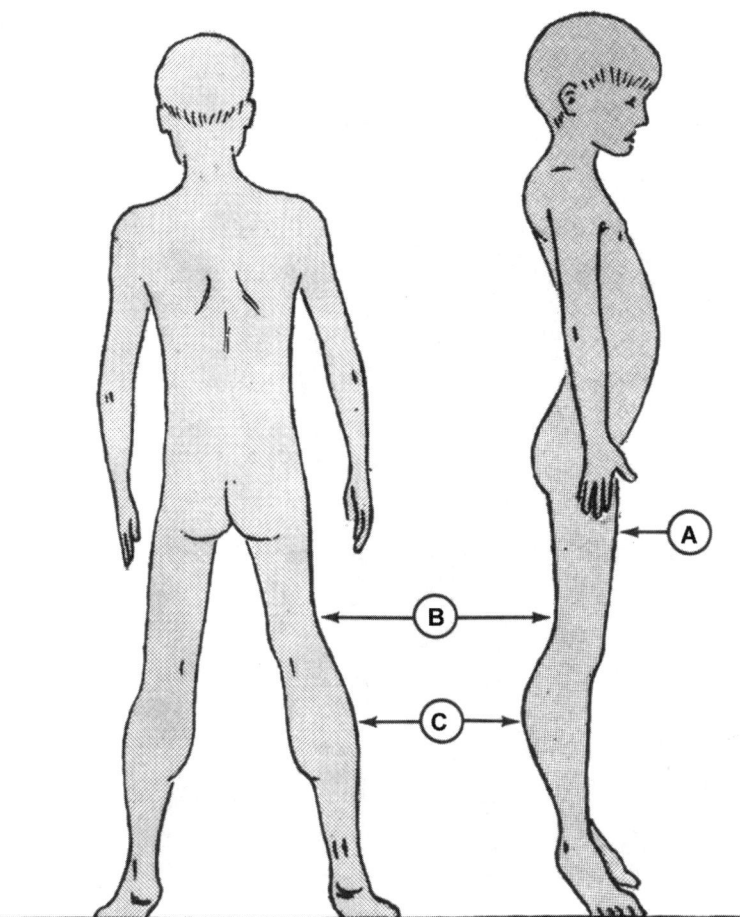

Figure 2 Contractures that inhibit orthograde posture. (**A**) Hip flexors, (**B**) tensor fasciae latae, and (**C**) gastrocsoleus.

and gait (3–6). Selective wasting of leg and foot musculature produces an equinovarus (clubfoot) deformity that, if untreated, further prevents the patient from maintaining an upright posture (Fig. 3). Although the spine is usually protected by ambulation, in DMD, the majority of patients with this disease who use wheelchairs develop scoliosis, which requires treatment.

MANAGEMENT

Orthopedic management in DMD requires a multidisciplinary approach, which includes physical and occupational therapy and the use of orthoses

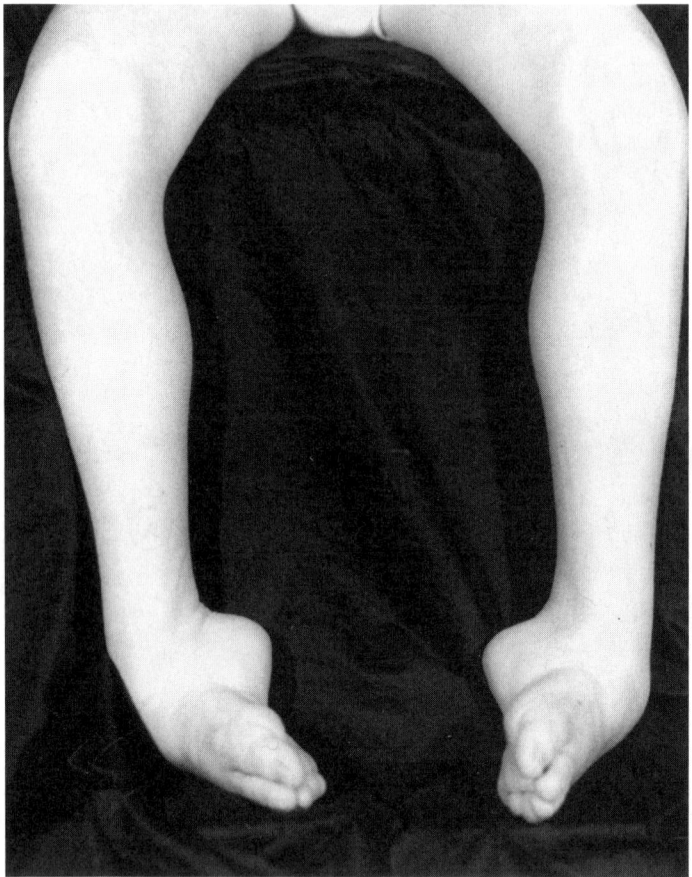

Figure 3 Advanced equinocavovarus in Duchenne muscular dystrophy.

(braces) and adaptive equipment. A variety of orthopedic procedures have proved successful in sustaining balance and mobility in selected patients. Reports on surgical management are in agreement regarding the fact that surgeries should permit early postoperative mobilization, because even brief bed rest can lead to rapid loss of strength. Because DMD is a relatively homogeneous condition with a course that is often predictable, interventions can be discussed on the basis of the patient's age.

STAGE I: DIAGNOSIS UNTIL 8 TO 9 YEARS OF AGE

During Stage I, the patient begins to develop heel cord contractures. The equinus (toe-walking) position of the foot during stance provides a ground

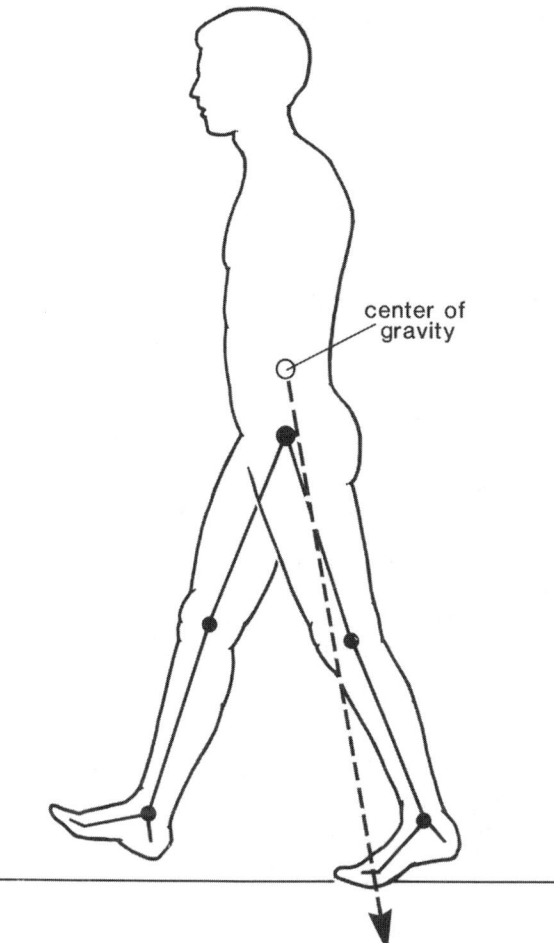

Figure 4 Ground reaction force vector.

reaction force (Fig. 4), which assists knee extension (straightening) and helps maintain the base of support under the center of gravity of the body (7). This keeps the weight-bearing force vector behind the axis of rotation of the hip and in front of the axis of rotation of the knee. This mild equinus, which helps the child balance, should not be discouraged. The development of severe toe-walking which threatens equilibrium can be delayed but not prevented by wearing a light tone-balancing orthosis (Fig. 5) which encourages dorsiflexion (bending up) while inhibiting plantar flexion (bending down) at the ankle, and supports the long arch stimulating heel cord

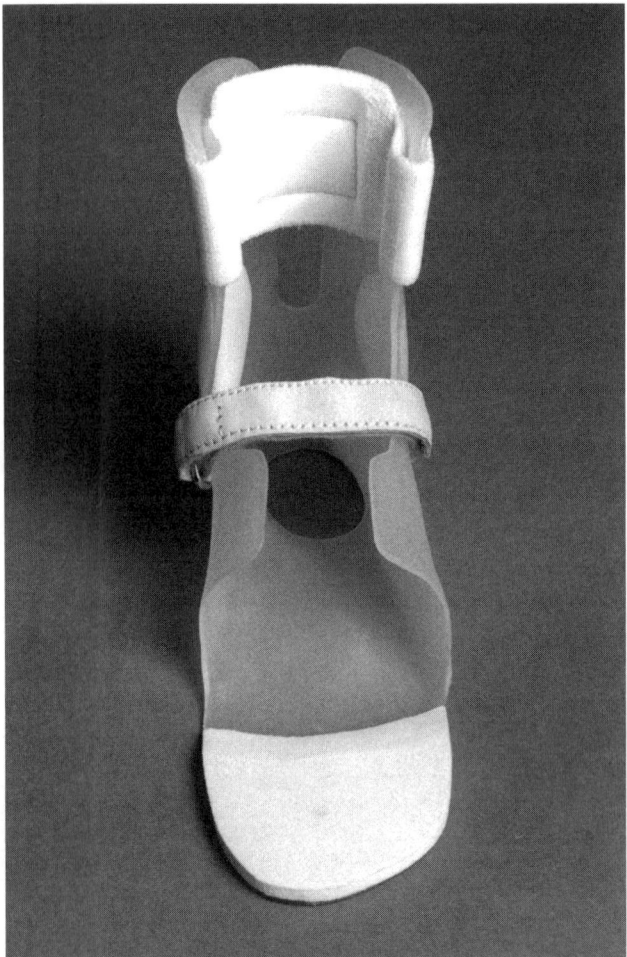

Figure 5 Tone-balance supramalleolar orthosis.

stretching during gait (8). Quadricep strength can be augmented with neoprene knee sleeves that incorporate anterior stays (Fig. 6).

There are no well-controlled studies demonstrating that either the use of orthotics or stretching prevents contractures. Although the Europeans (particularly Granata, Forst, Rideaux, and Goertzen) are performing surgical releases in an effort to prevent contracture, at even as young as four or five years of age, a randomized, closely controlled trial of early surgical treatment of contracture in 20 boys with DMD, aged four to six years, failed to show beneficial results (9–12). Although the deformities were corrected by surgery, strength and function were not improved (12). These investigators

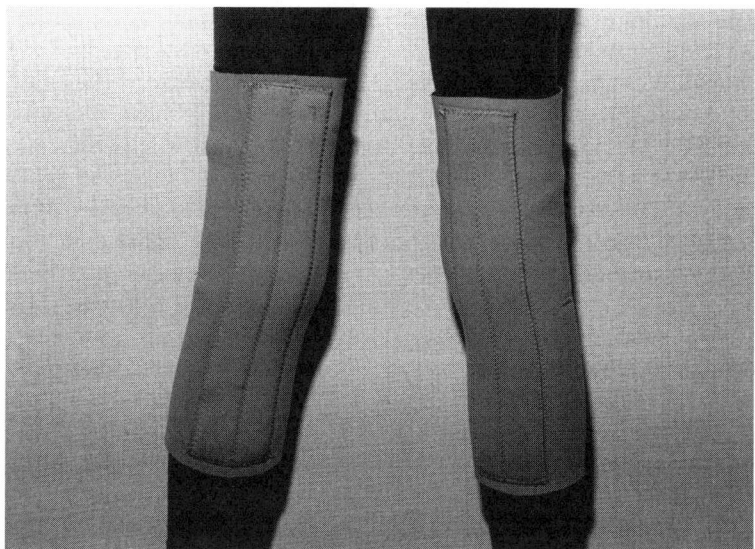

Figure 6 Neoprene knee sleeves with anterior stays.

noted that some of their subjects' conditions actually deteriorated more rapidly than those of children who did not undergo surgery. Therefore, early surgical treatment does not appear to be indicated.

FRACTURES

It has been noted that children with DMD, even those still ambulating, suffer from osteoporosis, thereby increasing their vulnerability to fracture. Because patients at complete rest lose strength at 3% to 5% a day, fractures, particularly of the lower extremities, should be treated conservatively but aggressively to maintain ambulation (13).

Almost half of such fractures are in the femur, 25% in the tibia, and the remainder in the upper extremities. The basis of these fractures is a marked decrease in bone mineral density in the axial skeleton, as measured in the upper femur, even in young patients with minimal functional impairment. Upper extremity fractures compromise balance and require aggressive conservative treatment to ensure that patients continue to ambulate.

Progressive muscle weakness in the younger, ambulatory child leads to a loss of balance and inability to move quickly enough to counteract an adverse force. When fractures occur, they need to be reduced and immobilized. Casting must be done with the extremity in a functional position so that walking and functional activities can be resumed as early as possible. For instance, with an ankle fracture, short leg casts should be applied with the ankle at neutral, even with tight heel cords. Casting in equinus position would lead to a permanent contracture. When long leg casts are used for more proximal fractures, the knee should be held in extension and the ankle at neutral. Some fractures do not require casting. These fractures have minimal forces tending to displace the fragments and they heal within the expected time (14).

Fractures in the wheelchair-dependent patient can be caused by a minimal sudden force applied at a contracted joint. The most common fractures occur around the knee joint at the distal femur or proximal tibia. Other sites include the proximal humerus, the distal tibia, and the wrist. Due to muscle atrophy, these fractures are generally minimally displaced. Initial immobilization can be accomplished by using a simple splint, such as a pillow (15).

STAGE II: 9 TO 12 YEARS OF AGE

Most DMD patients stop walking between 9 and 12 years of age. An ectomorphic patient usually walks (and reambulates after surgery) for a longer period than his endomorphic counterpart. In prognosticating loss of ambulation, it was found that the ability to rise from the seated position, ascend stairs, and ambulate are usually lost at yearly intervals in that sequence. With ankle equinus of 15° or more, if the sum of hip and knee extension lag reaches 90°, the child can no longer maintain an upright posture and ambulation soon ends (Fig. 7). However, the patient can usually tolerate knee extension lag better than extension lag of the hip because, with fixed ankle equinus, the knee, a hinge joint, can be passively locked into stable extension, whereas the hip, a ball and socket joint, cannot (1).

LOWER EXTREMITY SURGERY

For every surgical procedure, there are indications and conditions. In DMD, the indications are contractures that threaten upright posture and ambulation, and the condition for surgery is a cardiorespiratory status adequate to survive a general anesthetic.

A variety of procedures have been suggested. All studies utilize minimal surgery, permitting early ambulation. Spencer et al. (16,17) included release of lower extremity contractures and extremity bracing in a comprehensive muscular dystrophy rehabilitation program. They were able to increase the duration of walking, from the onset of symptoms, from an average of 4.4 years to an average of 8.7 years (18).

Siegel et al. (19) reported on 21 patients in the age group of 8 to 16 years, who were followed-up from 10 to 22 months postoperatively.

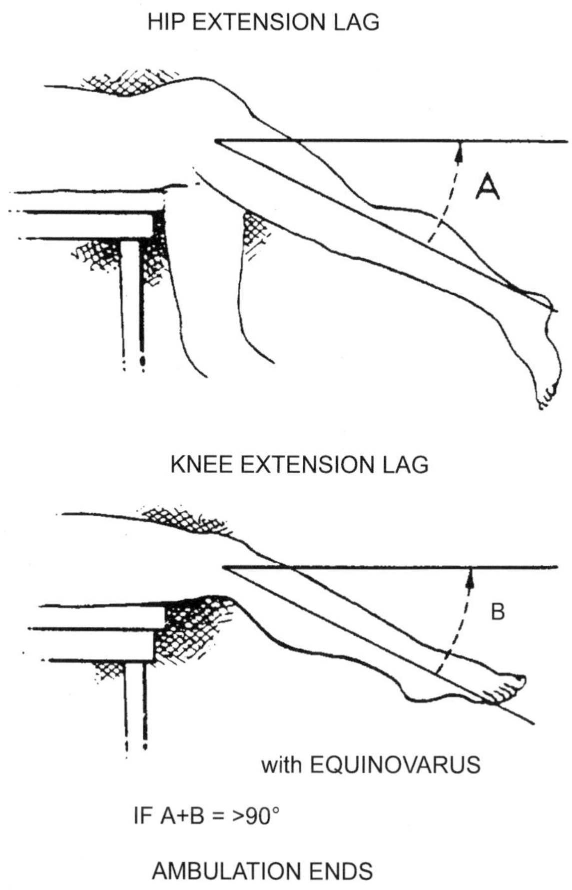

HIP EXTENSION LAG

KNEE EXTENSION LAG

with **EQUINOVARUS**

IF A+B = >90°

AMBULATION ENDS

Figure 7 Evaluation of hip and knee extension leg.

When last seen, all patients were able to stand without support and to walk for short distances without assistance.

Vignos et al. (20,21) reviewed the conditions of 144 boys who were followed for a mean of 8.9 years, managed with a combination of daily passive stretching exercises, and prescribed periods of standing and walking, Achilles tendon tenotomy (release), posterior tibial tendon transfer, and application of knee–ankle–foot orthoses (long leg braces). This program enabled patients to walk until a mean age of 13.6 years, with the ability to stand in orthoses after loss of walking, for an additional two years.

Bakker et al. (22) conducted a review of available literature on the effectiveness of knee–ankle–foot orthoses in the treatment of DMD. Operations on the lower limbs were performed on most patients, but a concomitant program of rehabilitation was not thoroughly described. Thirty articles describing 35 studies met the inclusion criteria for their review. They concluded that the scientific strength of the studies reviewed was poor. It appeared that the use of knee–ankle–foot orthoses can prolong assisted walking and standing, but they were uncertain as to whether it can prolong functional walking. The boys benefiting most had a relatively low rate of deterioration, were capable of enduring an operation, and were well motivated.

A study by Smith et al. (23) of 54 patients, of whom 29 underwent hip, knee, and ankle tenotomies and were followed for almost four years, revealed continued ambulation in braces until a mean age of almost 12 years 8 months and standing until an average of 13 years 5 months. A control group of 25 children who were not operated ceased ambulating at a mean age of 10 years and stopped standing at a mean age of 10 years 2 months.

Bach and McKeon (24) studied seven patients treated with musculotendinous surgery including posterior tibial transfer while ambulating with little difficulty, and six patients treated just before or after becoming wheelchair dependent. These authors observed that the prolongation of brace-free ambulation after treatment was a mean of 0.8 year greater than predicted for the group as a whole, but 0.93 year greater for the group treated early in comparison to 0.63 year for those treated according to the customary approach. The number of falls decreased significantly, and three patients who had posterior tibial transfers retained antigravity plus dorsiflexion strength and continued to wear normal footwear for up to four years after loss of ambulation.

Hsu (25) presented 24 patients who underwent hip, knee, and ankle tenotomies at a mean age of 10 years 2 months, and were followed, postoperatively, for an average of 3 years 9 months. These children continued ambulation and the use of long-leg braces to a mean age of 12 years 8 months and could stand up to an average of 13 years 5 months. A separate group of 25 children who were recommended to undergo surgery but declined to do so was followed, and it was found that they ceased ambulating at a mean age of 10 years and stopped standing at a mean age of 10 years 2 months.

Concerning tibialis posticus function, this muscle has a strength percentage that is second only to the gastrocsoleus complex. Continued strength in the face of weakness of other ankle musculature results in inversion (turning inward) contracture augmented by the tight Achilles, which rotates 30° to insert along the medial border of the os calcis. Transfer of the tibialis posterior tendon through the interosseous membrane has been described and successfully performed by Hsu (Fig. 8) (26,27).

Greene (28) compared transfer of the tibialis posterior tendon to the dorsum of the foot with lengthening of the tendon in 15 patients. His conclusion was that the unique prolongation of posterior tibialis strength in DMD makes transfer preferable for these patients.

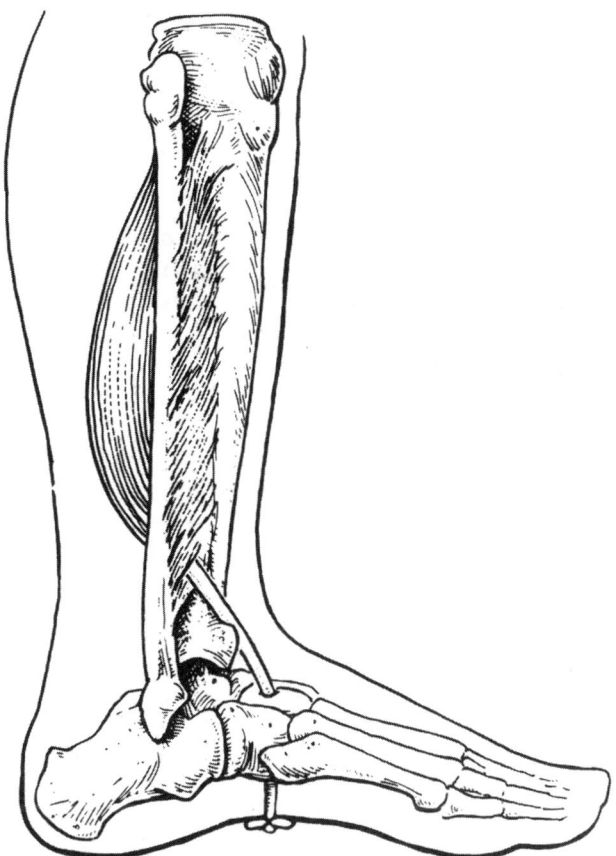

Figure 8 Posterior tibial transfer.

Sussman (29), in a small personal series of patients, offered an alternative approach to the correction of equinovarus that included tenotomy of the tibialis posterior, flexor digitorum longus, and flexor hallucis muscles at the level of the ankle at the time of Achilles tenotomy. Patients so treated demonstrated a decrease in subsequent equinovarus.

COMPARTMENT SYNDROME

Elevation of intracompartmental calf pressure in DMD can cause chronic compartment syndrome, which augments mechanical muscle damage, and may produce calf cramping. Relief of increased pressure by fasciotomy (releasing constricting fascia) inhibits this process. Intermittent pressure monitoring may prove of value in the routine orthopedic management of patients with this disease. Siegel (30) reported the use of this technique in 14 ambulatory and 8 nonambulatory DMD patients. Intracompartmental pressure was elevated in the majority of these patients and was reduced in patients who underwent percutaneous fasciotomy.

TALIPES EQUINOVARUS

Talipes equinovarus is a late deformity in DMD. This condition occurs secondary to selective weakening and contracture of foot musculature, augmented by tarsal deformity, and eventually prohibits standing and walking. Percutaneous tarsal medullostomy (enucleation) with soft tissue release has been successful in correcting the deformity (Fig. 9). An initial report was on seven feet (31). All were male, ranging in age from 9 to 13 years. Follow-up was 27 to 44 months postoperative. All patients were ambulatory without recurrence of deformity at that time. This program has enabled such patients to maintain independent pain-free ambulation and has significantly delayed wheelchair confinement with its inexorable downhill course.

The preferred surgical protocol in the severely contracted patient includes (i) hip, (ii) bipolar tensor fascia, and (iii) Achilles release performed percutaneously (Fig. 10) (19). In the average patient, percutaneous release of Achilles contracture is performed (32). A percutaneous tensor fascia release at the knee alone can also be done at the same time; this may prevent or at least decrease progression of hip flexion contracture. Below-knee plasters incorporating floor reaction (for toe–heel gait pattern) are applied if

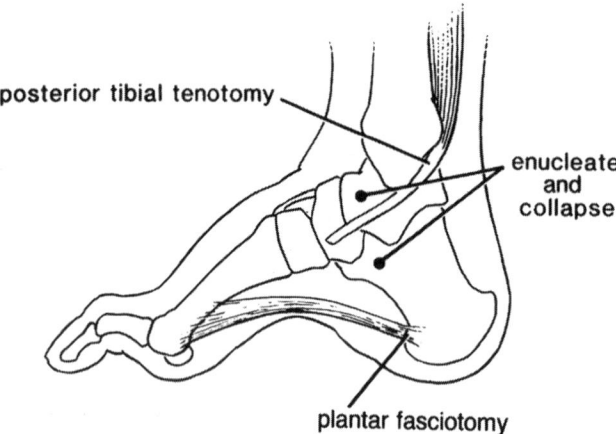

Figure 9 Surgical treatment (soft tissue release with tarsal medullostomy and brisement force collapse) of equinocavovarus deformity in Duchenne muscular dystrophy.

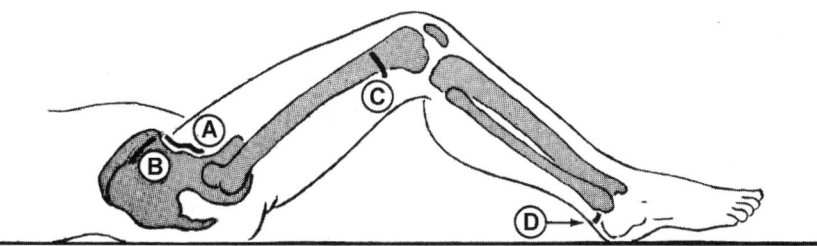

Figure 10 Sites for percutaneous tenotomy of lower extremity in DMD. (**A**) Hip flexors, (**B** and **C**) bipolar tensor fascia latae, and (**D**) triceps surae.

quadriceps strength is graded fair or better. Otherwise, long-leg plasters with the ankles at neutral are fitted. Orthoses incorporating these features are provided after three weeks. We prefer the closed cylinder design as it is lighter yet stronger in resisting superimposed torque stress (Fig. 11) (33). For children having quadriceps strength between that requiring a below-knee appliance and that requiring a knee–ankle–foot orthosis, a modified ankle–foot orthosis incorporating an attached neoprene wrap-around knee-support is available.

STAGE III: FULL-TIME SITTING

Wheelchair-bound patients develop hip and knee contractures, which are often greater than 30°. Release of these contractures in the patient who is sitting full time is not successful in permanently reducing deformity and therefore should not be performed.

The same is true of elbow contractures. The forearm is usually contracted in functional pronation, with the elbow in mild flexion. These contractures can usually be kept under control with assiduous stretching. Surgical release is contraindicated because the forearm is contracted in the position of function.

In the case of the wheelchair-confined patient who requires correction of severe equinovarus, a midtarsal closing wedge bone resection can be performed (Fig. 12) (1). For patients who cannot wear regular shoes, an alternative has again been suggested by Sussman (29). This includes Achilles tenotomy with resection of a 1- to 2-cm section of the tendon to prevent regrowth, along with tenotomy of the tibialis posticus and again of the flexor hallucis and flexor digitorum muscles. Hsu and Jackson (34) have written on the surgical release of contractures in these feet. Their indications for operative correction include severe pain, skin breakdown, and/or ulceration and the inability to fit reasonably costing and available shoes. Postoperative support by using ankle–foot orthosis/orthoses (AFOs) should help prevent recurrences.

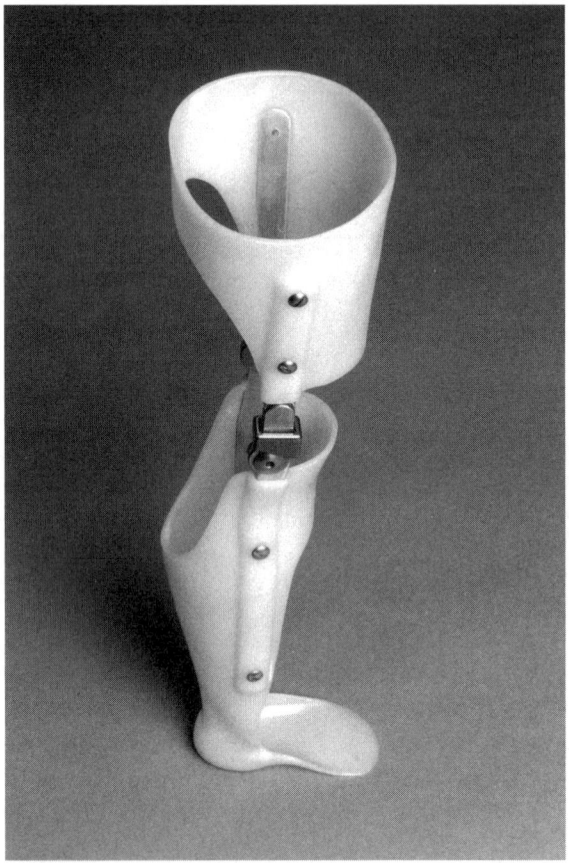

Figure 11 Cylindrical knee–ankle–foot orthosis with drop-ring locks.

Piriformis syndrome (nondiscogenic sciatica) has been reported in the wheelchair-confined patient with DMD (35). In this situation, the sciatic nerve is compressed by spasm of the piriformis muscle (Fig. 13). Massage of the piriformis and/or passive stretching exercises, local injections of steroid, or surgical release of the piriformis tendon are all ways of treating this annoying yet often underdiagnosed condition.

Wheelchair-confined DMD patients are predisposed to compression neuropathy of the upper extremities. Most commonly seen is ulnar neuropathy secondary to wheelchair armrest pressure on the forearm and elbow. In the normal elbow, the force for lifting the forearm is supplied by the biceps with a short lever distance from the muscle insertion to the fulcrum at the olecranon. When biceps function is lost, the forearm is "lifted" by applying downward force to tilt the elbow through a fulcrum supplied in the mid to

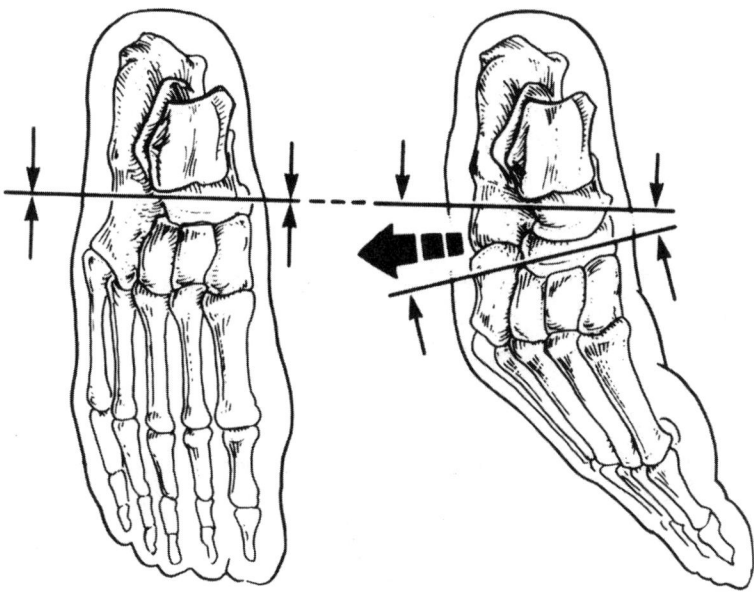

Figure 12 Midtarsal closing wedge osteotomy.

distal forearm by the armrest of the chair (Fig. 14). This lever arm is kept long to minimize the energy necessary to move the member, and pressure can be repeatedly imposed upon the ulnar nerve as it traverses the forearm. Relief is obtained by padding the armrest or providing a balanced forearm orthosis (Fig. 15) (36).

SCOLIOSIS

By far the most critical orthopedic issue in the wheelchair-confined DMD patient is the development of spinal deformity. This usually has its onset between the ages of 11 and 13. It is estimated that the majority of patients, whether braced or not, will develop significant scoliosis before they die.

In the thin patient, a fixed thoracolumbar lordosis locks the facet joints and inhibits the development of deformity in the coronal plane. However, severe lordosis in itself can be extremely debilitating. Although recommendations for surgical technique differ to some extent, most practitioners advise early spinal fusion with internal fixation in progressive curves. Ambulatory patients do not usually develop scoliosis because they maintain their pelvis level by performing alternating symmetrical and asymmetrical spinal exercise while shifting weight for torso balance during ambulation. Although any pattern of curve can be found, it is often a long C-shaped

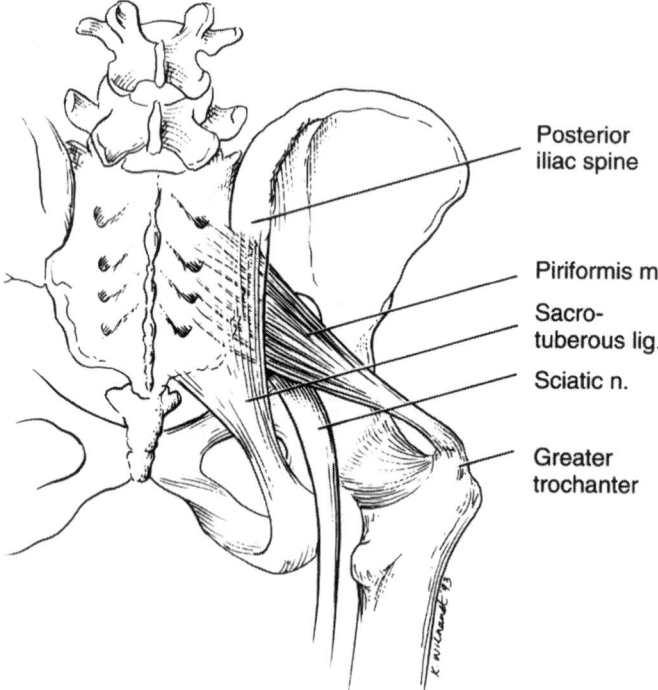

Figure 13 Anatomic relationship of sciatic nerve to piriformis muscle illustrating vulnerability of sciatic nerve due to piriformis pathology.

curve with the apex in the thoracolumbar region. The natural course of this deformity is usually relentless progression until the thorax is resting against the iliac crest (Fig. 16). Bracing with special seating systems (Fig. 17) may delay, but will not prevent, progression of scoliosis.

Studies by Hsu (37) have shown that approximately 90% of patients with DMD have a scoliosis curve of more than 20° and the curve progresses at about 10° a year (38). Patients lose approximately 7% of their pulmonary capacity for every 10° of curve and for every year after onset of scoliosis. These findings support the recommendation to consider performing a fusion when the scoliosis curve progresses beyond 20° and before pulmonary function significantly decreases.

Sufficient spinal growth will have occurred in the child with DMD by the age of 10 to 11, so that posterior fusion will not result in a marked loss of trunk height or the development of a crankshaft (twisting) deformity.

The older the patient is at the time of surgery, the greater is the risk of serious postoperative pulmonary complications. Patients with a forced vital

FORCES ABOUT THE ELBOW JOINT

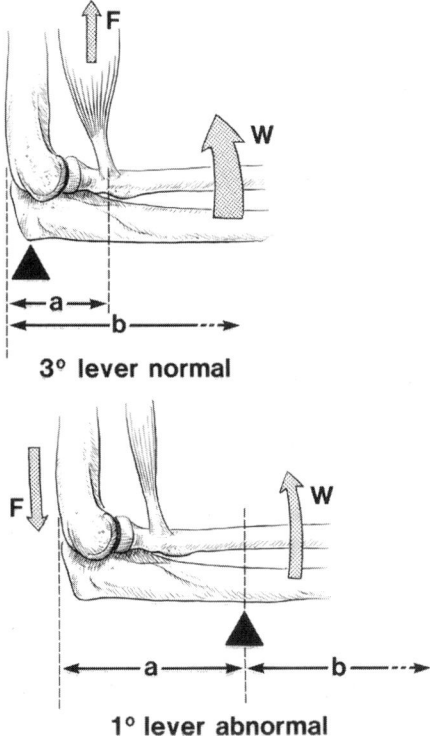

Figure 14 Biceps weakness causing shift from a third- to a first-degree lever system at the elbow, which can cause secondary ulnar nerve compression.

capacity of less than 30% may require prolonged intubation and possibly permanent tracheostomy.

Although most spinal surgeons say the earlier the better, the average acceptable curve for correction and fusion is 30° and the average acceptable forced vital capacity is 30% or greater.

The level and extent of arthrodesis is a matter of some discussion. Most surgeons agree that the fusion should extend at the upper level to the upper thoracic spine with care taken to ensure that thoracic kyphosis (convexity) is maintained such that the center of mass of the head is forward. This allows the patient to sustain head control because most patients retain strength in the neck extensors but lose it in the flexors.

The lowest level of fusion is also a topic of debate. If patients are stabilized before the onset of severe deformity, and pelvic obliquity is less than 10%, fixation to L5 may be sufficient. A balanced trunk over a level

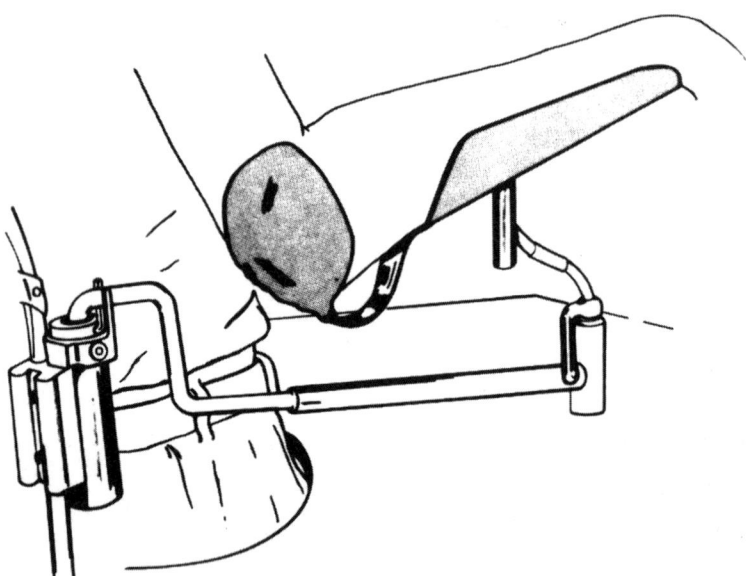

Figure 15 Balanced forearm orthosis.

pelvis is the surgical goal, which in certain patients can be achieved by fusion to L5. Nevertheless, some investigators disagree and have recommended that all spines be stabilized to the pelvis and arthrodesed to the sacrum.

A few studies have demonstrated that spinal fusion increases the patient's life span. However, according to a Toronto study that was well controlled for severity, there is absolutely no change in the life span if patients receive similar medical management. It is to be noted that although steroids can delay the onset and even decrease the severity of scoliosis, the child on steroid therapy will always have increased osteoporosis of the spine, which may compromise arthrodesis.

Patients who undergo spinal stabilization have a substantially enhanced quality of life compared to those who do not. Following spinal stabilization, they are better balanced in the wheelchair. An upright sitting posture is psychologically and physiologically desirable. The upper extremities can be freed from a supporting role and can be used for functional activities. Spinal fusion in the severely disabled older DMD-affected child with minimal arm strength can improve sitting stability enough to enable performance of tabletop tasks using the mobile arm support system (36). In a study of 68 patients from a clinical population of 183 patients with DMD, Miller et al. (39) concluded that a 35% normal forced vital capacity was a reliable indicator of pulmonary complication risk. Factors improving the patient's quality of life included segmental instrumentation and fusion from T2 to the pelvis,

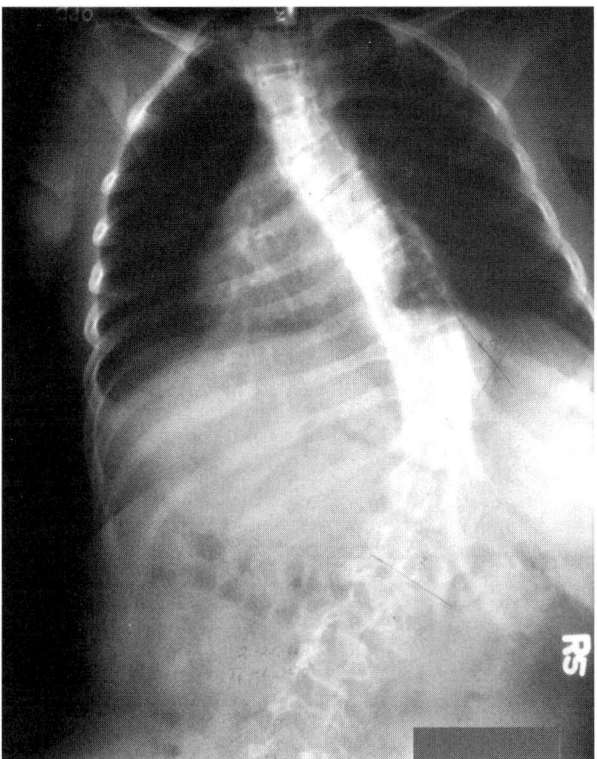

Figure 16 X-ray of advanced scoliosis in Duchenne muscular dystrophy.

correcting pelvic obliquity, and balancing the scoliosis, thus creating normal sagittal plane alignment. They concluded that life expectancy and the rate of deterioration of pulmonary function were unaffected by this procedure.

Bridwell et al. (40) sent questionnaires to evaluate function, self-image, cosmesis, pain, pulmonary status, patient care, quality of life, and satisfaction to 33 patients with DMD and 21 with spinal muscular atrophy who had undergone spinal fusion. Forty-eight patients returned the questionnaire and except for two who died within three months of surgery, all seemed to have benefited from the procedure. Cosmesis, quality of life, and overall satisfaction were rated highest.

Other studies that follow confirm the desirability of spinal stabilization.

Mubarak et al. (41) reported on 22 wheelchair-bound patients with DMD who underwent Luque segmental instrumentation and fusion. They concluded that if treatment is initiated early, segmental instrumentation and fusion from high thoracic vertebra to the fifth lumbar vertebra should be sufficient.

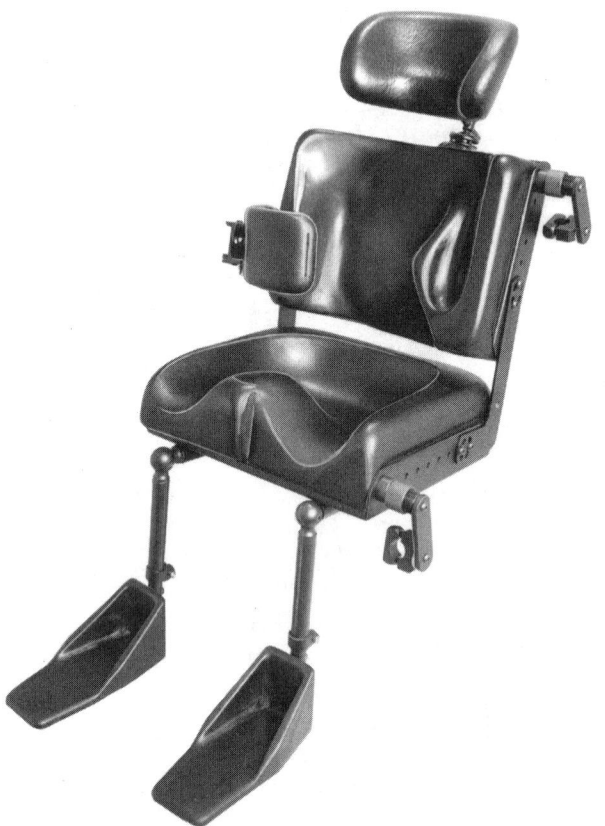

Figure 17 Customized external spinal containment wheelchair seating system.

Galasco et al. (42) reported on 55 patients with DMD, of whom 32 accepted surgical stabilization. These patients were compared on the basis of survival, forced vital capacity, peak expiratory flow, and severity of scoliosis. Scoliosis progressed rapidly in the nonoperated patients, as did respiratory deterioration. Spinal stabilization resulted in an improvement in the peak expiratory flow rate, which was maintained for up to five years.

Heller et al. (43), reporting on 31 patients, concluded that spinal stabilization should be carried out after loss of ambulation and as soon as a progressive curve of more than 20° is documented.

Hopf and Eysel (44) discussed the principles of operative treatment of neuromuscular scoliosis. They determined that the existing deterioration of vital capacity makes an anterior approach impossible, and that multisegmental instrumentation allows postoperative care without external support. However, there are surgeons doing anterior as well as posterior surgery where indicated on patients with DMD, and in many protocols, a light thoraco-lumbo-sacral orthosis is often worn for comfort for a brief interval in the postoperative period.

Finally, Kennedy et al. (45) studied the effect on subsequent respiratory function after spinal stabilization for scoliosis in DMD. Seventeen boys who underwent spinal stabilization at a mean age of 15 years were compared to 21 boys who had not undergone surgery. No difference was found between the arthrodesed and the nonsurgical group in the rate of deterioration of forced vital capacity, which was measured at 3% to 5% per year. There was no difference in life expectancy, and the conclusion was that although spinal stabilization in DMD improves quality of life, it does not alter the decline in pulmonary function or improve survival.

SUMMARY

In summary, surgery is indicated at appropriate times for the intelligent and aggressive management of DMD. Staged in a timely manner and performed properly, suitable surgeries can assist in enhancing performance and improving cosmesis, keeping the patient as functional as possible for as long as feasible.

REFERENCES

1. Siegel IM. Muscle and Its Diseases—An Outline Primer of Basic Science and Clinical Method. Chicago: Yearbook Medical Publishers, 1986.
2. Siegel IM, Glantz RH. Orthopaedic rehabilitation for standing and walking in selected neuromuscular diseases. J Neuro Rehab 1988; 2:131–136.
3. Johnson EW. Pathokinesiology of Duchenne muscular dystrophy: implications of management. Arch Phys Med Rehabil 1977; 58:4–7.
4. Siegel IM. Pathomechanics of stance in Duchenne muscular dystrophy. Arch Phys Med Rehabil 1972; 53:403–406.
5. Siegel IM, Weiss LA. Postural substitution in Duchenne's muscular dystrophy. JAMA 1982; 247:584.
6. Hsu JD, Furumasu J. Gait and posture changes in the Duchenne muscular dystrophy child. Clin Ortho Rel Res 1993; 288:122–125.
7. Sutherland DH, Olshen R, Cooper L, et al. The pathomechanics of gait in Duchenne muscular dystrophy. Dev Med Child Neurol 1981; 23:3–22.
8. Siegel IM, Bernardoni G. Orthotic management of equinus in early Duchenne muscular dystrophy using a supramalleolar tone-balancing orthosis. J Neuro Rehab 1997; 11:1–5.
9. Granata C, Giannini S, Ballestrazzi A, Merlini L. Early surgery in Duchenne muscular dystrophy. Experience at Istituto Ortopedico Rizzoli, Bologna, Italy. Neuromuscul Disord 1994; 4(1):87–88.
10. Forst J, Forst R. Lower limb surgery in Duchenne muscular dystrophy. Neuromuscul Disord 1999; 9(3):176–181.

11. Goertzen M, Baitzer A, Voit T. Clinical results of early orthopaedic management in Duchenne muscular dystrophy. Neuro Paed 1995; 26:257–259.
12. Manzur AY, Hyde SA, Rodillo E, Heckmatt JZ, Bentley G, Dubowitz V. A randomized controlled trial of early surgery in Duchenne muscular dystrophy. Neuromuscul Disord 1992; 2:379–387.
13. Siegel IM. Fractures of long bones in Duchenne muscular dystrophy. J Trauma 1977; 17:219–222.
14. Hsu JD. Extremity fractures in children with neuromuscular disease. Johns Hopkins Med J 1979; 195:89–93.
15. Gray B, Hsu JD, Furumasu J. Fractures caused by falling from a wheelchair in patients with neuromuscular disease. Dev Med Child Neurol 1992; 34:589–592.
16. Spencer GE Jr. Orthopedic care of progressive muscular dystrophy. J Bone Joint Surg 1967; 49a:1201–1204.
17. Spencer GE Jr, Vignos PJ Jr. Bracing for ambulation in childhood progressive muscular dystrophy. J Bone Joint Surg 1962; 44a:234–242.
18. Vignos PJ Jr, Archibald KC. Maintenance of ambulation in childhood muscular dystrophy. J Chronic Dis 1960; 12:273–290.
19. Siegel IM, Miller JE, Ray RD. Subcutaneous lower limb tenotomy in the treatment of pseudohypertrophic muscular dystrophy. J Bone Joint Surg 1968; 50(a):1437–1443.
20. Vignos PJ Jr, Wagner MB, Kaplan JS, Spenser GE. Predicting the success of reambulation in patients with Duchenne muscular dystrophy. J Bone Joint Surg 1983; 65a:719–728.
21. Vignos PJ Jr, Wagner MB, Karlinchak B, Katirji B. Evaluation of a program for long-term treatment of Duchenne muscular dystrophy. J Bone Joint Surg 1996; 78(12):1844–1852.
22. Bakker JP, de Groot IJ, Beckerman H, de Jong BA, Lankhorst GJ. The effects of knee-ankle-foot orthosis in the treatment of Duchenne muscular dystrophy: review of the literature. Clin Rehab 2000; 14:343–359.
23. Smith SE, Green NE, Cole RJ, Robison JD, Fenichel GM. Prolongation of ambulation in children with Duchenne muscular dystrophy by subcutaneous lower limb tenotomy. J Ped Ortho 1993; 13(3):336–340.
24. Bach JR, McKeon J. Orthopedic surgery and rehabilitation for the prolongation of brace-free ambulation of patients with Duchenne muscular dystrophy. Am J Phys Med Rehab 1991; 70(6):323–331.
25. Hsu JD. Surgical treatment of the child with Duchenne muscular dystrophy (DMD). In: Noble J, Galasko CSB, eds. Recent Developments in Orthopaedic Surgery. Manchester: University Press, 1987:135–142.
26. Hsu JD. Management of foot deformity in Duchenne's pseudohypertrophic muscular dystrophy. Orthop Clin North Am 1976; 79:984.
27. Hsu JD, Hoffer MM. Posterior tibial tendon transfer interiorly through the interosseous membrane: a modification of the technique. Clin Orthop 1978; 131:202–204.
28. Greene WB. Transfer versus lengthening of the posterior tibial tendon in Duchenne's muscular dystrophy. Foot Ankle 1992; 13(9):526–531.
29. Sussman M. Duchenne muscular dystrophy. J Am Acad Orthop Surg 2002; 10:138–151.

30. Siegel IM. Compartmental syndrome in Duchenne muscular dystrophy: early evaluation of an epiphenomenon leading to wasting, weakness and contracture. Med Hypothesis 1992; 38:339–345.
31. Siegel IM. Equinocavovarus in muscular dystrophy. Arch Surg 1974; 104:644–646.
32. Siegel IM. Triceps surae tether. Illinois Med J 1981; 160(6):432–435.
33. Siegel IM, Silverman O. Double cylinder plastic orthosis in the treatment of Duchenne muscular dystrophy. Phys Ther 1981; 15:1290–1291.
34. Hsu JD, Jackson R. Treatment of symptomatic foot and ankle deformities in the nonambulatory neuromuscular patient. Foot Ankle 1985; 5:238–244.
35. Siegel IM. Piriformis syndrome in the wheelchair-confined patient with neuromuscular disease. J Neuro Rehab 1993; 7:73–76.
36. Yasuda YL, Bowman K, Hsu JD. Mobile arm supports: criteria for successful use in muscle disease patients. Arch Phys Med Rehabil 1986; 67:253–256.
37. Hsu JD. The natural history of spine curvature progression in the nonambulatory Duchenne muscular dystrophy patient. Spine 1983; 8:771–775.
38. Hsu JD, Hall VM, Swank S, et al. Control of spine curvature in the Duchenne muscular dystrophy (DMD) patient. Orthop Transact 7; 24:1983.
39. Miller F, Moseley CF, Koreska J. Spinal fusion in Duchenne muscular dystrophy. Dev Med Child Neuro 1992; 34:775–786.
40. Bridwell KH, Baldus C, Iffrig TM, Lenke LG, Blanke K. Process measures and patient/parent evaluation of surgical management of spinal deformities in patients with progressive flaccid neuromuscular scoliosis (Duchenne muscular dystrophy and spinal muscular atrophy). Spine 1999; 24(13):1300–1309.
41. Mubarak SJ, Morin WD, Leach J. Spinal fusion in Duchenne muscular dystrophy—fixation and fusion to the sacropelvis? J Pediatr Orthop 1993; 13:752–757.
42. Galasco CS, Delaney C, Morris P. Spinal stabilization in Duchenne muscular dystrophy. J Bone Joint Surg 1992; 74(2):210–214.
43. Heller KD, Wirtz DC, Siebert CH, Forst R. Spinal stabilization in Duchenne muscular dystrophy: principles of treatment in record of 31 operative treated cases. J Pediatr Orthop B 2001; 10(1):18–24.
44. Hopf CG, Eysel P. One-stage versus two-stage spinal fusion in neuromuscular scoliosis. J Pediatr Orthop B 2000; 9(4):234–243.
45. Kennedy JD, Staples AJ, Brook PD, et al. Effect of spinal surgery on lung function in Duchenne muscular dystrophy. Thorax 1995; 50(11):1173–1178.

SECTION IV: EXPERIMENTAL THERAPEUTICS

10

Therapeutic Principles and Challenges in Duchenne Muscular Dystrophy

Dominic J. Wells

Gene Targeting Group, Department of Cellular and Molecular Neuroscience, Division of Neuroscience and Mental Health, Imperial College, Charing Cross Hospital, London, U.K.

INTRODUCTION

The development of therapies for Duchenne muscular dystrophy (DMD) is a daunting task. There are over 640 muscles in the human body and the majority of them are affected in this disorder with the intriguing exception of the extraocular muscles (1). DMD is caused by the absence or dysfunction of dystrophin, a subsarcolemmal protein that links the cytoskeleton of the muscle fiber to the extracellular matrix via proteins associated with the muscle membrane (2–4). Dystrophin attaches to the actin cytoskeleton at its amino terminus and to a series of proteins at its carboxy terminus, including some embedded in the cell membrane, in particular β-dystroglycan. The membrane-associated β-dystroglycan is in turn linked to merosin in the extracellular matrix via α-dystroglycan. Between the amino and carboxy termini, the majority of the dystrophin molecule is arranged as a long rod-like structure. In the absence of dystrophin, the muscle fibers are prone to damage, leading to cycles of muscle fiber necrosis and repair. The muscle damage is associated with fibrosis and loss of muscle fibers as repair fails. Consequently, there is muscle wasting and the development of joint contractures that lead to the loss of independent ambulation between the ages of 7 and 13, and subsequently to premature death from respiratory or cardiac failure. Additionally, not only are the skeletal muscles affected by the lack of dystrophin, but the cardiac and smooth muscles are also involved, and in some patients there is clear evidence of developmental abnormalities in the brain that lead to nonprogressive cognitive defects (5). A milder allelic variant of DMD is Becker muscular dystrophy (BMD). BMD has a very variable presentation, ranging from a DMD-like clinical progression to a much milder condition with significant muscle weakness developing much later in life. Although both conditions are due to mutations in the same gene, the difference in most cases relates to the effect of the mutation on the reading frame of the mRNA. In general, DMD results from mutations that disrupt the reading frame, leading to a failure to generate dystrophin protein. In contrast, BMD mutations generally retain the reading frame leading to the production of an in-frame but internally truncated dystrophin (6). Patients with BMD have been useful in understanding critical regions of the protein structure of dystrophin, and several cases have shown that large regions of the central rod domain part of the protein can be deleted while still retaining significant function of the molecule and thereby causing a mild clinical condition (7,8). Such observations have been important in the development of several of the gene therapy strategies.

The majority of experimental therapeutic approaches have concentrated on the treatment of skeletal muscle involvement, as this is the most marked manifestation of the disorder. These different approaches can be divided into genetic and pharmacological therapies (Table 1) and will be individually reviewed before concluding with an assessment of the current status and future challenges in the effective treatment of this fatal condition.

ANIMAL MODELS

The development of therapeutic strategies for DMD has benefited from the availability of both natural and induced mutations in the animal homologue of the DMD gene. The *mdx* mouse is a natural dystrophin mutant that was first detected in 1984 and was confirmed as the biochemical model of DMD in 1987 (3,9). The *mdx* mouse lacks dystrophin due to a point mutation in exon 23 that leads to a premature stop codon and the production of an unstable dystrophin peptide (10). As a result of this mutation, the muscle fibers are easily damaged and the mouse undergoes cycles of muscle fiber necrosis and regeneration from about two weeks of age (11). Subsequent to the discovery of the *mdx*, a number of additional mutant mice have been created. A series of induced dystrophin mutants were produced by Chapman et al. (12) following administration of a powerful mutagen (5ENU) to C57BL6 male mice, and these were named the mdx^{2cv}, mdx^{3cv}, mdx^{4cv}, and mdx^{5cv}. Each of these mice has a different mutation in the DMD gene, and in the case of the mdx^{3cv}, the mutation eliminates all the isoforms of dystrophin (13). The *mdx* has been crossed with several other gene knockouts to generate

Table 1 A Summary of Different Therapeutic Approaches to DMD

Therapeutic strategy	Detail
Genetic therapies	
Gene repair	Oligonucleotides and PCR products
Altered splicing	Antisense oligonucleotides
Gene delivery–cell transplants	Myoblasts and stem cells
Gene delivery–viral vectors	Retrovirus, lentivirus, adenovirus, adeno-associated virus, and herpes virus-based vectors
Gene delivery–nonviral vectors	Plasmid + physical methods of delivery
Pharmacological therapies	
Read-through	Gentamicin and related compounds
Gene upregulation	Utrophin and other genes
Corticosteroids	Prednisone and deflazacort
Protease inhibitors	Leupeptin
Myostatin	Blockade of inhibition of muscle growth
Supplements	Creatine monohydrate, coenzyme Q10, allopurinol and others

Abbreviation: DMD, Duchenne muscular dystrophy; PCR, polymerase chain reaction.

a mouse model that resembles the clinical course of DMD more closely. These include the *mdx*/utr double knockout and the *mdx*/MyoD double knockout mice (14–16).

The *mdx* mouse has been criticized as a model of DMD as it has a nearly normal lifespan and remains ambulatory throughout. Indeed it can be difficult to note significant differences when observing normal and *mdx* mice in the same cage, at least until the mice are more than 18 months old. Despite the clinical differences, the mouse is a good biochemical model as the lack of dystrophin leads to a failure to localize the other members of the dystrophin-associated protein complex to the muscle fiber membrane. This results in instability of the muscle fiber membrane and muscle necrosis. In contrast to the situation in established DMD pathology, the *mdx* mice show excellent regeneration in the majority of their skeletal muscles and only a limited increase in the density of the extracellular matrix. An important exception to this pattern is the diaphragm (Fig. 1B) which shows muscle fiber loss and increased fibrosis even from an early age (17). It seems possible that this difference in pathology compared to most of the other skeletal muscles may reflect a difference in the activity profile of the diaphragm, and it is notable that other frequently active muscles, such as the soleus, also show fiber loss and marked fibrosis as the mouse ages (18). Irradiation of the limbs of *mdx* mice, which impairs muscle regeneration, also results in muscle pathology that more closely resembles that of DMD (19). It is also

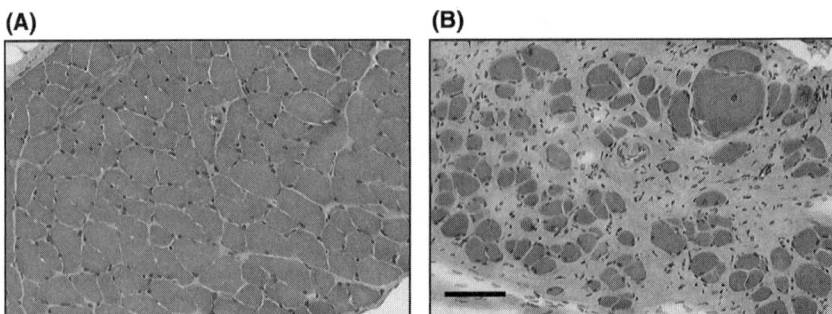

Figure 1 Micrographs of transverse sections of the diaphragm show marked differences between normal and dystrophic (*mdx*) mice. (**A**) The diaphragm of an eighteen-month-old C57BL10 mouse with the typical polygonal regular-sized muscle fibers with little connective tissue between fibers. (**B**) The diaphragm of an eighteen-month-old *mdx* mouse with pathological changes typical of Duchenne muscular dystrophy. The muscles fibers are of irregular size and are separated by marked accumulation of connective tissue and fat. There is evidence of muscle necrosis, regeneration, and inflammation. Scale bar indicates 100 µm.

important to note that the muscle histopathology in the *mdx* does not manifest until the mice are about two weeks old (11). This is in marked contrast to DMD where there is evidence of muscle necrosis in the last trimester of pregnancy (20). Hence experiments in neonatal mice are functionally equivalent to fetal gene therapy in man, a whole area that is subject to substantial ethical concerns (21).

Several cases among cats and dogs have been described that have muscular dystrophy associated with mutations in the species equivalent of the DMD gene (22–24). Feline muscular dystrophy is associated with specific enlargement of the tongue and diaphragm, and the primary complications relate to the intake of food and drink (25). Consequently, the cat has not been widely used as a model of DMD. In contrast, a number of colonies have been established worldwide for the golden retriever muscular dystrophy dog (GRMD, also known as the CXMD). The GRMD dog suffers a marked muscular dystrophy with severe symptoms at six months of age (26). It has been argued that the GRMD dog should be a part of any therapeutic development program because it belongs to a larger species and shows more severe muscle pathology. However, there are problems with this proposal. Unlike the condition in man, affected dogs present with variable symptoms including neonatal death due to massive muscle necrosis. Test treatments in the dog also require the development of canine-specific reagents to prevent the generation of immune responses to proteins from another species. It seems likely that muscular dystrophy due to the lack of dystrophin may arise in other mammalian species, but there have been no cases reported to date.

GENE THERAPEUTIC APPROACHES TO DMD

The underlying cause of the muscle wasting in DMD is the absence of dystrophin. Consequently, the majority of the proposed genetic therapies have aimed to restore expression of a functional version of dystrophin. Experimental approaches to this goal include direct repair of the DMD gene, modification of splicing of the primary transcript to eliminate stop mutations or restore the reading frame through the deletion of specific exons, and gene transfer of recombinant dystrophin cDNAs.

Gene Repair

DNA repair mechanisms are essential elements of a healthy cell. Mutations can arise as a result of the environment or as a consequence of imperfect DNA replication, and many of these are repaired before the problems are manifest. It is possible to direct such repair mechanisms to correct disease-causing mutations in cells in culture by the introduction of homologous sequences with the correct genetic code in the region of mutation (27). This has been demonstrated both in vitro and in vivo for the point mutation in the *mdx* mouse using chimeric RNA/DNA oligonucleotides (chimeraplasts) and PCR products for short fragment homologous recombination (28–30). The chimeraplast approach has also been tested in the GRMD dog (31). However, high efficiencies have only been reported in vitro, as delivery of sufficient amounts of the correcting DNA appears to be a significant limitation in vivo.

Modification of Splicing

An alternative to repairing the gene itself is to modify the splicing of the primary transcript in order to produce a modified mRNA. Splice site donors and acceptors can be blocked by sequence-specific antisense oligonucleotides, as can exonic splicing enhancer sequences (ESEs). A number of studies have demonstrated that this approach can lead to the skipping of mutant exons in both *mdx* and DMD cells in culture (32–34) and the restoration of dystrophin expression (32–36). Importantly, antisense oligonucieotide–directed exon skipping has been shown to work in vivo in the *mdx* mouse and results in the expression of an internally truncated murine dystrophin (37–41). One study has demonstrated an improvement in muscle strength in the *mdx* mouse following treatment, and expression of dystrophin up to three months following a single intramuscular treatment (39). More recently, the same group has shown the production of dystrophin following intravenous administration of antisense oligonucleotide (41). In DMD, such treatments could convert the phenotype to a BMD pathology, the severity of which would depend on which exons were missing from the internally truncated dystrophin. Thus, it has been calculated that this antisense therapy would be applicable to 65% of DMD cases (35). However, as only the mRNA is modified, and the dystrophin produced is only detectable for two to three months, the treatment will need to be repeated at these intervals. By modifying the chemistry of the oligonucleotides, it may be possible to increase the survival of these agents and so increase the period between treatments.

Gene Transfer

The whole body consequences of the transfer of recombinant dystrophin cDNAs have been assessed in transgenic *mdx* mice, an effective form of germ-line gene therapy. A number of studies have demonstrated that expression of full-length or a range of internally truncated dystrophin proteins can prevent the normal development of dystrophic pathology (42). However, the transgenic studies have all involved the expression of dystrophin prior to the onset of pathology in *mdx* mice and so are not informative as to the therapeutic potential of such recombinant dystrophins in muscle that has established dystrophic pathology. One study attempted to resolve this question by using an inducible dystrophin transgene and, although troubled by non-uniform expression of the transgene, appeared to show that the production of dystrophin can be beneficial in damaged muscle (43).

Gene therapy for DMD patients will not involve germ-line gene therapy, but rather requires the specific treatment of affected muscles (somatic gene therapy) and for ethical reasons must avoid the transmission of genetic changes to subsequent generations. The transfer of a functional dystrophin gene into skeletal muscle requires a vector to deliver the DNA to the myofiber. Such vectors can be broadly divided into three categories: cellular, viral, and nonviral.

Cell Transplants

Myogenic cells from the patient (after genetic modification) or from healthy donors can be injected into dystrophic muscles where they should be able to participate in the repair process, and so introduce dystrophin into the repaired muscle fibers. This process was first reported by Partridge et al. (44) in 1989 when they elegantly demonstrated the transfer of genetically matched myoblasts from healthy C57Bl10 mice into congenic *mdx* mice. The transplanted cells fused with the repairing cells to form muscle fibers that expressed dystrophin. This was repeated in other laboratories and then rapidly moved into clinical trials for DMD (45). The trials involved implantations of myoblasts grown in cultures from the biopsies of donors (mostly fathers), but results from these trials were disappointing (46–48). Subsequent investigations have revealed that poor uptake of transplanted cells was probably due to a combination of rapid cell death following delivery, immune responses to the transplanted cells, and possible loss of fusogenic capacity with prolonged culture (49). Although there have been substantial developments in understanding these processes as well as the use of stem cells from other tissues that differentiate to make myoblasts, the major limitation to successful therapeutic use of cell transplantation lies in the need to deliver cells locally to the muscle (50).

There was great excitement in 1998 when Ferrari et al. (51) demonstrated that bone marrow cells could contribute to muscle regeneration. This observation was followed by similar studies in the *mdx* mouse using a selected cell population from the bone marrow (52). However, the efficiencies seen in this study and in subsequent papers were too low to be of therapeutic value (53,54). Examination of a DMD patient who had received a bone marrow transplant for severe combined immunodeficiency (SCID) showed only a little contribution of the donor bone marrow to muscle regeneration (55). Thus bone marrow transplants seem unlikely to offer any therapeutic potential in DMD and have recently been shown to be ineffective in the GRMD dog (56). However, work on a stem cell derived from the dorsal aorta of mice shows that arterial delivery may allow a more efficient approach to cell transplants (57). The use of cells is discussed in greater detail in Chapters 13 and 14.

Viral Vectors for Gene Transfer

Viruses have evolved specifically to introduce the DNA or RNA that they carry into eukaryotic cells in order to replicate. By removing the viral genes required for replication, viruses can be used in the transfer of foreign DNA to effect the genetic modification of cells. To generate recombinant virus, viral genes are provided in trans, usually in the form of a viral packaging cell line. The concerns regarding the earlier generations of viral vectors were that they could recombine with wild-type virus in the patient and that the production systems were prone to the generation of replication competent virus. Such concerns have been largely eliminated through molecular engineering of viral vectors to ensure that residual viral sequences did not show significant homology to wild-type viruses and viral packaging genes provided in trans. [For a recent review of progress and problems with the use of viral vectors in gene therapy, readers are referred to Ref. (58)].

A variety of viral vectors have been tested in skeletal muscles in vivo, including those based on retrovirus, lentivirus, adenovirus, adeno-associated virus, and herpes simplex virus. The major features of these vectors are listed in Table 2 and the advantages and disadvantages of the individual vectors are discussed in the following sections.

Retroviral vectors: The majority of retroviral vectors are based on the murine Moloney leukemia virus. The cell specificity of these oncoretroviral

Table 2 A Summary of the Different Vector Systems for Gene Transfer into Skeletal Muscle

Vector	Genome	Packaging capacity	Inflammatory potential	Status of genome in cell	Main limitations	Main advantages
Retrovirus	RNA	8 kb	Low	Integrated	Only transduces dividing cells. May cause insertional oncogenesis	Persists in dividing cells. Can modify the satellite cell pool
Lentivirus	RNA	8 kb	Low	Integrated	May cause insertional oncogenesis	Transduces nondividing cells so suitable for muscle fibers
Adenovirus	dsDNA	8 kb[a] 30 kb[b]	High	Episomal	Capsid proteins induce a strong inflammatory response	Efficient, particularly in immature muscle
Adeno-associated virus	ssDNA	<5 kb	Low	>90% Episomal <10% Integrated	Small capacity for exogenous DNA	Very efficient and nonpathogenic
Herpesvirus	dsDNA	40 kb[a] 150 kb[c]	High	Episomal	Inflammatory and inefficient passage across connective tissue barriers	Large packaging capacity
Plasmid	DNA	>20 kb	Low	Episomal	Inefficient unless coupled with molecules to aid transfection or aided by physical methods	Vector contains no proteins so does not activate specific immune responses

[a] Replication defective.
[b] Extensively deleted viral genome (Gutted virus).
[c] Amplicon.
Abbreviations: dsDNA, double-stranded deoxyribonucleic acid; ssDNA, single-stranded deoxyribonucleic acid.

vectors is determined by the envelope protein and can be manipulated through the use of different retroviral producer cells that package the retrovirus with alternative envelope proteins (pseudotyping). Gene transfer with oncoretroviral vectors is dependent on cell division for efficient integration. This makes retroviral vectors ideal for the ex vivo treatment of cells from the patient before delivery to the muscle or the blood stream. The effectiveness of these vectors is limited with in vivo delivery, although there is evidence of transduction of some of the cells in the satellite cell pool (59). As retroviruses integrate into the host genome, there is a finite risk of insertional oncogenesis, although this appears to be a rare process except in cases where there is high selective pressure in favor of the transduced cells, as in the X-linked SCID treatments (60). At present, it seems likely that retroviral vectors will only be used in ex vivo gene transfer in DMD. Further considerations for using retroviral vectors for DMD are discussed in Chapter 18.

Lentiviral vectors: Lentiviral vectors are a different type of retroviral vectors that are based on human immunodeficiency virus (HIV) or equine infectious anemia virus (EIAV). Unlike the oncoretroviral vectors, they are able to integrate into nondividing cells such as the myonuclei of muscle fibers. As with the oncoretroviral vectors, different envelope proteins can be used to modify the efficiency and specificity of cell transduction. In vivo lentiviral gene transfer into mature skeletal muscle has been reported in a number of studies, but higher efficiencies of reporter gene expression have been reported following in utero gene transfer (61–66). If lentiviral vectors can also efficiently transduce the satellite cell population as well as the muscle fibers, then the benefits associated with a pool of genetically modified satellite cells might outweigh the risks associated with insertional mutagenesis. However, unless muscle-specific targeting can be achieved, in vivo administration carries a finite risk of insertion into cells of the germ line. As lentiviral vectors have not been as extensively studied as the adenoviral and adeno-associated viral (AAV) vectors, considerably more laboratory studies are required before this vector system can be considered for in vivo gene delivery in DMD.

Adenoviral vectors: A number of viral vectors carrying reporter genes or recombinant dystrophin cDNAs have been tested in the *mdx* mouse. Adenovirus-based vectors are highly efficient in the neonatal mouse, but efficiency falls as the muscle matures. This is due to the decreased expression of the coxsackie/adenoviral receptor (CAR) molecule. Reduced CAR levels can be overcome to some extent by delivering increased viral titers. Residual adenoviral genes present in the earlier generations of adenoviral vectors can also be expressed in some cell types, and this leads to the generation of a strong cellular immune response that can be cytotoxic to the transduced muscle. Such immune response limitations to expression in older mice have been overcome to some extent by the development of adenoviral vectors that have all the viral genes deleted. Gene transfer into mature muscle with these new generation vectors is much more stable than with the earlier generations. The gutted adenoviral vectors also have an increased packaging capacity for exogenous DNA. Early generation vectors were only able to accept a maximum of 8 kb of exogenous DNA, substantially less than the full coding sequence for dystrophin. In contrast, gutted adenoviral vectors can easily accommodate the full-length coding sequence for dystrophin, and indeed require additional "stuffer" DNA for optimal packaging of recombinant vectors. These vectors have shown promise with efficient dystrophin delivery into the muscles of juvenile and adult *mdx* mice and improvement in muscle function (67–69). However, following the relatively recent death of a teenage patient in a gene therapy dose escalation safety trial for ornithine transcarbamylase deficiency using an early generation adenoviral vector, increasing attention has been paid to issues of toxicity associated with adenoviral vectors and they are no longer regarded as the gene transfer vector of choice for all applications (70). Further considerations for using adenoviral vectors for DMD are discussed in Chapter 17.

AAV vectors: AAV vectors have proved to be very efficient in transducing both immature and mature skeletal muscle. However, the packaging capacity for exogenous DNA is limited to approximately 4.9 kb; thus, for dystrophin gene transfer, a highly modified version of the dystrophin cDNA is required. Harper et al. (71) have undertaken a comprehensive analysis of different dystrophin deletions using transgenic mice and have selected a microdystrophin that is capable of maintaining normal muscle structure. AAV-based gene transfer with this construct shows not only the restoration of the normal dystrophin-associated protein complex, but also an apparent stabilization of the muscle with a reduction in the proportion of centrally nucleated muscle fibers at six months compared to that of matched controls at the time of treatment. This suggests that, at least in the mouse, the microdystrophin is highly functional. Several other groups have also demonstrated efficient gene transfer in the mouse using AAV carrying various different microdystrophins and improvement in muscle function following treatment (72–74). AAV has also been used to deliver a short antisense RNA to induce exon skipping (75).

AAV vectors are generally associated with little immune response to the transgene product in comparison to adenoviral vectors, partly because of a reduced tendency to transduce antigen-presenting cells (76,77). Unfortunately, it has been shown that immune responses to transgene products from AAV vectors are enhanced in dystrophic muscles (78,79). Further considerations for using AAV vectors for DMD are discussed in Chapter 19.

Herpesvirus vectors: Herpes simplex virus (HSV) vectors can be used to transfer genes into neonatal mice, but have proved relatively inefficient for the transduction of adult muscle cells in vivo (80–82). This inefficiency appears to be largely due to the size of the virus leading to a failure to pass through the extracellular matrix and to access the muscle cell membrane (83). Thus it seems unlikely that such vectors would be useful in gene therapy for DMD.

Nonviral (Plasmid) Vectors

Nonviral vectors are based on plasmid DNA. A groundbreaking paper published by Wolff et al. (84) showed that naked plasmid DNA was taken up and expressed by muscle fibers after direct intramuscular injection. This was immediately followed by a paper showing that plasmids could be used to transfer recombinant dystrophin cDNAs into *mdx* mouse muscle (85). However, this process was very inefficient with less than 1% of fibers showing dystrophin expression. Recent developments in physical methods of delivery, such as in vivo electroporation, ultrasound, and pressure-mediated vascular delivery, have significantly improved the efficiency of plasmid gene transfer to clinically applicable levels (86–92). Complexing plasmid with block copolymers also enhances the efficiency of gene transfer following intramuscular injection (93). Plasmid DNA has a number of advantages compared to viral vectors: it is easy to manufacture and to control quality; it is easily stored; and as the vector does not contain proteins, it does not invoke specific acquired immune responses to the vector (94).

PHARMACOLOGICAL THERAPEUTIC APPROACHES TO DMD

As noted above, one of major problems of the genetic approach to the treatment of DMD is the need to target all the skeletal muscles. This is considered to be extremely difficult with gene therapy vectors (see Chapter 20). In contrast, pharmacological approaches in which the drug is taken orally or administered parenterally have the potential to treat all the affected muscles. While a gene therapy might be able to treat individual or groups of muscles to maintain function and thereby improve quality of life, pharmacological approaches involving systemic delivery are more likely to globally improve muscle function and thereby increase patient survival. Only one class of drugs, corticosteroids, is in routine clinical use for DMD, but a whole variety of other compounds are being tested, either in the *mdx* mouse or in limited human clinical trials (see Chapters 7 and 11).

Read-Through of Stop Mutations

Stop mutations account for about 5% to 15% of DMD cases. These mutations occur when deletion or substitution of individual DNA bases leads to the formation of a premature stop codon (95). Such signals terminate the translation of the protein, which is then rapidly degraded. In a dramatic study published in 1999, Barton-Davis et al. (96) demonstrated that administration of the aminoglycoside antibiotic gentamicin leads to read-through of the stop mutation in the *mdx* mouse and the production of significant quantities of dystrophin. Although the doses used in the mouse did not cause obvious toxicity, it was well recognized that lower doses could be toxic in man. Using the maximum permitted safe dose in humans, Wagner et al. (97) performed a short-term clinical trial in four DMD boys in the United States. Although they were unable to demonstrate any de novo production of dystrophin or a clear clinical benefit, they did demonstrate a reduction in serum creatine kinase. In contrast, a preliminary study report from a trial in Italy shows dystrophin expression in three out of four patients following treatment (98).

Other groups have been unable to validate the original findings in the *mdx* using gentamicin (99), although this difference may have been due to batch to batch variation in drug composition. PTC Therapeutics has developed a small molecule (PTC124) that appears to read-through stop mutations at much lower doses and with less toxic side effects than gentamiain. It should be noted that stop codons are an essential feature of normal genes and that such drugs may well lead to read-through and the production of abnormal proteins from other genes, althogh this does not appear to be a problem with PTC124. Non-target read-through would be a problem, as treatment will need to be repeated on a regular basis to replenish the dystrophin protein, and there is a possibility that any side effects will build up over time.

Upregulation of Compensating Genes

Transgenic studies using the *mdx* mouse have demonstrated that upregulation of a number of genes might be of benefit in the treatment of DMD. These include nitric oxide synthase, $\alpha 7\beta 1$ integrin, insulin-like growth factor 1, and calpastatin (100–103). The most promising candidate is utrophin, the autosomal homologue of dystrophin. Utrophin is localized to the same membrane complex as dystrophin during development, but as the muscle matures, utrophin becomes localized to the neuromuscular junction (104). Transgenic studies using recombinant utrophin have shown that it can compensate for the lack of dystrophin, and in the case of the full-length coding sequence, it can restore the normal phenotype of the muscles in the mouse (105,106). However, as with the dystrophin transgenics, these beneficial effects of utrophin upregulation are achieved with transgene expression preceding the normal onset of muscle pathology in the *mdx* mouse. Attempts to examine the effect of utrophin expression in pathological muscle through the use of an inducible utrophin transgene have not produced convincing data, due at least in part to the chimeric pattern of expression also seen in the inducible dystrophin transgenics (107,43).

Much is now known about the two major utrophin full-length promoters, and armed with this understanding, a high throughput screen is underway to identify molecules that can upregulate utrophin expression (108–110). Utrophin is also expressed in a wide variety of other tissues, and there were initial fears that upregulating the gene might lead to toxicity in nonmuscle tissues. Constitutive overexpression in a transgenic mouse suggests that this may not be a problem, but it should be noted that the promoter used in this experiment would have been active during embryogenesis, and so compensatory mechanisms may have been induced to counteract the consequences of utrophin overexpression (111). In contrast, a pharmacological approach to upregulate utrophin would be used postnatally, and any such compensating mechanisms either might not be available or might work less efficiently. Despite these concerns, if a drug that specifically upregulated utrophin expression was identified, such a therapy would be likely to make a major impact in the treatment of DMD.

Because utrophin is expressed at the neuromuscular and myotendinous junctions in muscles of DMD patients, it is unlikely to stimulate an immune response. Consequently, it has been proposed that, if it proves impossible to upregulate utrophin pharmacologically, then gene transfer approaches should utilize utrophin rather than dystrophin. There have been a few studies that demonstrate that utrophin can be transferred with the same range of vectors and that this leads to protection against the development of dystrophy and improves the function of dystrophic muscle (112–114). Additional details relating to the role of utrophin in DMD therapy are discussed in Chapter 12.

Corticosteroids

Corticosteroids have been used extensively and there is increasing evidence that they can substantially delay the muscle wasting and hence prolong ambulation (115). However, many reports are from open-label small trials or are anecdotal, and there is considerable variation in the regimes of administration as well as a debate about the relative benefits of prednisone (prednisolone) and deflazacort. There is a clear need for clinical trials that will critically assess the benefit of different treatment regimes, although it is debatable whether it is ethical to use a placebo group in such a trial. The use of steroids in delaying the loss of independent ambulation, even by a couple of years, may significantly reduce the respiratory complications that are associated with prolonged wheelchair use (116). These issues are reviewed in more detail in Chapter 7.

Protease Inhibitors

One of the consequences of dystrophin deficiency is an increase in the fragility of the muscle fiber membrane. This in turn allows the influx of calcium ions that initiate a number of cellular events including activation of proteases leading to further muscle damage. Leupeptin is a small trimeric amino acid that is a specific blocker of calpain, the calcium-activated protease specific to skeletal muscle. Leupeptin administration is reported to decrease the pathological pattern seen in *mdx* muscle and so has been proposed as a treatment for DMD (117). Other protease inhibitors are also being investigated (118).

Myostatin

Myostatin is a negative regulator of muscle growth, and the effects of blocking myostatin were first demonstrated in a knockout mouse, which showed dramatic increases in muscle mass compared to controls (119). Myostatin activity can also be inhibited by blocking its receptor binding using blocking antibodies, propeptide, or pseudoligands. Administration of blocking antibodies to *mdx* mice produced an increased muscle mass, reduced pathology, and an increase in muscle strength (120) as has administration of a propeptide sequence (121). These results suggest that myostatin blockade may help to increase muscle strength in DMD, although enlarging the remaining muscle fibers might make them more vulnerable to damage.

Supplements

There is a range of published studies investigating the potential for metabolic supplements to modify the disease process in DMD. A number of studies have demonstrated promising compounds in the *mdx* mouse (122). However, there are problems in comparing the results of studies in the *mdx* with DMD patients, as the two species commonly receive very different doses. In general, most studies in DMD have demonstrated limited benefit arising from the use of supplements such as creatine monohydrate, coenzyme Q10, or allopurinol (123–126). Current clinical trials are reviewed in Chapter 11.

POTENTIAL PROBLEMS IN TRANSLATING LABORATORY STUDIES INTO CLINICAL TREATMENTS

Many of the therapeutic approaches briefly reviewed above and in more detail elsewhere in this volume are still highly experimental and mostly have been developed in the mouse. There are a number of concerns associated with translating studies in a small, inbred laboratory animal into treatments for young boys with DMD. The most obvious difference is the size of the muscles. Reports from mouse studies commonly concentrate on the anterior tibial and quadriceps muscles, yet these muscles are rarely longer than 1.5 cm. Even at such short lengths, intramuscular injection rarely results in all of the muscle expressing a reporter gene let alone dystrophin. Studies in the much larger muscles of the GRMD dog confirm the limited diffusion of gene vectors injected directly into skeletal muscle (127). Thus treatment of DMD muscle by intramuscular injection will require a grid of injections probably spaced no further than 1 to 2 cm apart. So while intramuscular injections might be used in initial studies to demonstrate that particular vectors are safe in man and can deliver genes effectively, realistic treatments that yield clinical benefit will require delivery via the vasculature. In addition, treatment of individual muscles is unlikely to prove useful to the patient. A clinically valuable treatment will need to treat multiple muscle groups at the same time. Several teams have shown that it is possible to administer viral and nonviral vectors via the arterial route using vasoactive drugs to open up the muscle vascular bed and increase the permeability of the capillaries (91,92,128,129). More recently, efficient intravenous administration of viral and non-viral vectors has been reported (130–133).

The second problem facing clinical trials in man is the immunological response to the vector and the therapeutic gene product. Most of the viral vectors that show promise in murine studies, in particular adenoviral and AAV vectors, are based on viruses that commonly infect man. As a consequence, many people have developed immune responses to previous viral infections, and these pre-existing immune responses may limit the success of any treatment employing these vectors (134). Experiments in mice receiving multiple treatments show that the generation of a vector-specific immune response can reduce the efficiency of subsequent administrations of the same vector, although some studies did not report this problem (135–137). It is possible to use a range of different serotypes of the vector that can avoid this specific immune response, but this is likely to increase the regulatory and toxicity-testing burden of any protocol using viral vector-based gene transfer (138).

Many patients with DMD show a complete absence of dystrophin. Thus, their immune systems may view the de novo expression of dystrophin as a foreign protein following gene transfer, altered splicing, or read-through of stop mutations. This concern is highlighted by the observation of antidystrophin antibodies in DMD patients who have undergone myoblast transplantation and in a BMD patient who had received a cardiac transplant (48,139,140). There have been a number of studies addressing the potential of dystrophin to be immunogenic (141). The results of these studies and the more recent ones are conflicting. In all cases where it has been tested, human dystrophin provokes an immune response in the *mdx* that leads to loss of human dystrophin-positive fibers, unless gene transfer takes place in the early neonatal period (142,143). In contrast, we have noted no immune response to mouse dystrophin on using plasmid gene transfer (144,145). This may be due to the presence of rare dystrophin-positive revertant fibers that arise from endogenous exon skipping and/or the presence of the other isoforms of dystrophin that present much of the central rod domain and carboxy terminal in the *mdx* (146,147). However, other studies have reported immune responses to murine dystrophin (142,148). The presence of viral coat proteins and/or other foreign proteins may play a part in generating these immune responses to murine dystrophin, but the level of antigen presentation might also explain the differences between the different reports. It should also be noted that the *mdx* has a point mutation, and thus endogenous exon skipping can generate practically all the possible immunogenic epitopes of murine dystrophin. In DMD, the majority of mutations involve deletions, and even if endogenous exon skipping produces revertant fibers, these cannot present the full range of potential immunogenic epitopes. Hence, at least some patients are highly likely to generate immune responses to dystrophin gene transfer that involves regions deleted in the patient's dystrophin gene.

A third problem for the initial clinical trials is that the primary concern in early trials will be safety rather than efficacy. Protocols that have worked in laboratory studies may be too invasive when scaled up to human treatment. It is likely that even relatively benign protocols will be administered with reduced doses of the drug or vector system until these can be proved safe. In addition, informed ethical consent for experimental procedures will in most cases require that patients in the initial trials be at least 10 to 15 years old. By the later ages, DMD patients have very little remaining muscle, and it may be difficult to find sufficient muscle for treatment and biopsy to examine the effects of treatment. For maximum efficacy, treatment will need to commence prior to loss of the majority of muscle fibers. Thus, the initial clinical trials are unlikely to demonstrate the true potential of any therapeutic approach.

Finally, it is important to realize that the successful development of many of the proposed treatments will require considerable funds and, therefore, the involvement of commercial companies. But is it commercially viable for companies to develop treatments for DMD? DMD is thought to occur in all racial groups at a frequency in the order of 1 in 3500 male births. In the case of the United Kingdom, this only results in 100 new cases per year. Thus, the market within those countries where patients can afford the likely high cost of therapy is very small. It will not be economical for companies to develop fully approved clinical treatments unless the same therapeutic system can also be used in other diseases. For example, cell therapeutic approaches that are patient-specific are extremely unlikely to find a commercial sponsor. In contrast, development of a drug that can readthrough stop mutations, which occur in a whole range of genetic diseases, is a much more attractive commercial proposition.

CONCLUSIONS

A wide variety of therapeutic approaches are under development for the treatment of DMD. Although many of the genetic treatments offer the possibility of restoring dystrophin expression in dystrophic muscle, and thus correcting all the subsequent downstream events that lead to muscle wasting, they are in general limited to local or regional delivery, and so are more likely at present to provide an improved quality of life rather than increased patient longevity. A clear goal for those groups involved in the development of such therapies is to establish systems for efficient regional delivery to groups of muscles, such as the arms, that will lead to maintainance of function and preservation of a degree of independence for the patient. Intra-arterial pressure–mediated delivery of viral or nonviral vectors carrying recombinant dystrophin or utrophin is a promising development (91,92,128,129). Even more promising are the recents studies showing efficient intravenous delivery to multiple muscles, a much less invasive approach than arterial delivery (130–133).

In contrast, pharmacological approaches involve small compounds that can be given orally or by intravenous injection. As a result, they can reach the majority, if not all, of the affected skeletal muscles. There are a variety of drugs that have been shown to alter the pathological process in the *mdx* mouse, and these may be of benefit in DMD. However, great care needs to be taken when extrapolating from mouse to man, and doses tested in the mouse need to reflect those that can be realistically administered to humans. Recent improvements in antisense therapy leading to exon skipping in the splicing of the primary dystrophin transcript, and the production of internally truncated but functional dystrophin, may avoid many of the limitations on delivery associated with viral and nonviral vector systems (38–41). The small size of the antisense oligonucleotides should enable systemic delivery in a manner akin to the pharmacological therapies noted here. The diaphragm of the *mdx* mouse will serve as a critical assay for the beneficial effects of the systemic delivery of any of the above therapies.

It is commonly stated that there is no effective therapy for DMD. However, advances in medical care, in particular assisted ventilation, and the judicious use of corticosteroids have increased the lifespan of the average patient by 50% over the last 30 years (149). This improvement indicates that DMD is indeed a treatable disease, and the developments in novel therapies reviewed above and in more detail in other chapters of this volume promise additional improvements in longevity and an increased quality of life. However, it will be quite a few years before we are likely to have a cure for this debilitating and deadly genetic disorder. Few, if any, of the proposed treatments being developed at present will be able to do more than halt the course of the disease, and it will be important not to neglect the other aspects of the muscle pathology, in particular the fibrosis that accompanies the muscle damage. Early treatment of those affected will clearly result in the most beneficial outcome, not least because there will be more viable muscle in these patients, but also because the connective tissue proliferation will be less marked. In the long term, the ideal medical management will be early postnatal diagnosis, by tracking creatine kinase levels in blood samples from newborns, and rapid initiation of treatment. When we reach this stage we may well be closer to the cure for this devastating condition.

REFERENCES

1. Kaminski HJ, al-Hakim M, Leigh RJ, Katirji MB, Ruff RL. Extraocular muscles are spared in advanced Duchenne dystrophy. Ann Neurol 1992; 32:586–588.

2. Koenig M, Hoffman EP, Bertelson CJ, Monaco AP, Feener C, Kunkel LM. Complete cloning of the Duchenne muscular dystrophy (DMD) cDNA and preliminary genomic organization of the DMD gene in normal and affected individuals. Cell 1987; 50:509–517.
3. Hoffman EP, Brown RH Jr, Kunkel LM. Dystrophin: the protein product of the Duchenne muscular dystrophy locus. Cell 1987; 51:919–928.
4. Blake DJ, Weir A, Newey SE, Davies KE. Function and genetics of dystrophin and dystrophin-related proteins in muscle. Physiol Rev 2002; 82:291–329.
5. Emery A, Muntoni F. Duchenne Muscular Dystrophy. 3rd ed. Oxford University Press, 2003.
6. Monaco AP, Bertelson S, Liechti-Gallati S, Moser H, Kunkel LM. An explanation for the phenotypic differences between patients bearing partial deletions of the DMD locus. Genomics 1988; 2:90–95.
7. England SB, Nicholson LV, Johnson MA, et al. Very mild muscular dystrophy associated with the deletion of 46% of dystrophin. Nature 1990; 343:180–182.
8. Passos-Bueno MR, Vainzof M, Marie SK, Zatz M. Half the dystrophin gene is apparently enough for a mild clinical course: confirmation of its potential use for gene therapy. Hum Mol Genet 1994; 3:919–922.
9. Bulfield G, Siller WG, Wight PA, Moore KJ. X chromosome-linked muscular dystrophy (*mdx*) in the mouse. Proc Natl Acad Sci USA 1984; 81:1189–1192.
10. Sicinski P, Geng Y, Ryder-Cook AS, Barnard EA, Darlison MG, Barnard PJ. The molecular basis of muscular dystrophy in the *mdx* mouse: a point mutation. Science 1989; 244:1578–1580.
11. Coulton GR, Morgan JE, Partridge TA, Sloper JC. The *mdx* mouse skeletal muscle myopathy: I. A histological, morphometric and biochemical investigation. Neuropathol Appl Neurobiol 1988; 14:53–70.
12. Chapman VM, Miller DR, Armstrong D, Caskey CT. Recovery of induced mutations for X chromosome-linked muscular dystrophy in mice. Proc Natl Acad Sci USA 1989; 86:1292–1296.
13. Cox GA, Phelps SF, Chapman VM, Chamberlain JS. New *mdx* mutation disrupts expression of muscle and nonmuscle isoforms of dystrophin. Nat Genet 1993; 4:87–93.
14. Grady RM, Teng H, Nichol MC, Cunningham JC, Wilkinson RS, Sanes JR. Skeletal and cardiac myopathies in mice lacking utrophin and dystrophin: a model for Duchenne muscular dystrophy. Cell 1997; 90:729–738.
15. Deconinck AE, Rafael JA, Skinner JA, et al. Utrophin-dystrophin-deficient mice as a model for Duchenne muscular dystrophy. Cell 1997; 90:717–727.
16. Megeney LA, Kablar B, Garrett K, Anderson JE, Rudnicki MA. MyoD is required for myogenic stem cell function in adult skeletal muscle. Genes Dev 1996; 10:1173–1183.
17. Stedman HH, Sweeney HL, Shrager JB, et al. The mdx mouse diaphragm reproduces the degenerative changes of Duchenne muscular dystrophy. Nature 1991; 352:536–539.
18. Pastoret C, Sebille A. Further aspects of muscular dystrophy in *mdx* mice. Neuromuscul Disord 1993; 3:471–475.
19. Wakeford S, Watt DJ, Partridge TA. X-irradiation improves mdx mouse muscle as a model of myofiber loss in DMD. Muscle Nerve 1991; 14:42–50.

20. Turkel SB, Howell R, Iseri AL, Chui L. Ultrastructure of muscle in fetal Duchenne's dystrophy. Arch Pathol Lab Med 1981; 105:414–418.
21. Coutelle C, Rodeck C. On the scientific and ethical issues of fetal somatic gene therapy. Gene Ther 2002; 9:670–673.
22. Cooper BJ, Winand NJ, Stedman H, et al. The homologue of the Duchenne locus is defective in X-linked muscular dystrophy of dogs. Nature 1988; 334:154–156.
23. Carpenter JL, Hoffman EP, Romanul FC, et al. Feline muscular dystrophy with dystrophin deficiency. Am J Pathol 1989; 135:909–919.
24. Sharp NJ, Kornegay JN, Van Camp SD, et al. An error in dystrophin mRNA processing in golden retriever muscular dystrophy, an animal homologue of Duchenne muscular dystrophy. Genomics 1992; 13:115–121.
25. Gaschen FP, Hoffman EP, Gorospe JR, et al. Dystrophin deficiency causes lethal muscle hypertrophy in cats. J Neurol Sci 1992; 110:149–159.
26. Valentine BA, Cooper BJ, de Lahunta A, O'Quinn R, Blue JT. Canine X-linked muscular dystrophy. An animal model of Duchenne muscular dystrophy: clinical studies. J Neurol Sci 1988; 88:69–81.
27. Liu L, Parekh-Olmedo H, Kmiec EB. The development and regulation of gene repair. Nat Rev Genet 2003; 4:679–689.
28. Rando TA, Disatnik MH, Zhou LZ. Rescue of dystrophin expression in *mdx* mouse muscle by RNA/DNA oligonucleotides. Proc Natl Acad Sci USA 2000; 97:5363–5368.
29. Bertoni C, Rando TA. Dystrophin gene repair in *mdx* muscle precursor cells in vitro and in vivo mediated by RNA-DNA chimeric oligonucleotides. Hum Gene Ther 2002; 13:707–718.
30. Kapsa R, Quigley A, Lynch GS, et al. In vivo and in vitro correction of the mdx dystrophin gene nonsense mutation by short-fragment homologous replacement. Hum Gene Ther 2001; 12:629–642.
31. Bartlett RJ, Stockinger S, Denis MM, et al. In vivo targeted repair of a point mutation in the canine dystrophin gene by a chimeric RNA/DNA oligonucleotide. Nat Biotechnol 2000; 18:615–622.
32. Takeshima Y, Nishio H, Sakamoto H, Nakamura H, Matsuo M. Modulation of in vitro splicing of the upstream intron by modifying an intra-exon sequence which is deleted from the dystrophin gene in dystrophin Kobe. J Clin Invest 1995; 95:515–520.
33. Dunckley MG, Manoharan M, Villiet P, Eperon IC, Dickson G. Modification of splicing in the dystrophin gene in cultured *Mdx* muscle cells by antisense oligoribonucleotides. Hum Mol Genet 1998; 7:1083–1090.
34. Wilton SD, Lloyd F, Carville K, et al. Specific removal of the nonsense mutation from the mdx dystrophin mRNA using antisense oligonucleotides. Neuromuscul Disord 1999; 9:330–338.
35. van Deutekom JC, Bremmer-Bout M, Janson AA, et al. Antisense-induced exon skipping restores dystrophin expression in DMD patient derived muscle cells. Hum Mol Genet 2001; 10:1547–1554.
36. Takeshima Y, Wada H, Yagi M, et al. Oligonucleotides against a splicing enhancer sequence led to dystrophin production in muscle cells from a Duchenne muscular dystrophy patient. Brain Dev 2001; 23:788–790.

37. Mann CJ, Honeyman K, Cheng AJ, et al. Antisense-induced exon skipping and synthesis of dystrophin in the mdx mouse. Proc Natl Acad Sci USA 2001; 98:42–47.
38. Gebski BL, Mann CJ, Fletcher S, Wilton SD. Morpholino antisense oligonucleotide induced dystrophin exon 23 skipping in *mdx* mouse muscle. Hum Mol Genet 2003; 12:1801–1811.
39. Lu QL, Mann CJ, Lou F, et al. Functional amounts of dystrophin produced by skipping the mutated exon in the mdx dystrophic mouse. Nat Med 2003; 9:1009–1014.
40. Wells KE, Fletcher S, Mann CJ, Wilton SD, Wells DJ. Enhanced in vivo delivery of antisense oligonucleotides to restore dystrophin expression in adult *mdx* mouse muscle. FEBS Lett 2003; 552:145–149.
41. Lu Ql, Rabinowitz A, Chen YC, et al. Systemic delivery of antisense oligoribonucleotide restores dystrophin expression in body-wide skeletal muscles. Proc Natl Acad Sci USA 2005; 102:198–203.
42. Wells DJ, Wells KE. Gene transfer studies in animals: what do they really tell us about the prospects for gene therapy in DMD? Neuromuscul Disord 2002; 12:S11–S22.
43. Ahmad A, Brinson M, Hodges BL, Chamberlain JS, Amalfitano A. *Mdx* mice inducibly expressing dystrophin provide insights into the potential of gene therapy for duchenne muscular dystrophy. Hum Mol Genet 2000; 9:2507–2515.
44. Partridge TA, Morgan JE, Coulton GR, Hoffman EP, Kunkel LM. Conversion of *mdx* myofibres from dystrophin-negative to -positive by injection of normal myoblasts. Nature 1989; 337:176–179.
45. Karpati G, Pouliot Y, Zubrzycka-Gaarn E, et al. Dystrophin is expressed in mdx skeletal muscle fibers after normal myoblast implantation. Am J Pathol 1989; 135:27–32.
46. Gussoni E, Pavlath GK, Lanctot AM, et al. Normal dystrophin transcripts detected in Duchenne muscular dystrophy patients after myoblast transplantation. Nature 1992; 356:435–438.
47. Karpati G, Ajdukovic D, Arnold D, et al. Myoblast transfer in Duchenne muscular dystrophy. Ann Neurol 1993; 34:8–17.
48. Tremblay JP, Malouin F, Roy R, et al. Results of a triple blind clinical study of myoblast transplantations without immunosuppressive treatment in young boys with Duchenne muscular dystrophy. Cell Transplant 1993; 2:99–112.
49. Smythe GM, Hodgetts SI, Grounds MD. Immunobiology and the future of myoblast transfer therapy. Mol Ther 2000; 1:304–313.
50. Goldring K, Partridge T, Watt D. Muscle stem cells. J Pathol 2002; 197:457–467.
51. Ferrari G, Cusella-De Angelis G, Coletta M, et al. Muscle regeneration by bone marrow-derived myogenic progenitors. Science 1998; 279:1528–1530.
52. Gussoni E, Soneoka Y, Strickland CD, et al. Dystrophin expression in the mdx mouse restored by stem cell transplantation. Nature 1999; 401:390–394.
53. Ferrari G, Stornaiuolo A, Mavilio F. Failure to correct murine muscular dystrophy. Nature 2001; 411:1014–1015.
54. Corti S, Strazzer S, Del Bo R, et al. A subpopulation of murine bone marrow cells fully differentiates along the myogenic pathway and participates in muscle repair in the mdx dystrophic mouse. Exp Cell Res 2002; 277:74–85.

55. Gussoni E, Bennett RR, Muskiewicz KR, et al. Long-term persistence of donor nuclei in a Duchenne muscular dystrophy patient receiving bone marrow transplantation. J Clin Invest 2002; 110:807–814.
56. Dell'Agnola C, Wang Z, Strob R, et al. Hematopoietic stem cell transplantation does not restore dystrophin expression in Duchenne muscular dystrophy dogs. Blood 2004; 104:4311–4318.
57. Sampaolesi M, Torrente Y, Innocenzi A, et al. Cell therapy of alpha-sarcoglycan null dystrophic mice through intra-arterial delivery of mesoangioblasts. Science 2003; 301:487–492.
58. Thomas CE, Ehrhardt A, Kay MA. Progress and problems with the use of viral vectors for gene therapy. Nat Rev Genet 2003; 4:346–358.
59. Fassati A, Wells DJ, Sgro Serpente PA, et al. Genetic correction of dystrophin deficiency and skeletal muscle remodeling in adult MDX mouse via transplantation of retroviral producer cells. J Clin Invest 1997; 100:620–628.
60. Kohn DB, Sadelain M, Glorioso JC. Occurrence of leukaemia following gene therapy of X-linked SCID. Nat Rev Cancer 2003; 3:477–488.
61. Kafri T, Blomer U, Peterson DA, Gage FH, Verma IM. Sustained expression of genes delivered directly into liver and muscle by lentiviral vectors. Nat Genet 1997; 17:314–317.
62. Seppen J, Barry SC, Harder B, Osborne WR. Lentivirus administration to rat muscle provides efficient sustained expression of erythropoietin. Blood 2001; 98:594–596.
63. Kang Y, Stein CS, Heth JA, et al. In vivo gene transfer using a nonprimate lentiviral vector pseudotyped with Ross River Virus glycoproteins. J Virol 2002; 76:9378–9388.
64. O'Rourke JP, Hiraragi H, Urban K, Patel M, Olsen JC, Bunnell BA. Analysis of gene transfer and expression in skeletal muscle using enhanced EIAV lentivirus vectors. Mol Ther 2003; 7:632–639.
65. MacKenzie TC, Kobinger GP, Kootstra NA, et al. Efficient transduction of liver and muscle after in utero injection of lentiviral vectors with different pseudotypes. Mol Ther 2002; 6:349–358.
66. Waddington SN, Mitrophanous KA, Ellard FM, et al. Long-term transgene expression by administration of a lentivirus-based vector to the fetal circulation of immuno-competent mice. Gene Ther 2003; 10:1234–1240.
67. DelloRusso C, Scott JM, Hartigan-O'Connor D, et al. Functional correction of adult mdx mouse muscle using gutted adenoviral vectors expressing full-length dystrophin. Proc Natl Acad Sci USA 2002; 99:12,979–12,984.
68. Gilbert R, Dudley RW, Liu AB, Petrof BJ, Nalbantoglu J, Karpati G. Prolonged dystrophin expression and functional correction of *mdx* mouse muscle following gene transfer with a helper-dependent (gutted) adenovirus-encoding murine dystrophin. Hum Mol Genet 2003; 12:1287–1299.
69. Dudley RW, Lu Y, Gillbert R, et al. Sustained improvement of muscle function one year after full-length dystrophin gene transfer into mdx mice by a gutted helper-dependent adenoviral vector. Hum Gene Ther 2004; 15:145–156.
70. St George JA. Gene therapy progress and prospects: adenoviral vectors. Gene Ther 2003; 10:1135–1141.

71. Harper SQ, Hauser MA, DelloRusso C, et al. Modular flexibility of dystrophin: implications for gene therapy of Duchenne muscular dystrophy. Nat Med 2002; 8:253–261.
72. Wang B, Li J, Xiao X. Adeno-associated virus vector carrying human minidystrophin genes effectively ameliorates muscular dystrophy in *mdx* mouse model. Proc Natl Acad Sci USA 2000; 97:13,714–13,719.
73. Fabb SA, Wells DJ, Serpente P, Dickson G. Adeno-associated virus vector gene transfer and sarcolemmal expression of a 144 kDa micro-dystrophin effectively restores the dystrophin-associated protein complex and inhibits myofibre degeneration in nude/*mdx* mice. Hum Mol Genet 2002; 11:733–741.
74. Watchko J, O'Day T, Wang B, et al. Adeno-associated virus vector-mediated minidystrophin gene therapy improves dystrophic muscle contractile function in mdx mice. Hum Gene Ther 2002; 13:1451–1460.
75. Goyenvalle A, Vulin A, Fougerousse F, et al. Rescue of dystrophic muscle through U7 snRNA-mediated exon skipping. Science 2004; 306:1796–1799.
76. Jooss K, Yang Y, Fisher KJ, Wilson JM. Transduction of dendritic cells by DNA viral vectors directs the immune response to transgene products in muscle fibers. J Virol 1998; 72:4212–4223.
77. Jooss K, Chirmule N. Immunity to adenovirus and adeno-associated viral vectors: implications for gene therapy. Gene Ther 2003; 10:955–963.
78. Cordier L, Gao GP, Hack AA, et al. Muscle-specific promoters may be necessary for adeno-associated virus-mediated gene transfer in the treatment of muscular dystrophies. Hum Gene Ther 2001; 12:205–215.
79. Yuasa K, Sakamoto M, Miyagoe-Suzuki Y, et al. Adeno-associated virus vector-mediated gene transfer into dystrophin-deficient skeletal muscles evokes enhanced immune response against the transgene product. Gene Ther 2002; 9:1576–1588.
80. Huard J, Akkaraju G, Watkins SC, Pike-Cavalcoli M, Glorioso JC. LacZ gene transfer to skeletal muscle using a replication-defective herpes simplex virus type 1 mutant vector. Hum Gene Ther 1997; 8:439–452.
81. Akkaraju GR, Huard J, Hoffman EP, et al. Herpes simplex virus vector-mediated dystrophin gene transfer and expression in MDX mouse skeletal muscle. J Gene Med 1999; 1:280–289.
82. Wang Y, Mukherjee S, Fraefel C, Breakefield XO, Allen PD. Herpes simplex virus type 1 amplicon vector-mediated gene transfer to muscle. Hum Gene Ther 2002; 13:261–273.
83. Huard J, Feero WG, Watkins SC, Hoffman EP, Rosenblatt DJ, Glorioso JC. The basal lamina is a physical barrier to herpes simplex virus-mediated gene delivery to mature muscle fibers. J Virol 1996; 70:8117–8123.
84. Wolff JA, Malone RW, Williams P, et al. Direct gene transfer into mouse muscle in vivo. Science 1990; 247:1465–1468.
85. Acsadi G, Dickson G, Love DR, et al. Human dystrophin expression in mdx mice after intramuscular injection of DNA constructs. Nature 1991; 352:815–818.
86. Vilquin JT, Kennel PF, Paturneau-Jouas M, et al. Electrotransfer of naked DNA in the skeletal muscles of animal models of muscular dystrophies. Gene Ther 2001; 8:1097–1107.

87. Gollins H, McMahon J, Wells KE, Wells DJ. High-efficiency plasmid gene transfer into dystrophic muscle. Gene Ther 2003; 10:504–512.
88. Taniyama Y, Tachibana K, Hiraoka K, et al. Development of safe and efficient novel nonviral gene transfer using ultrasound: enhancement of transfection efficiency of naked plasmid DNA in skeletal muscle. Gene Ther 2002; 9: 372–380.
89. Danialou G, Comtois AS, Dudley RW, et al. Ultrasound increases plasmid-mediated gene transfer to dystrophic muscles without collateral damage. Mol Ther 2002; 6:687–693.
90. Lu QL, Liang HD, Partridge T, Blomley MJ. Microbubble ultrasound improves the efficiency of gene transduction in skeletal muscle in vivo with reduced tissue damage. Gene Ther 2003; 10:396–405.
91. Budker V, Zhang G, Danko I, Williams P, Wolff J. The efficient expression of intravascularly delivered DNA in rat muscle. Gene Ther 1998; 5:272–276.
92. Zhang G, Budker V, Williams P, Subbotin V, Wolff JA. Efficient expression of naked DNA delivered intraarterially to limb muscles of nonhuman primates. Hum Gene Ther 2001; 12:427–438.
93. Lu QL, Bou-Gharios G, Partridge TA. Non-viral gene delivery in skeletal muscle: a protein factory. Gene Ther 2003; 10:131–142.
94. Middaugh CR, Evans RK, Montgomery DL, Casimiro DR. Analysis of plasmid DNA from a pharmaceutical perspective. J Pharm Sci 1998; 87:130–146.
95. Roberts RG, Gardner RJ, Bobrow M. Searching for the 1 in 2,400,000: a review of dystrophin gene point mutations. Hum Mutat 1994; 4:1–11.
96. Barton-Davis ER, Cordier L, Shoturma DI, Leland SE, Sweeney HL. Aminoglycoside antibiotics restore dystrophin function to skeletal muscles of *mdx* mice. J Clin Invest 1999; 104:375–381.
97. Wagner KR, Hamed S, Hadley DW, et al. Gentamicin treatment of Duchenne and Becker muscular dystrophy due to nonsense mutations. Ann Neurol 2001; 49:706–711.
98. Politano L, Nigro G, Nigro V, et al. Gentamicin administration in Duchenne patients with premature stop codon. Preliminary results. Acta Myol 2003; 22:15–21.
99. Dunant P, Walter MC, Karpati G, Lochmuller H. Gentamicin fails to increase dystrophin expression in dystrophin-deficient muscle. Muscle Nerve 2003; 27:624–627.
100. Wehling M, Spencer MJ, Tidball JG. A nitric oxide synthase transgene ameliorates muscular dystrophy in *mdx* mice. J Cell Biol 2001; 155:123–131.
101. Burkin DJ, Wallace GQ, Nicol KJ, Kaufman DJ, Kaufman SJ. Enhanced expression of the alpha 7 beta 1 integrin reduces muscular dystrophy and restores viability in dystrophic mice. J Cell Biol 2001; 152:1207–1218.
102. Barton ER, Morris L, Musaro A, Rosenthal N, Sweeney HL. Muscle-specific expression of insulin-like growth factor I counters muscle decline in *mdx* mice. J Cell Biol 2002; 157:137–148.
103. Spencer MJ, Mellgren RL. Overexpression of a calpastatin transgene in *mdx* muscle reduces dystrophic pathology. Hum Mol Genet 2002; 11:2645–2655.
104. Lin S, Burgunder JM. Utrophin may be a precursor of dystrophin during skeletal muscle development. Brain Res Dev Brain Res 2000; 119:289–295.

105. Tinsley JM, Potter AC, Phelps SR, Fisher R, Trickett JI, Davies KE. Amelioration of the dystrophic phenotype of *mdx* mice using a truncated utrophin transgene. Nature 1996; 384:349–353.
106. Tinsley J, Deconinck N, Fisher R, et al. Expression of full-length utrophin prevents muscular dystrophy in mdx mice. Nat Med 1998; 4:1441–1444.
107. Squire S, Raymackers JM, Vandebrouck C, et al. Prevention of pathology in mdx mice by expression of utrophin: analysis using an inducible transgenic expression system. Hum Mol Genet 2002; 11:3333–3344.
108. Perkins KJ, Burton EA, Davies KE. The role of basal and myogenic factors in the transcriptional activation of utrophin promoter A: implications for therapeutic up-regulation in Duchenne muscular dystrophy. Nucleic Acids Res 2001; 29:4843–4850.
109. Chakkalakal JV, Stocksley MA, Harrison MA, et al. Expression of utrophin A mRNA correlates with the oxidative capacity of skeletal muscle fiber types and is regulated by calcineurin/NFAT signaling. Proc Natl Acad Sci USA 2003; 100:7791–7796.
110. Perkins KJ, Davies KE. Ets, Ap-1 and GATA factor families regulate the utrophin B promoter: potential regulatory mechanisms for endothelial-specific expression. FEBS Lett 2003; 538:168–172.
111. Fisher R, Tinsley JM, Phelps SR, et al. Non-toxic ubiquitous over-expression of utrophin in the mdx mouse. Neuromuscul Disord 2001; 11:713–721.
112. Wakefield PM, Tinsley JM, Wood MJ, Gilbert R, Karpati G, Davies KE. Prevention of the dystrophic phenotype in dystrophin/utrophin-deficient muscle following adenovirus-mediated transfer of a utrophin minigene. Gene Ther 2000; 7:201–204.
113. Ebihara S, Guibinga GH, Gilbert R, et al. Differential effects of dystrophin and utrophin gene transfer in immunocompetent muscular dystrophy (mdx) mice. Physiol Genomics 2000; 3:133–144.
114. Cerletti M, Negri T, Cozzi F, et al. Dystrophic phenotype of canine X-linked muscular dystrophy is mitigated by adenovirus-mediated utrophin gene transfer. Gene Ther 2003; 10:750–757.
115. Wong BL, Christopher C. Corticosteroids in Duchenne muscular dystrophy: a reappraisal. J Child Neurol 2002; 17:183–190.
116. Biggar WD, Gingras M, Fehlings DL, Harris VA, Steele CA. Deflazacort treatment of Duchenne muscular dystrophy. J Pediatr 2001; 138:45–50.
117. Badalamente MA, Stracher A. Delay of muscle degeneration and necrosis in *mdx* mice by calpain inhibition. Muscle Nerve 2000; 23:106–111.
118. Sawada H, Nagahiro K, Kikukawa Y, et al. Therapeutic effect of camostat mesilate on Duchenne muscular dystrophy in mdx mice. Biol Pharm Bull 2003; 26:1025–1027.
119. McPherron AC, Lawler AM, Lee SJ. Regulation of skeletal muscle mass in mice by a new TGF-beta superfamily member. Nature 1997; 387:83–90.
120. Bogdanovich S, Krag TO, Barton ER, et al. Functional improvement of dystrophic muscle by myostatin blockade. Nature 2002; 420:418–421.
121. Bogdanovich S, Perkins KJ, Krag TO, Whittemore LA, Khurana TS. Myostatin propeptide-mediated amelioration of dystrophic pathophysiology. FASEB J 2005; 19:543–549.

122. Granchelli JA, Pollina C, Hudecki MS. Pre-clinical screening of drugs using the *mdx* mouse. Neuromuscul Disord 2000; 10:235–239.
123. Walter MC, Lochmuller H, Reilich P, et al. Creatine monohydrate in muscular dystrophies: a double-blind, placebo-controlled clinical study. Neurology 2000; 54:1848–1850.
124. Louis M, Lebacq J, Poortmans JR, et al. Beneficial effects of creatine supplementation in dystrophic patients. Muscle Nerve 2003; 27:604–610.
125. Folkers K, Simonsen R. Two successful double-blind trials with coenzyme Q10 (vitamin Q10) on muscular dystrophies and neurogenic atrophies. Biochim Biophys Acta 1995; 1271:281–286.
126. Thomson WH. Clinical trials of allopurinol in Duchenne muscular dystrophy. Med Hypotheses 1985; 17:175–189.
127. O'Hara AJ, Howell JM, Taplin RH, et al. The spread of transgene expression at the site of gene construct injection. Muscle Nerve 2001; 24:488–495.
128. Greelish JP, Su LT, Lankford EB, et al. Stable restoration of the sarcoglycan complex in dystrophic muscle perfused with histamine and a recombinant adeno-associated viral vector. Nat Med 1999; 5:439–443.
129. Cho WK, Ebihara S, Nalbantoglu J, et al. Modulation of Starling forces and muscle fiber maturity permits adenovirus-mediated gene transfer to adult dystrophic (mdx) mice by the intravascular route. Hum Gene Ther 2000; 11:701–714.
130. Liang KW, Nishikawa M, Liu F, Sun B, Ye Q, Huang L. Restoration of dystrophin expression in mdx mice by intravascular injection of naked DNA containing full-length dystrophin cDNA. Gene Ther 2004; 11:901–908.
131. Hagstrom JE, Hegge J, Zhang G, et al. A facile nonviral method for delivering genes and siRNAs to skeletal muscle of mammalian limbs. Mol Ther 2004; 10:386–398.
132. Blankinship MJ, Gregorevic P, Allen JM, et al. Efficient transduction of skeletal muscle using vectors based on adeno-associated virus serotype 6. Mol Ther 2004; 10:671–678.
133. Wang Z, Zhu T, Qiao C, et al. Adeno-associated virus serotype 8 efficiently delivers genes to muscle and heart. Nat Biotechnol 2005; 23:321–328.
134. Chirmule N, Propert K, Magosin S, Qian Y, Qian R, Wilson J. Immune responses to adenovirus and adeno-associated virus in humans. Gene Ther 1999; 6:1574–1583.
135. Manning WC, Zhou S, Bland MP, Escobedo JA, Dwarki V. Transient immunosuppression allows transgene expression following readministration of adeno-associated viral vectors. Hum Gene Ther 1998; 9:477–485.
136. Parks R, Evelegh C, Graham F. Use of helper-dependent adenoviral vectors of alternative serotypes permits repeat vector administration. Gene Ther 1999; 6:1565–1573.
137. Chirmule N, Xiao W, Truneh A, et al. Humoral immunity to adeno-associated virus type 2 vectors following administration to murine and nonhuman primate muscle. J Virol 2000; 74:2420–2425.
138. Halbert CL, Rutledge EA, Allen JM, Russell DW, Miller AD. Repeat transduction in the mouse lung by using adeno-associated virus vectors with different serotypes. J Virol 2000; 74:1524–1532.

139. Huard J, Roy R, Bouchard JP, Malouin F, Richards CL, Tremblay JP. Human myoblast transplantation between immunohistocompatible donors and recipients produces immune reactions. Transplant Proc 1992; 24:3049–3051.
140. Bittner RE, Shorny S, Streubel B, Hubner C, Voit T, Kress W. Serum antibodies to the deleted dystrophin sequence after cardiac transplantation in a patient with Becker's muscular dystrophy. N Engl J Med 1995; 333:732–733.
141. Wells DJ, Ferrer A, Wells KE. Immunological hurdles in the path to gene therapy for Duchenne muscular dystrophy. Expert Rev Mol Med 2002; 4:1–23.
142. Gilchrist SC, Ontell MP, Kochanek S, Clemens PR. Immune response to full-length dystrophin delivered to DMD muscle by a high-capacity adenoviral vector. Mol Ther 2002; 6:359–368.
143. Ikezawa M, Cao B, Qu Z, et al. Dystrophin delivery in dystrophin-deficient DMD (mdx) skeletal muscle by isogenic muscle-derived stem cell transplantation. Hum Gene Ther 2003; 14:1535–1546.
144. Ferrer A, Wells KE, Wells DJ. Immune responses to dystropin: implications for gene therapy of Duchenne muscular dystrophy. Gene Ther 2000; 7:1439–1446.
145. Ferrer A, Foster H, Wells KE, Dickson G, Wells DJ. Long-term expression of full-length human dystrophin in transgenic mdx mice expressing internally deleted human dystrophins. Gene Ther 2004; 11:884–893.
146. Hoffman EP, Morgan JE, Watkins SC, Partridge TA. Somatic reversion/suppression of the mouse *mdx* phenotype in vivo. J Neurol Sci 1990; 99:9–25.
147. Lu QL, Morris GE, Wilton SD, et al. Massive idiosyncratic exon skipping corrects the nonsense mutation in dystrophic mouse muscle and produces functional revertant fibers by clonal expansion. J Cell Biol 2000; 148:985–996.
148. Ohtsuka Y, Udaka K, Yamashiro Y, Yagita H, Okumura K. Dystrophin acts as a transplantation rejection antigen in dystrophin-deficient mice: implication for gene therapy. J Immunol 1998; 160:4635–4640.
149. Eagle M, Baudouin SV, Chandler C, Giddings DR, Bullock R, Bushby K. Survival in Duchenne muscular dystrophy: improvements in life expectancy since 1967 and the impact of home nocturnal ventilation. Neuromuscul Disord 2002; 12:926–929.

11

Experimental Pharmacologic Therapies in Duchenne Dystrophy: Current Clinical Trials

Shannon L. Venance
Department of Clinical Neurological Sciences, University of Western Ontario, London, Ontario, Canada

Robert C. Griggs
Department of Neurology, University of Rochester Medical Center, Rochester, New York, U.S.A.

INTRODUCTION

Rationale

There is no cure currently available for Duchenne muscular dystrophy (DMD), a devastating and relentlessly progressive X-linked recessive muscle disease with an incidence of 1 in 3500 male births. In this condition, dystrophin is already absent in fetal muscle biopsies and creatine kinase (CK) levels are markedly elevated at birth, signifying active muscle degeneration and regeneration (1–3). Remarkably, affected boys are normal at birth and over the first one or two years of life, with overt clinical weakness often not evident for three or four years. Typically, weakness manifests before five years of age as difficulty in walking, running, or rising from the floor, followed by progression to the use of a wheelchair in the early teens and death due to cardiorespiratory failure in the second or third decade (see Chapter 1).

Despite the absence of dystrophin from all skeletal muscle, there is selective involvement of fast-twitch muscle fibers with relative sparing of the tongue musculature and complete sparing of extraocular muscles in DMD. In addition, the dystrophin-deficient *mdx* mouse and the dystrophin-deficient feline model have hypertrophied muscles, with little or no weakness. Taken together, these observations suggest that although dystrophin deficiency is present, it is not sufficient to cause the progressive weakness and wasting of DMD. The disease pathogenesis remains unknown. Unless molecular therapeutics are proven safe and efficacious, there is, and will continue to be, a need for pharmacological therapies that slow disease progression, improve functional muscle strength, and prolong ambulation. This chapter will briefly explore potential pharmacologic targets (covered in detail in Chapter 3) and discuss the relevance of animal models in clinical studies. The evolution of the clinical trials of corticosteroids in DMD will be highlighted as an early model for trial design. In addition, the rationale behind ongoing clinical trials and selected potential treatment strategies will be reviewed.

Potential Pharmacologic Therapeutic Targets

Dystrophin is a large cytoskeletal protein associated with a number of membrane-associated glycoproteins, forming the dystrophin–glycoprotein complex (DGC) which links the cytoskeleton to the extracellular matrix (4,5). Dystrophin and the DGC provide mechanical stabilization to the muscle fiber membrane, protecting against mechanical injury during contraction (6). The main consequence of dystrophin deficiency is thought to be muscle fiber membrane instability resulting in cycles of degeneration and regeneration until the regenerative capacity is exhausted and progressive weakness ensues (7). More recently, there is evidence to suggest that the DGC is involved in signal transduction pathways with abnormalities in cell survival signaling and in cellular defense cascades involving the neuronal nitric oxide synthase (nNOS), calmodulin, and Grb2 pathways (8). There are many additional secondary biochemical consequences to the primary dystrophin deficiency that are unexplained, such as abnormal calcium handling, abnormal localization of nNOS, metabolic and mitochondrial dysfunction, and muscle fiber necrosis and apoptosis (9–14). Immune responses are enhanced in concordance with the inflammation evident in DMD biopsies: predominantly T lymphocytes and macrophages, both peri/endomysial as well as invading nonnecrotic fibers (15,16). To date, there has been little benefit in translating experimental findings into successful drug therapy trials. Indeed, there are more negative clinical trials than positive clinical trials. Nevertheless, there is room for optimism with the recent rapid advances being made in the understanding of the molecular pathogenesis of dystrophin deficiency giving hope for successful therapies.

Glucocorticoids (See Chapter 7)

Prednisone and deflazacort, an oxazolone derivative of prednisolone, are the only currently available therapies for DMD, and they are not yet universally utilized. There is a rapid onset of action within 10 days, an improvement in functional muscle strength and a sustained slowing of disease progression for up to three years with daily oral prednisone (17,18). Prednisone treatment results in a rapid increase in muscle mass and reduced muscle breakdown (19).

Randomized, placebo-controlled, double-blind clinical trials have shown an improvement in muscle strength within one month, peaking at three months and maintained at six months (17–22). There were no significant differences between the low- and high-dose daily oral prednisone groups (0.75 and 1.5 mg/kg/day) treated for six months. However, there is a dose-dependent effect evident between 0.3 and 0.75 mg/kg/day oral prednisone, and the increase in functional muscle strength was not maintained when the boys were switched to an equivalent dosage, alternate day regimen (17,18,21,26). The most troublesome side effect of steroid treatment is weight gain, with up to a 25% mean increase in body weight in some patients; patients with weight gain had a lesser degree of improvement in muscle strength (27). Other side effects seen in the boys include Cushingoid features, change in behavior, hirsutism, short stature, and cataracts.

Studies with another glucocorticoid, deflazacort, aimed for a similar benefit but with fewer side effects (23–25,28,29). A randomized, double-blind, placebo-controlled trial of deflazacort (2 mg/kg alternate days) in 28 DMD boys with two-year follow-up data demonstrated an improvement in ability to rise from the floor and climb four stairs as well as a 13-month prolongation of independent ambulation in the treated group (24). It is not yet clear whether deflazacort has benefit comparable to prednisone or has lesser side effects (26).

Many questions remain on the use of corticosteroids in the treatment of DMD boys (27). Concern over corticosteroid side effects has limited the use of daily corticosteroids in DMD boys. Various intermittent dosing regimens have been suggested as an alternative to hopefully minimize some of the side effects of prednisone (30–33).

Moreover, many questions remain on the optimal use of corticosteroids and, in particular, on quality of life and risks of long-term side effects. These will need to be answered by well-designed clinical trials, either ongoing (Table 1) or in the future, to determine the best treatment to delay disease progression. There is a need for quality of life assessments as well as for instruments that address caregiver burden. Validated, internationally utilized functional outcome scores that directly measure disability (e.g., loss of ability to rise from the floor and loss of ability to walk) are required. What is the best treatment regimen to use (daily or intermittent pulsed, high

Table 1 Ongoing Clinical Trials

Design	Status	Age (yr)	Ambulatory	Target	Duration (months)	Steroid status	Primary outcome	Principal investigator	Site
Glucocorticosteroids									
Prednisone									
Randomized, unblinded (daily vs. weekly)	Closed	4–11	Ambulatory	60	15	Steroid naive	Muscle strength	D.M. Escolar	CINRMG, CNMC, Washington, D.C., U.S.
Randomized, double-blind, placebo-controlled	Complete	5–8	Yes	—	6	Steroid naive	Timed motor function	E.A.C. Beenakker, J.M. Fock	Arch Neurol 2005; 62:128–132
Prednisolone (intermittent)									
Randomized, double-blind, placebo-controlled	Active	<5	N/A	N/A	N/A	N/A	Muscle strength	A. Manzur	Hammersmith, U.K.
Deflazacort vs. prednisone									
Randomized, multicenter	Closed	>4	Yes	100	24	Steroid naive	Timed motor function; muscle strength	B.F. Reitter	University of Mainz, Germany
Anabolic agents									
Albuterol (β-adrenergic agonist)									
Double-blind, cross-over	Active	6–11	Yes	30	9	None for 3 months prior	Muscle strength and mass	M. Spencer	UCLA, Los Angeles, California, U.S.
Oxandrolone (anabolic steroid)									
Randomized, double-blind, placebo-controlled	Complete	5–10	Yes	51	6	Steroid naive	No benefit	G. Fenichel et al.	Neurol 2001; 56:1075–1079
Nutritional/metabolic supplements									
Creatine monohydrate									
Randomized, double-blind, cross-over	Complete	>8	2/30 nonambulatory	30	4	15/30 on steroids (dfz or pred)	Muscle strength and mass; muscle PCr content	M. Tarnopolsky	Neurol 2004; 62:1771–1777

Drug	Design	Status	Age		N	Duration	Inclusion	Outcome	PI	Site
Creatine monohydrate	Open label	Active	N/A	N/A	N/A	N/A	N/A	N/A	B.F. Reitter	University of Mainz, Germany
Glutamine and creatine	Randomized, double-blind	Closed	5–10	Yes	54	6	Steroid naive	Muscle strength score and QMT performance	DM Escolar et al.	Ann Neurol 2005; 58: 151–155
Coenzyme Q10	Open label, uncontrolled	Closed	5–11	Yes	15	6	Stable on pred or dfz > 6 months	Muscle strength/ safety and efficacy	D.M. Escolar	CINRMG, CNMC, Washington, D.C., U.S.
Mast cell stabilizer/anti-inflammatory										
Oxatomide (KUL0401)	Open label, uncontrolled	Closed	5–10	Yes	15	6	No steroids prior 12 months	Muscle strength/ safety and efficacy	D.M. Escolar; G. Buyse	CINRMG, CNMC, Washington, D.C., U.S.; University Hospitals, Leuven, Belgium
	Open label	Active	N/A	N/A	N/A	N/A	N/A	N/A	J.M. Fock	Groningen, The Netherlands
Stop codon readthrough										
Gentamicin 3	Open label, uncontrolled: stop codons	Closed	5–15	No	36	6	Steroid naive	N/A	J.R. Mendell	Ohio State, Columbus, U.S.
Gentamicin 2	Open label, uncontrolled: deletions	Closed	5–15	Yes	15	Closed	Steroid naive	N/A	J.R. Mendell	Ohio State, Columbus, U.S.
Gentamicin 1	Open label: stop codons	Closed	5–15	Approximately 50%	10	Closed	Steroid naive	N/A	J.R. Mendell	Ohio State, Columbus, U.S.

Abbreviation: PCr, phosphocreatine.

or low dose, prednisone or deflazacort)? When is the optimal time to initiate treatment (at the preclinical stage or in boys with early manifestations)? How long can independent ambulation be sustained? It is possible that once the mechanism of action of corticosteroids is clarified, rational polytherapy with drugs active at different points in the molecular pathophysiology of DMD may be suggested.

PRECLINICAL STUDIES

Animal Models

There are a variety of experimental animal models (mouse, cat, and dog), as well as genetically engineered murine models, used to study muscular dystrophies (34). The *mdx* mouse is the most widely used. The *mdx* mouse has a mild, relatively benign, dystrophic phenotype (35,36). The gene lesion is a premature termination of dystrophin translation resulting in the absence of dystrophin in the sarcolemma caused by a point mutation in the dystrophin gene on the X chromosome (37,38). The *mdx* mouse exhibits a great regenerative capacity with minimal interstitial fibrosis and adipose deposition with no gross impairment of motor functions, and muscle hypertrophy is effective in maintaining absolute force (35,36,39). The diaphragm in the *mdx* mouse, both at rest and after exercise, is more representative of the DMD dystrophic histopathology (40,41). Therefore, it is the exercised *mdx* mouse that manifests more severe weakness and has been used against control mice as a preclinical screening tool to identify drugs that enhance muscle strength (42–44).

One study used the exercised *mdx* mouse to screen 19 compounds: immunosuppressant and anti-inflammatory drugs (prednisone, pentoxifylline, oxatomide, cyclosporine, ebselen, acetaminophen, and ibuprofen), anabolic hormones [insulin-like growth factor (IGF-I) and growth hormone], protease inhibitors (pepstatin, calpain inhibitor-1), metabolites (creatinine, heme arginate), and several amino acids (alanine, glutamine, lysine, cysteine, and serine). Significant improvement was found with anabolic hormones (IGF-I), nutritional supplements (glutamine, creatinine), and the anti-inflammatory immunosuppressants (prednisone, pentoxifylline, oxatomide) (43). There remains a need for further experimental clarification of mechanisms and pathways that these compounds are involved with, and more importantly, regarding benefits, if any, that may be derived by their delivery to dystrophic and control muscles in animal models.

The golden retriever muscular dystrophy dog more closely resembles Duchenne dystrophy in humans, both clinically and pathologically (45,46). However, major phenotypic variability within and between litters as well as the lack of natural history data and reliable endpoints makes this model problematic for study (47,48).

Expression Profiling

Large-scale gene expression analyses are increasingly being used to explore molecular pathophysiology and identify differentially regulated mRNA expression in disease states (49–51). Messenger RNA expression profiles of pooled and individual muscle biopsies from patients with DMD versus normal controls showed significantly more overexpressed than underexpressed genes, possibly reflecting the increased protein turnover rate due to active muscle degeneration and regeneration (14,15,52). There was an overexpression of structural and developmental genes as expected with muscle regeneration in dystrophic muscle and an increase in immune response and extracellular matrix genes reflecting the inflammation and increased connective tissue (15). There was underexpression of genes involved with mitochondrial function and energy metabolism supporting generalized metabolic dysfunction, providing some evidence for metabolic/nutritional supplementation (Table 1) (14). DMD muscle expressed approximately 5% to 10% more of the genes in the genome than did nondystrophic muscle (52). The function of many of these differentially expressed genes is unknown. It remains to be determined, however, whether the alteration in expression reflects primary or secondary changes.

ACTIVE CLINICAL TRIALS

A number of clinical trials (Table 1) in North America and Europe aim at increasing muscle strength and slowing disease progression with an acceptable side-effect profile. High-throughput drug screening in the *mdx* mouse and DNA expression profiling have suggested possible therapies: creatine, coenzyme Q, oxatomide, and glutamine (14,15,43). These are currently being tested in human clinical trials. The rationale for each is given below.

Anabolic Agents That Increase Muscle Strength and/or Mass

β_2-Adrenoceptor Agonists

β_2-Adrenoceptor agonists may increase muscle protein synthesis rate in normal rats and in the *mdx* mouse (53–55). Treatment with clenbuterol, a β_2 agonist available in Europe, increased muscle force production and maximal shortening velocity, although muscle fatigue was increased in experimental animals, and endurance exercise training offset the treatment effects likely due to slow- to fast-twitch fiber type conversion (56,57). Clenbuterol treatment for 20 weeks in the *mdx* mouse did not increase absolute muscle force (58).

In healthy subjects voluntary muscle strength increased with short-term administration of salbutamol or albuterol (59,60). Clenbuterol has been administered to patients with atrophy due to orthopedic causes and used to enhance performance of athletes (61,62). In a short-term, open label pilot study, sustained-release albuterol (high dose, 16.0 mg/day) treatment for three months in 15 adults with facioscapulohumeral muscular dystrophy significantly increased the primary outcome measure, lean body mass determined by dual-energy X-ray absorptiometry (63). Currently, there is a double-blind cross-over design trial assessing the effects of oral albuterol on muscle strength and mass in 6- to 11-year-old ambulatory boys with DMD (Table 1).

Anabolic Corticosteroids

Anabolic corticosteroids have been assessed in the treatment of DMD to avoid the adverse effects of prednisone. Preliminary results suggested that stanozolol might increase muscle protein synthesis in muscular dystrophies (64). Oxandralone, a synthetic testosterone derivative, has been approved for treatment of weight loss. A three-month pilot study in steroid-naive boys with DMD, treated with oral oxandralone (0.1 mg/kg/day), demonstrated a significant improvement in the average muscle score of 0.315 units compared to an expected decline of 0.1 units in natural history controls (65). However, analysis of the RCT of ambulatory boys (age: 5–10 years, mean: 7.5 years) treated with oxandralone ($n = 26$) or placebo ($n = 25$) in a blinded fashion for six months, followed by a 12-month open label extension, failed to reveal any significant difference between the two groups in the primary outcome measure (change in average muscle strength), although there was improvement in the quantitative myometry testing, a secondary outcome measure (66). Oxandralone produced no adverse effects and was well tolerated in the boys with DMD.

Nutritional/Metabolic Supplements

Energy metabolism is impaired in DMD (67,68). Support for nutritional supplementation in DMD is given by the efficacy of supplementation in the rapid-screening exercised *mdx* mouse protocol, reduced metabolic and mitochondrial mRNA expression profiles in DMD biopsies, and small pilot studies using supplementation in patients with DMD or other neuromuscular diseases (14,43,69–72). However, all of the questions raised in the review of glucocorticoids (vide supra) that relate to clinical trial design, validated functional outcomes, appropriate dosing regimens, and pathophysiology are applicable to nutritional supplementation.

Creatine

Patients with DMD have a progressive metabolic deterioration that accompanies their muscle weakness (14,67,68). Creatine monohydrate, 95% residing in skeletal muscle, is produced in the liver and also consumed through meat products. Creatine has a role in skeletal muscle energy metabolism (as an immediate source of energy in the initial seconds of exercise) as a cellular energy buffer (of ATP/ADP) and is present at higher levels in type II muscle fibers. Early animal studies showed reduced creatine concentration in dystrophic muscle (73). Addition of creatine was found to increase phosphocreatine (PCr) in cultured *mdx* myotubes and reduce muscle necrosis in the *mdx* mouse muscle, raising the possibility of therapeutic benefit (74,75).

Young boys with DMD have an elevated intracellular pH and significantly lower intracellular PCr and PCr/Pi ratio compared to age-matched controls (67,68,76). Short-term creatine supplementation (5–10 g/day) has been shown to increase muscle strength and high intensity, but not low intensity, exercise performance in healthy volunteers and in patients with mitochondrial disorders and other neuromuscular diseases (72,77–79). The mechanism of action is unclear, and may be due to increased muscle PCr, enhancement of the ATP/ADP ratio, or perhaps stimulation of protein synthesis. Supplementation (1.5 g/day creatine) for one year in secondary creatine deficiency (gyrate atrophy of the choroid and retina associated with type II muscle fiber atrophy) resulted in a significant increase in the diameter of type II muscle fiber and an increase in body weight (80). A double-blind, placebo-controlled cross-over trial of oral creatine (5–10 g/day) for eight weeks reported mild improvement of muscle strength in 36 patients with a variety of muscular dystrophies, including eight patients with DMD (mean age: 10 years) (71). A single case was reported of a nine-year-old boy with DMD who showed improvement in muscle performance after 155 days of oral creatine (81). Creatine supplementation (3 g/day) for three months improved maximal voluntary contraction of elbow flexion with increased resistance to muscle fatigue and no change in lean body mass in 12 boys with DMD (mean age: 10.8 years; nine wheelchair dependent) (70). Clearly, these were preliminary studies with small samples, short duration, and variable dosages without the statistical power necessary to detect meaningful change, and more definitive trials are needed. The results of two recently completed, randomized, double-blind studies of creatine supplementation in boys with DMD are anticipated in the near future. A European trial is currently recruiting patients (Table 1).

Coenzyme Q10

Coenzyme Q10 (ubiquinone) is localized to the inner mitochondrial membrane, functioning as an essential cofactor of the electron transport chain, accepting electrons from complexes I and II, and transferring them to complex III and supporting ATP synthesis (82). The motivation to supplement with coenzyme Q10 arises from the belief that there may be metabolic, and in particular mitochondrial, dysfunction in diseases involving tissues with large concentrations of mitochondria, such as skeletal muscle. Little published data exist on coenzyme Q10 in the *mdx* mouse, and the impetus for clinical trials in DMD are small studies published on neurodegenerative and mitochondrial diseases (83–88). A larger prospective, randomized, double-blind clinical trial of coenzyme Q10 (300 mg bid) in early Huntington's disease, however, did not alter the primary endpoint, total functional capacity (89).

Patients with myotonic dystrophy have significantly reduced serum coenzyme Q10 levels relative to controls (90). Coenzyme Q10 supplementation for up to eight months in 16 patients with mitochondrial disease increased the serum coenzyme Q10 levels, but did not improve measures of oxidative metabolism (86). There are isolated case reports of benefit with supplementation in patients with a primary muscle coenzyme Q10 deficiency (91–93). Only one of eight patients with mitochondrial disease supplemented with coenzyme Q10 (150 mg/day) showed improvement in the PCr/Pi ratio on muscle magnetic resonance spectroscopy, and despite normalizing the resting venous lactate/pyruvate ratio, there was no improvement in muscle weakness (87,88,94). The support in the literature for the benefit from coenzyme Q10 supplementation in neuromuscular disease is equivocal at best. Dosage of coenzyme Q10 has ranged from 100 mg/day to 300 mg twice daily with little consensus (89,95). Additional studies looking at the scientific rationale for use of coenzyme Q10 specifically in DMD are necessary. Despite the lack of supporting data, recruitment is ongoing for an open-label clinical trial of coenzyme Q10 supplementation in ambulatory boys with DMD who are on a stable regimen of prednisone (Table 1).

Glutamine

Glutamine (10 mg/kg) and alanine were the only two of five amino acids assessed in the rapid screening exercised *mdx* mouse model to demonstrate a significant increase in muscle strength, although the mechanism of action was unclear (43). Concentrations of glutamine and alanine, as well as carnitine, are significantly lower in muscle from DMD patients when compared to controls by high-resolution proton NMR spectroscopy, and oral glutamine supplementation may have a protein-sparing effect in DMD (68,69). More experimental data to establish mechanism of action, dose–response curves, and relevant endpoints would be beneficial. A randomized, double-blind, placebo-controlled trial of glutamine therapy in steroid-naive, 5- to 10-year-old boys with DMD has been completed.

Anti-Inflammatory Agents that Stabilize Mast Cells

H1-Receptor Antagonist (Oxatomide)

Mast cell proliferation and activation have been proposed in the pathogenesis of fibrosis, which are marked in DMD, and may be a factor in the eventual failure of muscle regeneration and the progression of weakness (96–98). Increased numbers of mast cells are found in DMD muscle biopsies (99); content and localization of mast cells correlate with the clinical and histopathological presentation in dystrophin-deficient mice, dogs, and humans (98). Dystrophic muscle in the *mdx* mouse has an increased sensitivity to damage from mast cell histamines and proteases (100,101). Age-dependent differences in mast cells exist in DMD versus normal muscle, although fetal DMD and normal muscle show few non-degranulated mast cells (approximately 30/ mm^2) perivascularly in the perimysium (98). In DMD, beginning at birth, there is a rapid rise in mast cells by age 3 that peaks at age 5, persisting thereafter. The majority of the mast cells in the DMD samples are located in the endomysium, not the perimysium, and are often adjacent to areas of grouped necrosis, in significantly higher numbers (more than 250/mm^2) and with a degranulated, or activated, appearance (98). Two phase II, open-label studies of treatment with the H1-receptor antagonist oxatomide are underway. The primary outcome measures are safety and increase in muscle strength (Table 1).

Stop Codon Read-through and/or Membrane Stabilization

Aminoglycoside Antibiotics

The suppression of genetic mutations by drugs or small molecules, for example, by "skipping" a nonsense mutation or by manufacturing a "sense" codon through insertion of a single amino acid, may lead to functional dystrophin protein. Treatment of cultured cells with premature stop mutations (nonsense mutations) in the cystic fibrosis transmembrane conductance regulator (CFTR) with aminoglycoside antibiotics had previously been shown to restore synthesis of a full-length CFTR (102). The *mdx* mouse dystrophic phenotype arises from a point mutation that causes a premature stop codon (38). Nonsense mutations, causing early termination and absence of dystrophin are also found in 5% to 10% of boys with DMD (103). During a 14-day course of in vitro and in vivo gentamicin in the *mdx* mouse model, normalization of serum creatine kinase levels and 10% to 20% dystrophin positivity in skeletal muscle fibers, sufficient to prevent symptoms in the *mdx* mouse, was demonstrated (104,105). Furthermore, functional protection against mechanical injury in gentamicin-injected *mdx* muscle was demonstrated in isolated whole-muscle preparations using an eccentric contraction protocol (104). These results have led to further investigations in DMD, and are the impetus for the ongoing gentamicin clinical trials (Table 1). Recently, two groups published their collective and unsuccessful efforts to replicate the gentamicin treatment in the *mdx* mouse (106).

There is significant variability in the efficiency of aminoglycoside-induced read-through in cultured human embryo kidney cells which is dependent on the identity of the three different stop codons (UGA > UAG > UAA) and the nucleotide in the position immediately after the stop codon (107). The UAA (A) stop codon mutation, present in the *mdx* mouse and found to be responsive to in vivo aminoglycoside treatment, had the lowest read-through efficiency at approximately 1% suggesting a greater effectiveness of aminoglycoside treatment in DMD as the remaining stop codons showed a greater read-through frequency to treatment (104,107). The reason for the discrepancy between the results obtained in the *mdx* mouse and the tissue culture assay is not clear but may be related to elevated dystrophin mRNA levels.

Early reports in human studies are contradictory. Four Duchenne and Becker muscular dystrophy patients, with a nonsense mutation in the dystrophin gene, treated intravenously with 7.5 mg/kg gentamicin once daily for two weeks, failed to demonstrate any full-length dystrophin in posttreatment muscle biopsies (108). Preliminary results found that three of four DMD patients with the UGA stop codon had dystrophin-positive muscle fibers on biopsy after two six-day cycles of gentamicin (109). The serum CK values, which decreased in patients over the two-week trial period, were felt to be related to altered daily activities within the clinical trial routine, although a membrane stabilization effect has not been ruled out (108). The dose of gentamicin used was not associated with any nephrotoxicity or ototoxicity.

FUTURE DIRECTIONS

There are major barriers to the systemic delivery of gene- and cell-based therapies aimed at correction of dystrophin deficiency. Pharmacologic delivery of small molecules targeted directly to muscle, either alone or in combination with molecular techniques, is an attractive alternative. Rationale combinations of drugs acting through different biochemical pathways (e.g., IGF-I combined with myostatin inhibition to stimulate muscle hypertrophy and obstruct fibrosis; vide infra) may have a synergistic effect on dystrophic muscle. Several of these novel approaches will be briefly reviewed here and utrophin will be covered in Chapter 12.

Myostatin

A new strategy involves myostatin (GDF8), a muscle-specific member of the TGF-β family of growth and differentiation factors, which is highly conserved across species and functions as a negative regulator of skeletal muscle growth (110–112). Myostatin knockout mice and double-muscled cattle due to myostatin mutation have dramatically increased skeletal muscle mass due to hypertrophy or hyperplasia of muscle fibers (110,112,113). Conversely, overexpression of myostatin in Chinese hamster ovary-myostatin tumor–bearing nude mice resulted in considerable wasting (114). Myostatin regulates cell cycle progression of myoblasts by increasing the p21 cyclin–dependent kinase inhibitor which prevents the G_1–S transition (115). Myostatin mRNA levels were found to be significantly reduced in *mdx* mice but not in DMD, which may partially explain the hypertrophic phenotype in the *mdx* mouse (116–118). Functional improvement in muscle mass and strength was demonstrated in the *mdx* mouse with myostatin blocking antibodies and in a myostatin null *mdx* transgene (Fig. 1) (119,120). Weekly intraperitoneal injections of myostatin blocking antibodies for three months in a four-week-old male *mdx* mouse increased body weight, muscle mass, muscle size, and absolute muscle strength (119). A mutation in myostatin has been identified in a child

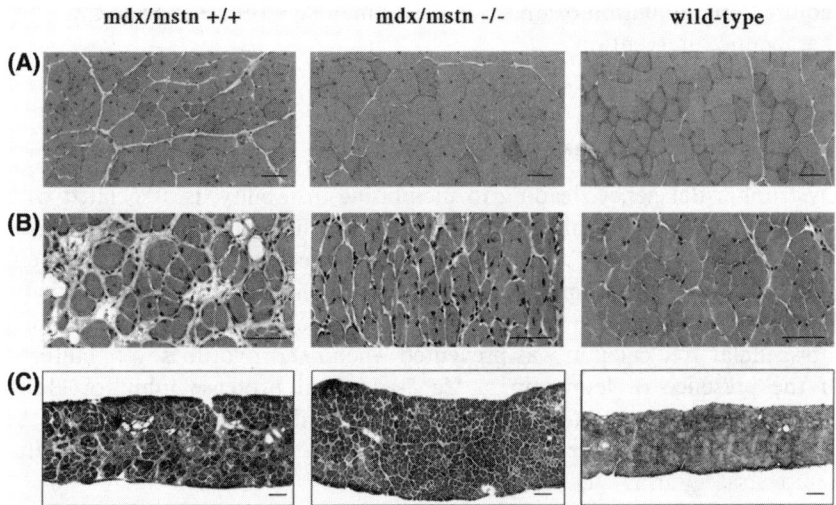

Figure 1 Histopathology of 9 month old mystostatin positive/*mdx* ($Mstn^{+/+}/mdx$), myostatin null/*mdx* ($Mstn^{-/-}/mdx$) and wild-type mice. (**A**) Tibialis muscle; (**B**) and (**C**) diaphragm. Scale bar: (A) and (B), 50 μm; (C), 100 μm. *Source*: From Ref. 120.

with muscle hypertrophy (121). The experimental work highlights the potential of myostatin inhibition as a therapeutic intervention, and clinical trials are currently underway.

Neuronal Nitric Oxide Synthase

Recently, the DGC has been found to be active in transmembrane signal transduction by acting as a scaffold to localize signaling proteins such as nNOS (121–124). nNOS is enriched in the fast-twitch muscle fibers that are selectively affected in DMD (125). Dystrophin deficiency results in loss of nNOS localization to the sarcolemmal membrane (13). nNOS knockout and *mdx* mice as well as boys with DMD have impaired attenuation of vasoconstriction during exercise, which was not seen in children with limb girdle muscular dystrophy and healthy controls (126,127). These findings support a role for nNOS in the regulation of blood flow in normal muscle and muscle ischemia in exercising dystrophic muscle (126). Others, however, have proposed an anti-inflammatory role for nitric oxide (NO) whereby nNOS deficiency promotes muscle damage through macrophage-mediated inflammation rather than ischemia (127). Transgenic restoration of NO production in the *mdx* mouse prevented muscle pathology, reduced serum CK levels, and had no effect on capillary density (127). Although further clarification of the role of nNOS and NO in dystrophin-deficient muscle is required, manipulation of nNOS and NO may be a future consideration for therapeutic intervention.

Calpain Inhibition/Calpastatin

Dystrophin deficiency, leading to membrane instability, is associated with influx of calcium and altered intracellular calcium homeostasis in muscle fibers (9). The influx of Ca^{2+}, perhaps through specific calcium-leak channels, may be involved in the pathogenesis of dystrophic muscle fiber necrosis by activating calcium-dependent proteases (calpains) (10). Elevation in resting intracellular free calcium was prevented when *mdx* myotubes were cultured in the presence of leupeptin, a Ca^{2+}-activated protease inhibitor (128). Calpain activity, reported as both reduced and increased in vivo in the *mdx* mouse, was inhibited by calpeptin and may prove to be a viable therapeutic strategy in DMD (129,130).

Short-term administration of calpeptin/leupeptin to the *mdx* mouse inhibited muscle degeneration, and there was a correlation between increased muscle size and decreased calpain activity (131). Calpastatin, a specific inhibitor of two of three skeletal muscle isoforms of calpain, was overexpressed in a transgenic *mdx* mouse and reduced muscle necrosis without any change in CK levels, providing a rationale for polytherapy using calpastatin possibly combined with a membrane stabilizing/repair compound (132,133).

IGF-I

There may be a role for IGF-I in stimulation of muscle regeneration in DMD. IGF-I stimulates skeletal muscle growth, inducing muscle hypertrophy by satellite cell activation and increased protein synthesis through calcineurin-mediated signaling (134–136). Subcutaneous IGF-I treatment for four weeks in laminin-deficient dystrophic mice improved muscle mass and absolute force with an increase in type IIb and IIa fibers (137). Transgenic mice with IGF-I expression restricted to skeletal muscle by the myosin light chain promoter sustained muscle hypertrophy in senescent skeletal muscle and produced hypertrophy with reduced fibrosis in the diaphragm of the *mdx* mouse (138,139). Transcriptional upregulation of IGF-I and IGF-II and two binding proteins involved in regulation of IGF were found in gene expression profiling studies in dystrophin-deficient DMD muscle (15,52). The gene profiling studies in combination with experimental data lend support to the concept of IGF-I stimulation of satellite cells as a possible therapeutic alternative, either alone or perhaps in combination with delivery of myostatin inhibitors or antibodies, to improve muscle strength and function in DMD (119).

CONCLUSIONS

The field of experimental pharmacologic therapeutics should continue to expand as scientific advancements offer new therapeutic targets to study. Surely the treatment options for DMD will follow, once we more fully understand the basic science underlying the pathophysiology of dystrophin deficiency and the regulation of muscle growth and development.

ACKNOWLEDGMENTS

The authors would like to thank Dr. R.T. Moxley for valuable comments and Drs. J. Kissel and R. Tawil for thoughtful review of the early drafts.

REFERENCES

1. Bieber FR, Hoffman EP, Amos JA. Dystrophin analysis in Duchenne muscular dystrophy: use in fetal diagnosis and in genetic counseling. Am J Hum Genet 1989; 45:362–367.
2. Dellamonica C, Collombel C, Cotte J, Addis P. Screening for neonatal Duchenne muscular dystrophy by bioluminescence measurement of creatine kinase in a blood sample on spotted paper. Clin Chem 1983; 29:161–163.
3. Greenberg CR, Jacobs HK, Nylen E, et al. Gene studies in newborn males with Duchenne muscular dystrophy detected by neonatal screening. Lancet 1988; 8608:425–427.
4. Hoffman EP, Brown RH Jr, Kunkel LM. Dystrophin: the protein product of the Duchenne muscular dystrophy locus. Cell 1987; 51:919–928.
5. Koenig M, Monaco AP, Kunkel LM. The complete sequence of dystrophin predicts a rod-shaped cytoskeletal protein. Cell 1988; 53:219–226.
6. Petrof BJ, Shrager JB, Stedman HH, Kelly AM, Sweeney HL. Dystrophin protects the sarcolemmal from stresses developed during muscle contraction. Proc Natl Acad Sci USA 1993; 90:3710–3714.
7. Mokri B, Engel AG. Duchenne dystrophy: electron microscopic findings pointing to a basic or early abnormality in the plasma membrane of the muscle fiber. Neurology 1975; 25:1111–1120.
8. Rando TA. The dystrophin–glycoprotein complex, cellular signaling, and the regulation of cell survival in the muscular dystrophies. Muscle Nerve 2001; 24:1575–1594.
9. Bodensteiner JB, Engel AG. Intracellular calcium accumulation in Duchenne dystrophy and other myopathies: a study of 567,000 muscle fibers in 114 biopsies. Neurology 1978; 28:439–446.
10. Fong PY, Turner PR, Denetclaw WF, Steinhardt RA. Increased activity of calcium leak channels in myotubes of Duchenne human and mdx mouse origin. Science 1990; 250:673–676.
11. Turner PR, Fong PY, Denetclaw WF, Steinhardt RA. Increased calcium influx in dystrophic muscle. J Cell Biol 1991; 115:1701–1712.
12. Ruegg UT, Gillis JM. Calcium homeostasis in dystrophic muscle. Trends Pharmacol Sci 1999; 20:351–352.

13. Grozdanovic Z, Gosztonyi G, Gossrau R. Nitric oxide synthase I (NOS-I) is deficient in the sarcolemma of striated muscle fibers in patients with Duchenne muscular dystrophy, suggesting an association with dystrophin. Acta Histochem 1996; 98:61–69.
14. Chen Y-W, Zhao P, Borup R, Hoffman EP. Expression profiling in the muscular dystrophies: identification of novel aspects of molecular pathophysiology. J Cell Biol 2000; 151:1321–1336.
15. Haslett JN, Sanoudou D, Kho AT, et al. Gene expression comparison of biopsies from Duchenne muscular dystrophy (DMD) and normal skeletal muscle. Proc Natl Acad Sci USA 2002; 99:15000–15005.
16. Arahata K, Engel AG. Monoclonal antibody analysis of mononuclear cells in myopathies. I. Quantitation of subsets according to diagnosis and sites of accumulation and demonstration and counts of muscle fibers invaded by T cells. Ann Neurol 1984; 16:193–208.
17. Griggs RC, Moxley RT III, Mendell JR, et al. Prednisone in Duchenne dystrophy. A randomized, controlled trial defining the time course and dose response. Arch Neurol 1991; 48:383–388.
18. Fenichel GM, Mendell JR, Moxley RT III, et al. A comparison of daily and alternate-day prednisone therapy in the treatment of Duchenne muscular dystrophy. Arch Neurol 1991; 48:575–579.
19. Rifai Z, Welle S, Moxley RT III, Lorenson M, Griggs RC. Effect of prednisone on protein metabolism in Duchenne dystrophy. Am J Physiol 1995; 268:E67–E74.
20. Mendell JR, Moxley RT, Griggs RC, et al. Randomized, double-blind six-month trial of prednisone in Duchenne's muscular dystrophy. N Engl J Med 1989; 320:1592–1597.
21. Fenichel GM, Florence JM, Pestronk A, et al. Long-term benefit from prednisone therapy in Duchenne muscular dystrophy. Neurology 1991; 41:1874–1877.
22. Griggs RC, Moxley RT III, Mendell JR, et al. Duchenne dystrophy: randomized, controlled trial of prednisone (18 months) and azathioprine (12 months). Neurology 1993; 43:520–527.
23. Mesa LE, Dubrovsky AL, Corderi J, Marco P, Flores D. Corticosteroids in Duchenne muscular dystrophy—deflazacort trial. Neuromuscul Disord 1991; 1:261–266.
24. Angelini C, Pegoraro E, Turella E, Intino MT, Pini A, Costa C. Deflazacort in Duchenne dystrophy: study of long-term effect. Muscle Nerve 1994; 17:386–391.
25. Biggar WD, Gingras M, Feblings DL, Harris VA, Steele CA. Deflazacort treatment of Duchenne muscular dystrophy. J Pediatr 2001; 138:45–50.
26. Manzur AY, Kuntzer T, Pike M, Swan A. Glucocorticoid corticosteroids for Duchenne muscular dystrophy. Cochrane Rev 2004; Issue 2.
27. Bushby K, Muntoni F, Uritzberea A, Hughes R, Griggs R. Report on the 124th ENMC International Workshop Treatment of Duchenne muscular dystrophy; defining the gold standards of management in the use of corticosteroids 2–4 April 2004, Naarden, The Netherlands. Neuromus Dis 2004; 14:526–534.
28. Schara U, Mortier J, Mortier W. Long-term steroid therapy in Duchenne muscular dystrophy—positive results versus side effects. J Clin Neuromusc Dis 2001; 2:179–183.

29. Silversides CK, Webb GD, Harris VA, Biggar DW. Effects of deflazacort on left ventricular function in patients with Duchenne muscular dystrophy. Am J Cardiol 2003; 91:769–772.
30. Sansome A, Royston P, Dubowitz V. Corticosteroids in Duchenne muscular dystrophy; a pilot study of a new low-dosage schedule. Neuromusc Disord 1993; 3:567–569.
31. Connolly AM, Schierbecker J, Renna R, Florence J. High dose weekly oral prednisone improves strength in boys with Duchenne muscular dystrophy. Neuromusc Disord 2002; 12:917–925.
32. Dubowitz V, Kinali M, Main M, Mercure E, Muntoni F. Remission of clinical signs in early Duchenne muscular dystrophy on intermittent low-dosage prednisolone therapy. Eur J Pediatr Neurol 2002; 6:153–159.
33. Kinali M, Mercuri E, Main M, Muntoni F, Dubowitz V. An effective, low-dosage, intermittent schedule of prednisolone in the long-term treatment of early cases of Duchenne dystrophy. Neuromusc Disord 2002; 12:S169–S174.
34. Allamand V, Campbell KP. Animal models for muscular dystrophy: valuable tools for the development of therapies. Hum Mol Genet 2000; 9:2459–2467.
35. Tanabe Y, Esaki K, Nomura T. Skeletal muscle pathology in X chromosome-linked muscular dystrophy (mdx) mouse. Acta Neuropathol (Berl) 1986; 69:91–95.
36. Coulton GR, Morgan JE, Partridge TA, Sloper JC. The mdx mouse skeletal muscle myopathy. I. A histological, morphometric and biochemical investigation. Neuropathol Appl Neurobiol 1988; 14:53–70.
37. Arahata K, Ishiura S, Ishiguro T, et al. Immunostaining of skeletal and cardiac muscle surface membrane with antibody against Duchenne muscular dystrophy peptide. Nature 1988; 333:861–863.
38. Sicinski P, Geng Y, Ryder-Cook AS, Barnard EA, Darlison MG, Barnard PJ. The molecular basis of muscular dystrophy in the *mdx* mouse: a point mutation. Science 1989; 244:1578–1580.
39. Lynch GS, Hinkle RT, Chamberlain JS, Brooks SV, Faulkner JA. Force and power output of fast and slow skeletal muscles from mdx mice 6–28 months old. J Physiol 2001; 535:591–600.
40. Stedman HH, Sweeney HL, Shrager JB, et al. The mdx mouse diaphragm reproduces the degenerative changes of Duchenne muscular dystrophy. Nature 1991; 352:536–539.
41. Brussee V, Tardif F, Tremblay JP. Muscle fibers of *mdx* mice are more vulnerable to exercise than those of normal mice. Neuromuscul Disord 1997; 7:487–492.
42. Hudecki MS, Pollina CM, Granchelli JA, et al. Strength and endurance in the therapeutic evaluation of prednisolone-treated MDX mice. Res Commun Chem Pathol Pharmacol 1993; 79:45–60.
43. Granchelli JA, Pollina C, Hudecki MS. Preclinical screening of drugs using the *mdx* mouse. Neuromuscul Disord 2000:235–239.
44. De Luca A, Pierno S, Liantonio A, Camerino DC. Pre-clinical trials in Duchenne dystrophy: what animal models can tell us about potential drug effectiveness. Neuromusc Disord 2002; 12:S142–S146.
45. Cooper BJ, Winand NJ, Stedman H, et al. The homologue of the Duchenne locus is defective in X-linked muscular dystrophy of dogs. Nature 1988; 334:154–156.

46. Kornegay JN, Tuler SM, Miller DM, Levesque DC. Muscular dystrophy in a litter of golden retriever dogs. Muscle Nerve 1988; 11:1056–1064.
47. Valentine BA, Winand NJ, Pradhan D, et al. Canine X-linked muscular dystrophy as an animal model of Duchenne muscular dystrophy: a review. Am J Med Genet 1992; 42:352–356.
48. Nonaka I. Animal models of muscular dystrophies. Lab Anim Sci 1998; 48:8–17.
49. Greenberg SA, Sanoudou D, Haslett JN, et al. Molecular profiles of inflammatory myopathies. Neurology 2002; 59:1170–1182.
50. Tsukahara T, Tsujino S, Arahata K. cDNA microarray analysis of gene expression in fibroblasts of patients with X-linked Emery–Dreifuss muscular dystrophy. Muscle Nerve 2002; 25:898–901.
51. Sanaudou D, Haslett JN, Kho AT, et al. Expression profiling reveals altered satellite cell numbers and glycolytic enzyme transcription in nemaline myopathy muscle. Proc Natl Acad Sci USA 2003; 100:4666–4671.
52. Bakay M, Zhao P, Chen J, Hoffman EP. A web-accessible complete transcriptome of normal human and DMD muscle. Neuromuscul Disord 2002; 12: S125–S141.
53. Hesketh JE, Campbell GP, Lobley GE, Maltin CA, Acamovic F, Palmer RM. Stimulation of actin and myosin synthesis in rat gastrocnemius muscle by clenbuterol; evidence for translational control. Comp Biochem Physiol C 1992; 102:23–27.
54. Rothwell NJ, Stock MJ. Modification of body composition by clenbuterol in normal and dystrophic (*mdx*) mice. Biosci Rep 1985; 5:755–760.
55. Dupont-Versteegden EE, Katz MS, McCarter RJ. Beneficial versus adverse effects of long-term use of clenbuterol in *mdx* mice. Muscle Nerve 1995; 18:1447–1459.
56. Dodd SL, Powers SK, Vrabas IS, Criswell D, Stetson S, Hussain R. Effects of clenbuterol on contractile and biochemical properties of skeletal muscle. Med Sci Sports Exer 1996; 28:669–676.
57. Lynch GS, Hayes A, Campbell SP, Williams DA. Effects of β_2-agonist administration and exercise on contractile activation of skeletal muscle fibers. J Appl Physiol 1996; 81:1610–1618.
58. Lynch GS, Hinkle RT, Faulkner JA. Power output of fast and slow skeletal muscles of mdx (dystrophic) and control mice after clenbuterol treatment. Exp Physiol 2000; 85:295–299.
59. Martineau L, Horan MA, Rothwell NJ, Little RA. Salbutamol, a beta 2-adrenoceptor agonist, increases skeletal muscle strength in young men. Clin Sci (Lond) 1992; 83:615–621.
60. Caruso JF, Signorile JF, Perry AC, et al. The effects of albuterol and isokinetic exercise on the quadriceps muscle group. Med Sci Sports Exer 1995; 27: 1471–1476.
61. Maltin DA, Delday MI, Watson JS, et al. Clenbuterol, a beta-adrenoceptor agonist, increases relative muscle strength in orthopaedic patients. Clin Sci (Lond) 1993; 84:651–654.
62. Prather ID, Brown DE, North P, Wilson JR. Clenbuterol: a substitute for anabolic corticosteroids? Med Sci Sports Exer 1995; 27:1118–1121.
63. Kissel JT, McDermott MP, Natarajan R, et al. Pilot trial of albuterol in facioscapulohumeral muscular dystrophy. Neurology 1998; 50:1402–1406.

64. Edwards RHT, Dworzak F, Gerber PP, et al. Stanozolol in patients with muscular dystrophy increases muscle protein synthesis measured *in vivo* with stable isotopes. Br J Clin Pharmacol 1985; 19:124–125.
65. Fenichel G, Pestronk A, Florence J, Robison V, Hemelt V. A beneficial effect of oxandrolone in the treatment of Duchenne muscular dystrophy: a pilot study. Neurology 1997; 48:1225–1226.
66. Fenichel GM, Griggs RC, Kissel J, et al. A randomized efficacy and safety trial of oxandrolone in the treatment of Duchenne dystrophy. Neurology 2001; 56:1075–1079.
67. Younkin DP, Berman P, Sladky J, Chee C, Bank W, Chance B. 31P NMR studies in Duchenne muscular dystrophy: age-related metabolic changes. Neurology 1987; 37:165–169.
68. Sharma U, Atri S, Sharma MC, Sarkar C, Jagannathan NR. Skeletal muscle metabolism in Duchenne muscular dystrophy (DMD): an in-vitro proton NMR spectroscopy study. Magn Reson Imaging 2003; 21:145–153.
69. Hankard RG, Hammond D, Morey W, Darmaun D. Oral glutamine slows down whole body protein breakdown in Duchenne muscular dystrophy. Ped Res 1998; 43:222–226.
70. Louis M, Lebacq J, Poortmans JR, et al. Beneficial effects of creatine supplementation in dystrophic patients. Muscle Nerve 2003; 27:604–610.
71. Walter MC, Lochmuller H, Reilich P, et al. Creatine monohydrate in muscular dystrophies: a double-blind, placebo-controlled clinical study. Neurology 2000; 54:1848–1850.
72. Tarnopolsky M, Martin J. Creatine monohydrate increases strength in patients with neuromuscular disease. Neurology 1999; 52:854–857.
73. Fitch CD, Moody LG. Creatine metabolism in skeletal muscle. V. An intracellular abnormality of creatine trapping in dystrophic muscle. Proc Soc Exp Biol Med 1969; 1:219–222.
74. Pulido SM, Passaquin AC, Leijendekker WJ, Challet C, Wallimann T, Regg UT. Creatine supplementation improves Ca^{2+} handling and survival in *mdx* skeletal muscle cells. FEBS Lett 1998; 439:357–362.
75. Passaquin AC, Renard M, Kay L, et al. Creatine supplementation reduces skeletal muscle degeneration and enhances mitochondrial function in *mdx* mice. Neuromuscul Disord 2002; 12:174–182.
76. Kemp GJ, Taylor DJ, Dunn JF, Frostick SP, Radda GK. Cellular energetics of dystrophic muscle. J Neurol Sci 1993; 116:201–206.
77. Harris RC, Soderlund K, Hultman E. Elevation of creatine in resting and exercised muscle of normal subjects by creatine supplementation. Clin Sci (Lond) 1992; 83:367–374.
78. Bosco C, Tihanyi J, Pucspk J, et al. Effect of oral creatine supplementation on jumping and running performance. Int J Sports Med 1997; 18:369–372.
79. Tarnopolsky MA, Roy BD, MacDonald JR. A randomized, controlled trial of creatine monohydrate in patients with mitochondrial cytopathies. Muscle Nerve 1997; 20:1502–1509.
80. Sipila I, Rapola J, Simell O, Vannas A. Supplementary creatine as a treatment for gyrate atrophy of the choroid and retina. N Engl J Med 1981; 304: 867–870.

81. Felber S, Skladal D, Wyss M, Kremser C, Koller A, Sperl W. Oral creatine supplementation in Duchenne muscular dystrophy a clinical and 31P magnetic resonance spectroscopy study. Neurol Res 2000; 22:145–150.
82. Crane FL, Sun IL, Sun EE. The essential functions of coenzyme Q. Clin Investig 1993; 71(suppl 8):S55–S59.
83. Koroshetz WJ, Jenkins BG, Rosen BR, Beal MF. Energy metabolism defects in Huntington's disease and effects of coenzyme Q10. Ann Neurol 1997; 41: 160–165.
84. Shults CW, Haas RH, Beal MF. A possible role of coenzyme Q10 in the etiology and treatment of Parkinson's disease. BioFactor 1999; 9:267–272.
85. Lodi R, Hart PE, Rajagopalan B, et al. Antioxidant treatment improves cardiac and skeletal muscle bioenergetics in patients with Friedreich's ataxia. Ann Neurol 2001; 49:590–596.
86. Matthews PM, Ford B, Dandurand RJ, et al. Coenzyme Q10 with multiple vitamins is generally ineffective in treatment of mitochondrial disease. Neurology 1993; 43:884–890.
87. Gold R, Seibel P, Reinelt G, et al. Phosphorus magnetic resonance spectroscopy in the evaluation of mitochondrial myopathies: results of a 6-month study with coenzyme Q. Eur Neurol 1996; 36:191–196.
88. Chan A, Reichmann H, Kogel A, Beck A, Gold R. Metabolic changes in patients with mitochondrial myopathies and effects of coenzyme Q_{10} therapy. J Neurol 1998; 245:681–685.
89. The Huntington Study Group. A randomize, placebo-controlled trial of coenzyme Q10 and remacemide in Huntington's disease. Neurology 2001; 57: 397–404.
90. Siciliano G, Mancuso M, Tedeschi D, et al. Coenzyme Q10, exercise lactate and CTG trinucleotide expansion in myotonic dystrophy. Brain Res Bull 2001; 56:405–410.
91. Ogasahara S, Engel AG, Frens D, Mack D. Muscle coenzyme Q deficiency in familial mitochondrial encephalomyopathy. Proc Natl Acad Sci USA 1989; 86:2379–2382.
92. Sobreira C, Hirano M, Shanske S, et al. Mitochondrial encephalomyopathy with coenzyme Q sub 10 deficiency. Neurology 1997; 48:1238–1243.
93. Di Giovanni S, Mirabella M, Spinazzola A, et al. Coenzyme Q10 reverses pathological phenotype and reduces apoptosis in familial CoQ10 deficiency. Neurology 2001; 57:515–518.
94. Bresolin N, Bet L, Binda A, et al. Clinical and biochemical correlations in mitochondrial myopathies treated with coenzyme Q10. Neurology 1988; 38:892–899.
95. Folkers K, Simonsen R. Two successful double-blind trials with coenzyme Q10 (vitamin Q10) on muscular dystrophies and neurogenic atrophies. Biochim Biophys Acta 1995; 1271:281–286.
96. Li QY, Raza-Ahmad A, MacAulay MA, et al. The relationship of mast cells and their secreted products to the volume of fibrosis in posttransplant hearts. Transplantation 1992; 53:1047–1051.
97. Aldenborg F, Nilsson K, Jarlshammar B, Bjermer L, Enerback L. Mast cells and biogenic amines in radiation-induced pulmonary fibrosis. Am J Respir Cell Mol Biol 1993; 8:112–117.

98. Gorospe, JRM, Tharp MD, Hinckley J, Kornegay JN, Hoffman EP. A role for mast cells in the progression of Duchenne muscular dystrophy? Correlations in dystrophin-deficient humans, dogs and mice. J Neurol Sci 1994; 122: 44–56.
99. Helliwell TR, Gunhan O, Edwards RH. Mast cells in neuromuscular disease. J Neurol Sci 1990; 98:267–276.
100. Granchelli JA, Hudecki MS, Pollina CM. Enhanced sensitivity of mdx mice to intramuscular injection of compound 48/80. Res Commun Chem Pathol Pharmacol 1994; 84:351–362.
101. Granchelli JA, Pollina C, Hudecki MS. Duchenne-like myopathy in double-mutant mdx mice expressing exaggerated mast cell activity. J Neurol Sci 1995; 131:1–7.
102. Howard M, Frizzell RA, Bedwell DM. Aminoglycoside antibiotics restore CFTR function by overcoming premature stop mutations. Nat Med 1996; 2: 467–469.
103. Prior TW, Bartolo C, Pearl DK, et al. Spectrum of the small mutations in the dystrophin coding region. Am J Hum Genet 1995; 57:22–33.
104. Barton-Davis ER, Cordier L, Shoturma DI, Leland SE, Sweeney HL. Aminoglycoside antibiotics restore dystrophin function to skeletal muscles of *mdx* mice. J Clin Invest 1999; 104:375–381.
105. Phelps SF, Hauser MA, Cole NM, et al. Expression of full-length and truncated dystrophin mini-genes in transgenic mdx mice. Hum Mol Genet 1995; 4: 1251–1258.
106. Dunant P, Walter MC, Karpati G, Lochmuller H. Gentamicin fails to increase dystrophin expression in dystrophin-deficient muscle. Muscle Nerve 2003; 27:624–627.
107. Howard MT, Shirts BH, Petros LM, Flanigan KM, Gesteland RF, Atkins JF. Sequence specificity of aminoglycoside induced stop codon readthrough: potential implications for treatment of Duchenne muscular dystrophy. Ann Neurol 2000; 48:164–169.
108. Wagner KR, Hamed S, Hadley DW, et al. Gentamicin treatment of Duchenne and Becker muscular dystrophy due to nonsense mutations. Ann Neurol 2001; 49:706–711.
109. Politano L, Nigro G, Nigro V, et al. Gentamicin administration in Duchenne patients with premature stop codon. Preliminary results. Acta Myol 2003; 22:15–21.
110. McPherron AC, Lawler AM, Lee SJ. Regulation of skeletal muscle mass in mice by a new TGF-beta superfamily member. Nature 1997; 387:83–90.
111. McLennan IS, Koishi K. The transforming growth-factor-betas: multifaceted regulators of the development and maintenance of skeletal muscles, motoneurons and Schwann cells. Int J Dev Biol 2002; 46:559–567.
112. McPherron AC, Lee SJ. Double muscling in cattle due to mutations in the myostatin gene. Proc Natl Acad Sci USA 1997; 94:12457–12461.
113. Grobet L, Martin LJ, Poncelet D, et al. A deletion in the bovine myostatin gene causes the double-muscled phenotype in cattle. Nat Genet 1997; 17:71–74.
114. Zimmers TA, Davies MV, Koniaris LG, et al. Induction of cachexia in mice by systemically administered myostatin. Science 2002; 296:1486–1488.

115. Thomas M, Langley V, Berry C, et al. Myostatin, a negative regulator of muscle growth, functions by inhibiting myoblast proliferation. J Biol Chem 2000; 275:40235–40243.
116. Zhu X, Hadhazy M, Wehling M, Tidball JG, McNally EM. Dominant negative myostatin produces hypertrophy without hyperplasia in muscle. FEBS Lett 2000; 474:71–75.
117. Tkatchenko AV, Le Cam G, Leger JJ, Dechesne CA. Large-scale analysis of differential gene expression in the hindlimb muscles and diaphragm of *mdx* mouse. Biochim Biophys Acta 2000; 1500:17–30.
118. Tseng BS, Zhao P, Pattison JS, et al. Regenerated *mdx* mouse skeletal muscle shows differential mRNA expression. J Appl Physiol 2002; 93:537–545.
119. Bogdanovich S, Krag TOB, Barton ER, et al. Functional improvement of dystrophic muscle by myostatin blockade. Nature 2002; 420:418–421.
120. Wagner KR, McPherron AC, Winik N, Lee SJ. Loss of myostatin attenuates severity of muscular dystrophy in *mdx* mice. Ann Neurol 2002; 52:832–836.
121. Schuelke M, Wagner KR, Stolz LE, et al. Myostatin mutation associated with gross muscle hypertrophy in a child. NEJM 2004; 350:2682–2688.
122. Kobzik L, Reid MB, Bredt DS, Stamler JS. Nitric oxide in skeletal muscle. Nature 1994; 372:546–548.
123. Brenman JE, Chao DS, Xia H, Aldape K, Bredt DS. Nitric oxide synthase complexed with dystrophin and absent from skeletal muscle sarcolemma in Duchenne muscular dystrophy. Cell 1995; 82:743–752.
124. Webster C, Silberstein L, Hays AP, Blau HM. Fast muscle fibers are preferentially affected in Duchenne muscular dystrophy. Cell 1988; 52:503–513.
125. Thomas GD, Sander M, Lau KS, Huang PL, Stull JT, Victor RG. Impaired metabolic modulation of α-adrenergic vasoconstriction in dystrophin-deficient skeletal muscle. Proc Natl Acad Sci USA 1998; 95:15090–15095.
126. Sander M, Chavoshan B, Harris SA, et al. Functional muscle ischemia in neuronal nitric oxide synthase-deficient skeletal muscle of children with Duchenne muscular dystrophy. Proc Natl Acad Sci USA 2000; 97:13818–13823.
127. Wehling M, Spencer MJ, Tidball JG. A nitric oxide synthase transgene ameliorates muscular dystrophy in mdx mice. J Cell Biol 2001; 155:123–131.
128. Turner PR, Schultz R, Ganguly B, Steinhardt RA. Proteolysis results in altered leak channel kinetics and elevated free calcium in mdx muscle. J Membr Biol 1993; 133:243–251.
129. Spencer MJ, Tidball JG. Calpain concentration is elevated although net calcium-dependent proteolysis is suppressed in dystrophin-deficient muscle. Exp Cell Res 1992; 203:107–114.
130. Alderton JM, Steinhardt RA. Calcium influx through calcium leak channels is responsible for the elevated levels of calcium-dependent proteolysis in dystrophic myotubes. J Biol Chem 2000; 275:9452–9460.
131. Badalamente MA, Stracher A. Delay of muscle degeneration and necrosis in mdx mice by calpain inhibition. Muscle Nerve 2000; 23:106–111.
132. Sorimachi H, Imajoh-Ohmi S, Emori Y, et al. Molecular cloning of a novel mammalian calcium-dependent protease distinct from both m- and mu-types. Specific expression of the mRNA in skeletal muscle. J Biol Chem 1989; 264:20106–20111.

133. Spencer MJ, Mellgren RL. Overexpression of a calpastatin transgene in *mdx* muscle reduces dystrophic pathology. Hum Mol Genet 2002; 11:2645–2655.
134. Engert JC, Berglund EB, Rosenthal N. Proliferation precedes differentiation in IGF-I-stimulated myogenesis. J Cell Biol 1996; 135:431–440.
135. Barton-Davis ER, Shoturma DI, Sweeney HL. Contribution of satellite cells to IGF-I induced hypertrophy of skeletal muscle. Acta Physiol Scand 1999; 167:301–305.
136. Musarò AN, McCullagh KJA, Naya FJ, Olson EN, Rosenthal N. IGF-1 induces skeletal myocyte hypertrophy through calcineurin in association with GATA-2 and NF-ATc1. Nature 1999; 400:581–585.
137. Lynch GS, Cuffe SA, Plant DR, Gregorevic P. IGF-I treatment improves the functional properties of fast- and slow-twitch skeletal muscles from dystrophic mice. Neuromuscul Disord 2001; 11:260–268.
138. Musarò A, McCullagh K, Paul A, et al. Localized Igf-1 transgene expression sustains hypertrophy and regeneration in senescent skeletal muscle. Nat Genet 2001; 27:195–200.
139. Barton ER, Morris L, Musaro A, Rosenthal N, Sweeney HL. Muscle-specific expression of insulin-like growth factor I counters muscle decline in *mdx* mice. J Cell Biol 2002; 157:137–147.

12

Utrophin: The Intersection Between Pharmacological and Genetic Therapy

Kelly J. Perkins
Department of Physiology and Pennsylvania Muscle Institute, University of Pennsylvania School of Medicine, Philadelphia, Pennsylvania, U.S.A.

Kay E. Davies
MRC Functional Genetics Unit, Department of Human Anatomy and Genetics, University of Oxford, Oxford, U.K.

INTRODUCTION

Dystrophin is a member of the spectrin superfamily of proteins and is closely related to the three proteins that constitute the dystrophin-related protein family, including the autosomal homologue, utrophin. The potential of utrophin to functionally compensate for dystrophin has been directly demonstrated in experiments using transgene and viral vector driven utrophin overexpression to ameliorate the dystrophic phenotype in *mdx* muscle (1–6). Thus, one potential approach for therapy of Duchenne muscular dystrophy (DMD) is to increase utrophin levels in muscle by increasing the transcriptional expression via promoter activation. In this chapter, we summarize the data that illustrates utrophin can compensate for the lack of dystrophin in dystrophic muscle, and is thus a desirable target for DMD therapeutic design. We review progress in methodologies for gene delivery, understanding control of endogenous expression, and strategies being utilized in the design and/or discovery of small pharmacological compounds for a utrophin-based upregulation strategy.

THE UTROPHIN GENE AND PROTEIN

Gene Structure

Dystrophin is a member of the spectrin super family of proteins that includes the dystrophin-related protein (DRP) utrophin, DRP2, and dystrobrevin (7–10). Utrophin has attracted particular interest because of its high similarity to dystrophin, at both the gene and protein levels (9,11). The utrophin gene encodes a 13 kb transcript and is localized on human chromosome 6q24 and on the proximal region of mouse chromosome 10 (7,12,13).

The utrophin gene, extending over 900 kb, contains more than 70 exons with an intron/exon structure similar to that of dystrophin, thereby suggesting that the two genes are related by an ancient genomic duplication event (14). Different isoforms of utrophin and dystrophin have been documented. Dystrophin consists of four full-length isoforms driven by different promoters that are expressed in a tissue-specific pattern. But only two full-length isoforms of utrophin have been described (see section "Promoter Studies of Utrophin"), which are designated as utrophin A and B and which differ by 31 amino acids at their N-terminal ends (11,15–18). Utrophin B is mainly expressed in endothelial cells whereas utrophin A is more ubiquitously expressed (19).

Shorter isoforms of both dystrophin and utrophin have been reported, which are driven from independent promoters that lie in the introns toward the C-terminal region of the genes. They are expressed in muscle and non-muscle tissues and have unique 5′ ends (20–24). Because these smaller protein products contain the binding sites for proteins associated with the dystrophin-associated protein complex (DAPC), they are probably linked with the extracellular matrix in non-muscle tissues. The presence of RNA corresponding to the utrophin products has been documented but the corresponding proteins have not been well described (21). Jimenez-Mallebrera et al. (25) have recently reported the presence of short isoforms in brain and testis by using immunocytochemistry, although translation was noted to be relatively inefficient. The functions of these various isoforms are not yet clear.

The actin-binding region of utrophin and dystrophin are very similar but there are some important differences. The first 250 amino acids at the N-terminal end of utrophin form a pair of calponin homology (CH) domains and bind F-actin with an affinity similar to that seen in the equivalent region of dystrophin, although the process is differentially regulated by Ca^{2+}/calmodulin (26–29). Crystallographic studies demonstrate structural similarities between utrophin and dystrophin, but atomic modeling suggests that the CH domain–actin interaction is more complex for dystrophin (30). Dystrophin binds actin in the rod domain but utrophin lacks this sequence (31). Utrophin has a short extension in the N-terminal region that is absent in dystrophin and results in greater binding affinity for actin (29,32,33). The cysteine-rich and C-terminal domains of utrophin show 80% identity with the corresponding domain of dystrophin (34). Not surprisingly, utrophin binds via its C-terminal domain to binding partners similar to that of dystrophin, called the DAPC, which includes dystroglycans, sarcoglycans, and syntrophins (35–38). However, colocalization studies suggest that utrophin associates with α-syntrophin whereas dystrophin associates with β2-syntrophin (39). In nonmuscle tissues, utrophin associates with similar complexes, although these vary between and within tissues (40).

The rod domain of utrophin and dystrophin is the least conserved region in these two proteins and consists of a number of spectrin-like repeats with proline-rich hinge regions (34). This region can be deleted in mildly affected patients and may therefore be under looser evolutionary constraints (41).

Tissue Distribution

Utrophin is expressed in many tissues. In addition to being expressed in the skeletal muscle, it is seen in the tissues of the lung, heart, smooth muscle, and brain and in retinal glial cells, platelets, Schwann cells of the peripheral nerves, and the kidney, in a variety of different complexes with diverse subcellular localization (40,42–49). In muscle, utrophin is found in intramuscular nerves, blood vessels, and myofibers, and is generally restricted to acetylcholine receptor (AChR)–rich crests at the neuromuscular junction (NMJ) in adult muscle, where it binds to components of the DAPC and the myotendinous junctions (36,46,50–53). Although the precise role of utrophin remains unclear, it is thought to play an important role in the structure of the postsynaptic cytoskeleton (54,55). The close association of AChRs and utrophin is found in developing muscle and in muscle cell culture, and utrophin is absent in myasthenias when autoantibodies against the AChR or mutations in the receptor are present (53,56–59).

It has been postulated that utrophin may be the autosomal fetal form of dystrophin because sarcolemmal localization of utrophin is detectable in early human fetal development at 11 weeks (60). At 23 weeks of gestation, utrophin disappears from the sarcolemma and is postnatally substituted by dystrophin. The molecular events giving rise to utrophin downregulation in a maturing muscle are not clear. The localization of utrophin at the sarcolemma in fetal muscle led to the hypothesis that utrophin may be able to functionally compensate for dystrophin in DMD patients, and perform complementing roles in normal functional or developmental pathways in muscle (61). In certain myopathies (including DMD), utrophin is found at the sarcolemma, although this has not been quantified using western blotting (62). Increased sarcolemmal utrophin levels are observed also in inflammatory myopathies (63).

As utrophin is extrasynaptically localized in recently regenerated muscle fibers which express protein isoforms reminiscent of those produced during myogenic development, it has been suggested that utrophin may give some form of structural rigidity to the developing myotubes (2,60,64–66). The presence of utrophin at the sarcolemma in regenerating fibers has been shown to be due to increased levels of utrophin A. However, this increase has been shown to be independent of the regeneration process itself and may be because of the stabilization of utrophin protein in the absence of dystrophin (67). Indeed, the onset of necrosis in *mdx* mice occurs only when the high levels of utrophin present in the fetal and perinatal period decline to the levels that are seen in adults, suggesting a protective role for utrophin in the absence of dystrophin (50). This delayed onset of DMD parallels observations in which high levels of fetal hemoglobin (Hb) at birth can compensate for defective adult Hb for a restricted time in β-thalassemia patients, delaying the onset of symptoms until fetal levels decline (68).

ANIMAL MODELS

Utrophin-Null Mutant Mice

The role of utrophin in muscle has been explored by creating a mutant mouse null for utrophin [*utrn* (54,55)]. An overt phenotype is not shown by *utrn* mice, although a reduction in the number of AChRs at the NMJ and in the postsynaptic folding has been observed. Thus, it has been proposed that utrophin plays a subtle but functionally important role in the stabilization of AChR clustering. A recent study has also suggested that utrophin may protect neurons in the central nervous system (CNS) against pathological insults as *utrn* mutant mice show increased vulnerability to kainite-induced seizures (69). Mild phenotypic changes seen in *mdx* and *utrn* mice may arise from functional redundancy, allowing each to compensate for the absence of the other. This hypothesis is supported by the observation that *utrn–mdx* (*dko*) mice have a very severe myopathic phenotype that can prove fatal within weeks of birth. These mice show many phenotypical signs such as progressive muscle weakness, contractures, and kyphoscoliosis, which are the same as those indicative of DMD (70,71).

Utrophin Overexpression in Muscle Rescues the *mdx* Phenotype

Direct evidence that utrophin could functionally compensate for dystrophin deficiency in muscle was provided in 1997 by the creation of the transgenic mouse line expressing a truncated utrophin transgene, under the control of the constitutive skeletal actin muscle promoter, on an *mdx* background (2).

A dramatic phenotypic improvement was observed, with histochemical analysis illustrating a striking decrease in fibrosis and necrosis, notably in the diaphragm (the most severely affected organ in the mouse model). A reduction in the proportion of myofibers in limb and diaphragm muscles with central nuclei was observed, thereby indicating a reduction in the amount of muscle regeneration compared with control *mdx* mice. In addition, serum creatine kinase (a marker of sarcolemmal permeability and cell damage) was reduced to near control levels. Immunohistology showed that the truncated utrophin protein had localized to the sarcolemma, where components of the DAPC had been restored (2). Several physiological parameters were also improved, including mean normalized tetanic force, force drop after sarcolemmal disruption, eccentric contraction, and Ca^{2+} homeostasis, all of which were also observed in a 1998 study of *mdx* mice expressing a full-length transcript (1,72). Both of the transgenic studies signified that utrophin levels required in a muscle are significantly less than endogenous utrophin levels that are normally observed in lung and kidney, and that the pathology depends on the amount of utrophin expression. The highest expressing lines (approximately 10-fold higher than endogenous levels) were able to affect almost complete phenotypic rescue when bred onto the *mdx* background, both in morphological and physiological tests (72). Quantitative analysis indicated that morphological and functional recovery was achieved with levels of muscle protein expression that were two- to threefold higher than wild-type muscle. This level of expression was about 50% of the normal wild-type level found in the kidney and approximately 25% of the endogenous level in the lung. More recent studies have shown that the overexpression of full-length recombinant utrophin by transgenic means can rescue the defective linkage between costameric actin filaments and the sarcolemma in *mdx* muscle, indicating that utrophin and dystrophin are functionally interchangeable actin binding proteins. Importantly from a potential therapeutic perspective, high-level ubiquitous expression of utrophin has no resultant toxicity (2,70,72–74).

PROMOTER STUDIES OF UTROPHIN

Control of Utrophin Expression

The first utrophin exon identified was non-coding, and separated from the second exon by a short genomic interval (18,75). This transcript was subsequently called "A," as a second independently regulated full-length isoform has been isolated [utrophin B (17)], giving rise to transcripts with unique 5′ exons that splice into a common mRNA at exon 3. Promoter A lies within an unmethylated CpG island at the 5′ end of the gene (14), whereas B resides immediately upstream of the large second exon of utrophin (17). Studies have indicated that although utrophin A and utrophin B are coexpressed, they are differentially regulated, responsive to different stimuli, and have distinct expression patterns (19,76). For example, in skeletal muscle, utrophin transcripts originating from the A promoter are located at the NMJ, while transcripts from the B promoter seem to be confined to endomysial capillaries and other blood vessels (19). This section will focus on current knowledge of the structure of the two promoters and transcriptional processes that command, control, and confer expression, including post-transcriptional mechanisms and *cis*-acting enhancer regions.

The Utrophin A Promoter

The initial observation that utrophin localizes to the NMJ indicated that at least one full-length promoter region may have the capacity to regulate transcription in a manner similar to synaptically expressed genes such as the AChR δ subunit, which is regulated during muscle cell differentiation and localized specifically at the NMJ (77). The genomic region surrounding utrophin A showed striking similarities; the first exon is untranslated, is transcribed from multiple start sites, lies within a CpG island, and shows an absence of TATA and CCAT motifs that are common to eukaryotic promoters (14,18). The minimal promoter element was identified (155 bp), and with the first exon the 900 bp upstream displays only 66% sequence conservation between human and mouse. Further definition of the core element revealed conserved cognate sequences for CG box binding transcription factors such as Ap2, Sp1, and Sp3, of which Ap2 and Sp1 have been implicated in optimal basal activity (18,78). The importance of these ubiquitously expressed factors in conferring a specific expression profile will be further discussed in the sections below.

Initial characterization of the utrophin A promoter by Dennis et al. (18) included the isolation of two important motifs within a 1 kb region upstream of the core promoter element. A consensus E-box (defined by the nucleotides CANNTG) is conserved between both species and is a helix-loop-helix factor–binding site involved in regulating muscle gene expression (79). In addition, the human and mouse utrophin 5′–flanking region contain the core sequence of the N-box (TTCCGG), an element shown to restrict the expression of the AChR δ subunit gene to the NMJ by enhancing expression at the endplate and by hypothetically acting as a silencer in extrajunctional areas. The N-box motif is also present in other AChR subunits and regulates the synaptic expression of at least some of these genes (77). The N-box is located at differing sites in the human and mouse utrophin sequence, which is consistent with previous observations that this motif is not necessarily conserved between the same AChR subunit gene in different species or between different subunit genes of the same species (77). The presence of both N- and E-motifs indicates that expression of the A transcript is subject to regulatory mechanisms similar to those previously described for other synaptic proteins such as the AChR during myogenic differentiation (80–86). In addition to this, a functional nuclear factor-activated T cell (NFAT) motif that has recently been delineated may be responsible for differential expression of this isoform, according to fiber type or response to oxidative capacity (76). The salient features of utrophin A promoter regulation as currently understood are summarized below and illustrated in (Fig. 1).

Synaptic Regulation Via the N-box

Expression of utrophin at the NMJ in adult muscle is partially attributable to enhanced transcription of the subsynaptic nuclei upon innervation, similar to the AChR receptor δ and ε subunit genes, which encode protein components essential for NMJ structure and function (77,87,88). The signaling cascade and binding factors, which lead to N-box dependent synaptic expression, appear conserved among genes expressed at the NMJ, and are thought to initiate the heregulin-elicited stimulation of Erk (and Jnk) MAP kinases, allowing phosphorylation of the ETS-related growth-associated binding protein (GABP) α/β class of transcription factors [although phosphorylation of the α subunit is essential, β-phosphorylation appears to be dispensable (89)]. The properties of the N-box motif present in the utrophin 5′ UTR were investigated and illustrated that utrophin experiences an N-box–mediated transcriptional response to heregulin and specifically to GABP, in vitro (90,91). GABP phosphorylation is thought to either aid interaction of the GABP complex with the overlapping utrophin N-box or ETS binding site (EBS; TTC*CGGA*; EBS italicized), or influence its ability to modify transcription (92,93). Initially, a reporter gene driven by a 1.3 kb promoter A fragment (containing the N-box) was preferentially expressed at postsynaptic nuclei in adult muscle (90). In vitro transcriptional activity by heregulin was abolished through N-box mutagenesis; overexpression of heregulin or GABP (α or β) in myotubes cultured from mice and human tissues caused an N-box–dependent increase in promoter activity, with a resultant 2.5-fold increase in utrophin mRNA levels, and protein–DNA assays performed with muscle extracts directly implicated GABP binding at the N-box. These findings were confirmed in vivo through direct gene transfer.

Importantly, interactions at the N-box are also modulated by interaction with elements bound to the core promoter element. This has been illustrated with Sp1 and Sp3, zinc finger-containing transcription factors which are able to cooperate with GABP α/β at the N-box to stimulate the utrophin promoter (94–96). Synergistic interaction between the Sp and ETS factors in muscle cells may be critical for the regulation of the utrophin promoter (96). As heregulin and GABP α/β are able to confer transcriptional activation of the utrophin A isoform in cultured muscle cells, upregulating in vivo endogenous A transcript in dystrophin-deficient muscle appears a promising therapeutic strategy (90,92). Conversely, the utrophin A promoter may be subject to transcriptional downregulation by repressors recognizing the

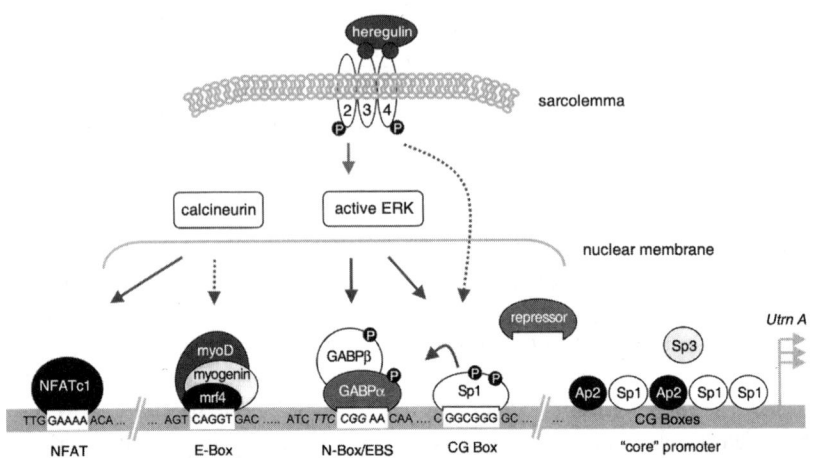

Figure 1 Transcriptional interactions identified within the human utrophin A promoter depicting current knowledge on transcriptional activation of the utrophin A isoform. The diagram shows the A promoter in interactive sections; the 1 kb upstream region containing the N- and E-boxes and the NFATc1 response region, and the core promoter element. For the core element, the binding ability of Ap2 and Sp1/3 has been demonstrated using a number of in vitro methods. Core promoter activity has been shown with Sp1, whereas Sp3 binds identical sites and is also implicated in interacting with GABP at the N-box. [*Note*: the binding site(s) of the Sp1/3 factors that associate with GABP are not confirmed]. The 1 kb region upstream of the core element of the A promoter contains an N-box that binds the ETS-related transcription factors GABPα/β. Binding motifs are delineated in white boxes. For the N-box signaling pathway, heregulin binds and stimulates its receptors HER2, 3, and 4 at the sarcolemma, and propagates a signal to Erk1/2 via HER2, a receptor tyrosine kinase. Erk1/2 phosphorylates GABPα/β (which binds to the promoter at the EBS) and Sp1 cooperatively interact (possibly directly) to activate the utrophin A promoter. This cascade may also act on unidentified binding factors of regulatory importance, such as the ETS family repressor ERF. This region also contains an E-box for binding of MRFs that act on the promoter during myogenesis. Characteristic factors that bind the N and E-boxes and confer transcriptional activation are as indicated, with the E-box illustrating individual myogenic factors that interact, sized according to their *trans*-activation ability. The recently defined NFAT response element is also illustrated. Dotted and full arrowed lines represent potential and defined signaling cascades, respectively; for more information, refer to section Promoter Studies of Utrophin. *Abbreviations*: EBS, ETS binding site; ERF, ETS2 repressor factor; MRF, myogenic regulatory factors; NFAT, nuclear factor-activated T cell. *Source*: From Refs. 18, 76, 78, 90, 92, 96, 97.

ETS site such as ETS2 repressor factor (ERF) or ERF-like molecules (97). Indeed, active repression may be a mechanism involved in the abrupt reduction of utrophin that occurs during the perinatal period, leading to relatively low levels (typically 0.01% of message) of utrophin encountered in adult skeletal muscle (98). As ERF is subject to regulation by MAP kinases, heregulin may influence utrophin expression by changing relative levels or activity of transcriptional repressors in addition to activators such as GABPα/β (92,97).

Myogenesis and the E-Box Element

Although signaling mechanisms determining synaptic regulation at the N-box have been well defined, little information was available until recently on the induction of utrophin expression that is observed during muscle differentiation. Initial characterization of the A promoter region identified a conserved E-box, a binding site for helix-loop-helix proteins of the MyoD family, including MyoD1, myogenin, myf5, and MRF4 (99–103). E-box motifs are found in the promoters of many muscle-specific genes, and enhance the in vitro transcriptional activity of the α, β, and γ AChR subunit genes (82,104,105). Clues of E-Box–mediated transcriptional regulation were initially outlined with the observation that the rate of total utrophin transcription increased approximately twofold during myogenesis in the mouse C2C12 muscle cell line (106). Direct evidence was provided in a study by Perkins et al. (78), in which an increase in endogenous utrophin A mRNA levels was paralleled by an increased expression of the transfected promoter construct that contained the conserved upstream muscle-specific E-box (78). MyoD, myogenin, and MRF4 are able to bind and *trans*-activate the A promoter up to 18-fold in myotubes in transient assays, in which the increases could be abolished by mutagenesis of the E-box. These studies confirmed that promoter A is regulated in a similar manner to other genes expressed in the muscle (107–110). Mechanistically, this type of positive regulation may involve a direct interaction between myogenic factors and basal factors that are bound to the core promoter (Fig. 1), analogous to the association of Sp1 and MyoD-myogenin factors required for activation of the human cardiac α-actin promoter in skeletal muscle cells (110). As myogenic factors respond differently to mechanisms that maintain cellular homeostasis, denervation, and acute electrical stimulation, it is not surprising that differences in *trans*-activation levels between individual MRFs have been observed for a number of synaptically expressed genes that contain functional E-boxes, such as the β (84) and ε AChR subunit genes, suggesting the existence of a MRF "rank order," in which individual factors show selective ability to activate target genes (111,112).

Using an approach similar to that postulated for N-box, E-box–mediated activation may be achieved through blocking the activity of "antimyogenic" basic helix-loop-helix proteins such as Dermo-1, Mtwist, Mist1, and MyoR, which use various modes of action, including the transcriptional repression of "promyogenic" factors such as MyoD, to specifically repress E-box–dependent gene expression (113–117). Alternatively, it may be possible to *trans*-activate utrophin promoter A in DMD muscle by delivery of pharmacological compounds that directly or indirectly alter myogenic factor levels and/or activity. In combination with the N-box, studies on the E-box underline the importance of these motifs and their interaction with elements in the core promoter in the developmental regulation of the utrophin gene in skeletal muscle.

Calcineurin and NFAT Signaling

Utrophin transcript levels have been shown to be three to four times more abundant in slow muscles than in fast muscles, which is attributed to an increased extrasynaptic utrophin A (118). Sustained calcium influx in slower, oxidative fibers allows the activation of calcium-dependent signaling pathways, such as the calcineurin or NFAT cascade (119,120). Calcineurin is a signaling molecule that is activated by increasing the cytosolic free calcium concentration, thereby inducing the transcription of hypertrophic response genes through dephosphorylation of NFAT molecules, which can exert positive effects on binding motifs present within target genes (120–123). A recent study has indicated that this cascade may regulate differences in utrophin A levels on a molecular level (76). Transgenic mice overexpressing calcineurin show increased utrophin mRNA levels, presumably through NFAT, a transcriptional effector of calcineurin. Inhibition of calcineurin resulted in an 80% decrease in utrophin A mRNA levels, and studies in transgenic mice expressing constitutively active calcineurin displayed fourfold higher levels of utrophin A transcript (76), illustrated through transfection and direct gene transfer. As calcineurin involves transcription factor binding of NFAT, a functional motif was delineated 5' to the E-Box within the 1 kb upstream human utrophin promoter region that bound NFATc1 in EMSA studies (Fig. 1) (119,120,124). Given the presence of a functional E-box motif within the A promoter, it is likely that this signaling pathway also directly affects the interaction of myogenic factors, in a similar fashion to that of myogenin promoter E-Box, which binds MyoD and is indirectly responsive to calcium and calcineurin via the decrease of the Id inhibitory proteins, possibly by downregulation of Egr-1 expression (125). This is supported by previous observations that NFATc1 is regulated in differentiated C2C12 myotubes, and calcineurin signaling is necessary for MyoD-induced myogenic differentiation of uncommitted fibroblasts (126).

The Utrophin B Promoter

In addition to the full-length utrophin A transcript and associated promoter region, in the year 1999, a second promoter that expresses a utrophin B isoform was identified within the large second intron, approximately 50 kb

3' to exon 2 for both human and murine sequences (17). The utrophin B transcript encodes a unique 31 amino acid first exon (1B), with human and mouse sequences showing 82% nucleotide and 77% translational identity. The A and B promoters are independently regulated and give rise to transcripts with unique 5' exons that splice into a common utrophin mRNA at exon 3 (17,18). Sequence analysis indicated that the promoter was of the TATA-Inr+ type, because of the absence of TATA or CAAT motifs; the presence of a short open reading frame within the 5' untranslated region prior to the start of the actual translation is similar to the structure of exon 2A. Similar to the approaches used for utrophin A, the 306 bp core promoter element was defined using a 5' to 3' deletion series and retained 70% activity of the full 1.5 kb construct in expressing cell lines (17,18). In addition, a 2 kb human and mouse alignment of the B locus shows limited overall homology (48%), with the only significant conserved region limited to exon 1B and 250 bp upstream from the 5' end of exon 1B, encompassing the minimal promoter region.

Isoform-specific murine antibodies to utrophin A and B have illustrated that utrophin B localizes to vascular endothelia (19). In a series of *trans*-activation experiments, individual members of the ETS and Ap-1 factor families were able to activate a human utrophin B reporter construct, similar to other vascular bed-specific genes such as endothelial cell-specific molecule-1 (127). Synergistic activation by GATA-2 and Ap-1 (c-jun) to the order of 20-fold was also observed, a phenomenon previously illustrated for human endothelin-1 and other endothelial-specific promoters (128–131). Present understanding of the transcriptional processes occurring within the core promoter element therefore indicates that the spatial restriction and enhanced function of the utrophin B promoter in endothelium may involve the formation of multiple protein complexes involving members of the ETS, GATA, Ap-1, and possibly Sp factor families (128).

Based on current knowledge of promoter activation and protein or transcript localization, the utrophin A isoform appears to be more relevant than utrophin B for a promoter activation strategy in DMD. Recent studies using RNase protection analysis on the expression of the two full-length utrophin isoforms in the *mdx* mouse indicated that the utrophin A protein is upregulated in dystrophin-deficient muscle, and is accompanied by a 50% increase (1.5×) in the utrophin A transcript, whereas utrophin B protein/transcript levels are unchanged (19). Given this relevance to an upregulation approach for a DMD therapy, the continued characterization of the transcriptional regulation of utrophin A is essential. Conversely, the observation that utrophin B levels remain constant does not necessarily indicate redundancy; this isoform may have a role in managing mechanical stress in endothelial cells and in dystrophin-deficient muscle.

Alternate Modulators of Utrophin Activity

Enhancer Elements and Additional Promoter Regions

The dystrophin locus contains a *cis*-acting enhancer that influences promoter activity, located 6.5 and 8.5 kb downstream from the muscle (M) promoter in the human and mouse sequences, respectively (132,133). The enhancer sequence is 65% conserved and approximately 200 bp in length for both species. The muscle-specific human dystrophin muscle enhancer [DME1 (132)] has a number of potential muscle-specific regulatory domains and increases M promoter activity in immature and mature skeletal muscle (133). The murine equivalent contains three functional E-boxes (of which two bind MyoD) and a serum response element (SRE); all are essential for enhancer activity in myotubes, although the SRE has also been implicated in transcriptional repression in myoblasts (133). Within the corresponding region of the human utrophin locus, a 128 bp orientation-independent *cis*-acting element called the downstream utrophin enhancer (DUE) has been identified, which enhances the utrophin A promoter in vitro (134). In contrast to DME1, no muscle-specific regulatory elements were localized and this region does not appear to confer increased activity during myogenic differentiation, suggesting that processes occurring via the E-box are DUE independent (134). Further investigation should elucidate whether consensus binding sites for the Ap1 and GATA transcription factor families are functional and if DUE activation is specific to the A promoter. Additional utrophin promoters giving rise to full-length isoforms may also be present within the 5' region, which may provide alternative targets for therapeutic manipulation.

Utrophin Post-Transcriptional Regulation and mRNA Stability

The majority of studies aimed at endogenous utrophin upregulation center primarily on transcriptional mechanisms; however, utrophin also appears to be subject to post-transcriptional control mechanisms in muscle fibers (135,136). Thus, targeting of mRNA stability is a potential means of achieving increased levels in muscle. In vitro studies have delineated specific regions within the 3' untranslated region which control transcript stability and targeting in cultured muscle cells; studies have also recently been performed in vivo, where post-transcriptional processing has a contributing role in increased utrophin transcript stability in slow versus fast muscle (118,136). It has been postulated that this process may be partially modulated by calcineurin levels, in addition to its recently defined role in enhancing transcriptional activity [see section "Calcineurin and NFAT Signaling" (76)]. These studies illustrate the importance of post-transcriptional events in the regulation and stability of utrophin in skeletal muscle cells and offer a promising avenue of research in providing targets for the development of pharmacological strategies designed to increase endogenous utrophin levels in DMD muscle fibers. This approach complements ongoing research into increasing utrophin levels via manipulation of transcriptional events within the 5' region.

OTHER EFFECTORS OF UTROPHIN UPREGULATION

In addition to effectors of utrophin regulation that act directly at the level of transcript initiation and/or stability, a number of promising transgenic approaches to compensate for dystrophin deficiency and indirectly increase utrophin levels have been reported. Ectopic expression of cytotoxic T cell (CT) GalNac transferase and overexpression of ADAM-12 promote survival and/or regeneration of the compromised muscle or affect post-transcriptional modification of proteins, including utrophin (137,138). Transgenic overexpression of the synaptic CT GalNAc transferase in *mdx* skeletal muscle leads to a 5.4-fold increase in full-length utrophin protein expression, in addition to upregulating many DAPs, including dystroglycans, sarcoglycans, and dystrobrevins equal to or above those of wild-type levels, along myofibers. ADAM-12 is an active transmembrane metalloproteinase required for myoblast fusion and for stimulation of myogenesis (139–142). Like utrophin, ADAM-12 is expressed in skeletal muscle during development, ceases after birth and reappears in skeletal muscle during regeneration (142–144). A 1.8-fold increase in utrophin A protein was observed in *mdx*/ADAM-12 mice compared to *mdx* controls; however, it was not accompanied by a corresponding increase in transcript levels, indicating the involvement of post-transcriptional events.

As illustrated by the studies in this section, remarkable progress has been made in the identification and characterization of mechanisms that regulate utrophin stability and transcription. These studies are essential in providing the necessary building blocks to understand utrophin regulation in muscle cells and represent a first step forward for drug design with the aim of an utrophin-based therapeutic strategy for DMD.

UTROPHIN-BASED THERAPEUTIC STRATEGIES

An observable degree of functional redundancy between dystrophin and utrophin indicates that their distinct functions relate more to discrete expression patterns rather than differences in biochemical or physical properties. This has been functionally demonstrated by the ability of utrophin overexpression to rescue the dystrophic phenotype in *mdx* muscle, and allows the consideration of possible therapeutic strategies.

Gene Delivery

The first strategy involves the direct delivery of utrophin protein to muscle. This approach may avoid the potential problems of an immune response associated with dystrophin delivery in patients and is consequently a more preferable option. Favorably, recent evidence has suggested that expression of an utrophin transgene is more prolonged than that of dystrophin, following adenoviral delivery to the muscles of immune-competent mice (145). Successful adenoviral delivery of utrophin to muscle has been demonstrated, with phenotypic improvement both in *mdx* and *dko* muscle (4,146). In the latter study, delivery of a first generation recombinant adenovirus containing an utrophin minigene to the limb muscle (tibialis anterior) of *dko* neonatal mice protected the muscle from subsequent dystrophic damage (4). Expression of the minigene was detectable in up to 95% of fibers 30 days postinjection and caused a significant decrease in necrosis. Importantly, these observations show that introducing the utrophin transgene after the onset of muscle necrosis and regeneration can correct the dystrophic phenotype.

Although studies mentioned in this chapter have been crucial in demonstrating the protective role of utrophin overexpression in transgenic *mdx* and *dko* mice (either in utero or via viral somatic transfer), several important insights are required for eventual therapeutic use. For example, it is necessary to understand whether expression of utrophin in muscle cells is equally effective at early and later stages of disease progression and if large quantities of utrophin in muscle results in short- or long-term benefits. An avenue of recent research that begins to address such uncertainties is the use of tetracycline-responsive transactivator analysis (147). This system allows the transcription of any gene to be somatically induced (or repressed) in multiple muscle groups at any point throughout the life of the mouse by the administration of tetracycline, and has been successful in determining the timing of controlled inducement of dystrophin in the *mdx* mouse to prevent dystrophic pathology (148). In this study, expression of dystrophin in utero was found to result in a more dramatic improvement in muscle morphology than its induction within a few days after birth. Importantly, induced dystrophin expression after four weeks of age did not result in obvious phenotypic improvement or positive morphological change in muscle. A similar study was undertaken for utrophin to determine the developmental period in which muscle-specific utrophin delivery is most effective in preventing the dystrophic phenotype (149). Less improvement was observed when utrophin was activated 30 days after birth, indicating that the stage at which utrophin therapy is initiated is crucial. If initiated at an early postnatal stage, utrophin therapy is effective and the extent of correction of dystrophic symptoms is dependent on utrophin expression levels.

Upregulation of Endogenous Utrophin

Based on analysis of the degree and type of improvement noted using transgene-mediated utrophin upregulation, pharmacological upregulation of utrophin is predicted to have a broad therapeutic benefit in DMD.

Importantly, as pre-existing cellular mechanisms are utilized, this approach would avoid many problems associated with conventional gene therapies. In principle, this could be achieved by a number of means in dystrophin-deficient muscle: the utrophin protein is known to be sensitive to intracellular degradation, and inhibition of proteases is a potential method of stabilizing preexisting utrophin within muscle. A promising approach involves the prevention of downregulation and/or upregulation of the endogenous utrophin gene in skeletal muscle sufficient to effect the two- to threefold increase in steady state protein levels that are necessary to prevent dystrophic pathology. This may be achieved through the use of small diffusible chemical compounds and has an inherent advantage of circumventing the challenge of conferring stable expression of transgenes in skeletal muscle. Such an approach has been successful in the treatment of β-thalassemia, which results from mutations in the β-globin gene. The fetal isoform γ-globin is downregulated after birth, such that a switch between fetal ($\alpha_2\gamma_2$) and adult ($\alpha_2\beta_2$) forms of Hb occurs by three to six months of age [reviewed in (150)]. Reactivation of transcription from the γ-globin locus in red cell precursors can functionally compensate for β-globin deficiency (151). Small compound treatments with butyrate derivatives are able to effect such reactivation through interaction with 5' regulatory elements of the γ-globin promoter (152–154). In some instances, changes in the patterns of DNA–protein interactions have been demonstrated in red cell precursors of patients, pre- and post-treatment (155). Early clinical trials have shown several beneficial, albeit variable, effects and illustrate an important principle with respect to validating a similar approach for utrophin (151,156,157). Patients have improved clinically following small compound transcriptional manipulation of genes encoding functionally similar proteins, achieving compensation for the absence of one protein by effecting upregulation of another. Importantly, pharmacological compounds do not necessarily require strict tissue-specific control and this is aided by the observation that ubiquitous overexpression of the target protein has no resulting toxicity in the *mdx* mouse (1,2,72,74).

Promoter Activation Strategies

As previously discussed, one potential approach to increasing utrophin levels in muscle for possible therapeutic purpose in humans is to increase the expression of the utrophin gene at a transcriptional level via promoter activation. This has lead to an interest in the identification and manipulation of important regulatory regions and/or molecules that increase the expression of utrophin and their delivery to dystrophin-deficient tissue. Research into the control of utrophin expression at the transcriptional level (as discussed in section "Promoter Studies of Utrophin") allows an opportunity to specifically design small compounds that interact with or target these processes (158). A systematic approach of investigating protein–DNA or protein–protein interactions of the proximal promoter regions and the use of in vitro reporter analysis have been successful in the recognition of a number of potential pathways for regulating expression via the N- and E-boxes of the utrophin A promoter. Further understanding of *trans*-acting factors and appropriate signaling pathways at these elements may assist in the design of specific molecules (such as heregulin) to target specific events to yield transcriptional activation. For example, current knowledge of transcriptional interactions at the N-box has led to the recent evaluation of L-arginine as an utrophin targeting compound for possible therapeutic use. This molecule is a limiting substrate for nitric oxide (NO) biosynthesis, which in turn mediates a signaling pathway that regulates agrin-induced aggregation of synapse-specific components at the NMJ, including utrophin (159). Studies of adult normal and *mdx* mice (and in corresponding myoblast lines in vitro) indicated that treatment with L-arginine, NO, or hydroxyurea (an intermediate compound in the L-arginine-NO pathway) increased utrophin levels and enhanced sarcolemmal localization (160,161). However, we are unable to recapitulate these findings using identical conditions, finding no such effect on utrophin transcription and/or protein levels upon delivery of either L-arginine or hydroxyurea in vitro (unpublished observations).

Methodologies for Small Compound Evaluation

An alternate approach to identifying suitable molecules that increase utrophin levels is the screening of random small compound libraries against an easily quantifiable automated assay. As an example, transcriptional upregulation of either of the utrophin full-length isoforms may be effected by the use of reporter gene–cell culture systems (described in Ref. 75). We are currently using this system in our laboratory as it has the inherent advantage of being able to rapidly identify additional compounds that positively interact via unknown mechanisms. A strategy that allows the analysis of greater genomic regions (>140 kb) and circumvents limitations of plasmid-based approaches involves BAC and PAC transgenesis. This homologous recombination-based method has been successful in the study of the myogenic genes myf5 and MRF4, where the resultant transgenic mice reproduced all known aspects of temporal and spatial expression from both loci (162). Importantly, novel elements were identified for myf-5 that were responsible for specific expression in individual cell populations and enabled the localization of multiple elements required for recapitulating the endogenous expression pattern of MRF4. We have recently constructed a 170 kb PAC, which encompasses both the A and B promoters including 35 kb of sequence 5' to exon 1A. This should enable us to delineate novel regulatory elements for utrophin expression and also to design a screening method to identify compounds which selectively upregulate utrophin A, B, or both.

Utrophin A and B antibodies will assist in confirming in vivo expression of the reporter proteins from the utrophin locus and provide a resource through which regions of transcriptional and protein distribution can be compared.

CONCLUSIONS

Given the ability of utrophin to serve as a functional replacement for the absence of dystrophin, this chapter has concentrated on studies of utrophin expression to identify the various mechanisms that give rise to the complex expression pattern in healthy and diseased tissue. Current knowledge on its transcriptional processes as a resource to enable identification of means to effect its upregulation in dystrophic tissue lends credence to the continued characterization of utrophin as an invaluable avenue of research for a definitive cure for DMD.

ACKNOWLEDGMENTS

This work was funded by the Muscular Dystrophy Campaign U.K., the Muscular Dystrophy Association, U.S.A., Association Francaise Contre les Myopathies (AFM), and the Medical Research Council, U.K. We would like to thank Tejvir Khurana for insightful suggestions and Helen Blaber for her help in typing the manuscript.

REFERENCES

1. Deconinck N, Tinsley J, De Backer F, et al. Expression of truncated utrophin leads to major functional improvements in dystrophin-deficient muscles of mice. Nat Med 1997; 3(11):1216–1221.
2. Tinsley JM, Potter AC, Phelps SR, Fisher R, Trickett JI, Davies KE. Amelioration of the dystrophic phenotype of mdx mice using a truncated utrophin transgene [see comments]. Nature 1996; 384(6607):349–353.
3. Cerletti M, Negri T, Cozzi F, et al. Dystrophic phenotype of canine X-linked muscular dystrophy is mitigated by adenovirus-mediated utrophin gene transfer. Gene Ther 2003; 10(9):750–757.
4. Wakefield PM, Tinsley JM, Wood MJ, Gilbert R, Karpati G, Davies KE. Prevention of the dystrophic phenotype in dystrophin/utrophin-deficient muscle following adenovirus-mediated transfer of a utrophin minigene. Gene Ther 2000; 7(3):201–204.
5. Kapsa R, Kornberg AJ, Byrne E. Novel therapies for Duchenne muscular dystrophy. Lancet Neurol 2003; 2(5):299–310.
6. Gilbert R, Nalbanoglu J, Tinsley JM, Massie B, Davies KE, Karpati G. Efficient utrophin expression following adenovirus gene transfer in dystrophic muscle. Biochem Biophys Res Commun 1998; 242(1):244–247.

7. Love DR, Hill DF, Dickson G, et al. An autosomal transcript in skeletal muscle with homology to dystrophin. Nature 1989; 339(6219):55–58.
8. Roberts RG, Freeman TC, Kendall E, et al. Characterization of DRP2, a novel human dystrophin homologue. Nat Genet 1996; 13(2):223–226.
9. Blake DJ, Tinsley JM, Davies KE. Utrophin: a structural and functional comparison to dystrophin. Brain Pathol 1996; 6(1):37–47.
10. Blake DJ, Nawrotski R, Peters MF, Froehner SC, Davies KE. Isoform diversity of dystrobrevin, the murine 87-kDa postsynaptic protein. J Biol Chem 1996; 271:7802–7810.
11. Blake DJ, Weir A, Newey SE, Davies KE. Function and genetics of dystrophin and dystrophin-related proteins in muscle. Physiol Rev 2002; 82(2):291–329.
12. Buckle VJ, Guenet JL, Simon Chazottes D, Love DR, Davies KE. Localisation of a dystrophin-related autosomal gene to 6q24 in man, and to mouse chromosome 10 in the region of the dystrophia muscularis (dy) locus. Hum Genet 1990; 85(3):324–326.
13. Guo WX, Nichol M, Merlie JP. Cloning and expression of full length mouse utrophin: the differential association of utrophin and dystrophin with AChR clusters. FEBS Lett 1996; 398(2–3):259–264.
14. Pearce M, Blake DJ, Tinsley JM, et al. The utrophin and dystrophin genes share similarities in genomic structure. Hum Mol Genet 1993; 2(11):1765–1772.
15. Sadoulet Puccio HM, Rajala M, Kunkel LM. Dystrobrevin and dystrophin: an interaction through coiled-coil motifs. Proc Natl Acad Sci USA 1997; 94(23):12,413–12,418.
16. Winder SJ. The membrane-cytoskeleton interface: the role of dystrophin and utrophin. J Muscle Res Cell Motil 1997; 18(6):617–629.
17. Burton EA, Tinsley JM, Holzfiend P, Rodrigues N, Davies KE. A second promoter provides an alternative target for therapeutic up-regulation of utrophin in Duchenne muscular dystrophy. Proc Natl Acad Sci USA 1999; 96(24): 14,025–14,030.
18. Dennis CL, Tinsley JM, Deconinck AE, Davies KE. Molecular and functional analysis of the utrophin promoter. Nucleic Acids Res 1996; 24(9): 1646–1652.
19. Weir AP, Burton EA, Harrod G, Davies KE. A- and B-utrophin have different expression patterns and are differentially up-regulated in mdx muscle. J Biol Chem 2002; 277(47):45,285–45,290.
20. Blake DJ, Schofield JN, Zuellig RA, et al. G-utrophin, the autosomal homologue of dystrophin Dp116, is expressed in sensory ganglia and brain. Proc Natl Acad Sci USA 1995; 92(9):3697–3701.
21. Wilson J, Putt W, Jimenez C, Edwards Y. Up71 and Up140, two novel transcripts of utrophin that are homologues of short forms of dystrophin. Hum Mol Genet 1999; 8:1271–1278.
22. Byers TJ, Lidov HG, Kunkel LM. An alternative dystrophin transcript specific to peripheral nerve. Nat Genet 1993; 4(1):77–81.
23. Howard PL, Dally GY, Wong MH, et al. Localization of dystrophin isoform Dp71 to the inner limiting membrane of the retina suggests a unique functional contribution of Dp71 in the retina. Hum Mol Genet 1998; 7(9):1385–1391.

24. Rodius F, Claudepierre T, Rosas Vargas H, et al. Dystrophins in developing retina: Dp260 expression correlates with synaptic maturation. Neuroreport 1997; 8(9–10):2383–2387.
25. Jimenez-Mallebrera C, Davies K, Putt W, Edwards YH. A study of short utrophin isoforms in mice deficient for full-length utrophin. Mamm Genome 2003; 14(1):47–60.
26. Winder SJ, Kendrick Jones J. Calcium/calmodulin-dependent regulation of the NH2-terminal F-actin binding domain of utrophin. FEBS Lett 1995; 357(2):125–128.
27. Winder SJ, Hemmings L, Maciver SK, et al. Utrophin actin binding domain: analysis of actin binding and cellular targeting. J Cell Sci 1995; 108(Pt 1):63–71.
28. Winder SJ. Structure–function relationships in dystrophin and utrophin. Biochem Soc Trans 1996; 24(2):497–501.
29. Morris GE, Nguyen TM, Nguyen TN, Pereboev A, Kendrick Jones J, Winder SJ. Disruption of the utrophin–actin interaction by monoclonal antibodies and prediction of an actin-binding surface of utrophin. Biochem J 1999; 337(Pt 1):119–123.
30. Sutherland-Smith AJ, Moores CA, Norwood FL, et al. An atomic model for actin binding by the CH domains and spectrin-repeat modules of utrophin and dystrophin. J Mol Biol 2003; 329(1):15–33.
31. Amann KJ, Guo AW, Ervasti JM. Utrophin lacks the rod domain actin binding activity of dystrophin. J Biol Chem 1999; 274(50):35,375–35,380.
32. Moores CA, Kendrick-Jones J. Biochemical characterisation of the actin-binding properties of utrophin. Cell Motil Cytoskeleton 2000; 46(2):116–128.
33. Moores CA, Keep NH, Kendrick-Jones J. Structure of the utrophin actin-binding domain bound to F-actin reveals binding by an induced fit mechanism. J Mol Biol 2000; 297(2):465–480.
34. Tinsley JM, Blake DJ, Roche A, et al. Primary structure of dystrophin-related protein. Nature 1992; 360(6404):591–593.
35. James M, Simmons C, Wise CJ, Jones GE, Morris GE. Evidence for a utrophin-glycoprotein complex in cultured cell lines and a possible role in cell adhesion. Biochem Soc Trans 1995; 23(3):398s.
36. Matsumura K, Ervasti JM, Ohlendieck K, Kahl SD, Campbell KP. Association of dystrophin-related protein with dystrophin-associated proteins in mdx mouse muscle. Nature 1992; 360(6404):588–591.
37. James M, Nguyen TM, Wise CJ, Jones GE, Morris GE. Utrophin-dystroglycan complex in membranes of adherent cultured cells. Cell Motil Cytoskeleton 1996; 33(3):163–174.
38. Peters MF, Adams ME, Froehner SC. Differential association of syntrophin pairs with the dystrophin complex. J Cell Biol 1997; 138(1):81–93.
39. Kramarcy NR, Sealock R. Syntrophin isoforms at the neuromuscular junction: developmental time course and differential localization. Mol Cell Neurosci 2000; 15(3):262–274.
40. Loh NY, Newey SE, Davies KE, Blake DJ. Assembly of multiple dystrobrevin-containing complexes in the kidney. J Cell Sci 2000; 113(Pt 15):2715–2724.
41. England SB, Nicholson LV, Johnson MA, et al. Very mild muscular dystrophy associated with the deletion of 46% of dystrophin. Nature 1990; 343(6254):180–182.

42. Matsumura K, Yamada H, Shimizu T, Campbell KP. Differential expression of dystrophin, utrophin and dystrophin-associated proteins in peripheral nerve. FEBS Lett 1993; 334(3):281–285.
43. Matsumura K, Shasby DM, Campbell KP. Purification of dystrophin-related protein (utrophin) from lung and its identification in pulmonary artery endothelial cells. FEBS Lett 1993; 326(1–3):289–293.
44. Pons F, Robert A, Fabbrizio E, et al. Utrophin localization in normal and dystrophin-deficient heart. Circulation 1994; 90(1):369–374.
45. Sewry CA, Man NT, Lynch T, Morris GE. Absence of utrophin in intercalated discs of human cardiac muscle. Histochem J 2001; 33(1):9–12.
46. Nguyen TM, Ellis JM, Love DR, et al. Localization of the DMDL gene-encoded dystrophin-related protein using a panel of nineteen monoclonal antibodies: presence at neuromuscular junctions, in the sarcolemma of dystrophic skeletal muscle, in vascular and other smooth muscles, and in proliferating brain cell lines. J Cell Biol 1991; 115(6):1695–1700.
47. Claudepierre T, Rodius F, Frasson M, et al. Differential distribution of dystrophins in rat retina. Invest Ophthalmol Vis Sci 1999; 40(7):1520–1529.
48. Earnest JP, Santos GF, Zuerbig S, Fox JE. Dystrophin-related protein in the platelet membrane skeleton. Integrin-induced change in detergent-insolubility and cleavage by calpain in aggregating platelets. J Biol Chem 1995; 270(45):27,259–27,265.
49. Raats CJ, van den Born J, Bakker MA, et al. Expression of agrin, dystroglycan, and utrophin in normal renal tissue and in experimental glomerulopathies. Am J Pathol 2000; 156(5):1749–1765.
50. Khurana TS, Watkins SC, Chafey P, et al. Immunolocalisation and developmental expression of dystrophin related protein in skeletal muscle. Neuromuscul Disord 1991; 1(3):185–194.
51. Nguyen TM, Le TT, Blake DJ, Davies KE, Morris GE. Utrophin, the autosomal homologue of dystrophin, is widely-expressed and membrane-associated in cultured cell lines. FEBS Lett 1992; 313(1):19–22.
52. Ohlendieck K, Ervasti JM, Matsumura K, Kahl SD, Leveille CJ, Campbell KP. Dystrophin-related protein is localized to neuromuscular junctions of adult skeletal muscle. Neuron 1991; 7(3):499–508.
53. Campanelli JT, Roberds SL, Campbell KP, Scheller RH. A role for dystrophin-associated glycoproteins and utrophin in agrin-induced AChR clustering. Cell 1994; 77(5):663–674.
54. Deconinck AE, Potter AC, Tinsley JM, et al. Postsynaptic abnormalities at the neuromuscular junctions of utrophin-deficient mice. J Cell Biol 1997; 136(4):883–894.
55. Grady RM, Merlie JP, Sanes JR. Subtle neuromuscular defects in utrophin-deficient mice. J Cell Biol 1997; 136(4):871–882.
56. Bewick GS, Young C, Slater CR. Spatial relationships of utrophin, dystrophin, beta-dystroglycan and beta-spectrin to acetylcholine receptor clusters during postnatal maturation of the rat neuromuscular junction. J Neurocytol 1996; 25(7):367–379.
57. Phillips W, Noakes P, Roberds S, Campbell K, Merlie J. Clutering and immobilization of acetylcholine receptors by the 43 kDa protein: a possible role for the dystrophin-related protein. J Cell Biol 1993; 123(3):729–740.

58. Sieb JP, Dorfler P, Tzartos S, et al. Congenital myasthenic syndromes in two kinships with end-plate acetylcholine receptor and utrophin deficiency. Neurology 1998; 50(1):54–61.
59. Slater CR, Young C, Wood SJ, et al. Utrophin abundance is reduced at neuromuscular junctions of patients with both inherited and acquired acetylcholine receptor deficiencies. Brain 1997; 120(Pt 9):1513–1531.
60. Clerk A, Morris GE, Dubowitz V, Davies KE, Sewry CA. Dystrophin-related protein, utrophin, in normal and dystrophic human fetal skeletal muscle. Histochem J 1993; 25(8):554–561.
61. Tinsley JM, Davies KE. Utrophin: a potential replacement for dystrophin? Neuromuscul Disord 1993; 3(5–6):537–539.
62. Karpati G, Carpenter S, Morris GE, Davies KE, Guerin C, Holland P. Localization and quantitation of the chromosome 6-encoded dystrophin-related protein in normal and pathological human muscle. J Neuropathol Exp Neurol 1932; 52(2):119–128.
63. Helliwell TR, Man NT, Morris GE, Davies KE. The dystrophin-related protein, utrophin, is expressed on the sarcolemma of regenerating human skeletal muscle fibres in dystrophies and inflammatory myopathies. Neuromuscul Disord 1992; 2(3):177–184.
64. Lin S, Gaschen F, Burgunder JM. Utrophin is a regeneration-associated protein transiently present at the sarcolemma of regenerating skeletal muscle fibers in dystrophin-deficient hypertrophic feline muscular dystrophy. J Neuropathol Exp Neurol 1998; 57(8):780–790.
65. Lanfossi M, Cozzi F, Bugini D, et al. Development of muscle pathology in canine X-linked muscular dystrophy. I. Delayed postnatal maturation of affected and normal muscle as revealed by myosin isoform analysis and utrophin expression. Acta Neuropathol (Berl) 1999; 97(2):127–138.
66. Takemitsu M, Ishiura S, Koga R, et al. Dystrophin-related protein in the fetal and denervated skeletal muscles of normal and mdx mice. Biochem Biophys Res Commun 1991; 180(3):1179–1186.
67. Weir AM, Morgan JE, Davies KE. A-utrophin up-regulation in mdx skeletal muscle is independent of regeneration. Neuromuscul Disord 2004; 14(1):19–23.
68. Vrettou C, Kanavakis E, Traeger-Synodinos J, et al. Molecular studies of beta-thalassemia heterozygotes with raised Hb F levels. Hemoglobin 2000; 24(3):203–220.
69. Knuesel I, Riban V, Zuellig RA, et al. Increased vulnerability to kainate-induced seizures in utrophin-knockout mice. Eur J Neurosci 2002; 15(9):1474–1484.
70. Deconinck AE, Rafael JA, Skinner JA, et al. Utrophin-dystrophin-deficient mice as a model for Duchenne muscular dystrophy. Cell 1997; 90(4):717–727.
71. Grady RM, Teng H, Nichol MC, Cunningham JC, Wilkinson RS, Sanes JR. Skeletal and cardiac myopathies in mice lacking utrophin and dystrophin: a model for Duchenne muscular dystrophy. Cell 1997; 90(4):729–738.
72. Tinsley J, Deconinck N, Fisher R, et al. Expression of full-length utrophin prevents muscular dystrophy in mdx mice. Nat Med 1998; 4(12):1441–1444.
73. Rybakova IN, Patel JR, Davies KE, Yurchenco PD, Ervasti JM. Utrophin binds laterally along actin filaments and can couple costameric actin with

sarcolemma when overexpressed in dystrophin-deficient muscle. Mol Biol Cell 2002; 13(5):1512–1521.
74. Fisher R, Tinsley JM, Phelps SR, et al. Non-toxic ubiquitous over-expression of utrophin in the mdx mouse. Neuromuscul Disord 2001; 11(8):713–721.
75. Dennis CL. Promoter Studies of the Utrophin Gene. Ph.D. Thesis, University of Oxford, Oxford, 1996.
76. Chakkalakal JV, Stocksley MA, Harrison MA, et al. Expression of utrophin A mRNA correlates with the oxidative capacity of skeletal muscle fiber types and is regulated by calcineurin/NFAT signaling. Proc Natl Acad Sci USA 2003; 100(13):7791–7796.
77. Koike S, Schaeffer L, Changeux J-P. Identification of a DNA element determining synaptic expression of the mouse acetylcholine receptor delta-subunit gene. Proc Natl Acad Sci USA 1995; 92:10,624–10,628.
78. Perkins KJ, Burton EA, Davies KE. The role of basal and myogenic factors in the transcriptional activation of utrophin promoter A: implications for therapeutic up-regulation in Duchenne muscular dystrophy. Nucl Acids Res 2001; 29(23):4843–4850.
79. Santoro IM, Yi TM, Walsh K. Identification of single-stranded-DNA-binding proteins that interact with muscle gene elements. Mol Cell Biol 1991; 11(4):1944–1953.
80. Buonanno A, Rosenthal N. Molecular control of muscle diversity and plasticity. Dev Genet 1996; 19(2):95–107.
81. Crowder CM, Merlie JP. Stepwise activation of the mouse acetylcholine receptor delta- and gamma-subunit genes in clonal cell lines. Mol Cell Biol 1988; 8(12):5257–5267.
82. Prody CA, Merlie JP. The 5′-flanking region of the mouse muscle nicotinic acetylcholine receptor beta subunit gene promotes expression in cultured muscle cells and is activated by MRF4, myogenin and myoD. Nucl Acids Res 1992; 20(9):2367–2372.
83. Hall ZW, Sanes JR. Synaptic structure and development: the neuromuscular junction. Cell 1993; 72(suppl):99–121.
84. Sanes JR, Hall ZW. Antibodies that bind specifically to synaptic sites on muscle fiber basal lamina. J Cell Biol 1979; 83(2 Pt 1):357–370.
85. Duclert A, Changeux JP. Acetylcholine receptor gene expression at the developing neuromuscular junction. Physiol Rev 1995; 75(2):339–368.
86. Burden SJ. The formation of neuromuscular synapses. Genes Dev 1998; 12(2):133–148.
87. Fromm L, Burden SJ. Synapse-specific and neuregulin-induced transcription require an ets site that binds GABPalpha/GABPbeta. Genes Dev 1998; 12:3074–3083.
88. Rimer M, Cohen I, Lomo T, Burden SJ, McMahan UJ. Neuregulins and erbB receptors at neuromuscular junctions and at agrin-induced postsynaptic-like apparatus in skeletal muscle. Mol Cell Neurosci 1998; 12(1–2):1–15.
89. Sunesen M, Huchet-Dymanus M, Christensen MO, Changeux JP. Phosphorylation-elicited quaternary changes of GA binding protein in transcriptional activation. Mol Cell Biol 2003; 23(22):8008–8018.

90. Gramolini AO, Angus LM, Schaeffer L, et al. Induction of utrophin gene expression by heregulin in skeletal muscle cells: role of the N-box motif and GA binding protein. Proc Natl Acad Sci USA 1999; 96(6):3223–3227.
91. Gramolini AO, Burton EA, Tinsley JM, et al. Muscle and neural isoforms of agrin increase utrophin expression in cultured myotubes via a transcriptional regulatory mechanism. J Biol Chem 1998; 273(2):736–743.
92. Khurana TS, Rosmarin AG, Shang J, Krag TO, Das S, Gammeltoft S. Activation of utrophin promoter by heregulin via the ets-related transcription factor complex GA-binding protein alpha/beta. Mol Biol Cell 1999; 10(6):2075–2086.
93. Fromm L, Burden SJ. Neuregulin-1-stimulated phosphorylation of GABP in skeletal muscle cells. Biochemistry 2001; 40(17):5306–5312.
94. Rosmarin AG, Luo M, Caprio DG, Shang J, Simkevich CP. Sp1 cooperates with the ets transcription factor, GABP, to activate the CD18 (beta2 leukocyte integrin) promoter. J Biol Chem 1998; 273(21):13,097–13,103.
95. Gegonne A, Bosselut R, Bailly RA, Ghysdael J. Synergistic activation of the HTLV1 LTR Ets-responsive region by transcription factors Ets1 and Sp1. EMBO J 1993; 12(3):1169–1178.
96. Galvagni F, Capo S, Oliviero S. Sp1 and Sp3 Physically interact and co-operate with GABP for the activation of the utrophin promoter. J Mol Biol 2001; 306(5):985–996.
97. Sgouras DN, Athanasiou MA, Beal GJ Jr, Fisher RJ, Blair DG, Mavrothalassitis GJ. ERF: an ETS domain protein with strong transcriptional repressor activity, can suppress ets-associated tumorigenesis and is regulated by phosphorylation during cell cycle and mitogenic stimulation. EMBO J 1995; 14(19):4781–4793.
98. Khurana T, Hoffman E, Kunkel L. Identification of a chromosome 6-encoded dystrophin-related protein. J Biol Chem 1990; 265:16,717–16,720.
99. Davis RL, Weintraub H, Lassar AB. Expression of a single transfected cDNA converts fibroblasts to myoblasts. Cell 1987; 51(6):987–1000.
100. Wright WE, Sassoon DA, Lin VK. Myogenin, a factor regulating myogenesis, has a domain homologous to MyoD. Cell 1989; 56(4):607–617.
101. Edmondson DG, Olson EN. A gene with homology to the myc similarity region of MyoD1 is expressed during myogenesis and is sufficient to activate the muscle differentiation program. Genes Dev 1989; 3(5):628–640.
102. Braun T, Gearing K, Wright WE, Arnold HH. Baculovirus-expressed myogenic determination factors require E12 complex formation for binding to the myosin-light-chain enhancer. Eur J Biochem 1991; 198(1):187–193.
103. Rhodes SJ, Konieczny SF. Identification of MRF4: a new member of the muscle regulatory factor gene family. Genes Dev 1989; 3(12B):2050–2061.
104. Jia HT, Tsay HJ, Schmidt J. Analysis of binding and activating functions of the chick muscle acetylcholine receptor gamma-subunit upstream sequence. Cell Mol Neurobiol 1992; 12(3):241–258.
105. Piette J, Bessereau JL, Huchet M, Changeux JP. Two adjacent MyoD1-binding sites regulate expression of the acetylcholine receptor alpha-subunit gene. Nature 1990; 345(6273):353–355.

106. Gramolini A, Jasmin B. Expression of the utrophin gene during myogenic differentiation. Nucl Acids Res 1999; 27:3603–3609.
107. Li Y, Camp S, Rachinsky TL, Bongiorno C, Taylor P. Promoter elements and transcriptional control of the mouse acetylcholinesterase gene. J Biol Chem 1993; 268(5):3563–3572.
108. Lassar AB, Buskin JN, Lockshon D, et al. MyoD is a sequence-specific DNA binding protein requiring a region of myc homology to bind to the muscle creatine kinase enhancer. Cell 1989; 58(5):823–831.
109. Donoviel DB, Shield MA, Buskin JN, Haugen HS, Clegg CH, Hauschka SD. Analysis of muscle creatine kinase gene regulatory elements in skeletal and cardiac muscles of transgenic mice. Mol Cell Biol 1996; 16(4):1649–1658.
110. Biesiada E, Hamamori Y, Kedes L, Sartorelli V. Myogenic basic helix-loop-helix proteins and Sp1 interact as components of a multiprotein transcriptional complex required for activity of the human cardiac alpha-actin promoter. Mol Cell Biol 1999; 19(4):2577–2584.
111. Neville CM, Schmidt M, Schmidt J. Response of myogenic determination factors to cessation and resumption of electrical activity in skeletal muscle: a possible role for myogenin in denervation supersensitivity. Cell Mol Neurobiol 1992; 12(6):511–527.
112. Sunyer T, Merlie JP. Cell type- and differentiation-dependent expression from the mouse acetylcholine receptor epsilon-subunit promoter. J Neurosci Res 1993; 36(2):224–234.
113. Gong XQ, Li L. Dermo-1, a multifunctional basic helix-loop-helix protein, represses MyoD transactivation via HLH domain, MEF2 interaction and chromatin deacetylation. J Biol Chem 2002; 277(14):12,310–12,317.
114. Spicer DB, Rhee J, Cheung WL, Lassar AB. Inhibition of myogenic bHLH and MEF2 transcription factors by the bHLH protein twist. Science 1996; 272(5267):1476–1480.
115. Lemercier C, To RQ, Carrasco RA, Konieczny SF. The basic helix-loop-helix transcription factor Mist1 functions as a transcriptional repressor of myoD. EMBO J 1998; 17(5):1412–1422.
116. Lu J, Webb R, Richardson JA, Olson EN. MyoR: a muscle-restricted basic helix-loop-helix transcription factor that antagonizes the actions of MyoD. Proc Natl Acad Sci USA 1999; 96(2):552–557.
117. Yu L, Mikloucich J, Sangster N, Perez A, McCormick PJ. MyoR is expressed in nonmyogenic cells and can inhibit their differentiation. Exp Cell Res 2003; 289(1):162–173.
118. Gramolini AO, Belanger G, Thompson JM, Chakkalakal JV, Jasmin BJ. Increased expression of utrophin in a slow versus a fast muscle involves posttranscriptional events Versus Am J Physiol Cell Physiol 2001; 281(4): C1300–C1309.
119. Serrano AL, Murgia M, Pallafacchina G, et al. Calcineurin controls nerve activity-dependent specification of slow skeletal muscle fibers but not muscle growth. Proc Natl Acad Sci USA 2001; 98(23):13,108–13,113.
120. Chin ER, Olson EN, Richardson JA, et al. A calcineurin-dependent transcriptional pathway controls skeletal muscle fiber ty,pe. Genes Dev 1998; 12(16):2499–2509.

121. Liu Y, Cseresnyes Z, Randall WR, Schneider MF. Activity-dependent nuclear translocation and intranuclear distribution of NFATc in adult skeletal muscle fibers. J Cell Biol 2001; 155(1):27–39.
122. Wu H, Naya FJ, McKinsey TA, et al. MEF2 responds to multiple calcium-regulated signals in the control of skeletal muscle fiber type. EMBO J 2000; 19(9):1963–1973.
123. Kubis HP, Scheibe RJ, Meissner JD, Hornung G, Gros G. Fast-to-slow transformation and nuclear import/export kinetics of the transcription factor NFATc1 during electrostimulation of rabbit muscle cells in culture. J Physiol 2002; 541(Pt 3):835–847.
124. Allen DL, Leinwand LA. Intracellular calcium and myosin isoform transitions. Calcineurin and calcium-calmodulin kinase pathways regulate preferential activation of the IIa myosin heavy chain promoter. J Biol Chem 2002; 277(47):45,323–45,330.
125. Friday BB, Mitchell PO, Kegley KM, Pavlath GK. Calcineurin initiates skeletal muscle differentiation by activating MEF2 and MyoD. Differentiation 2003; 71(3):217–227.
126. Delling U, Tureckova J, Lim HW, De Windt LJ, Rotwein P, Molkentin JD. A calcineurin-NFATc3-dependent pathway regulates skeletal muscle differentiation and slow myosin heavy-chain expression. Mol Cell Biol 2000; 20(17):6600–6611.
127. Tsai JC, Zhang J, Minami T, et al. Cloning and characterization of the human lung endothelial-cell-specific molecule-1 promoter. J Vasc Res 2002; 39(2):148–159.
128. Perkins KJ, Davies KE. Ets, Ap-1 and GATA factor families regulate the utrophin B promoter: potential regulatory mechanisms for endothelial-specific expression. FEBS Lett 2003; 538(1–3):168–172.
129. Lee ME, Bloch KD, Clifford JA, Quertermous T. Functional analysis of the endothelin-1 gene promoter. Evidence for an endothelial cell-specific cis-acting sequence. J Biol Chem 1990; 265(18):10,446–10,450.
130. Dorfman DM, Wilson DB, Bruns GA, Orkin SH. Human transcription factor GATA-2. Evidence for regulation of preproendothelin-1 gene expression in endothelial cells. J Biol Chem 1992; 267(2):1279–1285.
131. Kawana M, Lee ME, Quertermous EE, Quertermous T. Cooperative interaction of GATA-2 and AP1 regulates transcription of the endothelin-1 gene. Mol Cell Biol 1995; 15(8):4225–4231.
132. Klamut HJ, Bosnoyan Collins LO, Worton RG, Ray PN, Davis HL. Identification of a transcriptional enhancer within muscle intron 1 of the human dystrophin gene. Hum Mol Genet 1996; 5(10):1599–1606.
133. Marshall P, Chartrand N, Worton RG. The mouse dystrophin enhancer is regulated by MyoD, E-box-binding factors, and by the serum response factor. J Biol Chem 2001; 276(23):20,719–20,726.
134. Galvagni F, Oliviero S. Utrophin transcription is activated by an intronic enhancer. J Biol Chem 2000; 275(5):3168–3172.
135. Gramolini A, Karpati G, Jasmin B. Discordant expression of utrophin and its transcript in human and mouse skeletal muscles. J Neuropathol Exp Neurol 1999; 58(3):235–244.

136. Gramolini AO, Belanger G, Jasmin BJ. Distinct regions in the 3′ untranslated region are responsible for targeting and stabilizing utrophin transcripts in skeletal muscle cells. J Cell Biol 2001; 154(6):1173–1183.
137. Nguyen HH, Jayasinha V, Xia B, Hoyte K, Martin PT. Overexpression of the cytotoxic T cell GalNAc transferase in skeletal muscle inhibits muscular dystrophy in mdx mice. Proc Natl Acad Sci USA 2002; 99(8):5616–5621.
138. Moghadaszadeh B, Albrechtsen R, Guo LT, et al. Compensation for dystrophin-deficiency: ADAM12 overexpression in skeletal muscle results in increased alpha 7 integrin, utrophin and associated glycoproteins. Hum Mol Genet 2003; 12(19):2467–2479.
139. Blobel CP. Functional and biochemical characterization of ADAMs and their predicted role in protein ectodomain shedding. Inflamm Res 2002; 51(2):83–84.
140. Seals DF, Courtneidge SA. The ADAMs family of metalloproteases: multidomain proteins with multiple functions. Genes Dev 2003; 17(1):7–30.
141. Gilpin BJ, Loechel F, Mattei MG, Engvall E, Albrechtsen R, Wewer UM. A novel, secreted form of human ADAM 12 (meltrin alpha) provokes myogenesis in vivo. J Biol Chem 1998; 273(1):157–166.
142. Yagami-Hiromasa T, Sato T, Kurisaki T, Kamijo K, Nabeshima Y, Fujisawa-Sehara A. A metalloprotease-disintegrin participating in myoblast fusion. Nature 1995; 377(6550):652–656.
143. Kronqvist P, Kawaguchi N, Albrechtsen R, et al. ADAM12 alleviates the skeletal muscle pathology in mdx dystrophic mice. Am J Pathol 2002; 161(5):1535–1540.
144. Galliano MF, Huet C, Frygelius J, Polgren A, Wewer UM, Engvall E. Binding of ADAM12, a marker of skeletal muscle regeneration, to the muscle-specific actin-binding protein, alpha-actinin-2, is required for myoblast fusion. J Biol Chem 2000; 275(18):13,933–13,939.
145. Petrof B, Ebihara S, Guibinga G, et al. Differential effects of adenovirus-mediated dystrophin and utrophin gene transfer in dystrophic (mdx) mice. In: American Society of Gene Therapy, Washington, D.C., 1999 [p. abstract number 831].
146. Gilbert R, Nalbantoglu J, Petrof BJ, et al. Adenovirus-mediated utrophin gene transfer mitigates the dystrophic phenotype of mdx mouse muscles. Hum Gene Ther 1999; 10(8):1299–1310.
147. Gossen M, Bujard H. Tight control of gene expression in mammalian cells by tetracycline-responsive promoters. Proc Natl Acad Sci USA 1992; 89(12): 5547–5551.
148. Ahmad A, Brinson M, Hodges BL, Chamberlain JS, Amalfitano A. Mdx mice inducibly expressing dystrophin provide insights into the potential of gene therapy for Duchenne muscular dystrophy. Hum Mol Genet 2000; 9(17):2507–2515.
149. Squire S, Raymackers JM, Vandebrouck C, et al. Prevention of pathology in mdx mice by expression of utrophin: analysis using an inducible transgenic expression system. Hum Mol Genet 2002; 11(26):3333–3344.
150. Hoffbrand A, Pettit J. Essential Haematology. 2d ed. Oxford: Blackwell, 1984.
151. Faller DV, Perrine SP. Butyrate in the treatment of sickle cell disease and beta-thalassemia. Curr Opin Hematol 1995; 2(2):109–117.

152. Perrine SP, Miller BA, Faller DV, et al. Sodium butyrate enhances fetal globin gene expression in erythroid progenitors of patients with Hb SS and beta thalassemia. Blood 1989; 74(1):454–459.
153. Hudgins WR, Fibach E, Safaya S, Rieder RF, Miller AC, Samid D. Transcriptional upregulation of gamma-globin by phenylbutyrate and analogous aromatic fatty acids. Biochem Pharmacol 1996; 52(8):1227–1233.
154. Perrine SP, Dover GH, Daftari P, et al. Isobutyramide, an orally bioavailable butyrate analogue, stimulates fetal globin gene expression in vitro and in vivo. Br J Haematol 1994; 88(3):555–561.
155. Ikuta T, Kan YW, Swerdlow PS, Faller DV, Perrine SP. Alterations in protein–DNA interactions in the gamma-globin gene promoter in response to butyrate therapy. Blood 1998; 92(8):2924–2933.
156. Perrine SP, Ginder GD, Faller DV, et al. A short-term trial of butyrate to stimulate fetal-globin-gene expression in the beta-globin disorders [see comments]. N Engl J Med 1993; 328(2):81–86.
157. Cappellini MD, Graziadei G, Ciceri L, et al. Butyrate trials. Ann N Y Acad Sci 1998; 850:110–119.
158. Corbi N, Libri V, Fanciulli M, Tinsley JM, Davies KE, Passananti C. The artificial zinc finger coding gene 'Jazz' binds the utrophin promoter and activates transcription. Gene Ther 2000; 7(12):1076–1083.
159. Blottner D, Luck G. Just in time and place: NOS/NO system assembly in neuromuscular junction formation. Microsc Res Tech 2001; 55(3):171–180.
160. Chaubourt E, Fossier P, Baux G, Leprince C, Israel M, De La Porte S. Nitric oxide and l-arginine cause an accumulation of utrophin at the sarcolemma: a possible compensation for dystrophin loss in Duchenne muscular dystrophy. Neurobiol Dis 1999; 6(6):499–507.
161. Chaubourt E, Voisin V, Fossier P, Baux G, Israel M, De La Porte S. Muscular nitric oxide synthase (muNOS) and utrophin. J Physiol (Paris) 2002; 96(1–2):43–52.
162. Carvajal JJ, Cox D, Summerbell D, Rigby PW. A BAC transgenic analysis of the Mrf4/Myf5 locus reveals interdigitated elements that control activation and maintenance of gene expression during muscle development. Development 2001; 128(10):1857–1868.

13

Regenerative Therapy

J. E. Morgan, Karima Brimah, C. A. Collins, and T. A. Partridge
*Muscle Cell Biology Group, MRC Clinical Sciences Centre,
Imperial College, London, U.K.*

INTRODUCTION

Degeneration and regeneration of skeletal muscle fibers is a distinguishing feature of muscular dystrophies and is particularly conspicuous in Duchenne and Becker muscular dystrophies (DMD and BMD). Moreover, much of the clinical compromise of muscular function arising in these conditions is attributable to a progressive failure of the regenerative aspect of this process. This is manifest in two ways: first, there appears to be a diminution of myogenic potential resident in the muscles, and second, there is not merely a failure to produce sufficient muscle, but the muscle bulk is progressively replaced by fibrous scar and fatty tissue. Whether this second feature is mechanistically linked to the first, i.e., by derangement of the myogenic cell program toward fibrogenic and adipocytic fates, or is an opportunistic takeover of available space by independently determined fibrogenic and adipocytic cells, is a moot point (1,2). Resolution of this question is clearly important in determining the precise approach to be adopted to counteract the loss of muscle. In the former case, one would aim to block the transdifferentiation of myogenic cells, while in the second they would need to be supplemented in some way. Whatever the case, any comprehensive therapy for any but the youngest cases of DMD and BMD must address the issue of rescuing the failing myogenic response, but the precise means by which this can best be accomplished will depend on the exact nature of the disruption of the natural myogenic mechanisms. In addition, over the past few years, support has been provided for the argument that enhancing myogenesis in dystrophic muscles can be of benefit. This is made explicit in the notion that increasing the strength of muscles to above normal levels will reduce the stress placed on individual muscle fibers by day-to-day activity and thus reduce their susceptibility to necrosis, prolonging their average lifespan and reducing the inflammatory consequences of tissue injury (3,4).

HYPOTHETICAL MECHANISMS

By and large, the mechanisms that regulate the size of skeletal muscles, maintain them at a size appropriate to their workload, and repair them after minor injury are remarkably effective. This is to be expected, given the crucial impact of skeletal muscle function on survival. At the same time, the major metabolic price on the formation and maintenance of unnecessarily large muscles stresses the importance of mechanisms to constrain overactive myogenesis. At present, we have some broad understanding of the mechanisms behind the control of muscle size at the cellular level and some of the factors that regulate these cellular mechanisms, but not at a level of detail that would permit us to obtain precise control of the system (5,6). For many years, the chief source of myogenic cells has been held to be the satellite cell that lies between the surface of the muscle fiber and surrounding basement membrane, but it has become increasingly clear that this is not a homogeneous population in terms of its myogenic potential. Further confusion of the picture has been generated by recent demonstrations of an input into the myogenic population from the bone marrow derived "stem cells." Until now, the impact of these phenomena on the regeneration of skeletal muscle has not been determined, certainly in any quantitative way, though clearly each could impact the efficacy of myogenesis and is potentially open to manipulation for the purpose of improving muscle repair.

Likewise, a number of factors has been implicated in regulation of the size of muscles, most notably, insulin-like growth factors (IGF-1 and IGF-2), fibroblast growth factor-6 (FGF-6), and platelet-derived growth factor-BB (PDGF-BB) as promoters and TNFα and myostatin as inhibitors of muscle growth (7–12). Again, in no case has the mechanism by which this effect is achieved in vivo been clearly delineated. In fact, we do not even have a quantitative description that would permit us to interpret changes in terms of the relative contributions of change in myonuclear number versus change in the size of cytoplasmic domain of each myonucleus. Because the data gathered from tissue culture is remote from the stimuli and constraints that operate in vivo during muscle regeneration, it is important to gather information on what actually happens in vivo to gain some perspective on whether or not the tissue culture phenomena are relevant.

REGENERATION OF SKELETAL MUSCLE FROM MUSCLE PRECURSOR CELLS

The cell widely accepted as being largely, if not solely, responsible for the regeneration of skeletal muscle is the satellite cell, located under the basal lamina of the muscle fiber (13). Satellite cells are quiescent in undamaged muscle, but following an injury, they become activated and proliferate to create a pool of muscle precursor cells that can repair or replace damaged muscle.

Satellite cells are not a homogeneous population; the majority express M-cadherin, myf 5, and CD34, but a small number express none of these proteins, and it has been suggested that they may represent a less committed precursor or stem cell type (14,15).

Satellite cells are heterogeneous in their ability to form large clones in vitro, some being capable of forming only small colonies, whereas others are capable of extensive proliferation, implying that they are more stem cell–like (16,17). This may be due to different responses of individual satellite cells to mitogenic stimuli, fast-growing clones being more responsive to FGF-2 and expressing higher levels of FGF-2, FGF receptor-1, and heparan sulfate proteoglycans (18). Individual satellite cells may also have different capacities to divide asymmetrically. Only some may be true stem cells, able to give rise to a stem cell and a more committed myogenic cell, and this may be altered by environmental factors (19,20).

There is functional evidence that satellite cells are a heterogeneous population. Following an injury, some satellite cells proliferate prior to either differentiating into muscle or giving rise to more satellite cells. Other activated satellite cells proliferate little or not at all prior to fusion with damaged muscle fibers and are thought to be more committed precursor cells (16,21,22). In addition, a small population of "stem cell–like" muscle precursor cells in mouse muscle survives high doses of radiation (23).

Although the satellite cells present in a muscle of a young mouse appear to be capable of fully replacing that muscle following an injury, the regenerative capacity of muscle diminishes with age and rapidly declines in myopathic muscle (24). There is evidence that the capacity of myopathic muscle to successfully regenerate throughout the lifetime is hampered by the loss of regenerative capability of satellite cells (23,25–28). The reduced regenerative capacity of old human skeletal muscle may be due to either loss of satellite cells or reduction in their proliferation potential due to telomere shortening (29–31). Changes in the aged or diseased muscle environment, for example, reduction of notch in aged muscle, may also affect the capacity of satellite cells to regenerate (32). The poor regeneration of muscle in old animals may be due to poorly functioning old macrophages that do not produce sufficient growth factors and perhaps a general diminution of circulating growth factors in the aging individual (33–36).

Even when it is undergoing degeneration and regeneration as a result of an injury or a myopathy, skeletal muscle is not a particularly conducive environment for muscle regeneration from implanted muscle precursor cells or bone marrow stem cells (37,38). The majority of muscle precursor cells implanted into skeletal muscle die (39–45). At least part of the cause of this rapid cell death seems to be mediated by $CD4^+$, $CD8^+$, and NK cells and may be reduced by anti-LFA antibodies, but the final yield of muscle per implanted cell has not been markedly improved by such measures (43,46,47). It may be that the transplanted muscle cells that die may not be relevant to the regeneration of the muscle. Thus, the cells that survived transplantation were those that were not dividing in vitro immediately before grafting (40); stem cells often do not proliferate in culture (48). In vivo conditions selected for the survival of this stem cell–like subset of mpc whereas the non-stem cell–like donor muscle cells rapidly died. Under appropriate in vivo conditions, the surviving cells proliferated and made large amounts of donor muscle and gave rise to long-lived muscle precursor or stem cells (37,40,49–51).

Myoblast transplantation has been attempted in myopathic models, particularly the dystrophin-deficient *mdx* mouse and has been shown to increase the strength of regenerated mouse muscle (52–54).

The Effect of the Environment on Muscle Regeneration

Although regeneration in myopathic muscle from resident satellite cells may at first be effective, the cumulative changes that occur in the muscle as a result of the primary defect may eventually obstruct effective regeneration, either from endogenous or transplanted satellite cells.

Factors that affect conditions in regenerating dystrophic and aged skeletal muscle are complex and may have an impact on the survival, proliferation, and muscle forming capacity of either endogenous or transplanted mpc (55–60). In particular, changes in concentrations of chemokines, cytokines, and components of the complement pathway as well as genes involved in the immune response and extracellular matrix production in injured muscles may have profound effects on muscle regeneration (57–59,61). A change in gene expression that may promote muscle regeneration may be counteracted by other gene expression changes. For example, although IGF-1 is upregulated in DMD muscle, the beneficial effects of this growth factor may be offset by increased expression of IGF-binding proteins and insulin-like growth factor binding protein-5 (IGFBP-5) protease (62). Future work is therefore needed to determine the changes in injured or regenerating skeletal muscle that inhibit muscle regeneration.

One prominent change that occurs in dystrophic skeletal muscle is fibrosis (63–65). This increase in connective tissue may affect cell signaling and also physically impede the movement of satellite cells or implanted cells.

Although there is evidence that increased fibrosis of *mdx* muscle does not impair muscle regeneration, other changes in the fibrotic muscle environment may affect muscle regeneration (27,66). For example, transforming growth factor-beta1 (TGF-β1) is expressed at high levels in myopathic skeletal muscle and in the serum of DMD patients and is believed to play a pivotal role in skeletal muscle fibrosis (67,68). TGF-β1 stimulates deposition of collagens, resulting in the accumulation of fibrotic tissue (69). TGF-β1 inhibition by an anti-TGF-β human proteoglycan, decorin, or by gamma interferon, which inhibits TGF-β signaling, has been shown to reduce fibrosis and enhance endogenous muscle regeneration. But TGF-β appears to be beneficial to transplanted myoblasts, its anti-inflammatory activity reducing the death of the donor cells (70–72). Other direct effects of TGF-β on muscle cells may affect muscle regeneration. For example, TGF-β inhibits muscle differentiation by repressing myogenic regulatory factors (73). It is also a chemoattractant for muscle cells in vitro and is involved in control of myoblast migration in the development (74,75). Interactions between different signaling pathways that mediate the effects of growth factors involved in myoblast migration, proliferation, or differentiation, e.g., the reduction of IGFBP-5 by TGF-β, may modulate the actions of a particular growth factor on muscle regeneration (76).

Irradiation of skeletal muscle before implanting cells into it has a dramatic effect on the fate of the implanted cells. For example, the single mouse extensor digitorum longus (EDL) muscle fiber, bearing five to seven satellite cells, gave rise to large amounts of muscle following implantation into *mdx* nu/nu muscle that had been preirradiated with 18 Gy (Fig. 1). However, the EDL muscle fiber gave rise to no donor muscle following implantation into nonirradiated host muscle (77,78). Not only does preirradiation enhance the amount of muscle formed from normal muscle cells, but it has a profound effect on increasing the speed of tumor formation from the myogenic cell line C2C12 (37). Similar effects of an irradiated environment on implanted tumor cells have also been shown in irradiated mouse mammary glands (79). How the irradiated environment increases the amount of muscle formed by mpc implanted into it is not known. It may alter the amount of growth factor produced by the muscle; for example, irradiation increases the amount of IGF-1 produced by brain tumor cells and hepatocyte growth factor (HGF) receptor in pancreatic cancer cells (80,81).

GROWTH FACTORS AS REGENERATIVE THERAPY FOR MYOPATHIC OR AGED MUSCLES

The regeneration of skeletal muscle from either endogenous satellite cells or muscle precursor cells implanted into myopathic muscle may in theory be increased by the application of growth factors that have an effect on the proliferation, migration, or differentiation of myogenic cells in vitro.

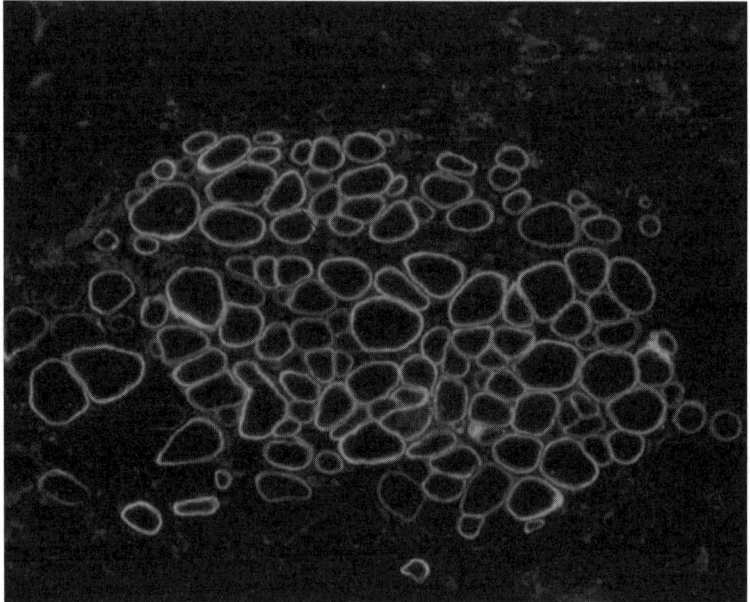

Figure 1 Satellite cells on one muscle fiber are capable of giving rise to large amounts of muscle. Cryostat section of an *mdx* nu/nu tibialis anterior muscle, which had been irradiated with 18 Gy and implanted with a single EDL muscle fiber from a normal donor mouse. Three weeks after implantation, the injected muscle contained 111 donor (dystrophin-positive) muscle fibers. *Abbreviation*: EDL, extensor digitorum longus.

However, such growth factors may not be effective in regenerating muscle. For example, although HGF, scatter factor, causes chemotaxis and proliferation of myogenic cells in culture and in ectopically grafted myogenic cells in vivo, it also inhibits muscle regeneration in vivo (74,82–85). Although several FGFs, including FGF-2, stimulate myoblast proliferation in vitro and in culture of mpc with FGF-2 prior to their implantation into *mdx* mice and increased the amount of donor muscle formed, FGF-2 did not augment endogenous muscle regeneration (9,86,87).

A number of factors may be manipulated to improve myopathic or aged muscle by promoting or restoring their regenerative capacity. Prominent among these are myostatin and IGF-1.

Myostatin, a member of the TGF-β superfamily, controls embryonic myoblast proliferation and negatively regulates satellite cell activation (88,89). Inhibition of myostatin increases mass and strength of adult skeletal muscle and, surprisingly, has been found to reduce the pathology and to improve function of *mdx* mouse muscle (4,12,90,91). Inhibition of myostatin might therefore act as a therapy by counteracting muscle loss as a consequence of disease, atrophy or aging, or other causes of sarcopoenia.

IGF-1 augments muscle growth and hypertrophy (7,92,93). IGF-1 expression improves the pathology and strength of *mdx* mouse muscle (3,94,95). IGF-1 overexpression in transgenic mice also significantly reduced fibrosis in the diaphragm (3). Circulating levels of IGF-1 decline with age and IGF-1 signaling is implicated in the degeneration of aging muscle (36,96). IGF-1 expression sustains mass in old mouse muscles and inhibits disuse atrophy (7,97). A muscle-specific variant of the IGF-1 gene may be responsible for the initial activation of quiescent satellite cells following an injury (98,99). However, the mechanism by which either myostatin or IGF-1 regulates muscle size, or by which any of these factors improve the *mdx* myopathy, is not known.

The ability of ADAM-12, a disintegrin and metalloproteinase involved in cell spreading and myoblast fusion, to ameliorate the *mdx* pathology may operate via two mechanisms: it is proposed that it acts to augment the adhesive force between the muscle fiber surface and the basal lamina by enhancing expression of utrophin and integrin $\beta 7$, but it may also act by cleaving IGFBPs-3 and -5, thus promoting the biological activity of IGF-1 and -2 (100–102).

STEM CELLS IN SKELETAL MUSCLE

The application of high doses of radiation to skeletal muscle kills the majority of satellite cells and as a consequence unmasks the ability of a radiation-resistant subpopulation of muscle cells to regenerate skeletal muscle and to give rise to satellite cells. Mature muscle fibers have nuclei that do not divide, so radiation has very little detrimental effect on muscle structure. However, if 16 to 18 Gy radiation is applied to growing or regenerating skeletal muscle, satellite cells are destroyed and the growth of young normal mouse muscle and regeneration of *mdx* mouse muscle is prevented (103–106). However, irradiated mouse muscle that is extensively damaged by injection of the snake venom, notexin, that destroys muscle fibers but spares single cells such as satellite cells, undergoes extensive regeneration (23,50). The radiation-resistant muscle precursor cells appear to be resident in skeletal muscle, as they are completely ablated by 25 Gy local irradiation (23). The restoration of the satellite cell pool in irradiated notexin-treated mouse muscles is, however, significantly reduced in dystrophic mdx compared to normal C57Bl/10 mice. The identity of these radiation-resistant skeletal muscle cells is not yet known. They may be a subset of satellite cells, or a more primitive stem cell present in skeletal muscle.

The ability to escape damage either by ionizing radiation or by toxic drugs is a feature of stem cells and may be used as a tool to enrich them. Side population (SP) cells that can exclude Hoescht dye may be purified from the bone marrow, muscle, and other organs and are enriched for stem cells (107). The SP cells derived from the bone marrow may participate, albeit rarely, in regeneration of skeletal muscle (15,108,109). However, it is not clear whether the bone marrow SP cells can reconstitute both the postmitotic muscle fibers and satellite cell compartment, or whether any individual cell can give rise to cells of both the hematopoetic and muscle lineages.

A similar SP cell may also be derived from skeletal muscle and can repopulate the hematopoetic system, giving rise to the three major blood lineages. Recent evidence suggests that the SP containing stem cells is not derived from satellite cells, but may be derived from the vasculature, migratory bone marrow cells, or mesenchyme stem cells (15,108,110,111). Although muscle SP cells do not differentiate into skeletal muscle in vitro, they do give rise to both skeletal muscle and satellite cells in vivo (112,113). It is possible that the radiation-resistant muscle cell is an SP cell; it may be the CD45+ stem cell that resides in skeletal muscle and is capable of reconstituting the hematopoetic system and contributing to muscle regeneration in injured muscles (114). The relationship between the SP, or the radiation-resistant or CD45+ cells, and the nonadherent cells that are present in adult muscle that appear to have extensive stem cell properties, remains to be established (115–117).

CONCLUSIONS

To effectively reverse or prevent loss of skeletal muscle that occurs as a consequence of a myopathy, disuse, or aging, the regenerative capacity of either the patient's own satellite cells or stem cells, or exogenously added satellite or stem cells, must be improved (118). The problem with both approaches is to modify the diseased or aged skeletal muscle environment to enable maximal muscle formation. Although growth factors have been shown to improve the *mdx* myopathy and to prevent atrophy in old mouse muscle, the mechanism of their action has not been elucidated, nor has their effect on implanted muscle cells been demonstrated.

The ability of a nonmyogenic stem cell, the mesangioblast, to extensively reconstitute alpha-sarcoglycan deficient mouse muscle after intra-arterial delivery suggests that systemic delivery of stem cells to treat myopathies is a real possibility (119). The possibility of systemically delivering muscle precursor or stem cells, together with a deeper understanding of how growth factor and cell signaling changes in damaged or aging skeletal muscle may lead to loss of regenerative capability, will help us to devise ways of counteracting the deleterious changes that occur in myopathic muscle.

ACKNOWLEDGMENTS

JEM and TP are funded by the MRC; KB is funded by a Muscular Dystrophy Campaign grant held by JEM; CAC is funded by the Engineering and Physical Sciences Research Council (EPSRC).

REFERENCES

1. Li Y, Huard J. Differentiation of muscle-derived cells into myofibroblasts in injured skeletal muscle. Am J Pathol 2002; 161(3):895–907.
2. Holst D, Grimaldi PA. New factors in the regulation of adipose differentiation and metabolism. Curr Opin Lipidol 2002; 13(3):241–245.
3. Barton ER, Morris L, Musaro A, Rosenthal N, Sweeney HL. Muscle-specific expression of insulin-like growth factor I counters muscle decline in mdx mice. J Cell Biol 2002; 157(1):137–148.
4. Bogdanovich S, Krag TO, Barton ER, et al. Functional improvement of dystrophic muscle by myostatin blockade. Nature 2002; 420(6914):418–421.
5. Horsley V, Friday BB, Matteson S, Kegley KM, Gephart J, Pavlath GK. Regulation of the growth of multinucleated muscle cells by an NFATC2-dependent pathway. J Cell Biol 2001; 153(2):329–338.
6. Horsley V, Jansen KM, Mills ST, Pavlath GK. IL-4 acts as a myoblast recruitment factor during mammalian muscle growth. Cell 2003; 113(4):483–494.
7. Musaro A, McCullagh KJ, Naya FJ, Olson EN, Rosenthal N. IGF-1 induces skeletal myocyte hypertrophy through calcineurin in association with GATA-2 and NF-ATc1. Nature 1999; 400(6744):581–585.
8. Wilson EM, Hsieh MM, Rotwein P. Autocrine growth factor signaling by insulin-like growth factor-II mediates MyoD-stimulated myocyte maturation. J Biol Chem 2003; 278(42):41109–41113.
9. Sheehan SM, Allen RE. Skeletal muscle satellite cell proliferation in response to members of the fibroblast growth factor family and hepatocyte growth factor. J Cell Physiol 1999; 181(3):499–506.
10. Yablonka-Reuveni Z, Rivera AJ. Influence of PDGF-BB on proliferation and transition through the MyoD-myogenin-MEF2A expression program during myogenesis in mouse C2 myoblasts. Growth Factors 1997; 15(1):1–27.
11. Reid MB, Li YP. Tumor necrosis factor-alpha and muscle wasting: a cellular perspective. Respir Res 2001; 2(5):269–272.
12. Grobet L, Pirottin D, Farnir F, et al. Modulating skeletal muscle mass by postnatal, muscle-specific inactivation of the myostatin gene. Genesis 2003; 35(4):227–238.
13. Mauro A. Satellite cell of skeletal muscle fibers. J Biophys Biochem Cytol 1961; 9:493–495.
14. Beauchamp JR, Heslop L, Yu DS, et al. Expression of CD34 and Myf5 defines the majority of quiescent adult skeletal muscle satellite cells. J Cell Biol 2000; 151(6):1221–1234.
15. Zammit P, Beauchamp J. The skeletal muscle satellite cell: stem cell or son of stem cell? Differentiation 2001; 68(4–5):193–204.
16. Schultz E. Satellite cell proliferative compartments in growing skeletal muscles. Dev Biol 1996; 175(1):84–94.

17. Mozdziak PE, McFarland DC, Schultz E. Telomeric profiles and telomerase activity in turkey satellite cell clones with different in vitro growth characteristics. Biochim Biophys Acta 2000; 1492(2–3):362–368.
18. McFarland DC, Liu X, Velleman SG, Zeng C, Coy CS, Pesall JE. Variation in fibroblast growth factor response and heparan sulfate proteoglycan production in satellite cell populations. Comp Biochem Physiol C Toxicol Pharmacol 2003; 134(3):341–351.
19. Conboy IM, Rando TA. The regulation of Notch signaling controls satellite cell activation and cell fate determination in postnatal myogenesis. Dev Cell 2002; 3(3):397–409.
20. Sherley JL. Asymmetric cell kinetics genes: the key to expansion of adult stem cells in culture. Stem Cells 2002; 20(6):561–572.
21. Grounds MD, McGeachie JK. Reutilisation of tritiated thymidine in studies of regenerating skeletal muscle. Cell Tissue Res 1987; 250(1):141–148.
22. McGeachie JK, Grounds MD. Initiation and duration of muscle precursor replication after mild and severe injury to skeletal muscle of mice. An autoradiographic study. Cell Tissue Res 1987; 248(1):125–130.
23. Heslop L, Morgan JE, Partridge TA. Evidence for a myogenic stem cell that is exhausted in dystrophic muscle. J Cell Sci 2000; 113(Pt 12):2299–2308.
24. Zammit PS Heslop L, Hudon V, et al. Kinetics of myoblast proliferation show that resident satellite cells are competent to fully regenerate skeletal muscle fibers. Exp Cell Res 2002; 281(1):39–49.
25. Endesfelder S, Krahn A, Kreuzer KA, et al. Elevated p21 mRNA level in skeletal muscle of DMD patients and mdx mice indicates either an exhausted satellite cell pool or a higher p21 expression in dystrophin-deficient cells per se. J Mol Med 2000; 78(10):569–574.
26. Reimann JA, Irintchev A, Wernig A. Regenerative capacity and the number of satellite cells in soleus muscles of normal and mdx mice. Neuromuscul Disord 2000; 10(4–5):276–282.
27. Luz MA, Marques MJ, Santo Neto H. Impaired regeneration of dystrophin-deficient muscle fibers is caused by exhaustion of myogenic cells. Braz J Med Biol Res 2002; 35(6):691–695.
28. Jejurikar S, Kuzon W. Satellite cell depletion in degenerative skeletal muscle. Apoptosis 2003; 8:573–578.
29. Renault V, Thornell LE, Eriksson PO, Butler-Browne G, Mouly V. Regenerative potential of human skeletal muscle during aging. Aging Cell 2002; 1(2):132–139.
30. Decary S, Hamida CB, Mouly V, Barbet JP, Hentati F, Butler-Browne GS. Shorter telomeres in dystrophic muscle consistent with extensive regeneration in young children. Neuromuscul Disord 2000; 10(2):113–120.
31. Cooper RN, Thiesson D, Furling D, Di Santo JP, Butler-Browne GS, Mouly V. Extended amplification in vitro and replicative senescence: key factors implicated in the success of human myoblast transplantation. Hum Gene Ther 2003; 14(12):1169–1179.
32. Conboy IM, Conboy MJ, Smythe GM, Rando TA. Notch-mediated restoration of regenerative potential to aged muscle. Science 2003; 302(5650):1575–1577.

33. Carlson BM, Faulkner JA. Muscle transplantation between young and old rats: age of host determines recovery. Am J Physiol 1989; 256(6 Pt 1): C1262–C1266.
34. Carlson BM, Dedkov EI, Borisov AB, Faulkner JA. Skeletal muscle regeneration in very old rats. J Gerontol A Biol Sci Med Sci 2001; 56(5):B224–B233.
35. Cannon JG. Intrinsic and extrinsic factors in muscle aging. Ann N Y Acad Sci 1998; 854:72–77.
36. Harridge SD. Ageing and local growth factors in muscle. Scand J Med Sci Sports 2003; 13(1):34–39.
37. Morgan JE, Gross JG, Pagel CN, et al. Myogenic cell proliferation and generation of a reversible tumorigenic phenotype are triggered by preirradiation of the recipient site. J Cell Biol 2002; 157(4):693–702.
38. Ferrari G, Cusella-De Angelis G, Coletta M, et al. Muscle regeneration by bone marrow-derived myogenic progenitors. Science 1998; 279(5356):1528–1530.
39. Beauchamp JR, Pagel CN, Partridge TA. A dual-marker system for quantitative studies of myoblast transplantation in the mouse. Transplantation 1997; 63(12):1794–1797.
40. Beauchamp JR, Morgan JE, Pagel CN, Partridge TA. Dynamics of myoblast transplantation reveal a discrete minority of precursors with stem cell-like properties as the myogenic source. J Cell Biol 1999; 144(6):1113–1122.
41. Fan Y, Maley M, Beilharz M, Grounds M. Rapid death of injected myoblasts in myoblast transfer therapy. Muscle Nerve 1996; 19(7):853–860.
42. Skuk D, Tremblay JP. Complement deposition cell death after myoblast transplantation. Cell Transplant 1998; 7(5):427–434.
43. Guerette B, Asselin I, Skuk D, Entman M, Tremblay JP. Control of inflammatory damage by anti-LFA-1: increase success of myoblast transplantation. Cell Transplant 1997; 6(2):101–107.
44. Guerette B, Skuk D, Celestin F, et al. Prevention by anti-LFA-1 of acute myoblast death following transplantation. J Immunol 1997; 159(5):2522–2531.
45. Skuk D, Caron NJ, Goulet M, Roy B, Tremblay JP. Resetting the problem of cell death following muscle-derived cell transplantation: detection dynamics and mechanisms. J Neuropathol Exp Neurol 2003; 62(9):951–967.
46. Skuk D, Caron N, Goulet M, Roy B, Espinosa F, Tremblay JP. Dynamics of the early immune cellular reactions after myogenic cell transplantation. Cell Transplant 2002; 11(7):671–681.
47. Hodgetts SI, Spencer MJ, Grounds MD. A role for natural killer cells in the rapid death of cultured donor myoblasts after transplantation. Transplantation 2003; 75(6):863–871.
48. Glimm H, Oh IH, Eaves CJ. Human hematopoietic stem cells stimulated to proliferate in vitro lose engraftment potential during their $S/G(2)/M$ transit and do not reenter $G(0)$. Blood 2000; 96(13):4185–4193.
49. Morgan JE, Beauchamp JR, Pagel CN, et al. Myogenic cell lines derived from transgenic mice carrying a thermolabile T antigen: a model system for the derivation of tissue-specific and mutation-specific cell lines. Dev Biol 1994; 162(2):486–498.
50. Gross JG, Morgan JE. Muscle precursor cells injected into irradiated mdx mouse muscle persist after serial injury. Muscle Nerve 1999; 22(2):174–185.

51. Blaveri K, Heslop L, Yu DS, Rosenblatt JD, Gross JG, Partridge TA, Morgan JE. Patterns of repair of dystrophic mouse muscle: studies on isolated fibers. Dev Dyn 1999; 216(3):244–256.
52. Partridge T. Myoblast transplantation. Neuromuscul Disord 2002; 12(suppl 1): S3–S6.
53. Arcila ME, Ameredes BT, DeRosimo JF, et al. Mass and functional capacity of regenerating muscle is enhanced by myoblast transfer. J Neurobiol 1997; 33(2):185–198.
54. DeRosimo JF, Washabaugh CH, Ontell MP, et al. Enhancement of adult muscle regeneration by primary myoblast transplantation. Cell Transplant 2000; 9(3):369–377.
55. Yan Z, Choi S, Liu X, et al. Highly coordinated gene regulation in mouse skeletal muscle regeneration. J Biol Chem 2003; 278(10):8826–8836.
56. Goetsch SC, Hawke TJ, Gallardo TD, Richardson JA, Garry DJ. Transcriptional profiling and regulation of the extracellular matrix during muscle regeneration. Physiol Genomics 2003; 14(3):261–271.
57. Summan M, McKinstry M, Warren GL, et al. Inflammatory mediators and skeletal muscle injury: a DNA microarray analysis. J Interferon Cytokine Res 2003; 23(5):237–245.
58. Porter JD, Khanna S, Kaminski HJ, et al. A chronic inflammatory response dominates the skeletal muscle molecular signature in dystrophin-deficient mdx mice. Hum Mol Genet 2002; 11(3):263–272.
59. Porter JD, Guo W, Merriam AP, et al. Persistent over-expression of specific CC class chemokines correlates with macrophage and T-cell recruitment in mdx skeletal muscle. Neuromuscul Disord 2003; 13(3):223–235.
60. Pattison JS, Folk LC, Madsen RW, Booth FW. Selected Contribution: identification of differentially expressed genes between young and old rat soleus muscle during recovery from immobilization-induced atrophy. J Appl Physiol 2003; 95(5):2171–2179.
61. Haslett JN, Sanoudou D, Kho AT, et al. Gene expression comparison of biopsies from Duchenne muscular dystrophy (DMD) and normal skeletal muscle. Proc Natl Acad Sci USA 2002; 99(23):15000–15005.
62. Bakay M, Zhao P, Chen J, Hoffman EP. A web-accessible complete transcriptome of normal human and DMD muscle. Neuromuscul Disord 2002; 12(suppl 1):S125–S141.
63. Morrison J, Lu QL, Pastoret C, Partridge T, Bou-Gharios G. T-cell-dependent fibrosis in the mdx dystrophic mouse. Lab Invest 2000; 80(6):881–891.
64. Best TM, Hunter KD. Muscle injury and repair. Phys Med Rehabil Clin N Am 2000; 11(2):251–266.
65. Pastoret C, Sebille A. Age-related differences in regeneration of dystrophic (mdx) and normal muscle in the mouse. Muscle Nerve 1995; 18(10):1147–1154.
66. Brussee V, Tardif F, Roy B, Goulet M, Sebille A, Tremblay JP. Successful myoblast transplantation in fibrotic muscles: no increased impairment by the connective tissue. Transplantation 1999; 67(12):1618–1622.
67. Yamazaki M, Minota S, Sakurai H, et al. Expression of transforming growth factor-beta 1 and its relation to endomysial fibrosis in progressive muscular dystrophy. Am J Pathol 1994; 144(2):221–226.

68. Ishitobi M, Haginoya K, Zhao Y, et al. Elevated plasma levels of transforming growth factor beta1 in patients with muscular dystrophy. Neuroreport 2000; 11(18):4033–4035.
69. Border WA, Noble NA. Transforming growth factor beta in tissue fibrosis. N Engl J Med 1994; 331(19):1286–1292.
70. Sato K, Foster W, Fukushima K, et al. Improvement of muscle healing through enhancement of muscle regeneration and prevention of fibrosis. Muscle Nerve 2003; 28(3):365–372.
71. Foster W, Li Y, Usas A, Somogyi G, Huard J. Gamma interferon as an antifibrosis agent in skeletal muscle. J Orthop Res 2003; 21(5):798–804.
72. Merly F, Huard C, Asselin I, Robbins PD, Tremblay JP. Anti-inflammatory effect of transforming growth factor-beta1 in myoblast transplantation. Transplantation 1998; 65(6):793–799.
73. Liu D, Black BL, Derynck R. TGF-beta inhibits muscle differentiation through functional repression of myogenic transcription factors by Smad3. Genes Dev 2001; 15(22):2950–2966.
74. Bischoff R. Chemotaxis of skeletal muscle satellite cells. Dev Dyn 1997; 208(4):505–515.
75. Olguin HC, Santander C, Brandan E. Inhibition of myoblast migration via decorin expression is critical for normal skeletal muscle differentiation. Dev Biol 2003; 259(2):209–224.
76. Rousse S, Lallemand F, Montarras D, et al. Transforming growth factor-beta inhibition of insulin-like growth factor-binding protein-5 synthesis in skeletal muscle cells involves a c-Jun N-terminal kinase-dependent pathway. J Biol Chem 2001; 276(50):46961–46967.
77. Collins CA, Partridge TA. Self-renewal of the adult skeletal muscle satellite cell. Cell Cycle 2005; 4(10). [Epub ahead of print]
78. Collins CA, Olsen I, Zammit PS, et al. Stem cell function, self-renewal, and behavioral heterogeneity of cells from the adult muscle satellite cell niche. Cell 2005; 122(2):289–301.
79. Park CC, Bissell MJ, Barcellos-Hoff MH. The influence of the microenvironment on the malignant phenotype. Mol Med Today 2000; 6(8):324–329.
80. Kim KU, Lallemand F, Montarras D, et al. Changes in expression of transferrin insulin-like growth factor 1, and interleukin 4 receptors after irradiation of cells of primary malignant brain tumor cell lines. Radiat Res 2003; 160(2):224–231.
81. Qian LW, Mizumoto K, Inadome N, et al. Radiation stimulates HGF receptor/c-Met expression that leads to amplifying cellular response to HGF stimulation via upregulated receptor tyrosine phosphorylation and MAP kinase activity in pancreatic cancer cells. Int J Cancer 2003; 104(5):542–549.
82. Corti S, Salani S, Del Bo R, et al. Chemotactic factors enhance myogenic cell migration across an endothelial monolayer. Exp Cell Res 2001; 268(1):36–44.
83. Sheehan SM, Tatsumi R, Temm-Grove CJ, Allen RE. HGF is an autocrine growth factor for skeletal muscle satellite cells in vitro. Muscle Nerve 2000; 23(2):239–245.
84. Barbero A, Benelli R, Minghelli S, et al. Growth factor supplemented matrigel improves ectopic skeletal muscle formation–a cell therapy approach. J Cell Physiol 2001; 186(2):183–192.

85. Miller KJ, Thaloor D, Matteson S, Pavlath GK. Hepatocyte growth factor affects satellite cell activation and differentiation in regenerating skeletal muscle. Am J Physiol Cell Physiol 2000; 278(1):C174–C181.
86. Kinoshita I, Vilquin JT, Roy T, Tremblay JP. Successive injections in mdx mice of myoblasts grown with bFGF. Neuromuscul Disord 1996; 6(3):187–193.
87. Mitchell CA, McGeachie JK, Grounds MD. The exogenous administration of basic fibroblast growth factor to regenerating skeletal muscle in mice does not enhance the process of regeneration. Growth Factors 1996; 13(1–2):37–55.
88. Sharma M, Langley B, Bass J, Kambadur R. Myostatin in muscle growth and repair. Exerc Sport Sci Rev 2001; 29(4):155–158.
89. McCroskery S, Thomas M, Maxwell L, Sharma M, Kambadur R. Myostatin negatively regulates satellite cell activation and self-renewal. J Cell Biol 2003; 162(6):1135–1147.
90. Whittemore LA, Song K, Li X, et al. Inhibition of myostatin in adult mice increases skeletal muscle mass and strength. Biochem Biophys Res Commun 2003; 300(4):965–971.
91. Wagner KR, McPherron AC, Winik N, Lee SJ. Loss of myostatin attenuates severity of muscular dystrophy in mdx mice. Ann Neurol 2002; 52(6): 832–836.
92. Fiorotto ML, Schwartz RJ, Delaughter MC. Persistent IGF-I overexpression in skeletal muscle transiently enhances DNA accretion and growth. Faseb J 2003; 17(1):59–60.
93. Glass DJ. Molecular mechanisms modulating muscle mass. Trends Mol Med 2003; 9(8):344–350.
94. Gregorevic P, Plant DR, Leeding KS, Bach LA, Lynch GS. Improved contractile function of the mdx dystrophic mouse diaphragm muscle after insulin-like growth factor-I administration. Am J Pathol 2002; 161(6):2263–2272.
95. De Luca A, Pierno S, Liantonio A, et al. Enhanced dystrophic progression in mdx mice by exercise and beneficial effects of taurine and insulin-like growth factor-1. J Pharmacol Exp Ther 2003; 304(1):453–463.
96. Grounds MD. Reasons for the degeneration of ageing skeletal muscle: a central role for IGF-1 signalling. Biogerontology 2002; 3(1–2):19–24.
97. Alzghoul MB, Gerrard D, Watkins BA, Hannon K. Ectopic expression of IGF-I and Shh by skeletal muscle inhibits disuse-mediated skeletal muscle atrophy and bone osteopenia in vivo. Faseb J 2004; 18(1):221–223.
98. Hill M, Goldspink G. Expression and splicing of the insulin-like growth factor gene in rodent muscle is associated with muscle satellite (stem) cell activation following local tissue damage. J Physiol 2003; 549(Pt 2):409–418.
99. Hill M, Wernig A, Goldspink G. Muscle satellite (stem) cell activation during local tissue injury and repair. J Anat 2003; 203(1):89–99.
100. Galliano MF, Huet C, Frygelius J, Polgren A, Wewer UM, Engvall E. Binding of ADAM12, a marker of skeletal muscle regeneration, to the muscle-specific actin-binding protein, alpha -actinin-2, is required for myoblast fusion. J Biol Chem 2000; 275(18):13933–13939.
101. Kronqvist P, Kawaguchi N, Albrechtsen R, et al. ADAM12 alleviates the skeletal muscle pathology in mdx dystrophic mice. Am J Pathol 2002; 161(5):1535–1540.

102. Loechel F, Fox JW, Murphy G, Albrechtsen R, Wewer UM. ADAM 12-S cleaves IGFBP-3 and IGFBP-5 and is inhibited by TIMP-3. Biochem Biophys Res Commun 2000; 278(3):511–515.
103. Wakeford S, Watt DJ, Partridge TA. X-irradiation improves mdx mouse muscle as a model of myofiber loss in DMD. Muscle Nerve 1991; 14(1):42–50.
104. Quinlan JG, Lyden SP, Cambier DM, Johnson SR, Michaels SE, Denman DL. Radiation inhibition of mdx mouse muscle regeneration: dose and age factors. Muscle Nerve 1995; 18(2):201–206.
105. Quinlan JG, Cambier D, Lyden S, et al. Regeneration-blocked mdx muscle: in vivo model for testing treatments. Muscle Nerve 1997; 20(8):1016–1023.
106. Pagel CN, Partridge TA. Covert persistence of mdx mouse myopathy is revealed by acute and chronic effects of irradiation. J Neurol Sci 1999; 164(2):103–116.
107. Alison M. Tissue-based stem cells: ABC transporter proteins take centre stage. J Pathol 2003; 200:547–550.
108. Seale P, Rudnicki MA. A new look at the origin function and "stem-cell" status of muscle satellite cells. Dev Biol 2000; 218(2):115–124.
109. Hawke TJ, Garry DJ. Myogenic satellite cells: physiology to molecular biology. J Appl Physiol 2001; 91(2):534–551.
110. Asakura A, Rudnicki MA. Side population cells from diverse adult tissues are capable of in vitro hematopoietic differentiation. Exp Hematol 2002; 30(11): 1339–1345.
111. Asakura A. Stem cells in adult skeletal muscle. Trends Cardiovasc Med 2003; 13(3):123–128.
112. Asakura A, Seale P, Girgis-Gabardo A, Rudnicki MA. Myogenic specification of side population cells in skeletal muscle. J Cell Biol 2002; 159(1):123–134.
113. Gussoni E, Soneoka Y, Strickland CD, et al. Dystrophin expression in the mdx mouse restored by stem cell transplantation. Nature 1999; 401(6751):390–394.
114. Polesskaya A, Seale P, Rudnicki MA. Wnt signaling induces the myogenic specification of resident CD45+ adult stem cells during muscle regeneration. Cell 2003; 113(7):841–852.
115. Qu-Petersen Z, Deasy B, Jankowski R, et al. Identification of a novel population of muscle stem cells in mice: potential for muscle regeneration. J Cell Biol 2002; 157(5):851–864.
116. Cao B, Zheng B, Jankowski RJ, et al. Muscle stem cells differentiate into haematopoietic lineages but retain myogenic potential. Nat Cell Biol 2003; 5(7): 640–646.
117. Jankowski RJ, Deasy BM, Huard J. Muscle-derived stem cells. Gene Ther 2002; 9(10):642–647.
118. Partridge TA. Stem cell route to neuromuscular therapies. Muscle Nerve 2003; 27(2):133–141.
119. Sampaolesi M, Torrente Y, Innocenzi A, et al. Cell therapy of alpha-sarcoglycan null dystrophic mice through intra-arterial delivery of mesoangioblasts. Science 2003; 301(5632):487–492.

14

Cellular Mediated Delivery: The Intersection Between Regenerative Medicine and Genetic Therapy

K. Liadaki, F. Montanaro, and L. M. Kunkel
Howard Hughes Medical Institute at the Children's Hospital, and Department of Pediatrics, Harvard Medical School, Boston, Massachusetts, U.S.A.

INTRODUCTION

Muscular dystrophies are a heterogeneous group of genetic disorders characterized by progressive muscle weakness and wasting. The most common and severe form of muscular dystrophy is Duchenne muscular dystrophy (DMD). DMD is an X-linked recessive disease characterized by a mutation in the gene encoding dystrophin, a myofiber stabilizing protein (1–3). A point mutation in exon 23 of the dystrophin gene causes a milder muscle wasting in mice (*mdx*) than that observed in humans (4). Dystrophin is a cytoskeletal protein mainly expressed in skeletal, cardiac, and smooth muscle, and in the brain, and is severely reduced or absent in DMD patients and *mdx* mice (4–7).

The delivery of normal dystrophin to all the muscles of DMD patients should be a potential means of treating the muscle wasting in DMD. A number of different experimental approaches are emerging and are the subject of other chapters in this book. In this chapter, we will focus on cell-based approaches that deliver dystrophin to diseased tissues. The rationale for cell-mediated therapy arose from the wealth of information available on the normal physiological mechanisms of muscle formation. Mature muscle cells of mammalian skeletal muscle, known as myofibers, are multinucleated syncytia formed by the fusion of mononucleated precursors named myoblasts. Successful delivery of normal myoblasts into dystrophic muscle should result in their fusion with host muscle fibers, allowing cells to contribute their normal gene products to the syncytial myofiber, thus replacing the missing or defective gene (e.g., dystrophin) of the host. Muscle is an attractive target for cell therapy, because it is likely that relatively few donor nuclei need to be incorporated per muscle fiber to restore functional levels of full-length dystrophin to the entire fiber. This chapter gives a detailed account of recent advances in the identification and characterization of different cell populations (muscle- and nonmuscle-derived) with therapeutic potential for treating DMD, as well as the disadvantages and possible risks associated with their use. In addition, emphasis is given to the different methods of delivery of donor cells, which constitute a significant factor for the efficiency of cell therapy, as has been clearly demonstrated in recent studies (8).

MUSCLE CELLS AVAILABLE FOR THERAPY OF DMD

Skeletal muscle is a tissue capable of sustained regeneration. The mechanisms underlying muscle repair and maintenance have been extensively studied (9,10). They involve a population of muscle precursor cells known as satellite cells. The main function of satellite cells involves the generation of myoblasts through asymmetric cell division, thus participating in the repair and maintenance of postnatal skeletal muscle (Fig. 1). They are normally mitotically quiescent and account only for 2% to 5% of the total nuclei present in the muscle fibers (11,12). However, during regeneration following muscle injury, satellite cells become activated and abandon their unique anatomical position between the basal lamina and the sarcolemma of the multinucleated muscle fibers. They proliferate extensively and produce sufficient mononuclear myoblasts to repair the damaged muscle, either by directly fusing with preexisting myofibers or by generating new myofibers by fusing with one another (13–15).

In mice, satellite cells first appear in the limbs of embryos at about 17.5 days postcoitum, but their developmental origin has not been fully established (11,16). Early experiments with quail chick chimeras indicated a possible somatic origin of satellite cells, while some recent studies suggest that satellite cells originate from endothelial precursors associated with the embryonic vasculature, including the dorsal aorta (17,18). Recent studies have indicated that satellite cells express the paired-domain transcription factor Pax7 and that the expression is required either for their myogenic specification, or for their self-renewal and maintenance of the quiescent state (9,19,20).

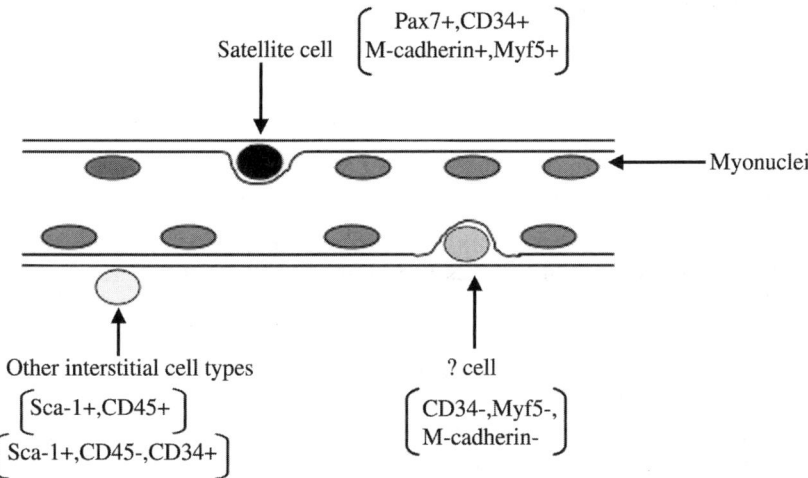

Figure 1 Normal muscle fiber with peripherally located myonuclei (*gray*) and satellite cells (*black*). The majority of satellite cells express Pax7, CD34, M-cadherin and Myf5. A minority of cells occupying a satellite cell–position (between the basal lamina and the sarcolemma of the muscle fiber) are negative for these markers, and might represent a population of cells with stem cell–like characteristics (*lighter gray*). Other cell populations, identified by cell surface markers, given in *brackets*, are located in the interstitial space of the muscle fiber (*white*).

In vitro, satellite cells separated from muscle fibers are capable of rapid proliferation and myogenesis (21,22). In addition, clones of myoblasts are capable of giving rise to new muscle and of self-renewing to give more satellite cells in vivo (23). Although it was believed for quite some time that satellite cells are a homogeneous population, recent studies have demonstrated the presence of at least two distinct cell populations within this group (Fig. 1). The major population exhibits high expression of M-cadherin, Pax7, CD34 (marker for vascular endothelial and myeloid progenitors), and c-Met [the receptor for hepatocyte growth factor (HGF)], and low expression of Myf5 (early marker of myogenic commitment). In the quiescent state, satellite cells express CD34 and Myf5, but expression of CD34 is lost after their activation (24). It is believed that CD34 is expressed by bone marrow (BM) precursors that are committed to a specific fate and have become arrested and held in reserve for subsequent activation; this could be the case for CD34-positive satellite cells in muscle (25). A minor cell population lies between the basal lamina and the sarcolemma of the muscle fiber, in a satellite cell–position, but does not express any of the previously mentioned surface markers (24). The heterogeneity in satellite–cell population possibly reflects several developmental origins within this population or different states of activation, and indicates that all satellite cells may not be equivalent (12,24,26). Interestingly, transplantation experiments have indicated that donor cells, derived from both muscle and nonmuscle tissues, can occupy a satellite cell–position upon engraftment in dystrophic muscles (27–31).

DELIVERY METHODS

Muscle is a major tissue spread throughout the organism and dystrophin is normally expressed in all muscles including cardiac, skeletal, and smooth muscle. Any effective cell therapy for muscular dystrophy must target delivery of functional donor cells to all areas of muscle regeneration. There are three major ways of delivering cells to damaged tissues: intramuscular, intravenous, and intraarterial injections.

Initial studies employed the intramuscular delivery of donor cells to specific muscle groups. This method favors the direct delivery of cells to the site of interest and therefore allows the evaluation of the ability of donor cells to fuse with existing myofibers and to produce gene products previously absent, such as dystrophin. In mice, there is clear evidence that normal muscle precursor cells can be injected into dystrophin deficient *mdx* muscle and in the best scenarios more than 90% of the myofibers have been shown to express dystrophin at their sarcolemmal membrane (32). Unfortunately, the therapeutic effect of intramuscular injections is often restricted to the injection site. There is no evidence that injected cells can transit outside the muscle to which they are delivered. Even if donor cells were extremely competent to survive and provide dystrophin expression, repeated intramuscular injections to multiple sites would be required to achieve an effective level of dystrophin myofiber expression throughout the muscle. In addition, intramuscular delivery remains a problem for muscle groups that are difficult to access, such as the diaphragm, the failure of which is the primary cause of death in DMD patients.

The circulatory system represents an attractive route for simultaneous delivery of cells to all damaged tissues, yet it was originally unclear if cells would be recruited from the circulation into the damaged tissues. Intravenous introduction of cells was first documented by Ferrari et al. (33) in a bone marrow transplantation (BMT) model of cell delivery. Subsequent studies have shown that the venous system will deliver cells to a damaged tissue, and that the degree of cellular uptake appears to correlate with the degree of damage. These studies indicate that venous delivery of cells is a practical and easy way of delivering cells in humans. Most of the studies presented later in this chapter involve intravenous transplantations of different populations of donor cells (derived from muscle, skin, and BM). These studies clearly demonstrated that intravenous injections allow the systemic delivery of donor cells to potentially all muscle groups. However, the low engraftment efficiency reported in all the studies (ranging from 1% to 9% depending on the cell population used) is the major disadvantage of intravenous delivery (27,29,33–35). A better knowledge of the molecular signals involved in the recruitment of injected cells and their incorporation into myofibers is essential to achieve therapeutic levels of donor cell engraftment. Such signals must be recognized by the donor cells and must be elevated in damaged tissues. Intravenous delivery has an additional major flaw in that the cells are dispersed through the heart and filtered through the lungs and liver before reaching the muscle, and this drawback may preclude future use.

Injection of cells into the iliac or femoral artery allows their direct delivery to the capillary beds of muscles, bypassing tissues of filtration such as liver and lungs. This recent approach has yielded promising early results with much higher efficiency of engraftment in the targeted muscle groups (8). Donor cells injected into a mouse femoral artery initially accumulate in the capillary bed, and from there they migrate into the interstitial tissue of downstream regenerating muscles. As early as 24 hours after transplantation, 30% of injected cells can be detected in the muscle downstream of the injected artery, while less than 3% of the same cell population is detected in the muscles when injected intravenously or intramuscularly. A single intraarterial delivery of cells into α-sarcoglycan null (α-SGnull) mice (model for limb-girdle muscular dystrophy) can be effective in restoring the expression of α-sarcoglycan (α-SG) protein and the other members of the dystrophin–glycoprotein complex in most leg muscles downstream of the injection site (36). In addition, repeated intraarterial injections seem sufficient to restore protein expression in more than 50% of the total muscle fibers even four months after injection (8). Therefore, the intraarterial delivery of a suitable cell population could enhance the efficiency of muscle regeneration in all muscle groups. Studies of intraarterial injections in mice are technically difficult to perform because they require a surgical procedure. In contrast, in larger animal models or in human patients, where the vessels are larger, intraarterial injections would be simpler and could theoretically be repeated frequently. The arterial delivery system has only recently been developed, yet it holds great promise for cell-based therapy. The nature of the cell-surface markers, which cause these cells to stick within the capillary beds and migrate into tissues, needs to be understood. The recent experiments took into account only a few muscles in the leg, and therefore delivery to and engraftment in other muscles must be studied.

INTRAMUSCULAR TRANSPLANTS OF MYOBLASTS

Early experiments indicated that transplantation of minced muscle or muscle precursor cells from one animal to another, results in the formation of hybrid myofibers which express the donor genes (37–40). Subsequent studies showed that injection of normal muscle precursor cells, either isolated from neonatal mice or derived from clonal cultures of normal human myoblasts, into *mdx* mice resulted in dystrophin expression in host muscles. These studies demonstrated that normal myoblasts were able to fuse with pre-existing or regenerating host dystrophic fibers and form mosaic muscle fibers, which express the full-length dystrophin gene (41,42). These early successful studies in mice led to a number of clinical trials of myoblast transfer therapy in humans. One of the first studies reported the expression of donor-derived dystrophin mRNA in three out of eight treated DMD patients who were analyzed one month after transplantation (43). However, dystrophin was detected at very low levels in only one case at six months after transplantation and no difference was reported in the force generation of the myoblast-injected muscles (43,44). Two other clinical trials also confirmed that only a small percentage of donor myoblasts could survive and fuse to form normal myotubes expressing dystrophin (45,46). An additional study reported only one DMD case (out of eight) that exhibited 5% dystrophin-positive fibers when analyzed eight weeks after myoblast injection (47). However, no dystrophin-positive fibers were detected one year later, nor was there an increase in the strength of the myoblast-injected muscles (47). A follow-up clinical trial did not detect dystrophin protein or mRNA expression in any of the three DMD patients examined three months after pure myoblast injections (48). In a larger study, 12 DMD patients were treated with a multiple myoblast injection protocol, but the authors reported no significant differences in the strength of the treated muscles (49). This study successfully overcame the problem of distinguishing the source of dystrophin protein in the transplanted regions by the use of peptide antibodies specific to the deleted exons of the dystrophin gene (49). Examination of the patients six months after the first myoblast transfer indicated that only one patient expressed donor-derived dystrophin in 10% of the patient's dystrophin-expressing muscle fibers, while the rest of the patients expressed donor-derived dystrophin in 0% to 1% of their muscle fibers (49). In addition, a large-scale human trial was reported which involved a relatively high number of patients (i.e., 21), but failed to detect dystrophin expression (50). These later findings are controversial and it is unclear whether any efficient engraftment was obtained (51). Apart from trials with DMD patients, one clinical trial was performed with patients with Becker muscular dystrophy, a milder form of muscular dystrophy also caused by dystrophin abnormalities. As in DMD cases, transplantation of myoblasts did not improve the strength of the implanted muscles, and no dystrophin expression was detected after four months of treatment (52).

The overall conclusions from the clinical trials were that myoblast transfer was a safe and feasible way to deliver cells capable of fusing with host muscle fibers and expressing donor-derived dystrophin. However, the efficiency of myoblast transfer was low and was attributed to rapid removal (due to limited survival or immune rejection) of the transplanted myoblasts. Gussoni et al. (53) later demonstrated that this might not be the case.

A re-evaluation of the biopsies of the same patients, analyzed in a previous study by the same group, revealed the presence of unexpectedly large numbers of donor-derived nuclei, many of which persisted as mononuclear cells, while others had become incorporated into mature myofibers, although a majority of them did not express dystrophin (43,53). In this study, and possibly in all the others, many injected cells escaped immune surveillance and persisted within the host muscle. Most of these cells did not lead to subsequent dystrophin expression, possibly because of environmental influences encountered in the diseased dystrophic muscle. Factors such as failure of dystrophin expression by donor cells, failure of donor myoblasts to differentiate or fuse with host myofibers, and the lack of sufficient numbers of regenerating fiber segments in the recipient muscle (patient age–dependent) were likely responsible for the poor overall therapeutic efficacy of myoblast transfer in humans.

Despite studies that failed to obtain therapeutic levels of dystrophin expression in humans, additional studies in *mdx* mice have been performed to improve the efficiency of engraftment of the injected cells. Host immunosuppression, induced by drugs such as FK506, cyclosporin A, and antilymphocyte serum, was successfully utilized to increase donor cell survival (54–57). Several host immune cell types, particularly T-cells, natural killer (NK) cells, macrophages, and mast cells, as well as the complement system were identified as the major components of the host immune system involved in the death of mismatched donor myoblasts (58). In addition, effective immunosuppression was shown to be required even for immunohistocompatible donors/recipients, and successful transplantation of human myoblasts was reported when immunodeficient *Scid* and *nude* mice were used as recipients (46,57,59–61). In addition, host irradiation, prior to myoblast transplantation, was tested and shown to increase the engraftment frequency of donor myoblasts (62–64). The effect of preirradiation was attributed to depletion of the majority of resident myogenic precursor cells (such as satellite cells), and/or to the production of growth factors that probably enhance donor cell proliferation within the graft site.

Like the human studies, the mouse studies pointed to the probable need for the use of less differentiated myogenic precursor cells, rather than terminally committed myoblasts. The identity of the populations of cells residing within the muscle was therefore reevaluated in an attempt to find a "muscle stem cell" better suited for cell-based therapy of DMD. Delivery methods were also an issue, because cells were not observed to migrate from the site of injection to other muscle groups or even adjacent fascia.

DONOR CELL SELECTION

An important issue that is to be addressed in cell transplantation is the selection of donor cells. It was clear from early studies in mice and humans that many of the donor cells were a composite of different cell types. Studies that involved transplantation of established myogenic cell lines or primary muscle cultures were not successful, while transplanted purified mouse myoblasts from primary cultures could persist up to six months (65–68). However, it was also reported that the in vitro expansion of myoblasts influences their subsequent in vivo survival (58). Studies of the early events following transplantation revealed markedly different fates for the injected myoblasts. The vast majority of donor myoblasts died immediately following transplantation, and donor-derived myofibers were formed from only a small proportion of the injected population. These latter cells appeared to retain the ability to proliferate in vivo, migrate into adjacent muscle groups, and differentiate into new myofibers for a considerable period of time after the original cell implant (32). Further studies (69,70) support the idea that loss of donor cells following transplantation involves two events; the first, as yet undefined, and to which different populations of donor myoblasts may be differentially susceptible, and the second, an inflammation-mediated event. Therefore, the minority of cells which survived after injection appear to be behaviorally distinct in that they are slowly dividing in culture, but rapidly proliferating after grafting into preirradiated muscle, thus suggesting the existence of a subpopulation of cells with stem cell–like characteristics (70). These observations prompted a search for other cells within muscle that would be better suited for transplantation.

MUSCLE SIDE POPULATION CELLS

Side population (SP) cells were first isolated from mouse BM via staining with the vital DNA dye Hoechst 33342, followed by analysis and purification using a fluorescence-activated cell sorter (71). BM-derived SP cells incorporate less Hoechst than other mononuclear cells [main population (MP)], and therefore appear less brightly stained with Hoechst. The low Hoechst staining of SP cells is thought to be because of their capacity to efflux Hoechst, mediated by the ABCG2/*brcp1* transporter (72,73). Using the same technique that is used to isolate BM SP cells, SP cells were isolated from skeletal muscle. Unlike previous studies using myoblasts, muscle SP cells have been tested by intravenous injection into lethally irradiated *mdx* mice to enhance incorporation into all muscle groups at once. Surprisingly, muscle SP cells were capable of reconstituting the hematopoietic lineage of lethally irradiated mice, albeit with considerably reduced ability compared to BM SP cells (27). In addition, muscle SP cells were able to home from the circulation into dystrophic muscle, fuse with existing myofibers, and produce dystrophin (maximum efficiency 9%) (27). Donor-derived nuclei were observed in centrally located positions within dystrophin-positive myofibers, suggesting that they had participated in the myofiber regeneration. Interestingly, a few donor-derived nuclei were detected at positions consistent with those of satellite cells, thus suggesting that muscle SP cells could give rise to muscle precursors. A recent study exploited the combination of gene- and cell-based DMD therapy in an autologous transplantation system using the *mdx5cv* mice (model of DMD with less revertant fibers than *mdx*) (74,75). Muscle SP cells isolated from *mdx5cv* donors were transduced with a lentivirus vector expressing human microdystrophin and were transplanted intravenously into noninjured *mdx5cv* recipients. The transduced cells were able to travel through the capillaries, enter into damaged muscle, and deliver human microdystrophin, albeit with low efficiency of engraftment (1%) (74).

The origin of SP cells in muscle was unclear from the early studies, but in several ways, they appeared distinct from BM SP cells. Characterization of muscle SP cells has demonstrated that more than 95% of the cells are positive for stem cell antigen-1 (Sca-1) and approximately 70% express CD34, but do not express hematopoietic restricted lineage markers, such as CD45 and c-kit (27,34). These marker analyses suggest, but do not prove, the nonhematopoietic origin of muscle SP cells. A recent study demonstrated that the parameters used during the isolation of muscle SP cells, including Hoechst concentration, play an important role in the SP cell homogeneity and viability (76). Therefore isolation of muscle SP cells, using low Hoechst concentrations (5 μg/mL) resulted in an increased percentage of CD45-positive SP cells (16%) (28). These muscle SP cells differentiated preferentially into hematopoietic lineages in vitro, but they were also capable of undergoing Pax7-independent myogenic specification upon coculture with primary myoblasts (28). These same muscle SP cells were able to engraft into regenerating muscles of immunodeficient *Scid/bg* mice with low engraftment efficiency (1.4% of donor-derived nuclei within muscle fibers), reported at two weeks following intramuscular injections. In addition, some injected muscle SP cells were found in positions characteristic of satellite cells, and expressed Pax7 (28). Analysis of cell surface markers and of the location within the muscle fiber demonstrated that muscle SP cells constitute a distinct population from satellite cells and may be associated with the vasculature within muscle (28). Muscle SP cells may form a reservoir of satellite cells during the latter stages of neonatal muscle development and may persist in adult skeletal muscle to maintain a steady state number of satellite cells.

OTHER MUSCLE-DERIVED CELLS AVAILABLE FOR CELL-MEDIATED THERAPY OF DMD

A variety of other methods have been used in attempts to identify myogenic stem cells. The "preplate" technique was used to isolate muscle-derived cells that do not adhere to collagen-coated flasks after a series of one-day platings in tissue culture dishes (69,77,78). This approach allowed the clonal expansion of single cells and identified a specific cell population, termed the muscle-derived stem cells (MDSC) that displayed unique characteristics commonly associated with noncommitted progenitor cells (78). MDSC express early myogenic markers (MyoD, myogenin) and stem cell markers (Sca-1, Flk-1), but are negative for hematopoietic markers (CD45, c-kit). MDSC are able to proliferate and retain their phenotype in vitro and further differentiate into muscle, neural, and endothelial lineages both in vitro and in vivo (78). Transplantation of MDSC obtained from newborn mice demonstrated dystrophin expression for 10 to 90 days after intramuscular injections into *mdx* mice. A recent study examined the intravenous injection of MDSC transduced with a human dystrophin expression cassette into *mdx* mice (79). Only low levels (0.18%) of donor cell incorporation into muscle were observed, which increased to 0.55% upon muscle injury. These engraftment levels are significantly lower compared to the levels obtained from intramuscular injections of MDSC, which suggests that the method of delivery of donor cells greatly influences the efficiency of their engraftment.

A rare population of cells, expressing both Sca-1 and the hematopoietic lineage marker CD45, was identified in skeletal muscle (28). These cells differ from satellite cells, which are negative for CD45 and Sca-1. However, in response to muscle damage, these resident (CD45+/Sca-1+) muscle cells become activated, proliferate, and their total number can be increased by tenfold (80). Polesskaya et al. (80) demonstrated that CD45+/Sca-1+ cells obtained from uninjured muscle were uniformly nonmyogenic and were not able to undergo myogenic differentiation in vitro. However, CD45+/Sca-1+ cells, purified from regenerating muscle, expressed myogenic markers and further differentiated into myosin heavy chain–expressing myocytes when cultured in muscle differentiation medium. In addition, this study was the first to demonstrate that Wnt signaling is implicated in the myogenic recruitment of muscle-derived CD45-positive cells (80). As in the case of embryonic precursor cells, Wnt signaling appears to be necessary and sufficient to induce and maintain the myogenic specification of adult muscle stem cells (81,82).

In an attempt to characterize multipotent stem cell populations derived from adult skeletal muscle, two independent groups identified Sca-1/CD34 double-positive cells. A slightly different protocol of preplating than that used by Qu et al. (69) and Qu-Petersen et al. (78) was used for the purification of Sca-1/CD34 double-positive cells from muscle of newborn mice (83). This was the first study that exploited intraarterial delivery of donor cells to achieve systemic delivery to all muscle groups. On intraarterial injection of Sca-1/CD34 double-positive cells, they firmly adhere to the endothelium of *mdx* muscles and further migrate from the circulation into all hind limb muscles of the *mdx* treated mice (83). The efficiency of engraftment, although low (1%), could be increased to a level of 12% when the muscles were damaged prior to injection. Another group identified CD34 and Sca-1 double-positive cell progenitors in the interstitial spaces of murine skeletal muscle (84). Clonal cultures of these cells could differentiate into the myogenic lineage, as well as endothelial cells and adipocytes. Intramuscular injections into immunodeficient *Scid/bg* mice demonstrated that donor cells were incorporated into the host muscle fibers and vascular endothelium in recipient muscles (84). Although these cells are distinct from satellite cells, they have the potential to become myoblasts, as indicated by the expression of Pax7, after three days in culture. These cells also expressed the ABCG2 transporter and might be a subpopulation of muscle SP cells (27).

The presence of functionally distinct populations of myogenic cells in skeletal muscle has been demonstrated by many groups (27,28,69,78,80,83). Most of these populations are sensitive to radiation. One study reported the presence of a small population of stem cell–like muscle precursors in normal mouse muscle, which survive high doses of radiation, such as 18 Gy (64). When normal and *mdx* muscles were irradiated and extensively damaged by injection of notexin, widespread muscle regeneration was still observed. Myogenic precursor cells, obtained from single myofibers isolated from treated muscles and cultured in vitro, proliferated more extensively when isolated from normal than from *mdx* mice (64). Therefore, this population of radiation-resistant muscle precursor cells survives as proliferative myogenic cells, and is called upon by extreme conditions of muscle damage, as it is markedly diminished in the muscles of dystrophic mice. Such a cell population, which is probably less prone to be rejected by the host immune system and is capable of achieving long-term repopulation of the host muscle tissue, has selective advantages for use in cell-mediated therapy of DMD.

It is clear from the above studies that a lot of progress has been made toward the identification of different stem cell populations residing in adult skeletal muscle which could be used for cell-mediated therapy of DMD. Muscle SP cells are able to home and contribute to dystrophin production in the regenerating muscle, as well as to the satellite cell pool, thus providing an autologous system of cell transplantation. MDSC, isolated by the preplating technique, are characterized by long-term proliferating capacity, strong self-renewal capabilities, multipotent differentiation, and immune-privileged behavior (incapable of developing tumors in immunodeficient *Scid* mice). MDSC and muscle SP cells share a majority of surface markers; however, their lineage commitment seems to be different. In addition, muscle SP cells have not yet been cultured successfully in vitro. We attempted to summarize the existing knowledge of characteristics and possible relationships of the different cell populations presented in this section and the hierarchy of cells in skeletal muscle, starting from a hypothetical muscle stem cell towards myoblasts and mature myofibers (Fig. 2). Further studies will be required to determine the exact relationships between these cell populations, and allow results from different groups to be directly compared, in order to proceed to the selection of the best suited population to be used for cell therapy of DMD.

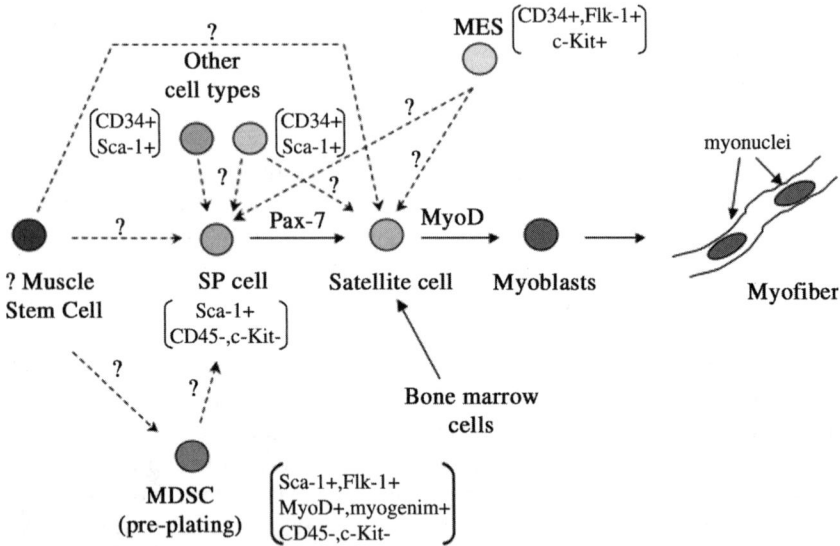

Figure 2 Schematic representation of relationships between cell populations with myogenic differentiation potential. An as yet undefined muscle stem cell might be the precursor of multiple different cell populations, which are characterized by the surface markers indicated in brackets, leading to the production of differentiated myocytes, which fuse to produce multinucleated myofibers. Dashed arrows denote to hypothetical relationships between cell populations, and solid arrows refer to experimentally demonstrated relationships. Only the surface markers that are expressed on more than 90% of the cells in a given population are shown in brackets.

NONMUSCLE-DERIVED CELLS PARTICIPATING IN MUSCLE REPAIR

The widespread muscle damage throughout the body of DMD patients requires an efficient and robust source of cells capable of long-term reconstitution after homing to the sites of lesions. The demonstration of the pluripotent nature of adult stem cells isolated from diverse tissues has raised the possibility of stem cell therapy for DMD. In the last five years, increasing interest has been shown in stem cells that are not normally resident within muscle but have the potential to give rise to skeletal muscle. Tissues such as BM, skin, and dorsal aorta provide alternative sources of myogenic cells. The existence of stem cells in the central nervous system, as well as in fetal liver and adipose tissue, which have the capacity to become directed towards myogenic differentiation, although under specific experimental conditions, have been demonstrated in other studies also (30,85–88).

STEM CELLS DERIVED FROM DORSAL AORTA (MESANGIOBLASTS)

Successful studies using stem cells isolated from dorsal aorta for cell-mediated therapy of muscular dystrophy have been described by Sampaolesi et al. (8), De Angelis et al. (18), and Minasi et al. (89). Initial characterization of fetal aorta-derived clones in vitro demonstrated coexpression of endothelial and myogenic markers (18). Further in vivo experiments demonstrated that myogenic progenitors from the dorsal aorta were able to participate in postnatal muscle growth and regeneration. When directly injected into the regenerating muscle of immunodeficient mice, genetically marked donor nuclei were incorporated into newly formed muscle fibers at low efficiency as indicated by a small number of clusters of donor-derived nuclei within regenerating fibers. A later study further characterized these embryonic aorta-derived cells, which were termed mesangioblasts (MES) (89). When expanded on a feeder layer of embryonic fibroblasts, MES could generate clones that became immortal and grew in vitro for more than one year. MES clones expressed hemoangioblastic markers (CD34, Flk-1, and c-kit) and maintained multipotency (differentiation into most mesodermal cell types such as hematopoietic) in culture or on transplantation into a chick embryo (89). In addition, grafts of quail or mouse embryonic aorta into host chick embryos demonstrated the presence of donor cells within the wall of intramuscular blood vessels, as well as within the muscle tissue, in differentiated muscle fibers (89). Interestingly, MES were able to contribute to regeneration of organs other than the transplantation site, such as cardiac muscle (89). Another study by the same group demonstrated that the intraarterial injection of MES into immunocompetent α-SGnull mice yielded the greatest reported efficiency of muscle engraftment (50%) (8). In addition, MES isolated from blood vessels of juvenile dystrophic mice and transduced ex vivo with α-SG–expressing lentivirus were able to reconstitute skeletal muscle in a manner similar to that seen with wild-type cells, following intraarterial injections into α-SGnull mice (8). A more recent study demonstrated that high mobility group box 1 protein (HMGB1), an abundant chromatin protein that is a signal of tissue damage, induces MES migration and proliferation in vitro (90). Although, the interaction of HMGB1 with its receptor is sufficient, it is not necessary for the in vivo MES homing to the muscles of the α-SGnull mice (90).

MES may represent a promising cell type for cell-mediated therapy of DMD. Autologous, genetically corrected vessel-associated stem cells have the ability to cross the endothelium and migrate into the tissue interstitium, where they are recruited by regenerating muscle fibers. If the donor cells express dystrophin, this can lead to reconstitution of the dystrophin–glycoprotein complex. MES have been isolated from human fetal vessels, an indication that similar cells with a potential for muscle regeneration could be found in humans; however, their fetal origin raises serious ethical concerns. Further work in this area might demonstrate whether it is feasible to isolate MES from the blood vessels of adult human patients.

BM-DERIVED CELLS WITH MYOGENIC POTENTIAL

The observation that BM-derived cells can home to muscle and differentiate into satellite cells has led to the hope that BMT could provide dystrophic muscle with a renewable source of myogenic progenitors. Initial experiments involved intravenous transplantation of whole BM cells into mice with dystrophic or regenerating normal muscles, and demonstrated the ability of BM-derived cells to migrate into damaged skeletal and cardiac muscle and participate in the regeneration process (33,91). Another study reported that transplantation of BM cells into normal mice contributes to muscle regeneration at a high frequency (3.5%), and that BM-derived cells were able to form satellite cells (29). However, irradiation-induced damage and subsequent exercise-induced damage were required for BM cells to participate in muscle regeneration. The same group also demonstrated a thousandfold range in the frequency with which diverse skeletal muscles incorporate BM-derived cells (92). Most striking was the finding of one specific muscle, the panniculus carnosus, in which up to 5% of myofibers incorporated BM-derived cells over a 16-month period in the absence of experimentally induced damage. This represents the highest reported frequency of muscle fibers incorporating BM cells (92). When BM side population (SP) cells were used in studies of intravenous transplantation of *mdx* mice, they were found to be capable of homing to muscles, fusing with the dystrophin-negative fibers of *mdx* mice and directing the expression of dystrophin within these fibers, albeit with low efficiency (up to 4%) (27). However, a study of long-term efficacy of BMT demonstrated that BM-derived muscle repair in the *mdx4cv* mouse (mouse model of DMD with less revertant fibers than *mdx*) could not exceed 1% of total muscle fibers, analyzed at 10 months following injection (35,75). Another study used the *c-xmd* canine model of DMD and demonstrated that BMT did not provide any clinical benefit, nor did it show any significant contribution of donor cells to the diseased skeletal muscle (93,94). These studies are in agreement with a recent study of a DMD patient who had received BMT at one year of age. BMT did not seem to be the cause of amelioration of the patient's dystrophic phenotype; however, the authors documented the ability of exogenous human BM cells to fuse into skeletal muscle and persist up to 13 years after transplantation (95). A recent study demonstrated that the myelomonocytic progenitors within hematopoietic cells constitute the BM-specific–cell type that contributes to skeletal muscle regeneration (96).

Despite the fact that BMT is a procedure already widely used to treat a variety of immunological human diseases, the above studies demonstrated that its application to DMD, due to its low efficiency, would first require extensive preclinical studies to establish ideal progenitor cells and conditions for transplantation. Further studies based on intraarterial delivery of BM cells might prove helpful towards increasing the efficacy of transplantation.

MESENCHYMAL STEM CELLS

BM contains mesenchymal stem cells (MSC) (also referred to as marrow stromal cells), which have the potential to differentiate into mesodermal lineages, including cartilage, bone, adipose tissue, and muscle (97–99). In vitro assays have shown that BM stroma-derived mesenchymal cells can differentiate into contractile myotubes under certain conditions (100). Moreover, implantation of MSC from adult mice into three-week-old *mdx* mice produced dystrophin-positive fibers (although at low frequency), which suggested that MSC have the potential to differentiate into myogenic cells in the *mdx* muscle (101). In another study, BM cells (labeled to express beta-galactosidase under the control of a muscle-specific promoter) were fractionated into adherent and nonadherent cells and used for intramuscular injections into immunodeficient *Scid/bg* regenerating mouse muscle (33). The presence of β-gal–positive nuclei in muscle fibers was observed only when mice were injected with the adherent fraction of BM-derived cells, which contained MSC progenitors. The authors concluded that MSC are able to migrate into the regenerating muscle, participate in the regeneration process, and give rise to fully differentiated myofibers. However, the contribution to the newly regenerated fibers was very low and took far longer to occur (six weeks after injection), compared to control mice implanted with muscle-derived myoblasts. More recently, mesodermal progenitor cells (MPC) were purified from postnatal human BM and expanded ex vivo (102). These MPC can differentiate at the single-cell level into MSC, as well as endothelium and skeletal myoblasts. Muscle-specific transcription factors (MyoD and myogenin) and other proteins were expressed within the MPC, following incubation in a defined medium specific for promotion of myogenic cell determination and differentiation. However, once directed into the myogenic pathway, these MPC lost multipotency and could not differentiate into other mesenchymal cell types (102). The therapeutic potential of MSC in primary muscle diseases such as DMD is promising, although the efficiency of muscle regeneration is still low and more studies are required to optimize the cell source, isolation, and expansion.

SKIN

Skin is a highly accessible source of cells that could be used for cell-mediated therapy, provided that the ability of skin cells to generate skeletal muscle is clearly demonstrated. Muscle fibroblasts appear incapable of efficiently contributing to muscle fiber formation without genetic modification (103,104).

However, dermal fibroblasts can convert to myogenesis when subjected to a "muscle environment" (grown in the presence of either normal or dystrophic myoblasts), or upon injection into either *mdx* or normal regenerating muscle (103,105–108). Interestingly, the conversion of fibroblasts to the myogenic lineage precedes their fusion with myoblasts (105). Recently, galectin-1, which is known to be secreted by muscle cells as they enter terminal differentiation, was identified as the factor capable of converting dermal fibroblasts to myogenic lineage (104,109,110).

SP cells have been isolated from epidermal preparations of adult mouse skin (34). Skin SP cells express markers similar to muscle SP cells, but differ from BM SP cells because they lack hematopoietic markers. When transplanted intravenously into nonirradiated *mdx* mice, skin SP cells were able to home to muscle and participate in muscle regeneration. Donor-derived nuclei were detected within up to 9% of dystrophin-positive myofibers analyzed three months after injection. Keratinocyte stem cells (of epidermal origin) have also been described as capable of excluding Hoechst dyes and contributing to all cell lineages when injected into blastocysts, although their myogenic potential has not been demonstrated (111). Earlier studies demonstrated that nuclear reprogramming can occur in keratinocytes upon fusion with muscle fibers in vitro, resulting in the expression of muscle genes (112).

Various studies have identified skin stem cells of epidermal and dermal origin, but their potential to differentiate into skeletal muscle has yet to be tested (111,113,114). Putative skin stem cells, such as skin SP cells, with the capability to give rise to muscle, need a more detailed biological characterization combined with different approaches for increasing their incorporation into dystrophic muscle to achieve therapeutically relevant levels of dystrophin expression.

CONCLUSIONS

Although the genetic defect responsible for DMD was identified approximately two decades ago, no effective therapy is currently available for the patients. Initial efforts were focused on myoblast transfer therapy, that is, transplantation of normal myoblasts into skeletal muscle, as a technique to provide a source of the normal dystrophin protein to the injured tissue. This technique was applied to deliver dystrophin to the muscles of the *mdx* mouse as well as DMD patients and was shown to be safe but inefficient. The low efficiency of myoblast transfer was attributed to poor survival of implanted myoblasts, failure to differentiate or fuse in the host environment, limited myoblast migration from the injection site, and/or elicitation of an immune response when donor myoblasts and host myofibers were not immunocompatible. The concept of stem cell therapy of DMD is a continuation of myoblast transfer, but with the use of cells that have a much broader differentiation capacity. Muscle stem cells with the potential for muscle repair include the SP cells, clonal expansions of muscle stem cells isolated by a preplating technique, and subpopulations of resident muscle cells identified by specific cell surface markers (including Sca-1, CD34, and CD45). In addition, BM, skin, and dorsal aorta offer a reservoir of stem cells capable of differentiating into skeletal muscle both in vitro and in vivo and participating in muscle regeneration, as has been successfully demonstrated in animal studies. Such stem cell populations need to be further explored to improve their isolation, ex vivo expansion, and in vivo engraftment in dystrophic human muscle.

Cell-mediated therapy of DMD relies on the efficient systemic delivery of donor cells with the potential of efficient long-term engraftment in all muscle groups, without eliciting immune rejection in the host environment. While further studies need to be performed to define the relationship between different muscle populations and the hierarchy of progenitors and stem cells in muscle tissue, the recent demonstration of significant therapeutic efficacy of donor cells upon intraarterial delivery has provided new insights for cell-mediated therapy. The advantage of cell transplantation relies on the fact that a normal cell could restore the physiological microenvironment of dystrophic muscle, which is not the case of targeted gene therapy approaches that are specifically directed to muscle fibers, and are mostly efficient for short-term reconstitution. Although the contribution to muscle repair of the different cell populations described in this chapter still remains too low to warrant clinical trials, it is encouraging (and not utopic) to believe that the combination of a suitable cell population with an efficient delivery method might prove to be the best approach for therapy of DMD.

ACKNOWLEDGMENTS

The authors would like to thank Dr. Emanuela Gussoni for careful reading and critical discussions, and the members of the Kunkel laboratory for helpful suggestions during the preparation of this manuscript. L.M.K. is an Investigator with the Howard Hughes Medical Institute. L.M.K. is supported by the Alva B. Gimbel Foundation.

REFERENCES

1. Hoffman EP, Brown RH Jr, Kunkel LM. Dystrophin: the protein product of the Duchenne muscular dystrophy locus. Cell 1987; 51:919–928.
2. Matsumura K, Campbell KP. Dystrophin-glycoprotein complex: its role in the molecular pathogenesis of muscular dystrophies. Muscle Nerve 1994; 17:2–15.
3. Ervasti JM, Campbell KP. Dystrophin and the membrane skeleton. Curr Opin Cell Biol 1993; 5:82–87.
4. Sicinski P, Geng Y, Ryder-Cook AS, Barnard EA, Darlison MG, Barnard PJ. The molecular basis of muscular dystrophy in the *mdx* mouse: a point mutation. Science 1989; 244:1578–1580.
5. Byers TJ, Kunkel LM, Watkins SC. The subcellular distribution of dystrophin in mouse skeletal, cardiac, and smooth muscle. J Cell Biol 1991; 115:411–421.

6. Nudel U, Robzyk K, Yaffe D. Expression of the putative Duchenne muscular dystrophy gene in differentiated myogenic cell cultures and in the brain. Nature 1988; 331:635–638.
7. Hoffman EP, Fischbeck KH, Brown RH, et al. Characterization of dystrophin in muscle-biopsy specimens from patients with Duchenne's or Becker's muscular dystrophy. N Engl J Med 1988; 318:1363–1368.
8. Sampaolesi M, Torrente Y, Innocenzi A, et al. Cell therapy of alpha-sarcoglycan null dystrophic mice through intra-arterial delivery of mesoangioblasts. Science 2003; 301:487–492.
9. Seale P, Sabourin LA, Girgis-Gabardo A, Mansouri A, Gruss P, Rudnicki MA. Pax7 is required for the specification of myogenic satellite cells. Cell 2000; 102: 777–786.
10. Morgan JE, Partridge TA. Muscle satellite cells. Int J Biochem Cell Biol 2003; 35:1151–1156.
11. Feldman JL, Stockdale FE. Temporal appearance of satellite cells during myogenesis. Dev Biol 1992; 153:217–226.
12. Goldring K, Partridge T, Watt D. Muscle stem cells. J Pathol 2002; 197:457–467.
13. Grounds MD. Age-associated changes in the response of skeletal muscle cells to exercise and regeneration. Ann NY Acad Sci 1998; 854:78–91.
14. Grounds MD, Yablonka-Reuveni Z. Molecular and cell biology of skeletal muscle regeneration. Mol Cell Biol Hum Dis Ser 1993; 3:210–256.
15. Seale P, Rudnicki MA. A new look at the origin, function, and "stem-cell" status of muscle satellite cells. Dev Biol 2000; 218:115–124.
16. Hartley RS, Bandman E, Yablonka-Reuveni Z. Skeletal muscle satellite cells appear during late chicken embryogenesis. Dev Biol 1992; 153:206–216.
17. Armand O, Boutineau AM, Mauger A, Pautou MP, Kieny M. Origin of satellite cells in avian skeletal muscles. Arch Anat Microsc Morphol Exp 1983; 72:163–181.
18. De Angelis L, Berghella L, Coletta M, et al. Skeletal myogenic progenitors originating from embryonic dorsal aorta coexpress endothelial and myogenic markers and contribute to postnatal muscle growth and regeneration. J Cell Biol 1999; 147:869–878.
19. Olguin HC, Olwin BB. Pax-7 up-regulation inhibits myogenesis and cell cycle progression in satellite cells: a potential mechanism for self-renewal. Dev Biol 2004; 275:375–388.
20. Oustanina S, Hause G, Braun T. Pax7 directs postnatal renewal and propagation of myogenic satellite cells but not their specification. Embo J 2004; 23: 3430–3439.
21. Rosenblatt JD, Lunt AI, Parry DJ, Partridge TA. Culturing satellite cells from living single muscle fiber explants. In Vitro Cell Dev Biol Anim 1995; 31:773–779.
22. Asakura A, Komaki M, Rudnicki M. Muscle satellite cells are multipotential stem cells that exhibit myogenic, osteogenic, and adipogenic differentiation. Differentiation 2001; 68:245–253.
23. Blaveri K, Heslop L, Yu DS, et al. Patterns of repair of dystrophic mouse muscle: studies on isolated fibers. Dev Dyn 1999; 216:244–256.
24. Beauchamp JR, Heslop L, Yu DS, et al. Expression of CD34 and Myf5 defines the majority of quiescent adult skeletal muscle satellite cells. J Cell Biol 2000; 151:1221–1234.

25. Sato T, Laver JH, Ogawa M. Reversible expression of CD34 by murine hematopoietic stem cells. Blood 1999; 94:2548–2554.
26. Zammit P, Beauchamp J. The skeletal muscle satellite cell: stem cell or son of stem cell? Differentiation 2001; 68:193–204.
27. Gussoni E, Soneoka Y, Strickland CD, et al. Dystrophin expression in the *mdx* mouse restored by stem cell transplantation. Nature 1999; 401:390–394.
28. Asakura A, Seale P, Girgis-Gabardo A, Rudnicki MA. Myogenic specification of side population cells in skeletal muscle. J Cell Biol 2002; 159:123–134.
29. LaBarge MA, Blau HM. Biological progression from adult bone marrow to mononucleate muscle stem cell to multinucleate muscle fiber in response to injury. Cell 2002; 111:589–601.
30. Fukada S, Miyagoe-Suzuki Y, Tsukihara H, et al. Muscle regeneration by reconstitution with bone marrow or fetal liver cells from green fluorescent protein-gene transgenic mice. J Cell Sci 2002; 15:1285–1293.
31. Heslop L, Beauchamp JR, Tajbakhsh S, Buckingham ME, Partridge TA, Zammit PS. Transplanted primary neonatal myoblasts can give rise to functional satellite cells as identified using the Myf5nlacZl+ mouse. Gene Ther 2001; 8:778–783.
32. Morgan JE, Pagel CN, Sherratt T, Partridge TA. Long-term persistence and migration of myogenic cells injected into pre-irradiated muscles of *mdx* mice. J Neurol Sci 1993; 115:191–200.
33. Ferrari G, Cusella-De Angelis G, Coletta M, et al. Muscle regeneration by bone marrow-derived myogenic progenitors. Science 1998; 279:1528–1530.
34. Montanaro F, Liadaki K, Volinski J, Flint A, Kunkel LM. Skeletal muscle engraftment potential of adult mouse skin side population cells. Proc Natl Acad Sci USA 2003; 100:9336–9341.
35. Ferrari G, Stornaiuolo A, Mavilio F. Failure to correct murine muscular dystrophy. Nature 2001; 411:1014–1015.
36. Duclos F, Straub V, Moore SA, et al. Progressive muscular dystrophy in alpha-sarcoglycan-deficient mice. J Cell Biol 1998; 142:1461–1471.
37. Partridge TA, Grounds M, Sloper JC. Evidence of fusion between host and donor myoblasts in skeletal muscle grafts. Nature 1978; 273:306–308.
38. Morgan JE, Watt DJ, Sloper JC, Partridge TA. Partial correction of an inherited biochemical defect of skeletal muscle by grafts of normal muscle precursor cells. J Neurol Sci 1988; 86:137–147.
39. Watt DJ, Morgan JE, Partridge TA. Use of mononuclear precursor cells to insert allogeneic genes into growing mouse muscles. Muscle Nerve 1984; 7:741–750.
40. Huard J, Labrecque C, Dansereau G, Robitaille L, Tremblay JP. Dystrophin expression in myotubes formed by the fusion of normal and dystrophic myoblasts. Muscle Nerve 1991; 14:178–182.
41. Partridge TA, Morgan JE, Coulton GR, Hoffman EP, Kunkel LM. Conversion of *mdx* myofibres from dystrophin-negative to -positive by injection of normal myoblasts. Nature 1989; 337:176–179.
42. Karpati G, Pouliot Y, Zubrzycka-Gaarn F, et al. Dystrophin is expressed in *mdx* skeletal muscle fibers after normal myoblast implantation. Am J Pathol 1989; 135:27–32.

43. Gussoni E, Pavlath GK, Lanctot AM, et al. Normal dystrophin transcripts detected in Duchenne muscular dystrophy patients after myoblast transplantation. Nature 1992; 356:435–438.
44. Miller RG, Sharma KR, Pavlath GK, et al. Myoblast implantation in Duchenne muscular dystrophy: the San Francisco study. Muscle Nerve 1997; 20:469–478.
45. Huard J, Bouchard JP, Roy R, et al. Human myoblast transplantation: preliminary results of 4 cases. Muscle Nerve 1992; 15:550–560.
46. Roy R, Tremblay JP, Huard J, Richards C, Malouin F, Bouchard JP. Antibody formation after myoblast transplantation in Duchenne-dystrophic patients, donor HLA compatible. Transplant Proc 1993; 25:995–997.
47. Karpati G, Ajdukovic D, Arnold D, et al. Myoblast transfer in Duchenne muscular dystrophy. Ann Neurol 1993; 34:8–17.
48. Morandi L, Bernasconi P, Gebbia M, et al. Lack of mRNA and dystrophin expression in DMD patients three months after myoblast transfer. Neuromuscul Disord 1995; 5:291–295.
49. Mendell JR, Kissel JT, Amato AA, et al. Myoblast transfer in the treatment of Duchenne's muscular dystrophy. N Engl J Med 1995; 333:832–838.
50. Law PK, Goodwin TG, Fang Q, et al. Feasibility, safety, and efficacy of myoblast transfer therapy on Duchenne muscular dystrophy boys. Cell Transplant 1992; 1:235–244.
51. Partridge T, Lu QL, Morris G, Hoffman E. Is myoblast transplantation effective? Nat Med 1998; 4:1208–1209.
52. Neumeyer AM, Cros D, McKenna-Yasek D, et al. Pilot study of myoblast transfer in the treatment of Becker muscular dystrophy. Neurology 1998; 51:589–592.
53. Gussoni E, Blau HM, Kunkel LM. The fate of individual myoblasts after transplantation into muscles of DMD patients. Nat Med 1997; 3:970–977.
54. Kinoshita I, Vilquin JT, Guerette B, et al. Immunosuppression with FK 506 insures good success of myoblast transplantation in *mdx* mice. Transplant Proc 1994; 26:3518.
55. Watt DJ, Morgan JE, Partridge TA. Long term survival of allografted muscle precursor cells following a limited period of treatment with cyclosporin A. Clin Exp Immunol 1984; 55:419–426.
56. Watt DJ, Partridge TA, Sloper JC. Cyclosporin A as a means of preventing rejection of skeletal muscle allografts in mice. Transplantation 1981; 31:266–271.
57. Huard J, Roy R, Guerette B, Verreault S, Tremblay G, Tremblay JP. Human myoblast transplantation in immunodeficient and immunosuppressed mice: evidence of rejection. Muscle Nerve 1994; 17:224–234.
58. Smythe GM, Hodgetts SI, Grounds MD. Immunobiology and the future of myoblast transfer therapy. Mol Ther 2000; 1:304–313.
59. Labrecque C, Roy R, Tremblay JP. Immune reactions after myoblast transplantation in mouse muscles. Transplant Proc 1992; 24:2889–2892.
60. Tremblay JP, Malouin F, Roy R, et al. Results of a triple blind clinical study of myoblast transplantations without immunosuppressive treatment in young boys with Duchenne muscular dystrophy. Cell Transplant 1993; 2:99–112.
61. Huard J, Roy R, Bouchard JP, Malouin F, Richards CL, Tremblay JP. Human myoblast transplantation between immunohistocompatible donors and recipients produces immune reactions. Transplant Proc 1992; 24:3049–3051.

62. Huard J, Tremblay G, Verreault S, Labrecque C, Tremblay JP. Utilization of an antibody specific for human dystrophin to follow myoblast transplantation in nude mice. Cell Transplant 1993; 2:113–118.
63. Morgan JE, Gross JG, Pagel CN, et al. Myogenic cell proliferation and generation of a reversible tumorigenic phenotype are triggered by preirradiation of the recipient site. J Cell Biol 2002; 157:693–702.
64. Heslop L, Morgan JE, Partridge TA. Evidence for a myogenic stem cell that is exhausted in dystrophic muscle. J Cell Sci 2000; 113:2299–2308.
65. Law PK, Goodwin TG, Li HJ. Histoincompatible myoblast injection improves muscle structure and function of dystrophic mice. Transplant Proc 1988; 20:1114–1119.
66. Morgan JE, Moore SE, Walsh FS, Partridge TA. Formation of skeletal muscle in vivo from the mouse C2 cell line. J Cell Sci 1992; 102:779–787.
67. Morgan JE. Myogenicity in vitro and in vivo of mouse muscle cells separated on discontinuous Percoll gradients. J Neurol Sci 1988; 85:197–207.
68. Rando TA, Blau HM. Primary mouse myoblast purification, characterization, and transplantation for cell-mediated gene therapy. J Cell Biol 1994; 125:1275–1287.
69. Qu Z, Balkir L, van Deutekom JC, Robbins PD, Pruchnic R, Huard J. Development of approaches to improve cell survival in myoblast transfer therapy. J Cell Biol 1998; 142:1257–1267.
70. Beauchamp JR, Morgan JE, Pagel CN, Partridge TA. Dynamics of myoblast transplantation reveal a discrete minority of precursors with stem cell-like properties as the myogenic source. J Cell Biol 1999; 144:1113–1122.
71. Goodell MA, Brose K, Paradis G, Conner AS, Mulligan RC. Isolation and functional properties of murine hematopoietic stem cells that are replicating in vivo. J Exp Med 1996; 183:1797–1806.
72. Zhou S, Schuetz JD, Bunting KD, et al. The ABC transporter Bcrp1/ABCG2 is expressed in a wide variety of stem cells and is a molecular determinant of the side-population phenotype. Nat Med 2001; 7:1028–1034.
73. Zhou S, Morris JJ, Barnes Y, Lan L, Schuetz JD, Sorrentino BP. Bcrp1 gene expression is required for normal numbers of side population stem cells in mice, and confers relative protection to mitoxantrone in hematopoietic cells in vivo. Proc Natl Acad Sci USA 2002; 99:12339–12344.
74. Bachrach E, Li S, Perez AL, et al. Systemic delivery of human microdystrophin to regenerating mouse dystrophic muscle by muscle progenitor cells. Proc Natl Acad Sci USA 2004; 101:3581–3586.
75. Danko I, Chapman V, Wolff JA. The frequency of revertants in *mdx* mouse genetic models for Duchenne muscular dystrophy. Pediatr Res 1992; 32:128–131.
76. Montanaro F, Liadaki K, Schienda J, Flint A, Gussoni E, Kunkel LM. Demystifying SP cell purification: viability, yield, and phenotype are defined by isolation parameters. Exp Cell Res 2004; 298:144–154.
77. Lee JY, Qu-Petersen Z, Cao B, et al. Clonal isolation of muscle-derived cells capable of enhancing muscle regeneration and bone healing. J Cell Biol 2000; 150:1085–1100.
78. Qu-Petersen Z, Deasy B, Jankowski R, et al. Identification of a novel population of muscle stem cells in mice: potential for muscle regeneration. J Cell Biol 2002; 157:851–864.

79. Cao B, Zheng B, Jankowski RJ, et al. Muscle stem cells differentiate into haematopoietic lineages but retain myogenic potential. Nat Cell Biol 2003; 5:640–646.
80. Polesskaya A, Seale P, Rudnicki MA. Wnt signaling induces the myogenic specification of resident CD45+ adult stem cells during muscle regeneration. Cell 2003; 113:841–852.
81. Cossu G, Borello U. Wnt signaling and the activation of myogenesis in mammals. Embo J 1999; 18:6867–6872.
82. Parker MH, Seale P, Rudnicki MA. Looking back to the embryo: defining transcriptional networks in adult myogenesis. Nat Rev Genet 2003; 4:497–507.
83. Torrente Y, Tremblay JP, Pisati F, et al. Intraarterial injection of muscle-derived CD34(+)Sca-1(+) stem cells restores dystrophin in *mdx* mice. J Cell Biol 2001; 152:335–348.
84. Tamaki T, Akatsuka A, Ando K, et al. Identification of myogenic-endothelial progenitor cells in the interstitial spaces of skeletal muscle. J Cell Biol 2002; 157:571–577.
85. Zuk PA, Zhu M, Mizuno H, et al. Multilineage cells from human adipose tissue: implications for cell-based therapies. Tissue Eng 2001; 7:211–228.
86. Rietze RL, Valcanis H, Brooker GF, Thomas T, Voss AK, Bartlett PF. Purification of a pluripotent neural stem cell from the adult mouse brain. Nature 2001; 412:736–739.
87. Galli R, Borello U, Gritti A, et al. Skeletal myogenic potential of human and mouse neural stem cells. Nat Neurosci 2000; 3:986–991.
88. Clarke DL, Johansson CB, Wilbertz J, et al. Generalized potential of adult neural stem cells. Science 2000; 288:1660–1663.
89. Minasi MG, Riminucci M, De Angelis L, et al. The meso-angioblast: a multipotent, self-renewing cell that originates from the dorsal aorta and differentiates into most mesodermal tissues. Development 2002; 129:2773–2783.
90. Palumbo R, Sampaolesi M, De Marchis F, et al. Extracellular HMGB1, a signal of tissue damage, induces mesoangioblast migration and proliferation. J Cell Biol 2004; 164:441–449.
91. Bittner RE, Schofer C, Weipoltshammer K, et al. Recruitment of bone-marrow-derived cells by skeletal and cardiac muscle in adult dystrophic *mdx* mice. Anat Embryol 1999; 199:391–396.
92. Brazelton TR, Nystrom M, Blau HM. Significant differences among skeletal muscles in the incorporation of bone marrow-derived cells. Dev Biol 2003; 262:64–74.
93. Sharp NJ, Kornegay JN, Van Camp SD, et al. An error in dystrophin mRNA processing in golden retriever muscular dystrophy, an animal homologue of Duchenne muscular dystrophy. Genomics 1992; 13:115–121.
94. Dell'Agnola C, Wang Z, Storb R, et al. Hematopoietic stem cell transplantation does not restore dystrophin expression in Duchenne muscular dystrophy dogs. Blood 2004; 104:4311–4318.
95. Gussoni E, Bennett RR, Muskiewicz KR, et al. Long-term persistence of donor nuclei in a Duchenne muscular dystrophy patient receiving bone marrow transplantation. J Clin Invest 2002; 110:807–814.
96. Doyonnas R, LaBarge MA, Sacco A, Charlton C, Blau HM. Hematopoietic contribution to skeletal muscle regeneration by myelomonocytic precursors. Proc Natl Acad Sci USA 2004; 101:13507–13512.

97. Pittenger MF, Mackay AM, Beck SC, et al. Multilineage potential of adult human mesenchymal stem cells. Science 1999; 284:143–147.
98. Piersma AH, Brockbank KG, Ploemacher RE, van Vliet E, Brakel-van Peer KM, Visser PJ. Characterization of fibroblastic stromal cells from murine bone marrow. Exp Hematol 1985; 13:237–243.
99. Prockop DJ. Marrow stromal cells as stem cells for nonhematopoietic tissues. Science 1997; 276:71–74.
100. Wakitani S, Saito T, Caplan AI. Myogenic cells derived from rat bone marrow mesenchymal stem cells exposed to 5-azacytidine. Muscle Nerve 1995; 18:1417–1426.
101. Saito MD, Dennis JE, Lennon DP, Young RG, Caplan AI. Myogenic expression of mesenchymal stem cells within myotubes of *mdx* mice in vivo and in vitro. Tissue Eng 1995; 1:327–343.
102. Reyes M, Lund T, Lenvik T, Aguiar D, Koodie L, Verfaillie CM. Purification and ex vivo expansion of postnatal human marrow mesodermal progenitor cells. Blood 2001; 98:2615–2625.
103. Gibson AJ, Karasinski J, Relvas J, et al. Dermal fibroblasts convert to a myogenic lineage in *mdx* mouse muscle. J Cell Sci 1995; 108:207–214.
104. Goldring K, Jones GE, Thiagarajah R, Watt DJ. The effect of galectin-1 on the differentiation of fibroblasts and myoblasts in vitro. J Cell Sci 2002; 115:355–366.
105. Breton M, Li ZL, Paulin D, et al. Myotube driven myogenic recruitment of cells during in vitro myogenesis. Dev Dyn 1995; 202:126–136.
106. Chaudhari N, Delay R, Beam KG. Restoration of normal function in genetically defective myotubes by spontaneous fusion with fibroblasts. Nature 1989; 341:445–447.
107. Pye D, Watt DJ. Dermal fibroblasts participate in the formation of new muscle fibres when implanted into regenerating normal mouse muscle. J Anat 2001; 198:163–173.
108. Relvas JB, Aldridge H, Wells KE, Wells DJ, Watt, DJ. Exogenous genes are expressed in *mdx* muscle fibres following the implantation of primary mouse skin cells. Basic Appl Myol 1997; 7:211–219.
109. Goldring K, Jones GE, Watt DJ. A factor implicated in the myogenic conversion of nonmuscle cells derived from the mouse dermis. Cell Transplant 2000; 9:519–529.
110. Goldring K, Jones GE, Sewry CA, Watt DJ. The muscle-specific marker desmin is expressed in a proportion of human dermal fibroblasts after their exposure to galectin-1. Neuromuscul Disord 2002; 12:183–186.
111. Liang L, Bickenbach JR. Somatic epidermal stem cells can produce multiple cell lineages during development. Stem Cells 2002; 20:21–31.
112. Blau HM, Pavlath GK, Hardeman EC, et al. Plasticity of the differentiated state. Science 1985; 230:758–766.
113. Toma JG, Akhavan M, Fernandes KJ, et al. Isolation of multipotent adult stem cells from the dermis of mammalian skin. Nat Cell Biol 2001; 3:778–784.
114. Taylor G, Lehrer MS, Jensen PJ, Sun TT, Lavker RM. Involvement of follicular stem cells in forming not only the follicle but also the epidermis. Cell 2000; 102:451–461.

15

Oligonucleotide-Mediated Exon Skipping and Gene Editing for Duchenne Muscular Dystrophy

Carmen Bertoni and Thomas A. Rando

*Department of Neurology and Neurological Sciences,
Stanford University School of Medicine, Stanford, California, and GRECC and
Neurology Service, VA Palo Alto Health Care System, Palo Alto,
California, U.S.A.*

INTRODUCTION

In the past decade, there has been increasing interest in the use of oligonucleotides as vectors for gene therapy for two major reasons. First, oligonucleotides have been found to have unique characteristics as drugs to modify the genome or the transcriptome. Investigators have capitalized on these characteristics to use oligonucleotides to alter genomic sequences and to regulate RNA processing. Second, oligonucleotides have distinct advantages over other gene therapy vectors, particularly viral vectors. Hurdles or limitations of virus-mediated gene therapy for Duchenne muscular dystrophy (DMD) (see Chapters 17–19) that are obviated by some or all oligonucleotide vectors include immune responses against viruses themselves and viral-encoded gene products, limitations of viral packaging size for such large cDNAs as dystrophin, non-sustained transgene expression for both non-integrating and integrating viruses, and the risk of insertional mutagenesis for integrating viral vectors. In addition, the cost of large-scale vector production for human gene therapy, including the cost of quality control, promises to be far less for non-viral vectors such as oligonucleotides than for viral vectors.

Oligonucleotide-mediated gene therapy for DMD currently encompasses two major approaches: modulation of pre-mRNA splicing by antisense oligonucleotides (AONs) (1), and gene editing by chimeric and nonchimeric oligonucleotides (2). This chapter will focus on the recent advances, major hurdles remaining, and future directions for each of these approaches. Other oligonucleotide-based approaches on the horizon are also discussed at the end of the chapter.

AONs

Structure and Mechanism of Action

AONs are oligonucleotides that are composed most commonly of RNA residues or their homologs, are complementary to pre-mRNA or mature transcripts, and thus act post-transcriptionally to modify gene expression. The activity of AONs to inhibit protein production is thought to relate either to the degradation of the targeted transcripts by RNase H or to the direct block of translation (3). The report that naturally occurring antisense RNAs in prokaryotes played a role in regulating the expression of their corresponding genes indicated that reverse complimentary nucleic acid was a "natural" mechanism for regulating gene expression (4,5). The demonstration that expression of antisense RNA could also modulate gene expression in eukaryotic cells stimulated the development of this technology for potential therapeutic applications (6). The use of AONs as therapeutic agents primarily in cancer and viral infections, where they are used to reduce expression of proteins that cause cellular dysfunction, has been studied; AONs are also under investigation for use in cardiovascular, hematological, and inflammatory disorders (7). There are dozens of ongoing AON-based clinical trials and the first FDA-approved antisense therapeutic, Vitravene™ (Isis Pharmaceuticals, Carlsbad, California, U.S.A.), is in use for the treatment of cytomegalovirus (CMV) retinitis in patients with acquired immune deficiency syndrome (AIDS).

The possibility that AONs could also be used to alter RNA splicing was first demonstrated by the pioneering work of Dominski and Kole (8) in 1993. They demonstrated that AONs could restore normal β-globin gene splicing in nuclear extracts of HeLa cells expressing mutants of human β-globin pre-mRNA with mutations in intronic regulatory regions. The skipping of an exon by AONs is accomplished by either targeting the AON to an intron/exon splice site or regulatory sequences within exons or introns that regulate splicing (Fig. 1), presumably by sterically interfering

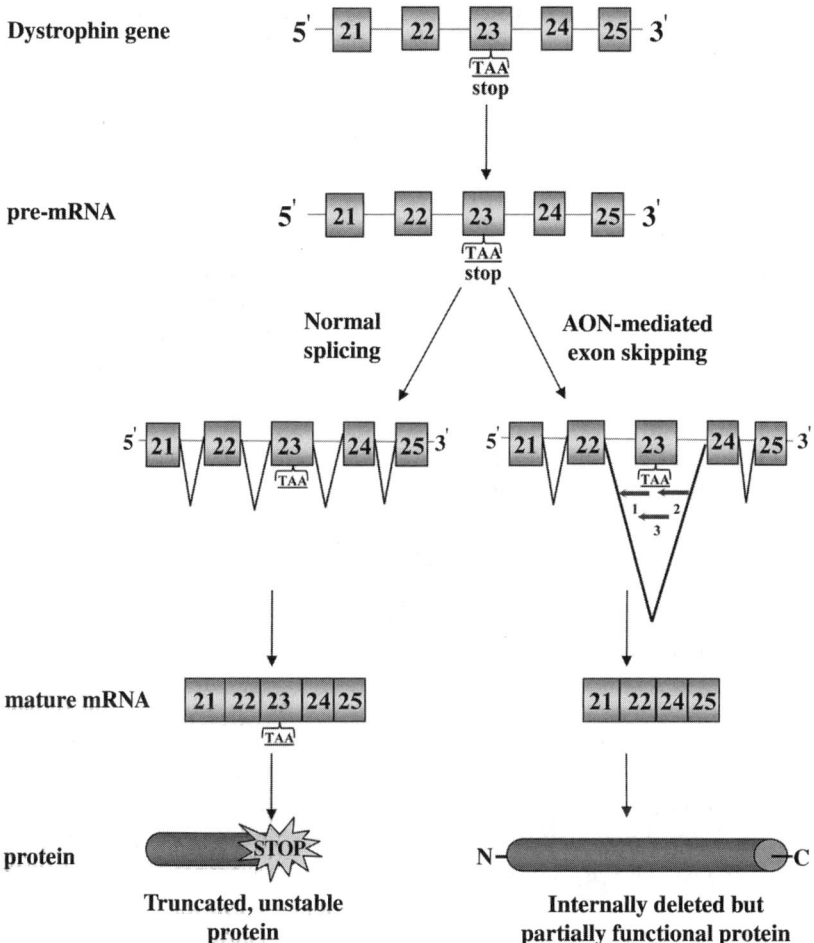

Figure 1 Antisense-mediated exon skipping in the *mdx* mouse. The *mdx* mouse has a stop codon in exon 23 of the dystrophin gene leading to the absence of any functional dystrophin production. AONs complementary to the premature mRNA of the dystrophin gene have been used to block the 5′ splice site (**1**), the 3′ splice site (**2**), or internal splicing regulatory regions (**3**) of exon 23 in the pre-mRNA. These blocking antisense constructs result in exon 22 being spliced directly to exon 24, thus producing an in-frame dystrophin transcript deleted for exon 23. The resulting protein is shorter than normal but retains most of the functional properties of full-length dystrophin. *Abbreviation*: AONs, antisense oligonucleotides.

with the spiceosome machinery and prompting the use of nearby, available splice sites (9). The modification of pre-mRNA splicing by AONs has been applied to numerous genes such as those encoding the cystic fibrosis transmembrane conductor regulator (CFTR) gene, tau, Bcl-x, c-myc, and the interleukin-5 receptor, whose aberrant expression is associated with degenerative, neoplastic, and inflammatory disorders (9).

Application of AON-Mediated Gene Therapy to DMD: Modification of Splicing

The rationale behind the use of AONs to redirect splicing of the dystrophin gene is the notion that the production of a shorter but in-frame transcript of the dystrophin gene could transform a severe DMD into a milder Bekker muscular dystrophy (BMD) phenotype. This approach is applicable to DMD because the majority of the patients have gene deletions that are deleterious not because of the deleted segment but because the mutation causes a shift of the translational reading frame (10). It is known that very large deletions can be associated with a very mild disease phenotype as long as the reading frame is preserved (11), which raises the possibility of a therapeutic approach aimed at reading frame restoration even in the setting of a large deletion. The goal is to alter splicing of the pre-mRNA to skip one or more exons, in addition to those already deleted, such that the resulting mature transcript is in-frame.

The first report of the application of AONs to restore dystrophin expression was published in 1995. Takeshima et al. (12) used 2'-O-methyl RNA oligonucleotides complementary to the first 31 nucleotides of exon 19 of the human dystrophin gene. The AON was specifically designed to block two exon recognition sequences (ERS) present in this region and was shown to efficiently induce skipping of exon 19 in an in vitro system as well as in transformed lymphoblastoid human cells (13). The reports that have followed these original observations have demonstrated the feasibility of AON-mediated modulation of gene expression for the treatment of DMD. In 1998, Dunckley et al. (14) reported the ability of 2'-O-methyl oligoribonucleotides to target and redirect splicing of the dystrophin gene in *mdx* muscle cells in culture. The *mdx* mouse has a nonsense point mutation in exon 23 of the dystrophin gene and the AON was designed to anneal to the acceptor splice site of exon 23. It was predicted that blocking of the region responsible for the recognition of the intron/exon splice consensus sequence would result in skipping of the entire exon to produce an in-frame transcript in which exon 22 was spliced directly to exon 24. Indeed the use of this AON resulted in the expression of truncated forms of dystrophin, which is detectable by immunostaining in cultured cells. Analysis at the mRNA level revealed the expression of a dystrophin transcript spliced from exon 22 directly into 30, thus lacking more than just exon 23 (14). Subsequent studies have demonstrated that other AONs can lead to the exclusion only of exon 23 from the *mdx* dystrophin gene by targeting the exon 23/intron 23 splice junction (15,16). No significant effects were detected when the 3' splice junction of intron 23 was targeted. Interestingly, additional splice variants were seen in the AON-treated cells in addition to the skipping of exon 23 only (15,16).

The effectiveness of AONs in redirecting splicing of the dystrophin pre-mRNA has also been demonstrated in cultured human cells. Cells from a Duchenne patient with an exon 45 deletion resulting in an out-of-frame transcript were used to test AONs targeting regulatory elements in exon 46 of the dystrophin gene. These AONs were capable of altering pre-mRNA splicing such that exon 44 was spliced to exon 47, skipping exon 46 and thus restoring the reading frame (17). AONs that target the regions within other exons were shown to lead to the skipping of those exons in the splicing of the normal dystrophin pre-mRNA (1). That targeting exonic sequences can restore dystrophin gene expression has been confirmed by studies performed in vitro on muscle cells derived from patients carrying various dystrophin mutations in different exons (18).

Recent studies have revealed that therapeutic levels of dystrophin can be achieved in single muscles of the *mdx* mouse which is injected with AONs. In vivo studies performed after intramuscular injections of AONs directed toward the exon 23/intron 23 splice site demonstrated the expression of functional levels of dystrophin (19). Remarkably, and attributing in large part to the transfection reagent used (the nonionic block copolymer F127), dystrophin expression was detected throughout the tibialis anterior muscle in approximately 20% of the fibers and at a level that was approximately 20% of that expressed in controls (19). This level of expression persisted for about four weeks and then began to decline, but was still above the previous level for three months after injection.

AONs: Hurdles/Future Directions

AON Modifications

Considerable attention has been paid to oligonucleotide design to promote stability and to increase target affinity. New generations of oligonucleotides, including 2'-*O*-methyl, 2'-*O*-methoxyethyl, and 2'-*O*-aminopropyl derivatives combined with phosphodiester or phosphorothioate internucleotide linkages, are being tested (Fig. 2). Morpholino oligomers with phosphoramidite linkages and peptide nucleic acids (PNAs) and with pseudo-peptide backbones have higher affinity for target sequences, are resistant to nucleases (and peptidases), and are uncharged and so they are expected to cross cell membranes easily (20). Morpholino AONs, annealed to oligonucleotide "leashes" to enhance uptake and delivery of the AONs to the nucleus, have recently been tested in *mdx* cells and have been found to induce exon skipping and dystrophin protein expression (21).

Systemic Delivery

Perhaps the greatest hurdle in translating gene therapy successes with oligonucleotides in cultured cells or experimental animal to clinical application in humans with DMD is the vector delivery throughout the musculature of the

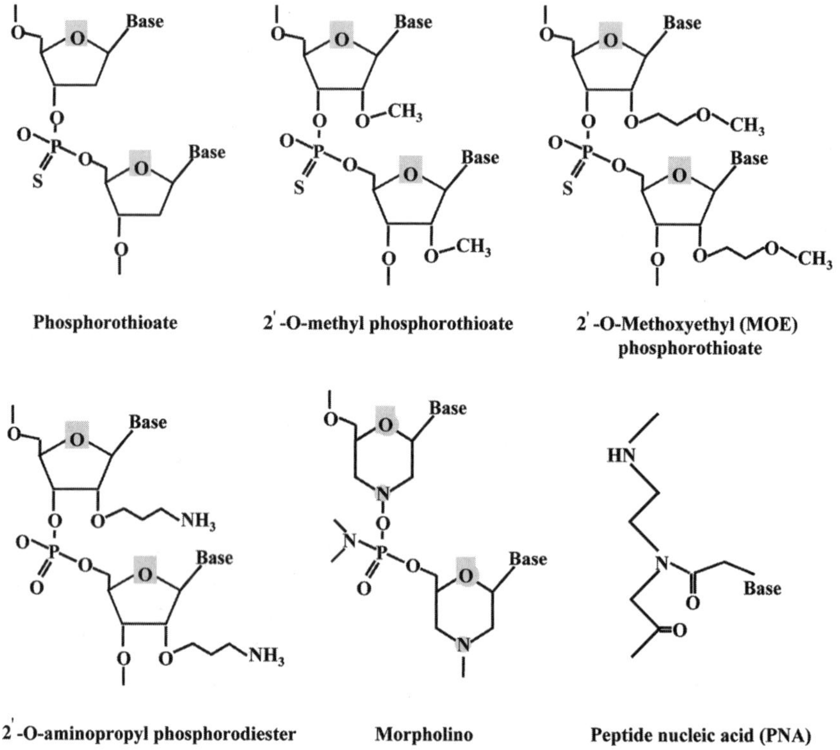

Phosphorothioate

2'-O-methyl phosphorothioate

2'-O-Methoxyethyl (MOE) phosphorothioate

2'-O-aminopropyl phosphorodiester

Morpholino

Peptide nucleic acid (PNA)

Figure 2 Oligonucleotide modifications. Multiple modifications of DNA and RNA bases have been tested in oligonucleotide vectors of various kinds. These modifications are generally used to increase resistance to degradation and enhance stability of the oligonucleotide vectors. Examples of nucleotide modifications that have been used to induce gene correction or AON-mediated exon skipping are shown. *Abbreviation*: AON, antisense oligonucleotide.

body. The ability of viruses to circulate in the blood and moreover to pass from the blood to the parenchymal cells of a tissue is a desirable characteristic of any gene therapy vector. It is unlikely that simple oligonucleotide vectors would be sufficiently stable in the blood following the intravenous injection, capable of passing across the endothelial barrier, and also able to reach the target tissues in sufficient quantity to be effective gene therapy vectors for gene editing. As such, virtually all work has been done with direct, intramuscular injection for the route of delivery. It is likely that for an intravenous delivery approach, oligonucleotides may require chemical modifications to promote stability in the blood, trans- or inter-endothelial cell passage, and cellular uptake. The development of systemic modes of delivery of oligonucleotide vectors is an active area of investigation by many laboratories, because it represents the single greatest challenge for application in human muscle diseases (22).

Spectrum of Clinical Application

An AON designed to target a specific splice site would be of therapeutic benefit to only a limited number of patients. However, one of the main advantages of AON-induced exon skipping as a therapeutic approach to DMD is that a large percentage of patients' deletions can theoretically be converted to in-frame transcripts by the skipping of only a few, restricted exons (18). This is because the mutations in the dystrophin gene are not randomly distributed along the length of the 2.5 Mb gene, but rather are concentrated in "hot spots," with specific regions being highly prone to having frame-shift deletions. For instance, skipping of exon 51 of the dystrophin gene would restore dystrophin expression in approximately 15% of all the DMD patients listed in the DMD-Leiden database (1,23,71). Thus, current approaches include developing a battery of a limited number of AONs that would be applicable for a majority of patients with frame-shift deletions.

Transient Efficacy

One of the main hurdles in the use of AONs to redirect splicing of a given gene is the need to continuously administer the oligonucleotides to achieve a sustained effect. As currently configured, the duration of effect is dependent on the stability of the AONs intracellularly and the stability of the protein product. From in vitro studies, AON-mediated redirection of splicing has been detectable only up to one week after transfection (18,24), whereas dystrophin expression in vivo was detectable several months after a single AON injection (19), presumably in part because of the stability of the dystrophin protein. This lack of sustained effect has led to the use of viral vectors to generate antisense constructs constitutively (9). Although it overcomes the problem of the transient effect of AONs, using viral vectors to constitutively express the constructs eliminates one of the main advantages of AON-mediated gene therapy, namely the avoidance of problems associated with viral-mediated gene therapy. Nevertheless, this type of hybrid approach of viral and non-viral approaches may reflect an inevitable trend in gene therapy. De Angelis et al. (24) have developed a unique virus-mediated system based on the expression of small nuclear RNAs (snRNAs) and their corresponding genes, to express antisense vectors to redirect splicing of the dystrophin gene (23). Portions of the antisense regions of U1, U7, and U2 snRNAs were replaced with sequences corresponding to the 5' and 3' splice sites of exon 51 in human dystrophin pre-mRNA (23). When expressed from retroviral constructs, these AON vectors were able to redirect splicing in cells with an exon 48 to 50 deletion, skipping exon 51 and restoring the reading frame. Data from *mdx* mouse muscle cells in culture supported the feasibility of the U7 expression system as an approach to inducing skipping of exon 23 in the *mdx* mouse, although the level of exon skipping was low (25). However, this approach was recently demonstrated to be highly efficacious in restoring the dystrophin expression in vivo in *mdx* mouse muscle (26).

Toxicity

Because there has been much more investigation of AONs as therapeutic vectors than other oligonucleotides, there is considerable data on toxicity from both local and systemic administration (7,27). While the nonspecific, toxic side effects are manageable, new generation AONs have led to better safety profiles. The collective experience with the use of AONs clinically will be of great benefit for developing this technology as a potential treatment for DMD.

Specificity

As noted above, AONs targeted to splice junctions may have more widespread effects on pre-mRNA splicing than just the desired skipping of a single exon (14–16). AONs targeted to internal exon sequences have also been reported to enhance, nonspecifically, alternative splicing of the dystrophin gene leading to multiple, aberrant transcripts of varying sizes (1). Advances in AON design may lead to an increase in the specificity of the targeting vectors and reduce the nonspecific effects on the splicing machinery.

OLIGONUCLEOTIDE-MEDIATED GENE EDITING

The use of oligonucleotides as gene editing vectors was due to the result of investigations in several different areas, but the success of homologous recombination was probably the most encouraging advance that inspired the notion that exogenous nucleic acid constructs could have the potential to modify the genome and replace mutant sequences with normal sequences. However, the low frequency of homologous recombination and the high frequency of non-homologous integration of such constructs clearly have limited the clinical applicability of this approach. As a result, interest turned to other oligonucleotide vectors that could be involved in homologous pairing reactions, thus ensuring the specificity of the reaction, but did not necessarily involve recombination or integration. Vectors currently under investigation initiate DNA repair mechanisms that have the ability to catalyze changes in single bases in genomic DNA. This approach, in which the genome might be modified in one base or only a few bases at a time, has been referred to as "gene editing." "Gene repair" is a form of gene editing when the modification is the conversion of a mutant base pair to a wild-type base pair for disease-causing point mutations. The use of oligonucleotides to edit the genome is appealing because of the relative simplicity of the vectors and also because the approach has broad theoretical applications, from site-directed mutagenesis of specific genes in embryonic stem cells to create animal models to therapeutic applications for human diseases.

Gene repair mediated by oligonucleotides has several advantages over traditional gene augmentation therapy, such as virus mediated gene delivery, in addition to the avoidance of untoward effects of viral vectors mentioned above. First, repair of the defective gene can be applied to both recessive and dominant disorders whereas gene augmentation is primarily applicable for recessive disorders. Second, the repair occurs at the genomic level, thus allowing the gene that has undergone correction to remain under its own regulatory mechanisms. Furthermore, this means that the correction is stable, thus avoiding the need for continuous delivery of the gene therapy vector to the tissue or organism.

Chimeric RNA/DNA Oligonucleotides

RNA/DNA Oligonucleotides: Structure and Mechanism of Action

The use of chimeric RNA/DNA oligonucleotides (RDOs, or chimeraplasts) for gene editing emerged from the study of the role of RecA and Rec2 proteins in DNA recombination and repair (28,29). In homologous pairing reactions, it appeared that recombination events could be promoted between DNA duplex molecules and homologous single stranded circular DNA depending on the structure of the duplex (29). This prompted the idea that the homologous pairing between an exogenous oligonucleotide vector and a genomic target could lead to the correction of a mutant genomic sequence through either recombination or induction of endogenous DNA repair activities (30). It was found that RNA/DNA chimeric molecules formed more stable homologous pairings with genomic targets than did all DNA duplexes (31). Thus, the first generation of oligonucleotides that were tested for gene editing properties were synthetic, chimeric oligonucleotides that consisted of both DNA and RNA moieties (30,32).

The original design was a contiguous stretch of 68 nucleotides containing both RNA and DNA residues (30), and the basic structure has remained essentially the same (Fig. 3). One region consists of a central pentameric bloc of DNA bases flanked on either side by RNA bases modified by $2'$-O-methylation to increase resistance to RNase H. An all-DNA sequence perfectly complementary to the RNA/DNA hybrid sequence allows for the formation of a stable duplex structure, with two polythymidine tracts creating double hairpin capped ends. A $3'$ GC clamp increases the stability of the duplex structure. In the hairpin loop structure, the $3'$ and $5'$ ends are juxtaposed but capped to minimize end-to-end ligation so that the strand break can permit the topological interwinding of the chimera with the DNA helix (33).

The RDOs are engineered to have a mismatch with a targeted base in either genomic or episomal DNA. The oligonucleotide is thus designed to bind to the endogenous sequence, produce helical distortion of the double

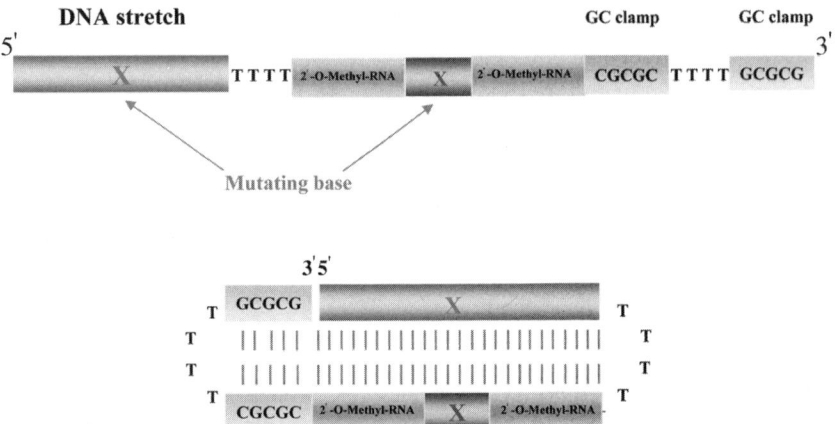

Figure 3 Structure of chimeric RDOs. The basic structure of an RDO consists of a stretch of DNA bases perfectly homologous to the region of the gene that is targeted for correction with the exception of a single base mismatch (the mutating base). A complementary region composed of 2'-O-methyl RNA interrupted by a pentameric block of DNA bases allows for internal pairing with the RDO, facilitated by polythymidine linkers forming hairpin loops. The GC clamp confers stability to the duplex structure. *Abbreviation*: RDOs, RNA/DNA oligonucleotides.

stranded DNA, and also activate the endogenous DNA repair processes to correct the mismatch (34,35). The current model of the process involves two distinct phases (Fig. 4). The first phase depends on proteins such as RecA or Rad51 (the mammalian or yeast homologue of RecA). These proteins promote strand invasion and the formation of stable displacement loops (D-loops) between the RDO and the targeted genomic sequence (36,37). The second phase involves the activation of endogenous mismatch repair systems responsible for the recognition of the mismatch present at the target base (34), as exemplified by the reduced gene correction activity in cells with diminished MSH2 activity (38). The mismatch repair activity results in the conversion of the targeted base, using the information provided by the DNA strand of the RDO (39). Clearly, in order to achieve base pair conversion, there must be a sequential process whereby the base on the complementary strand is modified.

Since their first application, RDOs have been investigated for their ability to target and to induce base pair conversions in a number of different cell types. To date, RDO-mediated gene editing has been successfully applied to eukaryotic and prokaryotic cells (35). Among eukaryotic cells, both plant and animal cells appear to be amenable to gene editing mediated by RDOs. The efficiency of gene correction appears to vary widely among cell types (40). This variability may relate to intrinsic differences in the activities of the enzymes involved in the pairing and repair

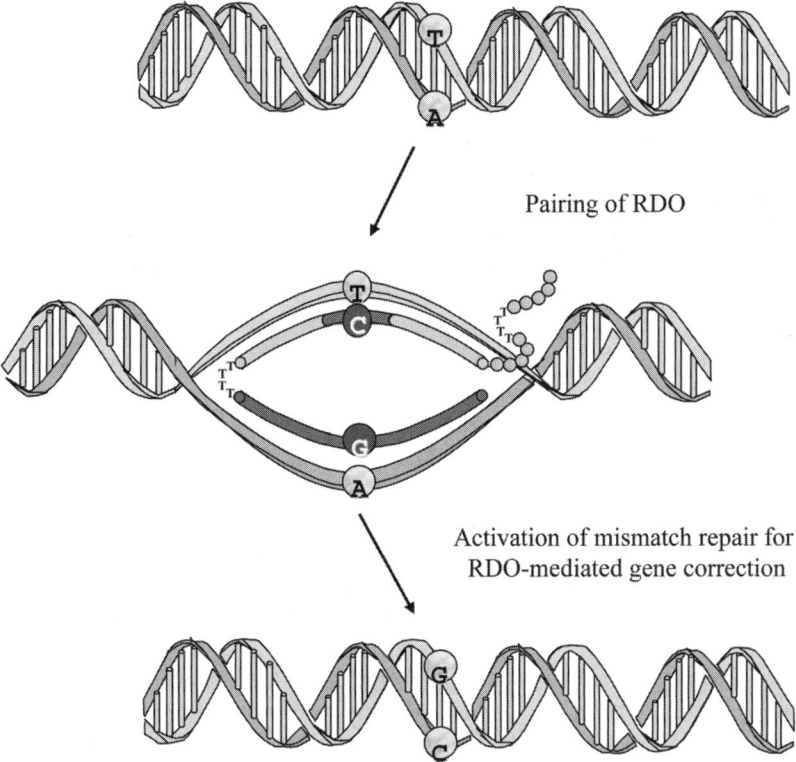

Figure 4 RDO-mediated gene repair. RDO-mediated gene editing is activated first by the pairing of the RDO with the genomic sequence targeted for correction. The creation of the mismatch between the RDO and the target sequence activates innate repair mechanisms present in the cell. Induction of mismatch repair activities can induce sequential base pair conversions in the genomic sequence, thus producing an "edited" sequence in the target gene. *Abbreviation*: RDOs, RNA/DNA oligonucleotides.

processes, primary and secondary structure of the specific RDO, chromatin folding and accessibility of the target gene, and the specific sequence of the target (41). Understanding the contribution of each of these variables in repair efficiencies will be important for rational development of subsequent generations of RDOs and for increasing the predictability necessary for clinical application.

Application of RDO-Mediated Gene Therapy to DMD:
Correction of Point Mutations

The initial studies of the use of RDOs to target and correct point mutations in the dystrophin gene were performed using the *mdx* mouse (42). As noted above, the *mdx* mouse has a nonsense point mutation in exon 23 of the dystrophin gene, and thus serves as an excellent model with which to test this gene repair technology. The targeting RDO was designed to pair perfectly with the region of the *mdx* dystrophin gene containing the point mutation, except for a mismatch engineered to occur with the point mutation itself. As a control, an identical RDO but lacking the mismatch was used. In vivo injection of the targeting RDO resulted in expression of dystrophin as early as four days after injection in mature myofibers clustered around the injection site (42). Gene correction was demonstrated at the genomic and transcript levels, consistent with the restoration of dystrophin expression. Furthermore, dystrophin expression was detectable up to three months after injection, demonstrating that the correction was stable after a prolonged period of time. The restoration of dystrophin expression occurred in approximately 5% to 10% of cells that took up the oligonucleotide after injection, but the uptake was limited to cells close to the injection site, thus limiting the overall efficacy (Fig. 5). Multiple injections would be a simple way to increase the efficacy, but distribution of RDOs throughout individual muscles and to muscles throughout the body remains a major area of technological development under investigation.

Beyond demonstrating the ability of RDOs to induce gene repair in multinucleated myofibers, it was also important to determine whether these vectors could correct the dystrophin mutation in muscle progenitor cells in the tissue. This is relevant for any gene therapy approach to DMD both because of the ongoing degeneration/regeneration of the tissue that occurs in the disease requiring the formation of new muscle from progenitor cells, but also because of the continuous turnover of myonuclei during the life of an individual even without a degenerative disorder of muscle. Thus, any strategy that targets only nuclei of the differentiated cell would be subject to gradual attenuation of the beneficial effect as those nuclei are replaced. Interestingly, gene correction was detectable in muscle progenitor cells from muscles injected with targeting RDOs (43). In vitro studies demonstrated that the efficacy of RDOs in correcting the *mdx* mutation in muscle precursor cells ranged between 2% and 15% (43).

RDO-mediated gene correction has been demonstrated also in the golden retriever muscular dystrophy (GRMD) dog. The GRMD model has a point mutation in the 3' consensus splice site of intron 6 of the dystrophin gene, causing a splicing alteration that deletes exon 7 from the mature transcript and results in a frame-shift mutation (44). Transcripts containing exon 7 of the dystrophin gene were detected six weeks after injection of a targeting RDO directly into muscles in vivo. The correction was demonstrated at the genomic level, and sequence analysis of the dystrophin transcripts further demonstrated correction of the GRMD mutation (45). Dystrophin protein expression was demonstrated by immunoblot and immunohistochemical analysis (45).

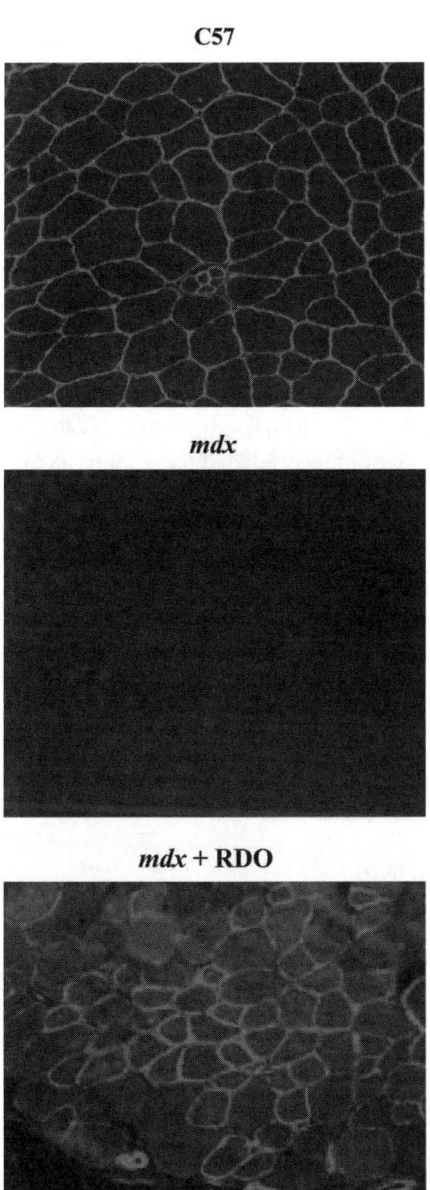

Figure 5 RDO-mediated gene correction in vivo. The panel labeled "C57" shows dystrophin expression in the wild-type strain, and the panel labeled "*mdx*" shows the complete absence of dystrophin in the *mdx* strain. Injection of a targeting RDO into *mdx* muscle results in restoration of dystrophin expression in mature myofibers clustered around the injection site (panel labeled "*mdx* + RDO"). The expression of dystrophin in these fibers is stable after correction. *Abbreviation*: RDO, RNA/DNA oligonucleotide.

Application of RDO-Mediated Gene Therapy to DMD: Modification of RNA Splicing

These results demonstrated the feasibility of using RDOs to target and correct point mutations in the dystrophin gene. Single point mutations, however, account for no more than about 15% of the mutations that cause DMD (46). Thus, recent studies have focused on RDOs for gene editing that may have broader applications for DMD patients with other kinds of mutations. Specifically, tests have been conducted on RDOs designed to alter consensus splice sites of the dystrophin gene to redirect splicing of the dystrophin pre-mRNA, which would have the therapeutic benefit described for AON-mediated exon skipping.

To test this possible application, the consensus sequence of the intron 22/exon 23 splice junction was targeted to skip exon 23 in the *mdx* mouse (47). As with AON-mediated exon skipping, this would be predicted to produce a truncated but in-frame transcript and restore dystrophin expression. Indeed, the targeting RDOs did alter the targeted base as predicted and did result in the expression of dystrophin missing exon 23 (47). Interestingly, alteration of the single splice site sequence had more widespread effects of splicing of the pre-mRNA, resulting in the production of multiple, alternatively spliced transcripts, several of which were in-frame, and thus multiple "dystrophins" of different sizes. As with the studies targeting the point mutations, these effects were stable over prolonged periods, confirming that the modification was at the genomic level (47). These results demonstrate that a gene editing approach can have applications well beyond the correction of point mutations and thus is theoretically applicable to most of the mutations causing DMD.

"Single Stranded" Oligodeoxyribonucleotides

Recent studies have indicated that the region of RDOs responsible for directing the nucleotide exchange is the all-DNA strand of the duplex (34,39). These results led to the development of a second generation of oligonucleotides with gene editing abilities. These oligonucleotides have been referred to as "linear" or "single stranded" because they appear to function without forming a duplex structure, and they are composed only of DNA residues, typically about 25 bases in length. Like RDOs, these single stranded oligodeoxyribonucleotides (ODNs) are completely homologous to the region of the target gene except for a central mismatch, and this mismatch is capable of creating genomic distortion at the targeted base to induce single base pair conversion (39). Although it is not certain that the mechanisms of action of ODNs are the same as RDOs, the proteins RAD51 and RAD52 seem to be required for pairing of the oligonucleotides to the genomic target (48). Because ODNs do not form duplexes, they can be designed to be complementary to either the transcribed or the nontranscribed strand of the genomic DNA (Fig. 6). To be effective, ODNs require the presence of unmodified

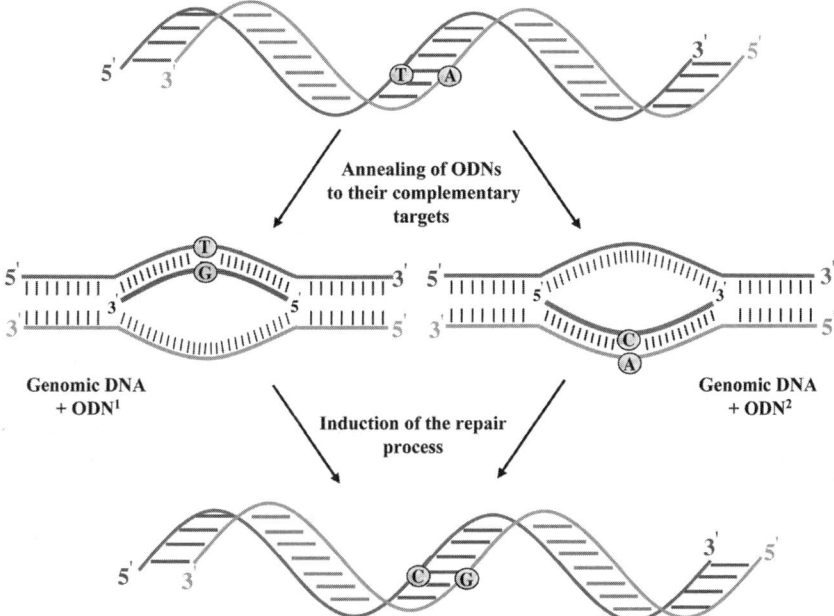

Figure 6 Pairing and gene correction with ODNs. Linear DNA oligonucleotides are a new generation of oligonucleotides with correction abilities designed to anneal with either the transcribed (ODN^1) or the nontranscribed strand (ODN^2) of the gene targeted for correction. Like RDOs, the mechanism of action is presumed to involve first a homologous pairing step and then a sequential mismatch repair process to lead to a single base pair conversion in the target sequence. Differences in repair efficiencies have been reported based on the strand of the DNA targeted by the ODN, suggesting that the repair process may be coupled to transcription. *Abbreviations*: ODNs, oligodeoxyribonucleotides; DNA, deoxyribonuleic acid; RDOs, RNA/DNA oligonucleotides.

bases in their core structure, while chemical modification of bases at the 5' and 3' ends substantially increases their stability (49). To date, the correction abilities of ODNs have been demonstrated in yeast and mammalian cells for both episomal and chromosomal targets (49–52).

Application of ODN-Mediated Gene Therapy to DMD: Gene Repair

In recent studies, the potential for ODNs to induce correction of point mutations in the dystrophin gene has been tested (53). Comparative analysis was initially performed using cultured muscle cells from the mdx^{5cv} mouse. This model for DMD has a point mutation in exon 10 of the dystrophin gene that creates a cryptic splice site. This cryptic splice site is selectively used in the splicing of the gene, resulting in a truncated message that is missing part of exon 10 and is out-of-frame, generating a nonsense codon in exon 11 of the mature transcript (54). This model is particularly suitable for performing quantitative analysis of the level of gene correction. ODNs were designed to correct the mdx^{5cv} mutation by targeting either the transcribed strand or the nontranscribed strand. Both targeting ODNs were capable of restoring dystrophin expression in vitro, while control ODNs had no effect (53). Gene correction was demonstrated at the genomic level by direct sequencing of polymerase chain reaction (PCR) products. Restoration of dystrophin expression was assessed at the mRNA level. Semiquantitative reverse transcription–polymerase chain reaction (RT–PCR) indicated that the level of gene correction varied between 0.2% and 5% in those cells. Restoration of dystrophin expression was also demonstrated at the protein level, and revealed full-length dystrophin in cells treated with ODNs targeted to either strand. Intriguingly, the ODN that was designed to target the nontranscribed strand was more effective than that targeted to the transcribed strand (53). Strand bias in ODN-mediated gene editing has been observed in other systems (39,49,50,55), suggesting that the mechanism of action can discriminate between a transcribed strand and a nontranscribed strand. The strand bias observed in myoblasts is particularly interesting in this regard because the dystrophin gene is not transcribed until after the cells are induced to undergo terminal differentiation (53). Thus, the strand bias is not likely to be directly related to the process of transcription or the transcriptional machinery itself. Direct injection of ODNs in vivo also resulted in the correction of the mdx^{5cv} mutation as determined by the restoration of dystrophin protein expression. The expression of dystrophin was assessed as early as two weeks after injection, was localized in mature myofibers clustered around the injection site, and was stable for at least three months after injection (53).

RDOs and ODNs: Hurdles/Future Directions

Oligonucleotide Uptake and Translocation

It is almost certainly the case that an increase in oligonucleotide uptake, nuclear translocation, and stability would enhance the efficiency of gene editing. It is presumed that the efficiency of base exchange is related to mass action, and that the more homologous pairing events that occur, the more frequently a genomic modification is likely to occur. Other than using standard transfection reagents, no specific modifications have been made to RDOs or ODNs to promote cellular uptake or nuclear translocation. Likewise, no specific modifications, such as coupling to nuclear translocation sequences, have been tested to increase translocation to the nucleus.

Systemic Delivery

The issues for delivering RDOs and ODNs to the musculature of the body are virtually the same as those described for AONs. Ultimately, the translation of

ODN-mediated gene editing from studies in cell culture or after intramuscular injection to clinical trials will require systemic delivery. However, unlike AON-mediated exon skipping, the effects of ODNs are permanent and thus would not require repeated injections for sustained therapeutic effect.

As an alternative to an in vivo delivery approach, ODNs may be excellent vectors for ex vivo gene therapy because they induce permanent gene correction. Although most cellular vehicles that have myogenic potential contribute only minimally to muscle via vascular delivery (56), the recent demonstration of high level of engraftment of mesangioblasts in an animal model of muscular dystrophy, delivered via the vasculature, is very encouraging (57). If it is possible to isolate and grow mesangioblasts from patients, then gene repair could be carried out ex vivo. The cellular vehicle containing a corrected gene could then be introduced into the patient's circulation to promote systemic delivery through an intraarterial route to the major muscle groups, and perhaps the heart and diaphragm.

Spectrum of Clinical Application

A major limitation of oligonucleotide-mediated gene correction is currently represented by their ability to efficiently induce only single base pair alterations at the genomic level. Targeting key base pairs in regions controlling splicing, as described above, has the potential to expand greatly the spectrum of patients who could theoretically benefit from a gene editing approach with RDOs, ODNs, or newer generation oligonucleotide vectors. However, a better understanding of how RNA splicing can be broadly affected by changes in single splice sites would be important for reliable use in clinical applications. As another alternative, oligonucleotide-mediated editing may be capable of inserting or deleting a single base pair in the genomic sequence rather than just inducing a change of a base pair (38,50). Because every frame-shift mutation can be converted to an in-frame transcript by either the addition or deletion of a single base, this approach would have broad applicability to the vast majority of DMD patients. Unfortunately, at this point, the current vectors appear to have only limited capabilities to add or delete bases to genomic DNA. Improved vector design with more efficient pairing characteristics or capacities to induce DNA repair processes more efficiently may render oligonucleotides more effective as mediators of base pair addition or deletion, and this will greatly expand the spectrum of application of ODN-mediated gene editing.

OTHER TECHNOLOGIES

Short Fragment Homologous Recombination

This technology involves the use of single stranded short DNA fragments derived from PCR amplicons of length ranging from 400 to 800 bp. The fragments are homologous to the region of the gene containing the mutation except that they code for the normal sequence. When introduced in cells undergoing cell division, they have been shown to correct mutations or deletions of up to three nucleotides in length (58,59). To date this technology has been applied to the CFTR gene of cystic fibrosis as well as several episomal targets (60,61). The mechanism of action of short fragment homologous recombination (SFHR) seems to involve homologous recombination and may rely also on the activation of repair mechanisms.

SFHR has been applied for restoring the normal dystrophin sequence in the *mdx* mouse, and correction at the genomic level has been reported in vitro using standard PCR-based methods, although corresponding increases in normal transcript and protein production was not observed (62). Positive results using this technology were also obtained in vivo, although the level of gene correction appeared to be much lower. Like RDOs and ODNs, SFHR vectors can be applied to ex vivo gene therapy using a cell therapy approach after gene correction (63).

Triplex-Forming Oligonucleotides

Although not yet applied to mutations of the dystrophin gene, triple helix (triplex)-forming oligonucleotides (TFOs) have been shown to have multiple activities in modulating gene expression, including targeted base conversion when the TFO is conjugated to a mutagen (64). In that regard, TFOs would be applied similarly to RDOs or ODNs to correct point mutations. One of the limitations of TFOs is the requirement to bind to polypurine sequences, thus perhaps limiting their application across a full range of point mutations in the dystrophin gene. TFOs have also been found to increase the rates of recombination between homologous sequences in close proximity and thus may have the potential to mediate gene repair through recombination (64), similar to the conceptual approach of SFHR.

Trans-Splicing Oligonucleotides

Trans-splicing group I intron ribozymes and spliceosome-mediated RNA *trans*-splicing (SMaRT) oligonucleotides have been studied as therapeutic vectors for modifying RNA splicing (65,66). In each case, mutant pre-RNAs have been induced to generate functional RNAs by modifying the splicing process, and in that regard would be analogous to that of AONs in the treatment of mutations in the dystrophin gene. Neither of these approaches has been applied to model systems related to DMD at this time.

Homologous Recombination

The development of homologous recombination technology has profoundly changed the field of molecular genetics and initially offered hope as the ultimate gene repair technology. However, the frequency of homologous recombination has generally been considered to be too low to be viable therapeutically, particularly because the rate on non-homologous recombination exceeds that of homologous recombination (67). However, there has been renewed interest in this approach for ex vivo gene therapy, providing encouragement that this may yet have viable therapeutic applications (68,69).

CONCLUSIONS

Substantial progress has been made in the development of oligonucleotide-mediated gene therapies in the past decade. These technologies are new and thus are likely to evolve significantly in the coming years. As viral vectors move toward increased simplicity, oligonucleotide vectors are likely to move toward increased complexity to combine the nucleotide-based specificity with other features necessary to clinically applicable therapeutics such as modifications to improve targeting and delivery. Furthermore, some oligonucleotide-based therapies may be combined with viral based systems to take advantage of the unique properties of each. Analysis of toxicity will be a key aspect of trials in both animal models and humans, and specific and non-specific toxic effects will have to be balanced with the potential benefits of genetic therapy. As oligonucleotide-mediated gene therapy approaches move from the bench to the bedside, cost of vector production will become an increasingly pressing concern. Advances in synthetic chemistry and the development of synthesizers capable of generating hundreds of grams of purified oligonucleotides in single runs are making the use of oligonucleotides as gene therapy vectors a reality (70). In general, there is reason for optimism that a new class of oligonucleotide "drugs" will emerge in the next decade to be added to the pharmacopoeia to complement current and emerging conventional agents in the treatment of DMD.

ACKNOWLEDGMENT

This work was supported by grants from the Muscular Dystrophy Association to CB and to TAR.

REFERENCES

1. Aartsma Rus A, Bremmer Bout M, Janson AA, den Dunnen JT, van Ommen GJ, van Deutekom JC. Targeted exon skipping as a potential gene correction therapy for Duchenne muscular dystrophy. Neuromuscul Disord 2002; 12:S71–S77.
2. Rando TA. Oligonucleotidemediated gene therapy for muscular dystrophies. Neuromuscul Disord 2002; 12:S55–S60.
3. Good L. Translation repression by antisense sequences. Cell Mol Life Sci 2003; 60:854–861.

4. Simons RW, Kleckner N. Translational control of IS10 transposition. Cell 1983; 34:683–691.
5. Mizuno T, Chou MY, Inouye M. A unique mechanism regulating gene expression: translational inhibition by a complementary RNA transcript (micRNA). Proc Natl Acad Sci USA 1984; 81:1966–1970.
6. Izant JG, Weintraub H. Inhibition of thymidine kinase gene expression by antisense RNA: a molecular approach to genetic analysis. Cell 1984; 36:1007–1015.
7. Pirollo KF, Rait A, Sleer LS, Chang EH. Antisense therapeutics: from theory to clinical practice. Pharmacol Ther 2003; 99:55–77.
8. Dominski Z, Kole R. Restoration of correct splicing in thalassemic pre-mRNA by antisense oligonucleotides. Proc Natl Acad Sci USA 1993; 90:8673–8677.
9. Vacek M, Sazani P, Kole R. Antisense-mediated redirection of mRNA splicing. Cell Mol Life Sci 2003; 60:825–833.
10. Koenig M, Beggs AH, Moyer M, Scherpf S, Heindrich K, Bettecken T, et al. The molecular basis for Duchenne versus Becker muscular dystrophy: correlation of severity with type of deletion. Am J Hum Genet 1989; 45:498–506.
11. Love DR, Flint TJ, Genet SA, Middleton Price HR, Davies KE. Becker muscular dystrophy patient with a large intragenic dystrophin deletion: implications for functional minigenes and gene therapy. J Med Genet 1991; 28:860–864.
12. Takeshima Y, Nishio H, Sakamoto H, Nakamura H, Matsuo M. Modulation of in vitro splicing of the upstream intron by modifying an intra-exon sequence which is deleted from the dystrophin gene in dystrophin Kobe. J Clin Invest 1995; 95:515–520.
13. Pramono ZA, Takeshima Y, Alimsardjono H, Ishii A, Takeda S, Matsuo M. Induction of exon skipping of the dystrophin transcript in lymphoblastoid cells by transfecting an antisense oligodeoxynucleotide complementary to an exon recognition sequence. Biochem Biophys Res Commun 1996; 226:445–449.
14. Dunckley MG, Manoharan M, Villiet P, Eperon IC, Dickson G. Modification of splicing in the dystrophin gene in cultured Mdx muscle cells by antisense oligoribonucleotides. Hum Mol Genet 1998; 7:1083–1090.
15. Wilton SD, Lloyd F, Carville K, Fletcher S, Honeyman K, Agrawal S, et al. Specific removal of the nonsense mutation from the mdx dystrophin mRNA using antisense oligonucleotides. Neuromuscul Disord 1999; 9:330–338.
16. Mann CJ, Honeyman K, Cheng AJ, Ly T, Lloyd F, Fletcher S, et al. Antisense-induced exon skipping and synthesis of dystrophin in the mdx mouse. Proc Natl Acad Sci USA 2001; 98:42–47.
17. van Deutekom JC, Bremmer Bout M, Janson AA, Ginjaar IB, Baas F, den Dunnen JT, et al. Antisense-induced exon skipping restores dystrophin expression in DMD patient derived muscle cells. Hum Mol Genet 2001; 10:1547–1554.
18. Aartsma Rus A, Janson AA, Kaman WE, Bremmer Bout M, den Dunnen JT, Baas F, et al. Therapeutic antisense-induced exon skipping in cultured muscle cells from six different DMD patients. Hum Mol Genet 2003; 12:907–914.
19. htpp://www.dmd.nl.
20. Lu QL, Mann CJ, Lou F, Bou Gharios G, Morris GE, Xue SA, et al. Functional amounts of dystrophin produced by skipping the mutated exon in the mdx dystrophic mouse. Nat Med 2003; 9:1009–1014.
21. Sazani P, Vacek MM, Kole R. Short-term and long-term modulation of gene expression by antisense therapeutics. Curr Opin Biotechnol 2002; 13:468–472.

22. Gebski BL, Mann CJ, Fletcher S, Wilton SD. Morpholino antisense oligonucleotide induced dystrophin exon 23 skipping in mdx mouse muscle. Hum Mol Genet 2003; 12:1801–1811.
23. Lu QL, Rabinowitz A, Chen YC, Yokota T, Yin H, Alter J, et al. Systemic delivery of antisense oligoribonucleotide restores dystrophin expression in body-wide skeletal muscles. Proc Natl Acad Sci USA 2005; 102:198–203.
24. De Angelis FG, Sthandier O, Berarducci B, Toso S, Galluzzi G, Ricci E, et al. Chimeric snRNA molecules carrying antisense sequences against the splice junctions of exon 51 of the dystrophin pre-mRNA induce exon skipping and restoration of a dystrophin synthesis in Delta 48-50 DMD cells. Proc Natl Acad Sci USA 2002; 99:9456–9461.
25. Mann CJ, Honeyman K, McClorey G, Fletcher S, Wilton SD. Improved antisense oligonucleotide induced exon skipping in the mdx mouse model of muscular dystrophy. J Gene Med 2002; 4:644–654.
26. Brun C, Suter D, Pauli C, Dunant P, Lochmuller H, Burgunder JM, et al. U7 snRNAs induce correction of mutated dystrophin pre-mRNA by exon skipping. Cell Mol Life Sci 2003; 60:557–566.
27. Goyenvalle A, Vulin A, Fougerousse F, Leturcq F, Kaplan JC, Garcia L, et al. Rescue of dystrophic muscle through U7 snRNA-mediated exon skipping. Science 2004; 306:1796–1799.
28. Kurreck J. Antisense technologies. Improvement through novel chemical modifications. Eur J Biochem 2003; 270:1628–1644.
29. Kmiec EB, Cole A, Holloman WK. The REC2 gene encodes the homologous pairing protein of Ustilago maydis. Mol Cell Biol 1994; 14:7163–7172.
30. Kotani H, Kmiec EB. DNA cruciforms facilitate in vitro strand transfer on nucleosomal templates. Mol Gen Genet 1994; 243:681–690.
31. Yoon K, Cole-Strauss A, Kmiec EB. Targeted gene correction of episomal DNA in mammalian cells mediated by a chimeric RNA.DNA oligonucleotide. Proc Natl Acad Sci USA 1996; 93:2071–2076.
32. Kotani H, Germann MW, Andrus A, Vinayak R, Mullah B, Kmiec EB. RNA facilitates RecA-mediated DNA pairing and strand transfer between molecules bearing limited regions of homology. Mol Gen Genet 1996; 250:626–634.
33. Cole Strauss A, Yoon K, Xiang Y, Byrne BC, Rice MC, Gryn J, et al. Correction of the mutation responsible for sickle cell anemia by an RNA-DNA oligonucleotide. Science 1996; 273:1386–1389.
34. Ye S, Cole Strauss AC, Frank B, Kmiec EB. Targeted gene correction: a new strategy for molecular medicine. Mol Med Today 1998; 4:431–437.
35. Gamper HB Jr, Cole Strauss A, Metz R, Parekh H, Kumar R, Kmiec EB. A plausible mechanism for gene correction by chimeric oligonucleotides. Biochemistry 2000; 39:5808–5816.
36. Andersen MS, Sorensen CB, Bolund L, Jensen TG. Mechanisms underlying targeted gene correction using chimeric RNA/DNA and single-stranded DNA oligonucleotides. J Mol Med 2002; 80:770–781.
37. Gamper HB, Hou YM, Kmiec EB. Evidence for a four-strand exchange catalyzed by the RecA protein. Biochemistry 2000; 39:15,272–15,281.
38. Drury MD, Kmiec EB. DNA pairing is an important step in the process of targeted nucleotide exchange. Nucleic Acids Res 2003; 31:899–910.

39. Cole Strauss A, Gamper H, Holloman WK, Munoz M, Cheng N, Kmiec EB. Targeted gene repair directed by the chimeric RNA/DNA oligonucleotide in a mammalian cell-free extract. Nucleic Acids Res 1999; 27:1323–1330.
40. Gamper HB, Parekh H, Rice MC, Bruner M, Youkey H, Kmiec EB. The DNA strand of chimeric RNA/DNA oligonucleotides can direct gene repair/conversion activity in mammalian and plant cell-free extracts. Nucleic Acids Res 2000; 28:4332–4339.
41. Santana E, Peritz AE, Iyer S, Uitto J, Yoon K. Different frequency of gene targeting events by the RNA-DNA oligonucleotide among epithelial cells. J Invest Dermatol 1998; 111:1172–1177.
42. Parekh-Olmedo H, Czymmek K, Kmiec EB. Targeted gene repair in mammalian cells using chimeric RNA/DNA oligonucleotides and modified single-stranded vectors. Sci STKE 2001; 2001:L1.
43. Rando TA, Disatnik MH, Zhou LZ. Rescue of dystrophin expression in mdx mouse muscle by RNA/DNA oligonucleotides. Proc Natl Acad Sci USA 2000; 97:5363–5368.
44. Bertoni C, Rando TA. Dystrophin gene repair in mdx muscle precursor cells in vitro and in vivo mediated by RNA-DNA chimeric oligonucleotides. Hum Gene Ther 2002; 13:707–718.
45. Sharp NJ, Kornegay JN, Van Camp SD, Herbstreith MH, Secore SL, Kettle S, et al. An error in dystrophin mRNA processing in golden retriever muscular dystrophy, an animal homologue of Duchenne muscular dystrophy. Genomics 1992; 13:115–121.
46. Bartlett RJ, Stockinger S, Denis MM, Bartlett WT, Inverardi L, Le TT, et al. In vivo targeted repair of a point mutation in the canine dystrophin gene by a chimeric RNA/DNA oligonucleotide. Nat Biotechnol 2000; 18:615–622.
47. Amalfitano A, Rafael JA, Chamberlain JS. Structure and mutation of the dystrophin gene. In: Brown SC, Lucy JA, eds. Dystrophin. Cambridge: Cambridge University Press, 1996:1–26.
48. Bertoni C, Lau C, Rando TA. Restoration of dystrophin expression in mdx muscle cells by chimeraplast-mediated exon skipping. Hum Mol Genet 2003; 12:1087–1099.
49. Liu L, Cheng S, van Brabant AJ, Kmiec EB. Rad51p and Rad54p, but not Rad52p, elevate gene repair in *Saccharomyces cerevisiae* directed by modified single-stranded oligonucleotide vectors. Nucleic Acids Res 2002; 30:2742–2750.
50. Igoucheva O, Alexeev V, Yoon K. Targeted gene correction by small single-stranded oligonucleotides in mammalian cells. Gene Ther 2001; 8:391–399.
51. Liu L, Rice MC, Kmiec EB. In vivo gene repair of point and frameshift mutations directed by chimeric RNA/DNA oligonucleotides and modified single-stranded oligonucleotides. Nucleic Acids Res 2001; 29:4238–4250.
52. Parekh-Olmedo H, Drury M, Kmiec EB. Targeted nucleotide exchange in *Saccharomyces cerevisiae* directed by short oligonucleotides containing locked nucleic acids. Chem Biol 2002; 9:1073–1084.
53. Kren BT, Wong PY, Steer CJ. Short, single-stranded oligonucleotides mediate targeted nucleotide conversion using extracts from isolated liver mitochondria. DNA Repair 2003; 2:531–546.
54. Bertoni C, Morris GE, Rando TA. Strand bias in oligonucleotide-mediated dystrophin gene editing. Hum Mol Genet 2005; 14:221–233.

55. Im WB, Phelps SF, Copen EH, Adams EG, Slightom JL, Chamberlain JS. Differential expression of dystrophin isoforms in strains of mdx mice with different mutations. Hum Mol Genet 1996; 5:1149–1153.
56. Liu L, Rice MC, Drury M, Cheng S, Gamper H, Kmiec EB. Strand bias in targeted gene repair is influenced by transcriptional activity. Mol Cell Biol 2002; 22:3852–3863.
57. Partridge TA. Stem cell route to neuromuscular therapies. Muscle Nerve 2003; 27:133–141.
58. Sampaolesi M, Torrente Y, Innocenzi A, Tonlorenzi R, D'Antona G, Pellegrino MA, et al. Cell therapy of alpha-sarcoglycan null dystrophic mice through intra-arterial delivery of mesoangioblasts. Science 2003; 301:487–492.
59. Kunzelmann K, Legendre JY, Knoell DL, Escobar LC, Xu Z, Gruenert DC. Gene targeting of CFTR DNA in CF epithelial cells. Gene Ther 1996; 3:859–867.
60. Goncz KK, Kunzelmann K, Xu Z, Gruenert DC. Targeted replacement of normal and mutant CFTR sequences in human airway epithelial cells using DNA fragments. Hum Mol Genet 1998; 7:1913–1919.
61. Sangiuolo F, Bruscia E, Serafino A, Nardone A, Bonifazi E, Lais M, et al. In vitro correction of cystic fibrosis epithelial cell lines by small fragment homologous replacement (SFHR) technique. BMC Med Genet 2002; 3:8.
62. Colosimo A, Goncz KK, Novelli G, Dallapiccola B, Gruenert DC. Targeted correction of a defective selectable marker gene in human epithelial cells by small DNA fragments. Mol Ther 2001; 3:178–185.
63. Kapsa R, Quigley A, Lynch GS, Steeper K, Kornberg AJ, Gregorevic P, et al. In vivo and in vitro correction of the mdx dystrophin gene nonsense mutation by short-fragment homologous replacement. Hum Gene Ther 2001; 12:629–642.
64. Kapsa RM, Quigley AF, Vadolas J, Steeper K, Ioannou PA, Byrne E, et al. Targeted gene correction in the mdx mouse using short DNA fragments: towards application with bone marrow-derived cells for autologous remodeling of dystrophic muscle. Gene Ther 2002; 9:695–699.
65. Seidman MM, Glazer PM. The potential for gene repair via triple helix formation. J Clin Invest 2003; 112:487–494.
66. Sullenger BA, Cech TR. Ribozyme-mediated repair of defective mRNA by targeted, trans-splicing. Nature 1994; 371:619–622.
67. Puttaraju M, Jamison SF, Mansfield SG, Garcia Blanco MA, Mitchell LG. Spliceosome-mediated RNA trans-splicing as a tool for gene therapy. Nat Biotechnol 1999; 17:246–252.
68. Roth DB, Wilson JH. Relative rates of homologous and nonhomologous recombination in transfected DNA. Proc Natl Acad Sci USA 1985; 82:3355–3359.
69. Hatada S, Nikkuni K, Bentley SA, Kirby S, Smithies O. Gene correction in hematopoietic progenitor cells by homologous recombination. Proc Natl Acad Sci USA 2000; 97:13,807–13,811.
70. Chamberlain JR, Schwarze U, Wang PR, Hirata RK, Hankenson KD, Pace JM, et al. Gene targeting in stem cells from individuals with osteogenesis imperfecta. Science 2004; 303:1198–1201.
71. Akhtar S, Agrawal S. In vivo studies with antisense oligonucleotides. Trends Pharmacol Sci 1997; 18:12–18.

16

The Intravascular Delivery of Naked DNA for Treating Duchenne Muscular Dystrophy

Jon A. Wolff

Departments of Pediatrics and Medical Genetics, Waisman Center, University of Wisconsin–Madison, Madison, Wisconsin, U.S.A.

Hans Herweijer

Mirus Bio Corporation, Madison, Wisconsin, U.S.A.

INTRODUCTION

Duchenne Muscular Dystrophy: A Need for Therapy

Duchenne muscular dystrophy (DMD) is an important candidate for gene therapy because of its prevalence and life-threatening nature. Although population-based screening programs have been developed for Tay-Sachs disease and cystic fibrosis, this approach is of limited value in DMD since one-third of all cases arise de novo without carrier status in the mother (1,2). Newborn screening is possible and enables early intervention (3–5).

"Proof-of-Principle" for Developing a Gene Therapy for DMD

There are several components that are required for developing a gene therapy for a disease. The first step is establishing the "proof-of-principle" for the approach. This involves determining the expression of a certain gene in target cells that would likely prevent the pathologic process and help the patient. For DMD, the molecular and cellular rationale for gene therapy has been provided by transgenic studies in the *mdx* mouse model for DMD in which prenatal expression of full-length dystrophin was ameliorative (6–9). Full-length and truncated dystrophins localize to the sarcolemma and also induce the localization of a dystrophin-associated glycoprotein to the sarcolemma in dystrophin-positive myofibers, thus preventing the degeneration and loss of myofibers. Dystrophin expression is also associated with an increased proportion of peripheral nuclei (a sign of normal, well-differentiated muscle). Using an inducible expression system in transgenic mice, postnatal expression of full-length mouse dystrophin (mDys) also attenuated the *mdx* mouse muscle pathology (10). Postnatal gene transfer studies using adenoviral and adeno-associated vectors and other types of viral vectors have also found that the exogenous dystrophin expression is sufficient to prevent muscle dystrophy (11–15).

Loss of muscle fibers is also prevented by naked DNA transfer (16,17). Naked plasmid DNA (pDNA) injections of a mini-dystrophin construct attenuated muscle necrosis and loss of muscle force contractions in the diaphragm of *mdx* mice (18).

The Amount of Gene Expression Required for Treating DMD

Although these studies have established proof-of-principle, gene therapy for DMD is particularly challenging because the large dystrophin gene must be delivered to many muscle groups throughout the body. The amount of dystrophin expression that is necessary to substantially alleviate the disease is an open question (1,19). The extent of foreign dystrophin expression needs to be assessed based upon the number of dystrophin-positive fibers (e.g., by immunohistochemistry) and the amount of dystrophin protein (e.g., by immunoblot). Based on the transgenic and postnatal gene transfer studies in mice and the natural history of human patients, there is a consensus that at least 10% to 20% of normal dystrophin protein expression is required to alleviate the disease. The restriction of dystrophin protein to nuclear domains along a myofiber (range 100–300 µm) also complicates gene therapy (20). There is some concern that dystrophin expression needs to be along the entire myofiber to prevent increased stress on dystrophin-negative regions. However, this remains a theoretical concern without any experimental data. The fact that the number of dystrophin-positive fibers is stable over time after pDNA or adenoviral delivery in *mdx* mouse muscle argues that this outcome is unlikely (17,21). Also, there appears to be a positive bystander effect in which dystrophin-negative myofibers adjacent to dystrophin-positive ones are protected to a small extent from degeneration (22). Gene transfer is likely not uniform but spotty, thereby leading to high levels of transfection in specific muscle groups or regions of muscles.

In DMD patients, this may prevent degeneration of specific muscles in these high expressing regions, thereby preserving sufficient function of the muscle at least for routine activities that do not require much strength.

PLASMID DNA DELIVERY

The primary challenge in developing most gene therapies at this time is the ability to obtain sufficient gene expression in the target cells long enough to attenuate the disease state. This has been the hurdle in muscular dystrophy gene therapy as well, and a variety of vectors are being developed for the delivery of genes to muscles (15,23). These include viral vectors such as adenoviral and adeno-associated vectors, and nonviral vectors such as naked DNA. Our studies suggest that the method of intravascular delivery of naked pDNA could be used for delivering the normal human dystrophin gene to the peripheral limbs of patients with DMD to preserve limb function. Preventing the loss of limb muscle use would help maintain quality of life such as the use of hands for many self-care and communication (e.g., computer) skills. This chapter focuses on the delivery and stability of expression of our proposed intravascular/naked pDNA strategy (Fig. 1). While viral-derived delivery systems have held the most sway, the intravascular delivery of naked nucleic acids under increased pressure is gaining more favor because of its simplicity, ease-of-use, and utility for effectively delivering nucleic acids to hepatocytes and striated myofibers in vivo.

Nonviral Vectors

Nonviral approaches go by a variety of descriptive names, such as synthetic delivery systems and physical–chemical methods, that emphasize different aspects of the approach. The types of nonviral methods that are being developed for the delivery of naked DNA include lipoplexes (cationic lipids), polyplexes [e.g., polyethylenimine (PEI)], lipopolyplexes (polymer/lipid mixtures), electroporation, and particle acceleration (also known as gene gun). Synthetic vectors have a number of advantages and disadvantages in comparison to viral vectors. Most nonviral systems are relatively less efficient than viral vectors and this dampens enthusiasm for their use. This tenet needs to be reconsidered as continual improvements in synthetic vectors are bridging the gap between the two gene transfer approaches. In cells in culture, transfection efficiencies are approaching 100% using the new cationic lipid reagents. High efficiencies of gene transfer and expression can also be achieved from nonviral vectors under certain conditions for in vivo delivery to animal cells. The intravascular delivery of naked DNA under elevated pressure leads to high levels of expression in liver, muscle, and other tissues that approach the expression levels achievable with viral vectors (see below).

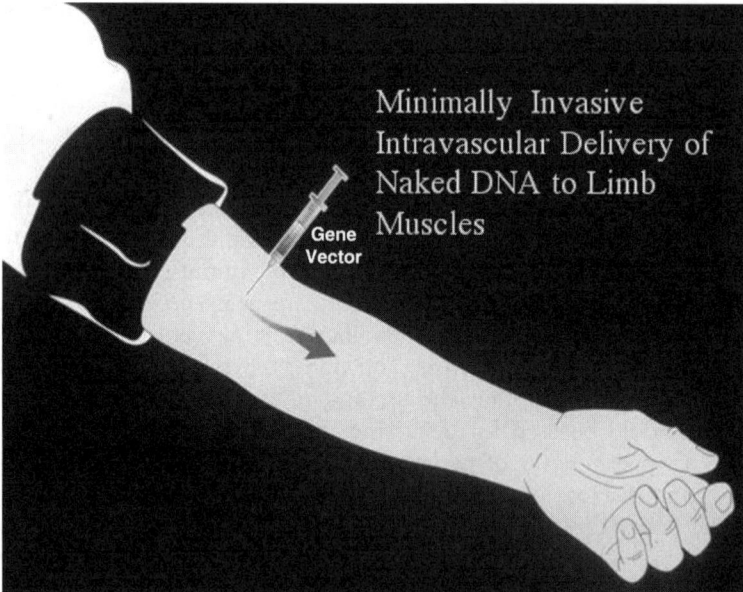

Figure 1 Diagrammatic representation of how the intravascular procedure would be applied in humans. This approach would entail a blood pressure cuff being placed and inflated on a limb, and then naked DNA would be injected rapidly into a limb vessel in a relatively large volume.

The injection of pDNA expression vectors complexed with either cationic lipids or PEI into a peripheral vein can enable high levels of expression in the lung (24,25). These encouraging results suggest that the nonviral delivery systems can enable foreign gene expressions in levels that are comparable to viral vectors. Further progress will blur this commonly invoked distinction between nonviral and viral vectors.

Although there is little chance of having preexisting neutralizing antibodies against nonviral vectors, repetitive administrations could induce an immune response against components of the synthetic vectors. Innate or inflammatory responses to nonviral vector administration may be more problematic. As transfection reagents are being increasingly used for in vivo delivery, it is being increasingly appreciated that acute toxic responses may also be elicited by cationic lipids and polycations (25).

Potential Advantages of Naked DNA

There are several advantages of using pDNA for treating DMD; the major advantage, besides its simplicity, is its ability to express the full-length dystrophin. Although relatively large amounts of clinical grade pDNA are required, it is still much easier and less expensive to produce when compared to viral vectors. Naked pDNA is also safer as there is no chance of administering replication-competent viruses. Also, our preliminary data indicate that aberrant expression (in nonmuscle tissues) is less likely with the intravascular delivery of naked pDNA than with viral vectors (26). Aberrant expression of dystrophin is probably not harmful, but should be avoided if possible.

Another major advantage is that repetitive administrations of naked pDNA have not led to the production of anti-DNA antibodies (27). Repetitive DNA intravascular administrations of pDNA were possible with no loss of gene expression in the liver (28). Similar results have been obtained after repetitive intravascular injections into muscle (unpublished data). Repeat administrations may be valuable in treating DMD. Different muscle groups could be targeted at different times. Also, as the exogenous dystrophin DNA sequences reside in myofiber nuclei, which may be slowly lost over years, repeat administrations over the lifetime of the individual will likely be required to maintain dystrophin expression.

Injection of Naked DNA in Muscle Results in Transfection of Cells In Vivo

Direct in vivo gene transfer with naked DNA was first demonstrated when efficient transfection of myofibers was observed following the injection of mRNA or pDNA into skeletal muscle (29). Expression was found in all types of striated muscle cells, including type I and type II skeletal myofibers and cardiac muscle cells (27,30–33). Muscles such as the rectus femoris or tibialis anterior that are circumscribed by a well-defined epimysium may enable the highest expression levels since they provide the best distribution and retention of the injected pDNA. However, the efficiency of gene transfer into skeletal or cardiac muscle is relatively low and variable. This is especially problematic for larger animals including nonhuman primates (27). Attempts to increase pDNA uptake, for instance, by inducing muscle regeneration, have not increased efficiency to a level that would allow for clinical use in gene therapy protocols.

Electroporation Enhances Uptake of Injected pDNA into Muscle and Skin

In the recent past, there has been a marked increase in the number of studies employing intramuscular or intradermal injection of naked DNA followed by electroporation. Gene transfer efficiency and safety have increased because of technical improvements in electroporation equipment as well as better methodology (34). Gene transfer to a variety of different cell types in vivo has been demonstrated. Expression levels in muscle are at least 10-fold higher compared to injection of pDNA without electroporation, but are accompanied by elevation of serum creatine kinase levels (35). It is not clear whether these increases in transgene expression (especially of secreted proteins) are due to enhanced gene transfer into myofibers, or to simultaneous transfer into different cell types (e.g., endothelial cells). Although expression levels are considered sufficient to warrant further investigation of this method for gene therapy, for instance in chronic anemia or the muscular dystrophies (36,37), they are not as high as that achieved following intravascular delivery (see below) (38).

INTRAVASCULAR DELIVERY OF NAKED PLASMID DNA

Intravascular Delivery of Plasmid DNA into Liver

Intravascular delivery of genes is attractive because there is no necessity for multiple intraparenchymal injections into the target tissue. The gene is disseminated throughout the tissue as the vascular system accesses every cell. Vascular delivery could be systemic or regional, wherein injections are given into specific vessels that supply the target tissue (39). The intravascular delivery of adenoviruses or cationic lipid–DNA complexes in adult animals mostly results in their expression in vascular-accessible cells such as the endothelial cells or the hepatocytes reached via the sinusoid fenestrae. Our first evidence for the expression of intravascularly delivered naked pDNA was obtained from the liver. Following delivery of naked pDNA via the portal vein, the hepatic vein, or the bile duct in mice and rats, efficient transgene expression was obtained in hepatocytes throughout the liver (28,40,41). The expression levels were substantially increased by the use of hyperosmotic injection solutions and on occlusion of the blood outflow from the liver, although it was later shown that a hyperosmotic solution was not absolutely necessary.

In small and large animals, the rapid injection of nucleic acids into either liver vessels or the tail vein (in rodents only) enabled foreign gene expression from pDNA-based expression vectors or inhibition of targeted mRNA expression by siRNA's (40–44). The simplicity and effectiveness of this increased pressure tail vein (also known as hydrodynamic) technique is popularizing the use of naked DNA and is increasingly being adopted by many laboratories for a variety of molecular and cellular biologic studies.

Intravascular Delivery of Plasmid DNA into Muscle

For intrinsic muscle disorders such as DMD in which many muscles have to be targeted, the intravascular delivery of naked pDNA to several different muscle groups is essential. Also, the limited distribution of pDNA through the interstitial space that follows intramuscular injection is avoided on using the intravascular approach. Increased efficiency of gene delivery should be anticipated by the intimate association of muscle cells with capillaries. Muscle has a high density of capillaries that are in close contact with the myofibers. Delivery of pDNA to muscle via capillaries places the pDNA in more direct contact with the myofibers and substantially decreases the interstitial space that the pDNA has to traverse to access a myofiber. However, the endothelium in muscle capillaries is of the continuous, nonfenestrated type and has low solute permeability, especially to large macromolecules. Nonetheless, rapid delivery of relatively large volumes of pDNA solutions (10 mL injected into rat iliac artery) resulted in very efficient gene transfer into myofibers (45). Under the optimal injection condition, up to 50% of myofibers expressed β-galactosidase in many areas of the muscles. These transfection efficiencies are comparable to what can be achieved using viral vectors.

Experiments on the intravascular delivery of pDNA, although technically difficult, have successfully been performed in mice (46). This is contrary to the usual predicament in a gene therapy approach, wherein it is difficult to extend a procedure from small animal models to large ones (27). The use of dystrophin expression vectors in the *mdx* mouse is discussed below. Intravascular delivery to skeletal muscles in the limbs has successfully been performed in large animals including rabbits, dogs, and rhesus monkeys (47). Several alternative methods for delivering the pDNA solution and blocking limb blood flow have been evaluated. Delivery via a catheter to limb target muscle groups, in combination with blocking blood flow with a tourniquet or blood pressure cuff, is very effective in larger animals. In rhesus monkeys, transfection efficiencies of 40% have been observed (Fig. 2) (26). Most importantly for human therapeutic relevance, the ability of the procedure to work not only in rodents, but also in larger animals including nonhuman primates, is an important measure of the clinical potential of a gene delivery technique (26).

Comparison of Intravascular/Naked DNA Delivery Approach With Viral Vectors

We performed the same intravascular injection procedure into the femoral artery of adult rats using 10^{12} recombinant adeno-associated viral vector type 2 (rAAV2) particles expressing luciferase under control of the cytomegalovirus (CMV) promoter (Table 1) (25). Using the rAAV2 vector, we were able to obtain 10 to 20 µg of luciferase per limb, which is similar to that achieved using the intravascular/naked DNA approach. Although it is difficult to compare expression levels using different amounts of different vectors, it is still noteworthy that expression levels from the use of naked pDNA were similar to that from rAAV. We have also injected adenoviral vectors intra arterially and have observed luciferase levels much less than that obtained with naked pDNA. These preliminary results suggest that expression levels from the use of intravascular/naked pDNA technique are close to the levels that can be achieved from viral vectors.

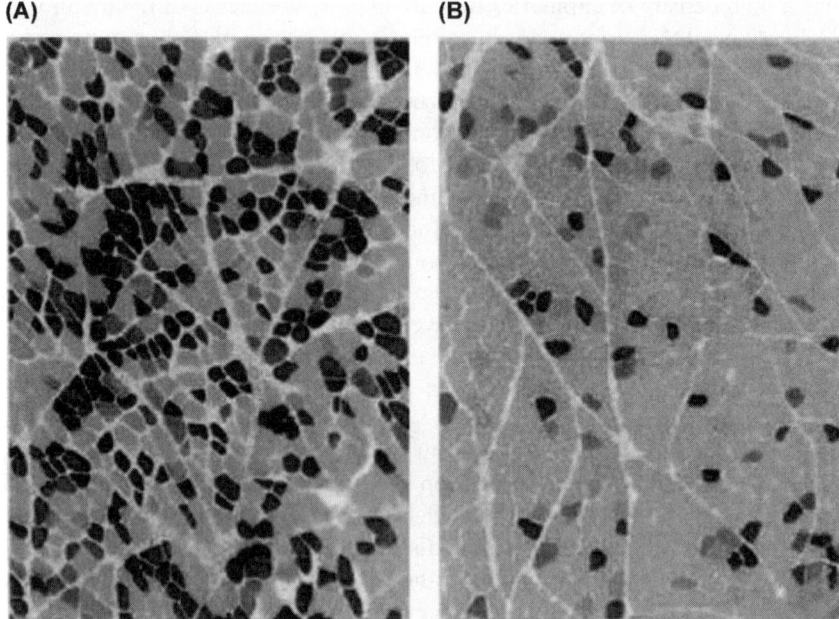

Figure 2 Photomicrographs of rhesus monkey muscle sections histochemically stained for β-galactosidase expression. (**A**) A muscle (pronator teres) with a high level of expression; (**B**) a muscle (abductor pollicis longus) with an average level of expression. The muscles were taken from limbs injected intra-arterially with a plasmid DNA solution containing 100 μg/mL of pCMV-LacZ (a pDNA vector expressing β-galactosidase under transcriptional control of the cytomegalovirus promoter). *Source*: From Ref. 26.

Effect of Plasmid DNA Size on Expression

The effect of plasmid size on the efficiency of luciferase expression was determined because plasmid expression vectors with the full-length dystrophin construct would be larger than most other plasmid vectors (Fig. 3) (46).

Table 1 Luciferase Expression (μg/Muscle Group) in Rat Leg Muscle Injected with 10^{12} Particles of rAAV2 Vectors Expressing Luciferase Using the Increased-Pressure Intravascular Injection Procedure

Time postinjection (wk)	Mean luciferase (μg/total leg)	Luciferase range	n
2	6.3	1.8–13.9	4
4	17.4	8.1–26.4	2
8	10.3	9.4–11.3	2

Abbreviation: rAAV2, recombinant adeno-associated viral vector type 2.

Stuffer DNA of different sizes from lambda phage was inserted 3' to the polyadenylation site of pCILuc (a pDNA vector expressing luciferase under transcriptional control of the cytomegalovirus promoter) to create luciferase expression vectors of increasing sizes. The same number (moles) of pDNA molecules was injected for each expression vector into the tail vein or the saphenous vein of ICR mice. Liver and muscle tissues were analyzed for luciferase expression one week after injection. Using tail vein injections, which deliver DNA mostly to liver, we found that vector size per se or the lambda DNA sequences did not affect liver luciferase expression (Fig. 3A). However, on intravascular delivery of pDNA to muscle, there appeared to be a small effect in which the 17.1 kb pDNA expressed approximately two-fold less in muscle tissues than the 5.7 kb pDNA (Fig. 3A). A similar size effect was seen in *mdx* mice as well (data not shown). In addition, a similar effect of pDNA size on expression efficiency was also observed when the pDNA was injected directly into mouse muscle (intramuscular) or transfected into HeLa cells in vitro (Fig. 3B and C).

One possible reason for the different pDNA size effects in liver and muscle is that the vascular system of liver has large fenestrae that muscle

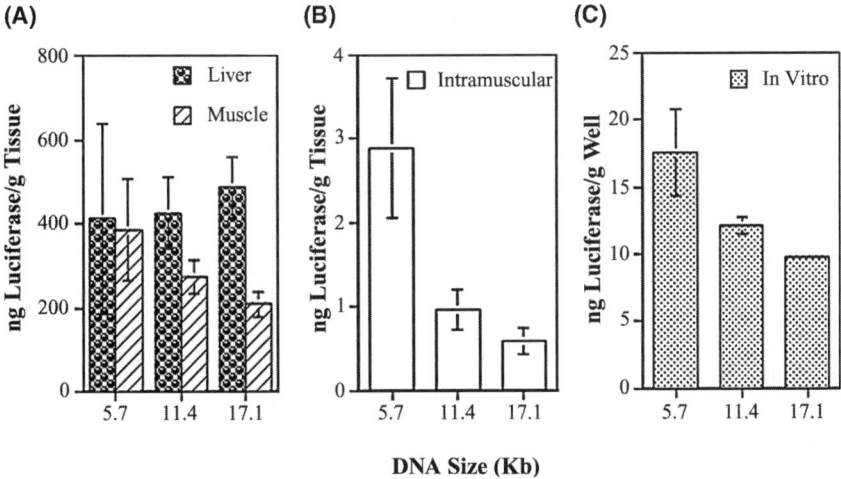

Figure 3 Mean expression of luciferase following the intravascular delivery of three plasmids of different sizes to either liver or muscle in ICR mice (**A**), directly injected into quadriceps muscles of C57 mice (**B**), or transfected using *Trans*IT®-LT1 transfection reagent (Mirus Bio Corp., Madison, WI, U.S.) into HeLa cells in vitro (**C**). The plasmids have the same expression cassette as pCILuc. 40 µg of pCILuc (5.7 kb in size), 80 µg of pCILuc-11.4, and 120 µg of pCILuc-17.1 were injected to deliver the same molar amount of each pDNA. Liver and HeLa cell expression were analyzed one day after injection, while the muscles were analyzed one week afterward. $n = 3$ to 5 for each data point; T bars indicate standard error. *Source*: From Ref. 46.

does not. The lack of fenestrae in the muscle vasculature could impede extravasation of the larger pDNA. However, the larger pDNA expressed less luciferase even after direct intramuscular injection (Fig. 3B) (17). This suggests that extravascular elements such as the extracellular matrix or intracellular barriers in myofibers impede delivery of large pDNA. The effect of pDNA size on transfection into cultured cells suggests the presence of an intracellular hurdle (Fig. 3C). Similarly, an effect of plasmid size on expression following electrotransfer into skeletal muscle or cationic lipid–mediated transfection of cultured cells has been observed previously (37,48–50).

Safety of the Intravascular Procedure for Muscle

Although the transfection efficiencies obtained in these intravascular studies were unprecedented for a nonviral vector, concerns about clinical viability remain as a consequence of the use of a tourniquet, the large volumes injected, the high rates of injection, and the use of an artery as the route of administration. The short time required for occluding blood flow to skeletal muscle should be well tolerated in a human clinical setting as ischemia can be tolerated by muscles for two to three hours. In fact, a common anesthetic procedure for distal limb surgery (e.g., carpal tunnel repair) involves the placement of a tourniquet to block both venous and arterial blood flow and the intravenous administration of a local anesthetic (e.g., lidocaine) distal to the tourniquet. Surgery in humans can be performed for several hours using these anesthetic procedures. Similarly, histologic analyses of the muscles from rats, dogs, and rhesus monkeys in our experiments indicated that the ischemia did not cause myofiber damage. However, transient increases in serum creatine kinase levels up to several thousand units per liter of blood were observed, which resolved within a few days. These levels are within the range observed after exercising (51). Histologic analysis and radiographic studies also did not reveal any damage to the limb blood vessels.

Postulated Mechanisms of Naked DNA Transport and Uptake

Blood vessels have a large number of small pores (approximately 4 nm diameter) and only few large pores (approximately 20–30 nm) (52). The gyration radius for pDNA molecules is in the order of approximately 100 nm (53). Yet, supercoiled pDNA in plectonemic form has a super helix dimension of approximately 10 nm (54). This implies that pDNA is capable of crossing microvascular walls by stringing through the large pores. As elevated pressure appears to be very important in the transfection of liver and skeletal muscle, we hypothesize that this enhances pDNA transfer by opening the endothelial barrier. Raising the intravascular hydrostatic pressure transiently increases water flow through the large pores and thereby forces the extravasation of pDNA.

Our unpublished studies using fluorescent-labeled DNA indicate that increased intravascular pressure is required for extravasation of the delivered pDNA. Based on cell localization and competition experiments, we hypothesize that muscle and liver cells have an intrinsic ability to take up naked pDNA by an active process. The injection process may activate this intrinsic process.

mdx MOUSE STUDIES

Dystrophin Expression in *mdx* Mice

Two different, full-length mDys expression vectors were constructed: using a desmin control region (DCR), pDCR-mDys linked to the desmin enhancer/promoter (26.6 kb), and pCMV-mDys using the CMV promoter (21.8 kb). The hind limbs of either the mdx^{4cv} or the mdx^{5cv} mice were injected intra-arterially with approximately 300 µg of these plasmid constructs and the muscles were analyzed at various times afterward (Fig. 4; only data with DCR shown). Low- and high-power views are shown from sections with relatively high percentages of dystrophin-positive myofibers (Fig. 4). Quantitative analyses indicated that the procedure enabled up to 5% of entire muscle groups and limbs to be positive for dystrophin (Fig. 5). The DCR promoter construct yielded similar percentages of positive cells as the CMV promoter construct. The percentage of dystrophin-positive cells was similar in the mdx^{4cv} and mdx^{5cv} strains.

Given the phenomenon of rare revertant dystrophin-positive myofibers in *mdx* muscle, two controls were used. In the mice injected with the dystrophin constructs, the contralateral muscle was not injected. The average percentage of dystrophin-positive myofibers in these noninjected muscles was around 0.2%. The percentage of dystrophin-positive cells was significantly greater in the experimental muscles injected with dystrophin constructs than in the noninjected control muscles (p values < 0.005). The number of revertants in control muscles did not increase over the time of this study. This is consistent with our previous observation that the mdx^{4cv} and mdx^{5cv} strains have far fewer revertants than other *mdx* strains (55). As a second control, hind limbs were injected with pCILuc in order to determine whether the injection process itself can lead to an increased number of revertants. Quantitative analyses indicated that these pCILuc-injected muscles had similar numbers of dystrophin-positive (revertant) fibers as the uninjected control muscles.

Stable mDys Expression in *mdx* Mice

The time course of dystrophin expression was also determined. In the mdx^{4cv} strain, the percentage of dystrophin-positive cells was stable for at least six months following injection with the pDCR-mDys construct and for at least

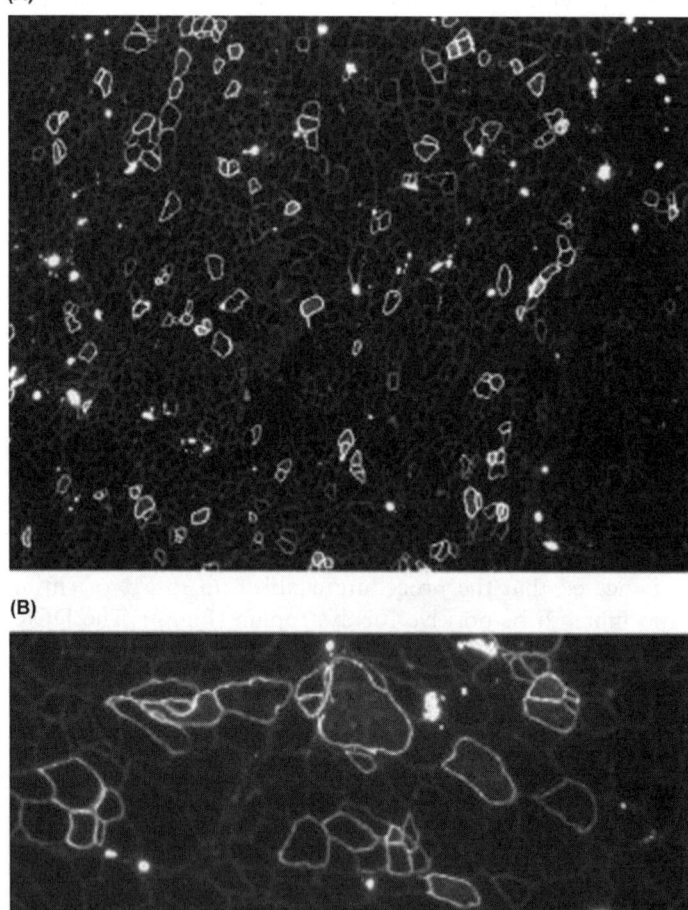

Figure 4 Immunohistochemical staining for mDys expression in mdx^{4cv} mouse muscle one month after intra-arterial injection of approximately 300 µg of pDCR-mDys. (**A**) Images were captured with a 4× objective and (**B**) 10× objective. *Abbreviations*: mDys, mouse dystrophin; pDCR, plasmid expression vector with desmin control region. *Source*: From Ref. 46.

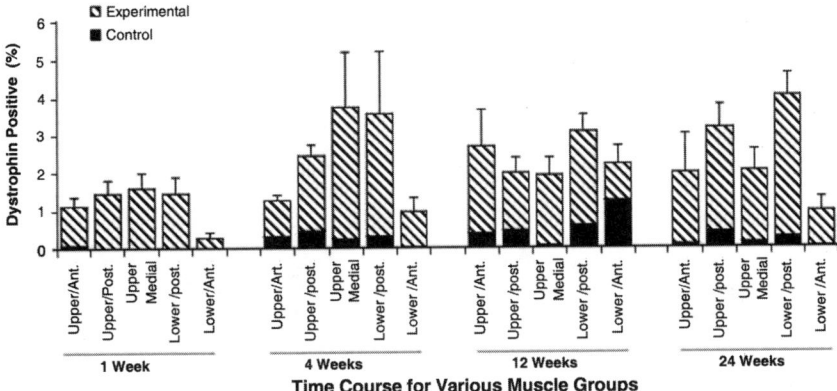

Figure 5 Mean percentage of dystrophin-positive cells in the indicated hind limb muscle groups at various times after intra-arterial injection of approximately 300 μg of pDCR-mDys into mdx^{4cv} mice. The mice were three to six months in age at the time of injection. The black areas indicate the number of dystrophin-positive fibers (revertants) in the control muscles (from the contralateral, uninjected muscles). $n = $ 3 to 5 for each data point; T bars indicate standard error. *Abbreviations*: mDys, mouse dystrophin; pDCR, plasmid expression vector with desmin control region. *Source*: From Ref. 46.

three months following injection with the pCMV-mDys construct (Fig. 5; only data with DCR shown). Similar results were obtained in the mdx^{5cv} strain.

Stable expression of mDys in *mdx* mice requires that a number of molecular and cellular processes must take place (Table 2). One requirement is that the pDNA persists in the postmitotic nuclei of myofibers. Our previous studies have shown that long-term foreign gene expression from naked pDNA is possible even without chromosome integration, if the target cell is postmitotic (as in muscle) or slowly mitotic (as in hepatocytes). pDNA is lost from nuclei that divide (56). In nonmitotic nuclei, the pDNA is treated basically like chromosomal DNA, but remains episomal, does not replicate, and is not expunged from an intact nucleus (Fig. 6).

Table 2 Requirements for Stable pDNA-Mediated Dystrophin Expression in Dystrophic Muscle

---
pDNA persistence in postmitotic nuclei of myofibers
    Transcription from pDNA promoters is not shut down in muscle
    Dystrophin expression prevents muscle degeneration
    Absence of a cellular immune response against myofibers expressing exogenous dystrophin

---

Abbreviation: pDNA, plasmid DNA.

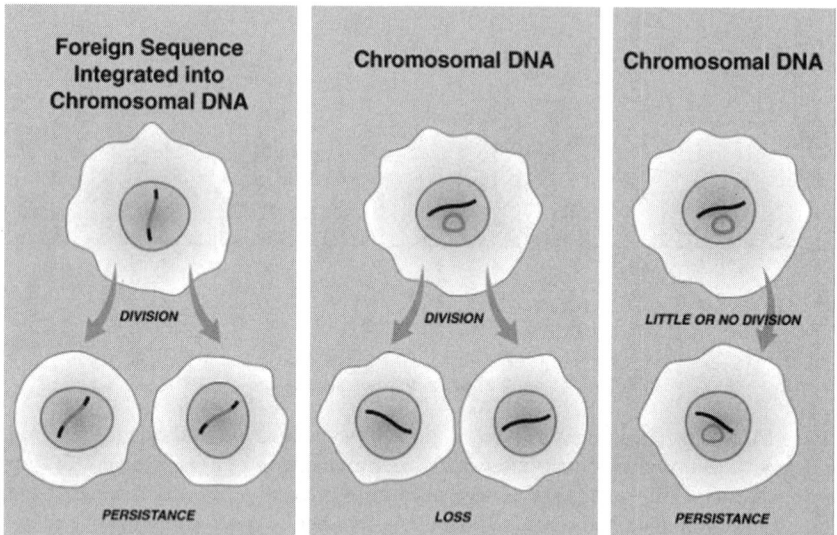

Figure 6 Possible scenarios for the fate of transfected DNA and the effect of cell division on its persistence. (*Left panel*) Transfected DNA inserts into chromosomal DNA and persists after cell division. (*Middle panel*) Transfected DNA remains extrachromosomal and is lost upon cell division. (*Right panel*) Transfected DNA remains extrachromosomal and persists if there is no (or little) cell division.

Another requirement for stable expression is that there be no shutdown of promoters within pDNA. As this is a phenomenon that occurs after the intravascular delivery of pDNA to the liver, it does not appear to occur in muscle (26,47,57).

The observed stable expression of dystrophin in *mdx* mice also requires that dystrophin expression prevents *mdx* myofibers from degenerating. Naked pDNA only transfects myofibers and not satellite cells (58). Previously, we had shown that low levels of luciferase could be stably expressed after direct intramuscular injection in normal mice, but not in *mdx* mice (17). A plasmid construct that expressed both luciferase and dystrophin enabled persistent luciferase expression in *mdx* muscle (17). This suggested that pDNA dystrophin expression prevented the muscle degeneration that occurs in adult *mdx* mice. In addition, pDNA delivery leads to dystrophin expression within a limited region of the myofibers due to the effect of nuclear domains and the fact that pDNA only enters a few of the myonuclei. Thus, this limited dystrophin expression within one myofiber is sufficient to prevent loss of myofiber nuclei.

Finally, stable expression requires that foreign mDys expression within *mdx* muscle does not lead to a cellular immune response that destroys the dystrophin-expressing myofibers (46). In the *mdx* mice injected intra-arterially with either pCMV-mDys or pDCR-mDys, the presence of a cellular immune response was analyzed by costaining the muscle sections for dystrophin-positive myofibers and either CD4- or CD8-positive cells. None of the muscles at one, three, or six months after injection had an increased number of such T cells around dystrophin-positive myofibers or other myofibers. In addition, hematoxylin/eosin histologic analysis revealed that none of the muscles had evidence of increased myofiber damage. Without a cellular immune response, it is unlikely that a cytotoxic immune response would kill the dystrophin-expressing myofibers.

However, more than half the mice had detectable antimouse dystrophin antibodies by one month. The incidence of a humoral response was similar in both *mdx* strains and did not correlate with the amount of dystrophin expression. It is of interest that the elicitation of antibodies against mDys did not lead to loss of dystrophin expression. Most likely, the intracellular location of dystrophin makes it inaccessible to antibody-mediated immune effects. The occurrence of persistent dystrophin expression despite the presence of antidystrophin antibodies has also been observed following histocompatible myoblast transplantation in immunocompetent *mdx* mice (59,60).

Previous studies have shown that the direct intramuscular injection of pDNAs expressing full-length human dystrophin led to the development of antihuman dystrophin antibodies and clustering of CD8-positive cells around dystrophin-positive myofibers (61,62). However, neither a humoral nor a cellular response was detected following multiple injections of constructs expressing mini- or full-length mDys from the muscle-specific muscle creatine kinase (MCK) promoter (62). Accordingly, these studies reported stable expression of mDys in immunocompetent *mdx* mice. Most likely antidystrophin antibodies were observed in our study because the intravascular procedure led to higher levels of dystrophin. Our results also differed from the previous studies in other ways. We used the mdx^{4cv} and mdx^{5cv} mice, whereas the previous study used the original *mdx* strain. The mdx^{4cv} and mdx^{5cv} mice may be more immune responsive to foreign dystrophin expression because they express less of the truncated, nonmuscle dystrophin isoforms and have fewer revertant fibers (55,63).

In our *mdx* mouse study, stable dystrophin expression was observed with constructs containing either the CMV or DCR promoter. Previously, we found that the muscle-specific MCK promoter enabled more prolonged luciferase expression than the CMV promoter after intra-arterial pDNA delivery to immunosuppressed rats (26). After the direct intramuscular injection of pDNA, persistent expression of low levels of luciferase is possible with all types of promoters (64). Yet, with the high levels of expression achieved after intravascular delivery of pDNA, long-term expression of reporter genes such as luciferase required that the animal be immunosuppressed (26). Presumably, the higher levels of expression lead to a cellular immune response against the cells expressing the transfected gene. If a muscle-specific promoter was used, long-term expression only required immunosuppression to be transiently employed around the time of pDNA administration (26). Similar effects caused by transient immunosuppression or muscle-specific promoters on the proclivity of an immune response have also been observed on using viral vectors (65–67). The use of muscle-specific promoters may be especially important in reducing the immune response in muscle degeneration that accompanies muscle dystrophy (67,68).

The relevance of immune studies in mice to the human situation has been debated in the context of vaccine development and other gene therapies for single gene defects such as hemophilia (69,70). Interestingly, a recent study used a human leukocyte antigen (HLA) class I humanized mouse model to explore the immune effects of human dystrophin expression (71). The mouse model is H-2 negative and transgenically expresses the HLA-A*0201 class I allele that is present in 50% of the Caucasian population. Following injection of a naked pDNA expressing full-length human dystrophin from the CMV promoter into notexin-treated muscles of the mouse model, $CD8^+$ T cells were induced to recognize a specific dystrophin epitope present in dystrophin's spectrin-like repeat 9 domain. This human epitope is not present in either mDys or utrophin. Perhaps most importantly, no cellular response against shared epitopes in Becker-like dystrophins, short dystrophin isoforms, or utrophin were induced, suggesting that an "auto-immune" process is unlikely to be initiated.

FUTURE PROSPECTS

While our studies to date suggest that the intravascular approach is promising, a variety of additional studies are in progress to determine if and how this approach could be used in the clinic. For one, we are optimizing the basic delivery approach to reduce the required volumes and injection speeds to increase the safety of the approach. Recently, we have discovered that naked pDNA can be delivered efficiently to limb muscles using an intravenous route of administration (72).

In addition, we are working to extend the intravascular approach to deliver genes to the diaphragm and respiratory muscles to prevent the loss of respiratory function. A previous study reported expression of full-length mDys in the diaphragm muscle of *mdx* mice after a naked pDNA expression vector was injected under low pressure into the tail vein and the inferior vena cava was briefly clamped (73). The other set of target muscles would include the back muscles to prevent the scoliosis and kyphosis that typically accompany muscular dystrophy. The intravascular approach can express naked pDNAs in cardiac myocytes but the efficiency is much lower than that for skeletal muscle. It could be used to treat myocardial ischemia but it is unlikely to be effective in the treatment of intrinsic cardiac muscle disorders. We have initiated a series of studies in the canine Duchenne model in golden retrievers, using pDNAs that express the canine dystrophin gene. Our preliminary results indicate that we can express dystrophin in at least 10% of the myofibers in some muscle groups.

In summary, the intravascular delivery of naked pDNA is an attractive approach for treating patients with DMD. Within several years, clinical studies should be initiated to determine its utility in preventing muscular dystrophy in limbs.

REFERENCES

1. Davies KE. Challenges in Duchenne muscular dystrophy. Neuromuscul Disord 1997; 7:482–486.
2. Biggar DW, Klamut HJ, et al. Duchenne muscular dystrophy: current knowledge, treatment, and future prospects. Clin Orthop Relat Res 2002; 401:88–106.
3. van Ommen GJ, Scheuerbrandt G. Neonatal screening for muscular dystrophy. Consensus recommendation of the 14th workshop sponsored by the European Neuromuscular Center (ENMC). Neuromuscul Disord 1993; 3(3):231–239.
4. Parsons EP, Clarke AJ, et al. Newborn screening for Duchenne muscular dystrophy: a psychosocial study. Arch Dis Child Fetal Neonatal Ed 2002; 86(2):F91–F95.
5. Parsons EP, Bradley DM, et al. Newborn screening for Duchenne muscular dystrophy [comment]. Arch Dis Child 2003; 88(1):91–92.
6. Cox GA, Cole NM, et al. Overexpression of dystrophin in transgenic mdx mice eliminates dystrophic symptoms without toxicity. Nature 1993; 364(6439):725–729.
7. Lee CC, Pons F, et al. Mdx trangenic mouse: restoration of recombinant dystrophin to the dystrophic muscle. Hum Gene Ther 1993; 4:273–281.
8. Phelps SF, Hauser MA, et al. Expression of full-length and truncated dystrophin mini-genes in transgenic mdx mice. Hum Mol Genet 1995; 4(8):1251–1258.
9. Wells DJ, Wells KE, et al. Expression of human full-length and minidystrophin in transgenic mdx mice: implications for gene therapy of Duchenne muscular dystrophy. Hum Mol Genet 1995; 4:1245–1250.
10. Ahmad A, Brinson M, et al. Mdx mice inducibly expressing dystrophin provide insights into the potential of gene therapy for Duchenne muscular dystrophy. Hum Mol Genet 2000; 9:2507–2515.
11. Wang B, Li J, et al. Adeno-associated virus vector carrying human minidystrophin genes effectively ameliorates muscular dystrophy in mdx mouse model. Proc Natl Acad Sci USA 2000; 97:13714–13719.
12. Dickson G, Roberts ML, et al. Recombinant micro-genes and dystrophin viral vectors. Neuromuscul Disord 2002; 12:S40–S44.
13. Scott JM, Li S, et al. Viral vectors for gene transfer for micro-, mini-, or full-length dystrophin. Neuromuscul Disord 2002; 12:S23–S29.
14. Watchko J, O'Day T, et al. Adeno-associated virus vector-mediated minidystrophin gene therapy improves dystrophic muscle contractile function in mdx mice. Hum Gene Ther 2002; 13:1451–1460.
15. Wells DJ, Wells KE. Gene transfer studies in animals: what do they really tell us about the prospects for gene therapy in DMD. Neuromuscul Disord 2002; 12:S11–S22.

16. Acsadi G, Dickson G, et al. Human dystrophin expression in mdx mice after intramuscular injection of DNA constructs. Nature 1991; 352(6338):815–818.
17. Danko I, Fritz J, et al. Dystrophin expression improves myofiber survival in *mdx* muscle following intramuscular plasmid DNA injection. Hum Mol Genet 1993; 2:2055–2061.
18. Decrouy A, Renaud JM, Davis HL, et al. Mini-dystrophin gene transfer in mdx diaphragm muscle fibers increases sarcolemmal stability. Gene Ther 1997; 4:401–408.
19. Hauser MA, Chamberlain JS. Progress towards gene therapy for Duchenne muscular dystrophy. J Endocrinol 1996; 149(3):373–378.
20. Gussoni E, Blau HM, et al. The fate of individual myoblasts after transplantation into muscles of DMD patients. Nat Med 1997; 3(9):970–977.
21. Dudley R, Lu Y, et al. Sustained improvement of muscle function one year after full-length dystrophin gene transfer into mdx mice by a gutted helper-dependent adenoviral vector. Hum Gene Ther 2004; 15:145–156.
22. Dunant P, Iarochelle N, et al. Promoter ameliorates muscular dystrophy in fast, but not in slow muscles of transgenic mdx mice. Mol Ther 2003; 8:80–89.
23. Lu QL, Bou-Gharios G, et al. Non-viral gene delivery in skeletal muscle: a protein factory. Gene Ther 10:131–142.
24. Goula D, Benoist C, et al. Polyethylenimine-based intravenous delivery of transgenes to mouse lung. Gene Ther 1998; 5(9):1291–1295.
25. Trubeskoy VS, Wong SC, et al. Recharging cationic DNA complexes with highly charged polyanions for in vitro and in vivo gene delivery. Gene Ther 2003; 10:261–271.
26. Zhang G, Budker V, et al. Efficient expression of naked DNA delivered intraarterially to limb muscles of nonhuman primates. Hum Gene Ther 2001; 12:427–438.
27. Jiao S, Williams P, et al. Direct gene transfer into nonhuman primate myofibers in vivo. Hum Gene Ther 1992; 3(1):21–33.
28. Zhang G, Vargo D, et al. Expression of naked plasmid DNA injected into the afferent and efferent vessels of rodent and dog livers. Hum Gene Ther 1997; 8(15):1763–1772.
29. Wolff JA, Malone RW, et al. Direct gene transfer into mouse muscle in vivo. Science 1990; 247(4949 Pt 1):1465–1468.
30. Lin H, Parmacek MS, et al. Expression of recombinant genes in myocardium in vivo after direct injection of DNA. Circulation 1990; 82(6):2217–2221.
31. Acsadi G, Jiao S, et al. Direct gene transfer and expression into rat heart in vivo. New Biol 1991; 3(1):71–81.
32. Buttrick PM, Kass A, et al. Behavior of genes directly injected into the rat heart in vivo. Circ Res 1992; 70(1):193–198.
33. Gal D, Weir L, et al. Direct myocardial transfection in two animal models. Evaluation of parameters affecting gene expression and percutaneous gene delivery. Lab Invest 1993; 68(1):18–25.
34. Somiari S, Glasspool-Malone J, et al. Theory and in vivo application of electroporative gene delivery. Mol Ther 2000; 2(3):178–187.
35. Hartikka J, Sukhu L, et al. Electroporation-facilitated delivery of plasmid DNA in skeletal muscle: plasmid dependence of muscle damage and effect of poloxamer 188. Mol Ther 2001; 4(5):407–415.

36. Terada Y, Tanaka H, et al. Efficient and ligand-dependent regulated erythropoietin production by naked dna injection and in vivo electroporation. Am J Kidney Dis 2001; 38(4 suppl 1):S50–S53.
37. Vilquin JT, Kennel PF, et al. Electrotransfer of naked DNA in the skeletal muscles of animal models of muscular dystrophies. Gene Ther 2001; 8(14):1097–1107.
38. Jiang J, Yamato E, et al. Intravenous delivery of naked plasmid DNA for in vivo cytokine expression. Biochem Biophys Res Commun 2001; 289(5):1088–1092.
39. Zhang G, Budker V, et al. Surgical procedures for intravascular delivery of plasmid DNA to organs. Meth Enzymol 2002; 346:125–133.
40. Budker V, Zhang G, et al. Naked DNA delivered intraportally expresses efficiently in hepatocytes. Gene Ther 1996; 3(7):593–598.
41. Zhang G, Budker V, et al. High levels of foreign gene expression in hepatocytes after tail vein injections of naked plasmid DNA. Hum Gene Ther 1999; 10(10):1735–1737.
42. Liu F, Song Y, Liu D. Hydrodynamics-based transfection in animals by systemic administration of plasmid DNA. Gene Ther 1999; 6:1258–1266.
43. Lewis DL, Hagstrom JE, Loomis AG, Wolff JA, Herweijer H. Efficient delivery of siRNA for inhibition of gene expression in postnatal mice. Nat Genet 2002; 32:107–108.
44. McCaffrey AP, Meuse L, Pham TT, Conklin DS, Hannon GJ, Kay MA. RNA interference in adult mice. Nature 2002; 418:38–39.
45. Budker V, Zhang G, et al. The efficient expression of intravascularly delivered DNA in rat muscle. Gene Ther 1998; 5(2):272–276.
46. Zhang G, Ludtke JJ, Thioudellet C, et al. Intraarterial delivery of naked plasmid DNA expressing full-length mouse dystrophin in the mdx mouse model for Duchenne muscular dystrophy. Hum Gene Ther 2004; 15(8):770–782.
47. Herweijer H, Zhang G, et al. Time course of gene expression after plasmid DNA gene transfer to the liver. J Gene Med 2001; 3(3):280–291.
48. Kreiss P, Cameron B, et al. Plasmid DNA size does not affect the physicochemical properties of lipoplexes but modulates gene transfer efficiency. Nucl Acids Res 1999; 27:3792–3798.
49. Campeau P, Chapdelaine P, et al. Transfection of large plasmids in primary human myoblasts. Gene Ther 2001; 8:1387–1394.
50. Kamiya H, Yamazaki J, et al. Size and topology of exogenous DNA as determinant factors of transgene transcription in mammalian cells. Gene Ther 2002; 9:1500–1507.
51. Nosaka K, Clarkson PM. Variability in serum creatine kinase response after eccentric exercise of the elbow flexors. Int J Sports Med 1996; 17(2):120–127.
52. Rippe B, Haraldsson B. Transport of macromolecules across microvascular walls: the two-pore theory. Physiol Rev 1994; 74(1):163–219.
53. Fisherman DM, Patterson GD. Light scattering studies of super coiled and nicked DNA. Biopolymers 1996; 38:535–552.
54. Rybenkov VV, Vologodskii AV, et al. The effect of ionic conditions on the conformations of super coiled DNA. 1. Sedimentation analysis. J Mol Biol 1997; 267(2):299–311.
55. Danko I, Chapman V, et al. The frequency of revertants in mdx mouse genetic models for Duchenne muscular dystrophy. Ped Res 1992; 32:128–131.

56. Ludtke JJ, Sebestyen MG, et al. The effect of cell division on the cellular dynamics of microinjected DNA and dextran. Mol Ther 2002; 5(5 Pt 1):579–588.
57. Herweijer H, Wolff JA. Progress and prospects: naked DNA gene transfer and therapy. Gene Ther 2003; 10(6):453–458.
58. Wolff J, Dowty M, et al. Expression of naked plasmids by cultured myotubes and entry of plasmids into T tubules and caveolae of mammalian skeletal muscle. J Cell Sci 1992; 103:1249–1259.
59. Bittner RE, Shorny S, et al. Serum antibodies to the deleted dystrophin sequence after cardiac transplantation in a patient with Becker's muscular dystrophy. New Engl J Med 1995; 333:732–733.
60. Vilquin J-T, Wagner E, et al. Successful histocompatible myoblast transplantation in dystrophin-deficient mdx mouse despite the production of antibodies against dystrophin. J Cell Biol 1995; 131:975–988.
61. Braun S, Thioudellet C, et al. Immune rejection of human dystrophin following intramuscular injections of naked DNA in mdx mice. Gene Ther 2000; 7(17):1447–1457.
62. Ferrer A, Wells KE, et al. Immune responses to dystrophin: implications for gene therapy of Duchenne muscular dystrophy. Gene Ther 2000; 7:1439–1446.
63. Im WB, Phelps SF, et al. Differential expression of dystrophin isoforms in strains of mdx mice with different mutations. Hum Mol Genet 1996; 5(8): 1149–1153.
64. Wolff JA, Ludtke JJ, et al. Long-term persistence of plasmid DNA and foreign gene expression in mouse muscle. Hum Mol Genet 1992; 1(6):363–369.
65. Lochmuller H, Petrof BJ, et al. Transient immunosuppression by FK506 permits a sustained high-level dystrophin expression after adenovirus-mediated dystrophin minigene transfer to skeletal muscles of adult dystrophic (mdx) mice. Gene Ther 1996; 3(8):706–716.
66. Jooss K, Turka LA, et al. Blunting of immune responses to adenoviral vectors in mouse liver and lung with CTLA4Ig. Gene Ther 1998; 5(3):309–319.
67. Cordier L, Gao GP, et al. Muscle-specific promoters may be necessary for adeno-associated virus-mediated gene transfer in the treatment of muscular dystrophies. Hum Gene Ther 2001; 12(2):205–215.
68. Hartigan-O'Connor D, Kirk CJ, et al. Immune evasion by muscle-specific gene expression in dystrophic muscle. Mol Ther 2001; 4:525–533.
69. Hein WR, Griebel PJ. A road less traveled: large animal models in immunological research. Nat Rev Immunol 2002; 3:79–84.
70. Walsh CE. Gene therapy progress and prospects: gene therapy for the hemophilia's. Gene Ther 2003; 10:999–1003.
71. Ginhoux F, Doucet C, et al. Identification of an HLA-A*0201-restricted epitopic peptide from human dystrophin; Application in Duchenne muscular dystrophy gene therapy. Mol Ther 2003; 8:274–283.
72. Hagstrom JE, Hegge J, et al. A facile non-viral method for delivering genes and siRNA to skeletal muscle of mammalian limbs. Mol Ther 2004; 10:386–398.
73. Liu F, Nishikawa M, et al. Transfer of full-length Dmd to the diaphragm muscle of Dmd(mdx/mdx) mice through systemic administration of plasmid DNA. Mol Ther 2001; 4(1):45–51.

17

Adenoviral-Mediated Gene Therapy

Laura Goldberg and Paula R. Clemens
*Department of Neurology,
University of Pittsburgh, Pittsburgh,
Pennsylvania, U.S.A.*

INTRODUCTION

Adenoviruses (Ad) have been the subject of intense study since their isolation in the early 1950s (1). Over the past five decades, this study has greatly contributed to our understanding of many facets of Ad biology including fundamental aspects of the Ad life cycle, the dynamic interplay between Ad infection and the host immune response, and clinical disease associated with Ad infection. The discovery of the ability of Ad to deliver large amounts of DNA to the nucleus of an infected cell in a remarkably efficient manner prompted research aimed at developing Ad vectors for use as gene delivery vehicles. Ad vectors have long been recognized as particularly well suited for gene delivery in the therapy of genetic deficiency diseases such as Duchenne muscular dystrophy (DMD), given their broad tropism, large insert capacity, and their ability to infect quiescent cells. Ongoing studies delineating the molecular details of Ad infection and the host immune response continue to promote and guide innovative strategies designed to harness Ad for successful gene delivery to muscle. The purpose of this chapter is to summarize the major advances in Ad vector development, to present the progress in Ad-mediated gene transfer to dystrophin-deficient muscle, and to discuss the key hurdles that need to be overcome before Ad vector–mediated gene therapy becomes a viable clinical therapeutic agent for the treatment of DMD.

ADENOVIRAL CAPSID STRUCTURE

There are over 50 distinct human Ad serotypes that are distinguished by type-specific neutralization studies (2). These serotypes have been classified into six subgroups (subgroups A–F) based on differential hemagglutination patterns, oncogenic potential, and DNA G+C content (2). The serotypes are associated with a variety of relatively benign clinical disease processes including respiratory disease, gastroenteritis, and epidemic conjunctivitis.

Ad are nonenveloped, regular icosahedrons with diameters ranging from 70 to 100 nm (2). The Ad capsid (Fig. 1), composed of 252 capsomeres, has 20 triangular facets with 12 vertices. Each triangular facet is comprised of 12 capsomeres called hexons. Each vertex is a capsomere called penton base. Extending out from each penton base protein is a fiber protein, which is composed of three identical polypeptide chains. The trimeric fiber protein contains a shaft domain that inserts into the penton base protein and a globular knob domain responsible for mediating cell attachment. In addition to these three capsid components, the Ad icosahedron contains several other capsid proteins including polypeptides VI, VIII, and IX that likely play a role in stabilizing the capsomeres. In addition to the capsomere proteins, there are several proteins that reside in the core of the viral particle along with the linear, double-stranded DNA. The core proteins include (*i*) a viral

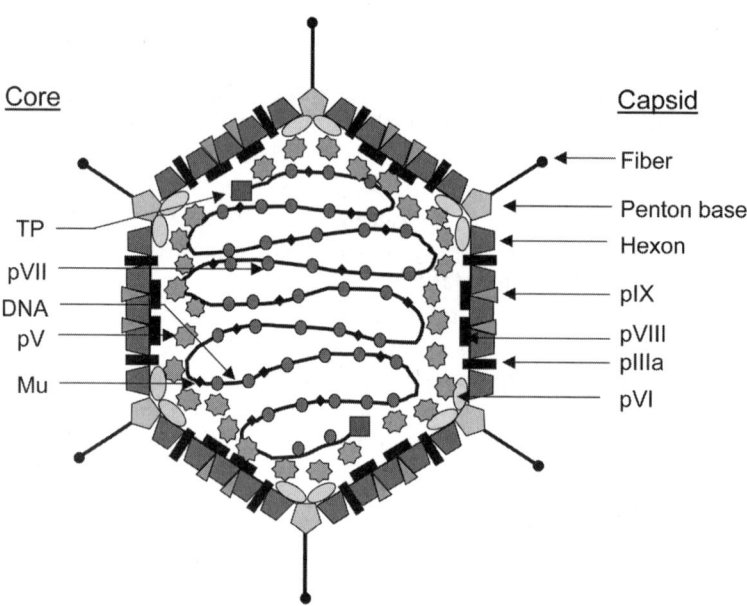

Figure 1 The Ad capsid structure. *Source*: Adapted from Ref. 48.

protease that plays a role in viral assembly and disassembly, (*ii*) polypeptide VII, which is tightly associated with the core DNA, (*iii*) mu, another DNA-associated core protein, and (*iv*) polypeptide V, which helps to link the core to the capsid. Ad DNA is covalently associated with the terminal protein and linked to the capsid via protein VI (2).

PATHWAY OF INFECTION

Tremendous progress has been made in elucidating the molecular mechanisms involved in the pathway of Ad infection responsible for the efficient delivery of Ad DNA to the nucleus of an infected cell. The first step in Ad infection is attachment of the viral particle to the cell surface (Fig. 2).

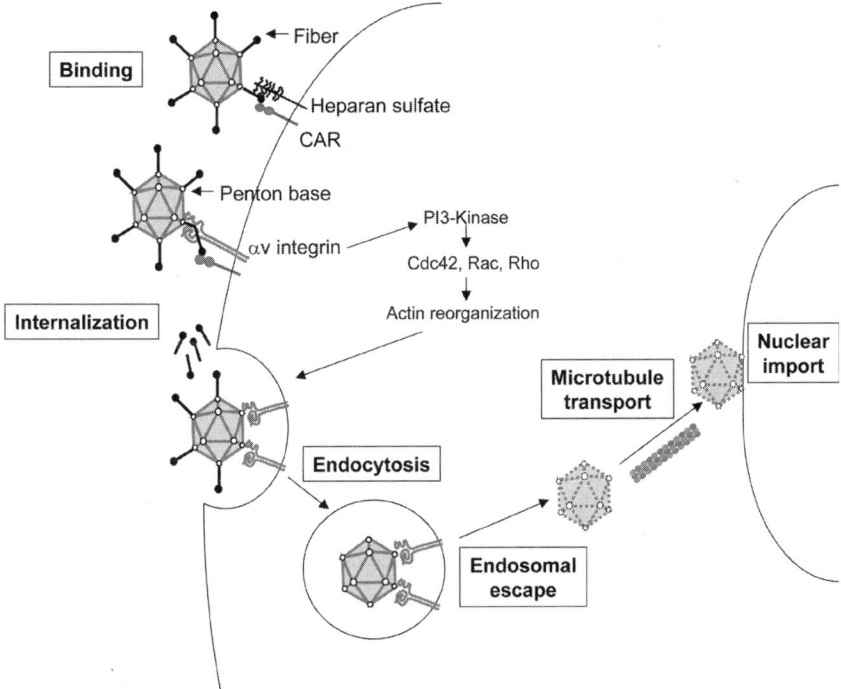

Figure 2 The pathway of Ad infection. A high-affinity interaction between Ad fiber protein and cellular CAR, and a lower-affinity interaction between Ad penton base and cell-surface $\alpha v \beta 3$- and $\alpha v \beta 5$-integrins mediate binding and internalization, respectively. Ad subsequently enters the cell in a clathrin-coated endosome, rapidly gains access to the cytoplasm, and using the microtubule cytoskeleton, trafficks to the nucleus where it engages components of the NPC to translocate the Ad DNA into the host nucleus. *Abbreviations*: Ad, adenoviruses; CAR, coxsackievirus–adenovirus receptor; NPC, nuclear pore complex.

The protruding fiber protein mediates this critical step. For most Ad subgroups (A, C, E, and F), the distal knob domain of the fiber protein mediates attachment by binding with high affinity to the coxsackievirus–adenovirus receptor (CAR) on the cell surface (3–5). CAR is a 46 kDa member of the immunoglobulin (Ig) family and has two Ig-like domains, a single-pass transmembrane domain and a cytoplasmic domain (4). Several research groups have shown that CAR is able to mediate Ad infection even in the absence of its cytoplasmic domain, suggesting that it primarily serves as a docking site for Ad attachment to the cell surface (6–8). It has recently been shown that CAR is a component of tight junctions located at the basolateral surface of epithelium (9). CAR is expressed in a wide variety of tissues, with high levels in liver, kidney, and heart, and lower levels in spleen and skeletal muscle (10). The widespread expression of CAR likely contributes to the wide array of cell types susceptible to Ad infection. Alternative binding receptors, including the major histocompatibility complex (MHC) class I $\alpha 2$ domain, sialic acid (for Ad serotype 37), $\alpha m\beta 2$ integrins, and heparin sulfates have been implicated in Ad infection of various cell types (11–19).

CAR expression is relatively low in mature muscle, and it has been shown that CAR overexpression in muscle cells increases their susceptibility to Ad infection, indicating that Ad infection is greatly facilitated by the presence of a highly prevalent CAR pathway (4,20,21). However, in the natural setting of relatively low CAR expression, it remains unclear what role CAR actually plays in Ad infection of muscle tissue in vivo. Indeed, Einfeld et al. (22) showed that an Ad vector ablated for fiber–CAR interactions transduced muscle as well as the unmodified Ad vector following intramuscular injection in adult mice, suggesting that the classical fiber–CAR interactions may not be important for Ad muscle infection. Using the same Ad vector ablated for fiber–CAR interactions, we observed similar findings in primary muscle cell culture demonstrating that the findings are, at least in part, muscle cell autonomous (Goldberg and Clemens, unpublished). Further research is required to explore the importance of CAR and the alternate binding receptors in Ad infection of muscle cells in the dystrophin-normal and -deficient settings.

Subsequent to cell binding, Ad internalization is triggered by a lower affinity interaction between the arginine–glycine–aspartic acid (RGD) motif in Ad penton base, the capsid protein located at the base of each fiber, and cell surface $\alpha v\beta 3$ and $\alpha v\beta 5$ integrins (23). Other integrins have also been implicated in the pathway of Ad infection including $\alpha v\beta 1$ and $\alpha 5\beta 1$ (24–26). Studies by Nakano et al. (27) indicate that fiber release occurs at the cell surface after CAR binding, and following penton base–αv integrin binding, the remaining Ad capsid undergoes endocytosis in clathrin-coated pits (28). Internalization, a process that requires dynamin, occurs rapidly with a $t_{1/2}$ of 2.5 minutes (29,30). Integrin clustering, caused by Ad penton base binding, activates phosphotidylinositol-3-OH kinase and a subsequent signaling cascade, including the Rho family

GTPases and p130^{CAS} (31–33). The exact mechanisms by which the signal cascade facilitates Ad internalization are unknown but they likely involve downstream effects on the actin cytoskeleton (31). Interestingly, studies showing the ability of the pentameric penton base protein to engage over four integrins suggest that the structure of the penton base maximizes the potential for integrin clustering and subsequent cell signaling (34).

Following endocytosis, the Ad particle rapidly escapes from the early endosome and gains access to the cytoplasm. Although both $\alpha v\beta 3$ and $\alpha v\beta 5$ integrins promote Ad internalization, several studies suggest that the binding of Ad penton base specifically with the $\alpha v\beta 5$ integrins mediates this unique feature of endosomal disruption (35,36). In addition, it has been proposed that this process requires low pH (29,37,38). The Ad cysteine protease (L3/p23), which is required for DNA uncoating, is activated by both the binding of penton base to cell surface integrins and the reducing environment of the endosome and cytoplasm (39,40). Once the Ad particle escapes from the endosome, additional capsid proteins dissociate including penton base proteins, pIIIa, pVIII, and pIX, and the partially uncoated Ad particle trafficks to the nucleus using the microtubule cytoskeleton and the microtubule-dependent motor protein, dynein (29,41). Ad docks at the nuclear pore complex (NPC) and utilizes the NPC machinery to translocate its DNA into the host nucleus (42,43). Many of the details of this step are yet to be determined, but studies suggest that the hexon coat protein may play a key role in DNA entry into the nucleus (44).

Following Ad entry and delivery of DNA to the nucleus, there occurs a highly regulated cascade of events that leads to DNA replication and capsid production. Ad DNA remains as an episome in the nucleus. The Ad genome is a 36 kilobase (kb), linear, double-stranded DNA that can be functionally divided into an early region and a late region flanked by

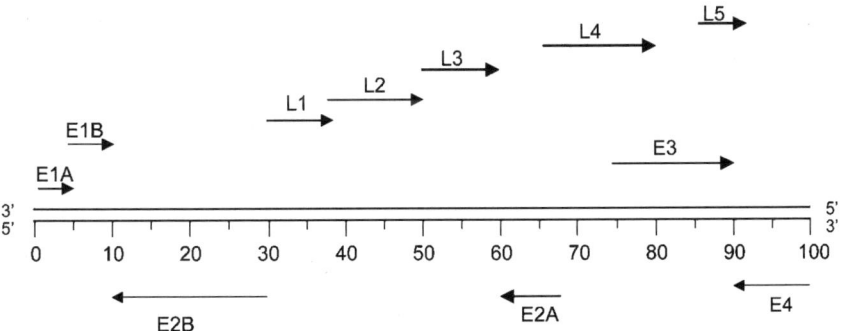

Figure 3 A transcription map of the Ad genome. The early gene cassettes are designated E and the late gene cassettes are designated L. Arrows indicate the direction of transcription.

inverted terminal repeat (ITR) sequences (Fig. 3). The left ITR contains the packaging signal that is required for packaging of the DNA into a capsid. The early region contains genes encoding proteins involved in the early steps of Ad infection and includes E1a, E1b, E2, E3, and E4 (2,45). The E1 proteins are the first ones to be expressed during infection, and they serve to activate transcription of the other viral genes and to modulate the host cell cycle. The E2 proteins are involved in Ad DNA replication and include DNA binding protein and DNA polymerase (45). The E3 proteins are involved in reducing the host antiviral immune mechanisms and the E4 region encodes proteins involved in diverse activities including viral RNA metabolism and control of host protein synthesis (46,47). The late region genes primarily encode the structural capsid components (1,48).

The stepwise process of infection starting with Ad attachment to the cell surface and culminating in Ad DNA delivery to the nucleus is extremely efficient. Studies tracking fluorescently labeled Ad particles show that over 80% of the fluorophore localizes to the nucleus within 60 minutes (29). Less than 5% of the infecting virus is lost through trafficking to the lysosome (49). The ability of Ad to transfer large amounts of DNA to the nucleus of the host cell in such an efficient manner makes it a particularly promising vector for gene therapy applications.

ADENOVIRAL VECTORS

To generate Ad vectors, Ad has been genetically engineered to capitalize on its efficient gene delivery mechanisms, while disabling its ability to generate infectious particles after in vivo use. The attractive features of Ad vector therapeutic gene delivery include infection of many cell types, relatively easy genome manipulation and vector production in the laboratory, and the efficient generation of high titer vector stocks. Ad vectors infect nondividing cells such as postmitotic muscle fibers in mature muscle. Furthermore, their capacity to carry large therapeutic DNA makes them particularly well suited for delivery of the large complementary DNA (cDNA) that encodes dystrophin.

The extensive knowledge of the Ad life cycle coupled with the detailed characterization of the Ad genome have been exploited to engineer Ad for gene therapy applications. The main goals of vector development have been to maximize safety by rendering Ad replication-incompetent, increase transgene insert capacity, and reduce the immunogenicity of the Ad vector. Incredible progress has been made in optimizing virus production protocols to facilitate these goals and has yielded three major generations of Ad vectors (Fig. 4).

First-Generation Vectors

These vectors, most often based on subgroup C Ad (Ad2 and Ad5 serotypes), are rendered replication-incompetent by deletions of the E1 region (50). The E1

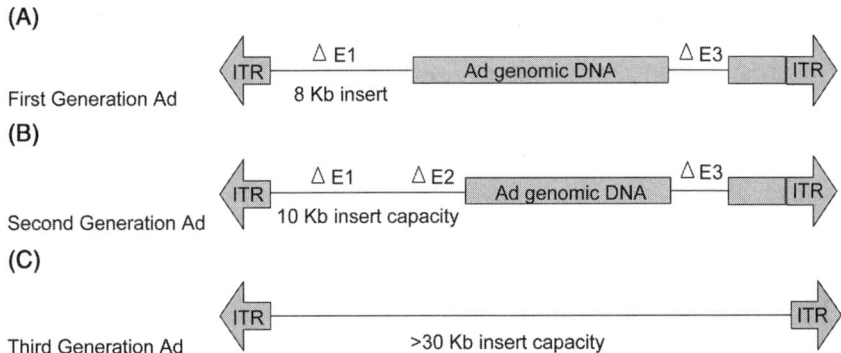

Figure 4 A schematic diagram of the three generations of Ad vectors. (**A**) A first-generation Ad vector with deletions of the E1 and E3 genes allowing an 8-kb carrying capacity. (**B**) A second-generation Ad vector with deletion of the E1 and E2 genes. Second-generation Ad vectors can accommodate approximately 10 kb of transgene DNA. (**C**) A third-generation Ad vector (also called high-capacity, gutted, or helper-dependent Ad) deleted of all viral genes allowing for approximately 30 kb of transgene carrying capacity. All generations of Ad vectors contain the packaging signal and ITRs as these elements are essential for viral production. *Abbreviations*: Ad, adenoviruses; ITR, inverted terminal repeats.

deletion interferes with the replication capability of the Ad vector because, as discussed earlier, viral transcription is dependent on E1 proteins. In the absence of E1 proteins, the cascade of viral transcription is halted, and so, the remaining early and late genes are not expressed. These vectors can be easily propagated in 293 packaging cell lines that are stably transduced with the 5′ end of the Ad genome containing the E1 region. The E1 protein produced in the packaging cell line acts in trans to activate viral transcription from the recombinant vector (51). First-generation Ad vectors also generally have a deletion of the E3 region, because E3 is nonessential for Ad vector propagation in vitro, and its deletion provides space for larger transgene inserts. The maximum packaging capability of Ad vectors is believed to be limited to approximately 2% more than the native DNA length of 36 kb.

First-generation Ad vectors have been successfully used to deliver the dystrophin gene. When a first-generation Ad vector carrying a Becker muscular dystrophy–like minidystrophin construct was delivered to muscle of newborn *mdx* mice, dystrophin expression was present in up to 50% of the myofibers of the injected muscle and persisted for up to three months (52). Another study using the same vector showed transgene expression up to six months and found a reduction in the number of muscle fibers harboring centrally-placed nuclei (a histologic feature of muscle degeneration and regeneration) and in other dystrophic histopathology in injected versus uninjected muscle (53). First-generation Ad vector–mediated delivery of the dystrophin minigene to newborn *mdx* muscle also led to reduced susceptibility to eccentric contraction–induced muscle damage, and dystrophin delivery to muscle of immunosuppressed adult *mdx* mice reduced the loss of force-generating capacity, indicating that Ad-mediated delivery of dystrophin is capable of providing functional benefit to dystrophin-deficient muscle (54,55).

Although dystrophin delivery mediated by first-generation Ad vectors can lead to improvement of the muscle cell at both the histological and the functional levels, there are two major drawbacks that limit the clinical utility of these first-generation vectors. First, they have a carrying capacity of only 8 kb of transgene coding region, which is not sufficient to accommodate the 11 kb coding region of dystrophin. Although the minidystrophin constructs with rod-domain deletions that preserve reading frame can provide significant benefit to muscle and are easily accommodated by first-generation Ad vectors, several reports suggest that full-length dystrophin is preferable (56–60). Second, there is a detrimental immune response mounted against the Ad-infected cells that significantly hinders the long-term transgene expression from these vectors (61–64). Despite the deletion of E1 and E3 genes in the first-generation Ad vector, there is likely to be leaky transcription from the viral promoters that produces Ad antigens that are able to elicit an immune response (48,61,65). Indeed, studies have shown that first-generation Ad-mediated delivery of transgenes encoding self-proteins elicited a damaging immune response, thus assuring that viral antigens themselves play a significant role in triggering the immune system (66,67). To overcome the limitations of the first-generation Ad vectors, additional deletions in Ad early genes have been made, resulting in the production of second-generation Ad vectors.

Second-Generation Vectors

Second-generation vectors carry disabling mutations or deletions in the remaining early genes encoded by the E2 and/or E4 cassettes. The dual goals of the second-generation vector design are to increase the DNA carrying capacity and to decrease the immunogenicity shown by the first-generation Ad vectors. Further attenuation of the Ad vector could reduce viral protein synthesis, thereby leading to a diminished immune response directed against viral antigens. In addition, multiple deletions in the Ad genome theoretically reduce the risk of recombination leading to replication-competent Ad during vector propagation.

Second-generation Ad vectors containing temperature-sensitive mutations in the E2 gene were shown to achieve more persistent transgene expression and induce less immune response than first-generation Ad vectors (68,69). However, such benefits were not always seen with the temperature-sensitive mutation, and second-generation Ad vectors containing E2 deletions were constructed to maximize the attenuating effects of further early gene disruption (70–72). Although these vectors were more difficult to grow to the high titers typical of first-generation Ad vectors, they displayed decreased "leaky" viral protein expression and, compared to first-generation Ad vector–mediated delivery, enabled more prolonged expression of a transgene encoding a neoantigen when delivered in vivo (71–74). Following in vivo delivery, a second-generation vector deleted for E1 and E4 was also shown to have reduced viral protein synthesis and increased stability in mouse liver as compared to first-generation Ad vectors. However, in contrast to the studies by Gao et al. (75), increased stability of transgene expression was only observed in the context of a transgene encoding a self-protein. To our knowledge, there are no published reports of the use of second-generation Ad vectors for dystrophin gene delivery.

Third-Generation Vectors

To circumvent the continued problem of leaky Ad gene expression and the resulting unfavorable immune response as well as to further increase the transgene insert capacity, third-generation Ad vectors (also referred to as gutted, gutless, high-capacity, or helper-dependent Ad vectors) were developed containing only the ITRs and the packaging signal but no viral genes (76–78). The reduced immunogenicity and very large transgene insert capacity (greater than 30 kb) make this an extremely promising Ad vector for delivering full-length dystrophin gene to muscle and achieving long-term expression. Because this vector contains no viral genes, vector production requires all the necessary viral proteins to be provided in trans. Therefore, production of third-generation Ad vectors is technically more demanding and typically requires coinfection of packaging cell lines with a first-generation Ad vector (helper virus) that can supply all the viral proteins essential for replication and encapsidation of the third-generation Ad vector. Following propagation, purification of the third-generation Ad vector requires separation from the helper virus, which is one of the major limitations of this system. Because a major goal of third-generation Ad vectors is to eliminate all immunogenic viral protein–coding sequences, any contamination with first-generation Ad vector could potentially reduce the benefit of these vectors. Significant enhancement of vector production was achieved by flanking the helper virus packaging signal with loxP sites and stably transducing the packaging cell line with the *Cre* gene (79). Cre protein expression during viral vector propagation results in excision of the helper virus–packaging signal by Cre-mediated loxP recombination. Loss of the packaging signal from the helper virus genome enriches the packaging of the recombinant vector and limits the packaging of helper virus particles. Further development of strategies to overcome the difficulties in producing the helper-dependent high-capacity Ad vectors will greatly help in their clinical use (79–83).

Successful expression of full-length dystrophin delivered by third-generation Ad vectors has been demonstrated in *mdx* muscle cells in vitro and in *mdx* mouse muscle in vivo (76–78,84–89). Intramuscular delivery of a third-generation Ad vector containing full-length dystrophin into newborn *mdx* mice led to biochemical restoration of the dystrophin-associated complex at the muscle membrane and an improvement in muscle histology (89). In the absence of expression of neoantigens encoded by the vector transgenes, third-generation Ad vector DNA was shown to persist in the muscle tissue for up to five months (90,91). In addition to biochemical improvements, functional improvement following third-generation Ad vector–mediated delivery of full-length dystrophin to adult *mdx* mice was demonstrated by an increased resistance of transduced muscle to contraction-induced injury (85). Similarly, dystrophin gene transfer to neonatal and juvenile *mdx* mice by third-generation Ad vectors containing two full-length murine dystrophin coding sequences led not only to restoration of the dystrophin-associated protein complex and improved muscle histology, but also decreased susceptibility to contraction-induced muscle damage and, for the neonatally treated mice, decreased muscle hypertrophy and increased maximal force–generating capacity (88). These studies demonstrate the tremendous therapeutic potential of third-generation Ad vector–mediated dystrophin delivery for DMD therapy. Interestingly, a number of studies have shown that some Ad proteins enhance transgene expression (84,87,92,93), suggesting that incorporation of select viral genes back into the third-generation Ad vector could enhance transduction by these vectors.

IMMUNITY INDUCED BY ADENOVIRAL VECTORS

The host immune response triggered by Ad vector–mediated gene delivery is arguably the most significant hindrance to the successful application of Ad vector gene therapy for the treatment of DMD. Immune-mediated clearance mechanisms limit both the efficiency and persistence of transgene expression from Ad vectors, and it has been reproducibly demonstrated that transgene expression following vector administration is improved in animals with immature or suppressed and compromised immune systems (54,61–64, 67,86,94–96). Studies indicate that both the transgene and the vector play a role in triggering the immune system (64,86).

Ad vector–mediated gene delivery induces both the innate and the adaptive arms of the immune system. Acute inflammation is rapidly triggered by the Ad vector particle in a dose-dependent manner and in the absence of gene transcription [recently reviewed in Ref. (97)]. A host of cytokines and chemokines including IL-6 (interleukin-6), macrophage inflammatory protein-2, tumor necrosis factor α (TNF-α), IL-8, IL-10, IP-10, and the C-C chemokine RANTES are induced upon Ad vector delivery (98–103). It has been shown that interactions between Ad capsid components and cell-surface receptors activate proinflammatory cell signaling cascades including the p38/MAPK pathway (99). This innate immune response to Ad vector delivery activates professional antigen-presenting cells such as dendritic cells, which then initiate the adaptive immune response.

In the setting of Ad vector–mediated dystrophin gene delivery, activated dendritic cells carrying Ad and dystrophin antigens traffic to peripheral lymphoid tissue such as the regional lymph nodes, and then activate antigen-specific CD4+ and CD8+ T cells by presentation of antigen peptides on MHC class II and I molecules, respectively. Engagement of the T cell receptor and costimulation by the same dendritic cell results in activation of the antigen-specific T cell to produce IL-2 and proliferate. Activated effector T cells then circulate and can participate in the cellular and humoral components of adaptive immunity (104).

In the context of Ad vector–mediated gene delivery to liver, the humoral response primarily prevents vector readministration by the production of neutralizing antibodies (105,106). This inability to readminister the Ad vector has also been shown in the context of muscle gene delivery in mouse models (107). The same study demonstrated that impairment of costimulation of T cells through gene transfer of a CTLA4Ig gene restored the ability to readminister the Ad vector to muscle (107). Presumably, impaired activation of CD4+ T cells diminished activation of B cells and thereby their ability to produce antibody and also interfered with the T cell–mediated processes that normally lead to the specific development of neutralizing antibodies. These studies highlighted the participation of humoral immunity in Ad vector–mediated muscle gene transfer.

The second major component of adaptive immunity is the cellular response that removes infected cells. This is principally mediated by CD8+ T cells that are activated to become cytotoxic T lymphocytes (CTLs). In the context of muscle gene delivery, therapeutic impairment of T cell activation by CTLA4Ig or CD40Ig resulted in prolonged transgene expression in muscle and diminished histological and cytokine evidence for a cellular immune response in transduced muscle (107–110).

In the majority of patients with DMD, large deletions in the dystrophin gene lead to a loss of protein expression and therefore, in these patients, dystrophin may be perceived as a neoantigen (111). Gilchrist et al. (86) demonstrated the development of antidystrophin antibodies at a time long after a single Ad vector–mediated gene delivery to neonatal *mdx* mouse skeletal muscle. An antidystrophin response was demonstrated in a dystrophin-deficient mouse model that received a dystrophin-expressing myogenic cell transplantation (111). As the therapeutic application of dystrophin gene transfer to DMD patients would require life-long expression of dystrophin, it is clear that these issues will need to be addressed in clinical applications of dystrophin gene transfer.

The tremendous progress made in elucidating the nature of the immune response triggered by Ad vector–mediated transgene delivery has greatly facilitated efforts to abrogate this detrimental inflammatory response. The strategies employed by researchers to limit the immune response can be divided into two general approaches: (*i*) alteration of the input vector to reduce its immunogenicity and (*ii*) modulation of the host immune system to reduce its response to transgene delivery. Manipulation of the input vector has led to striking reductions in the inflammatory responses of Ad vector–mediated gene delivery. Because cellular and humoral adaptive immune responses are mounted against the viral gene products and input capsid proteins as well as the transgene products, efforts to reduce Ad immunogenicity have focused on both vector and transgene manipulations. As described in the section on third-generation Ad vectors, deletion of all viral genes in concert with improved methods of vector propagation has significantly reduced the role of viral gene products in triggering the immune response. Researchers have also explored the use of alternate Ad serotypes, both human (112,113) and nonhuman (114–119), to circumvent the Ad neutralizing antibodies triggered by the input capsid components which prevent efficient vector readministration. In addition to manipulating the Ad vector, researchers have modified the transgene in an effort to reduce its immunogenicity. Studies have shown that placing the dystrophin transgene under the control of a muscle-specific promoter can reduce its antigenicity, an effect that is likely accomplished by minimizing dystrophin expression in professional antigen-presenting cells such as dendritic cells (120). In addition, utrophin, a structural and functional homolog of dystrophin capable of providing benefit to dystrophic muscle when delivered by Ad vectors (121–123), has been studied as a potentially less inflammatory alternative to dystrophin, given that it is normally expressed in muscle cells and should therefore be perceived as a self-antigen. Indeed, it was shown that utrophin delivery led to prolonged expression and decreased inflammation compared to dystrophin delivery in immunocompetent *mdx* mice (124). Although these strategies help to limit the adaptive immune response, the innate immunity triggered by the Ad particle and the continued problem of transgene antigenicity, especially in the heightened inflammatory mileu of dystrophic muscle (125), make it necessary to combine the strategy of vector and transgene manipulation with host immunosuppression.

Numerous studies have shown that suppression of the host immune system improves the efficacy of Ad vector–mediated dystrophin delivery. Transient immunosuppression by FK506 (96) alone and in combination with an immunomodulatory IgG, CTLA4Ig, have been shown to increase Ad vector–mediated dystrophin expression in *mdx* mice (110). In the latter study, a reduction in the anti-Ad humoral response facilitated repeat vector administration (110). Codelivery of an Ad vector carrying a marker gene, enhanced green fluorescent protein (eGFP), to muscle and a third-generation Ad vector carrying immunosuppressive genes CTLA4Ig and/or CD40Ig to either muscle or liver of immunocompetent C57BL/10 mice led to a decreased immune response and prolonged transgene expression (107,108).

In addition to modulating the immune system of the host, several groups have researched in utero gene transfer to fetuses as a promising means of reducing immune-mediated clearance of transgene expression by taking advantage of the relatively immature state of the fetal immune system. To date, it appears that this strategy does not induce tolerance to Ad vector proteins, but does permit a single readministration of Ad vector postnatally (126).

TARGETING ADENOVIRAL VECTORS

General Development

Work in the field of vector development has greatly advanced the utility of Ad vectors in the delivery of full-length dystrophin to muscle. However, Ad vector–mediated dystrophin delivery to muscle still remains a daunting task for a variety of reasons. DMD is a disease of biochemical deficiency making it important to deliver dystrophin to a vast majority of myofibers (127). Given that skeletal muscle represents over 30% of body mass, the target tissue for DMD gene therapy is enormous. Although it has been estimated that dystrophin levels as low as 20% of normal levels will impart some muscle protection, these dystrophin-positive fibers will obviously need to be well distributed throughout the body to provide therapeutic benefit (58). For these reasons, the clinical utility of Ad vector delivery via intramuscular injection is greatly limited and successful gene therapy for DMD will likely require systemic delivery approaches. Another significant challenge in applying Ad vectors in DMD gene therapy is the inability of Ad to infect mature muscle efficiently. The observation that as muscle matures, it becomes refractory to Ad infection has been made both in vitro and in vivo (128–131). The mechanisms underlying this maturation-dependent decrease in Ad transduction remain unclear, but likely involve changes in the extracellular matrix (132–134) and a decrease in the levels of the classical Ad binding (CAR) and internalization (αv integrin) receptors associated with muscle maturation (21,129). An encouraging strategy for overcoming these challenges is to impart Ad vectors with muscle-specific targeting moieties so that they may transduce muscle in an efficient and specific manner following systemic administration.

The main goals of vector targeting are to limit the transduction of nontarget tissues while concomitantly increasing efficiency of target tissue transduction. These dual objectives will facilitate systemic administration, a prerequisite for successful gene therapy protocols for use in many disease processes including DMD. In addition to facilitating systemic delivery, targeting the Ad vector to a receptor highly prevalent on muscle cells may

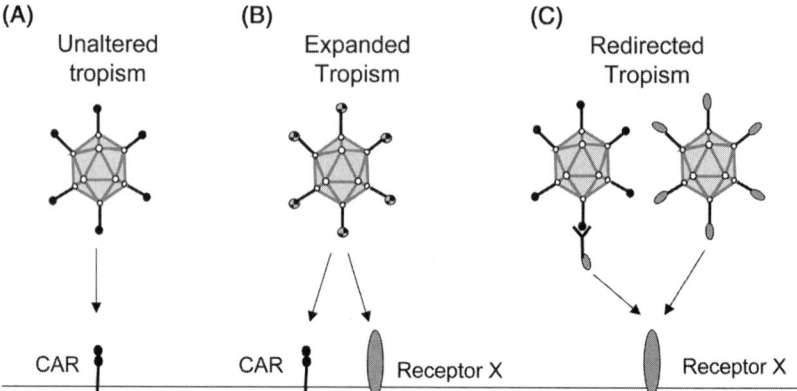

Figure 5 Targeting Ad vectors to tissue-specific receptors through Ad capsid modifications. (**A**) Unmodified Ad. (**B**) Ad with expanded tropism in which a targeting moiety incorporated into the Ad fiber protein directs binding to an additional tissue-specific receptor but does not interfere with CAR binding. (**C**) Ad with tissue-specific binding in which modifications to the Ad capsid abolish native tropism and redirect Ad binding to a tissue-specific receptor. The modifications can involve genetic manipulation and/or the postassembly use of bispecific targeting molecules. *Abbreviations*: Ad, adenovirus; CAR, coxsackievirus–adenovirus receptor.

circumvent the low level of CAR and potentially increase transduction efficiency. Finally, redirecting Ad vectors to a muscle-specific receptor may reduce the immunogenicity of the targeted Ad vector by limiting transduction of antigen-presenting cells and reducing the vector's ability to trigger cellular proinflammatory signal transduction pathways normally induced by classical Ad capsid–cell receptor interactions (101).

The twin goals of targeting, to ablate native tropism and to reroute the vector to a new tissue-specific receptor, have been achieved by two general methods (Fig. 5). The first method involves modifications that are genetically engineered into the Ad capsid. The development of Ad vectors genetically ablated for native tropism has been greatly facilitated by the characterization of Ad capsid structure and the molecular detailing of its interactions with host cell receptors (34,135–138). A number of research groups have used this information to introduce ablating mutations into the CAR-binding domain of the fiber and into the αv integrin–binding domain of the penton base (22,136,139,140). In addition, the identification of flexible protruding loops in the fiber protein has enabled researchers to genetically modify these regions to display targeting peptides (141,142). A number of groups have shown targeting benefits with heterologous peptides incorporated into the Ad fiber (142–149). In addition to modifications of the fiber protein, targeting ligands incorporated into other capsid components, including penton base (150), hexon (151), and pIX coat protein (152), have similarly shown increased knob-independent infection. The major advantage of this targeting strategy is that once the modifications are engineered, the end product is a stable, relatively simple, single-component targeting reagent. However, several disadvantages of this strategy exist. Because the targeting results from genetic manipulation of the Ad DNA, it is necessary to re-engineer each new targeting vector. The vectors can be hard to grow and much effort has been directed at creating new packaging cell lines to compensate for the genetic ablations and capsid modifications (153,154). Finally, because the targeting peptides are displayed within the context of the capsid proteins, the targeting ligand must be compatible with proper capsid assembly. This may restrict the choice of ligands that can be suitably incorporated into the coat proteins, and ongoing efforts are being made to further delineate the requirements for successful peptide incorporation (155).

The second general approach for targeting Ad to specific cells is to link targeting moieties to the Ad capsid after viral assembly. For this strategy, bispecific molecules are employed which bind to the Ad capsid and the target receptor. The bispecific molecule contains an Ad-binding component, typically an antibody recognizing the Ad particle, linked to the targeting component, usually a ligand or an antitarget receptor antibody. Because the targeting constructs in this method are added to the Ad particle postassembly, they are not restricted by capsid constraints and therefore do not interfere with normal propagation methods, making this an attractive approach for its ease of manipulation and adaptability to a myriad of desired targets. Many research groups have successfully employed the bispecific targeting strategy to redirect Ad vectors to a variety of cell surface receptors including the folate receptor (156), fibroblast growth factor receptor (157), αv integrins (158), CD3 (159), E-selectin (160), EpCAM (161), and epidermal growth factor receptors (162). Importantly, targeting efficacy using bispecific moieties has also been shown in vivo (163–165).

Targeting Adenoviral Vectors to Muscle

Only a few studies of Ad targeting to skeletal muscle have been reported in the literature. Bouri et al. (166) demonstrated that targeting the Ad vector to heparan sulfate through a polylysine moiety genetically engineered into Ad fiber protein improved the transduction of myoblasts, myotubes, and isolated myofibers in vitro as well as mature myofibers in vivo. These results indicate that the low transduction efficiency of mature muscle can be overcome by directing Ad to a more prevalent receptor on muscle cells, and therefore provide important proof-of-principle demonstration of the feasibility of enhancing muscle transduction through targeting. In studies by Volpers et al. (167), an Ad vector displaying the Ig domain of staphylococcal protein A dramatically enhanced transduction of primary human myoblasts and myotubes in vitro when preincubated with an anti-α7 integrin or antineuronal cell adhesion molecule (NCAM) antibody. Of note, the protein A–modified vector still retained CAR-binding and an intact penton base. Thus, defining the role of the classical pathways of Ad binding and internalization in the infectious route of entry of the $\alpha 7$- and NCAM-targeted Ad vectors will broaden our understanding of the mechanisms leading to target-mediated enhanced transduction.

In contrast to the two studies just discussed, Bilbao et al. (168) determined that targeting high-capacity Ad vectors to αv integrins through an RGD motif engineered into the fiber protein did not increase transduction of fetal muscle in vivo or in vitro despite the high cell-surface expression of αv integrins in the target tissue. It was shown that the targeting moiety actually reduced the transduction efficiency in cells positive for CAR and αv integrin when compared to untargeted control vector. The RGD-modified Ad vector retained CAR binding, and the experiments performed to dissect out the contributions of CAR and αv integrins in the pathway of the RGD-modified Ad infection indicated that the targeting moiety was competing for cell attachment and, as a consequence, redirecting Ad away from the efficient CAR-mediated pathway. The inability of the RGD–αv integrin interaction to compensate for the loss in CAR binding led to reduced transduction of the target cells. In summary, the targeting studies performed in muscle indicate that redirecting Ad vectors to muscle-specific receptors can greatly enhance muscle transduction efficiency, but as studies by Bilbao et al. suggest, attention to the mechanism of transduction by the modified Ad vector will be crucial for optimizing the targeting strategy.

FUTURE CHALLENGES

Since the discovery of dystrophin over a decade ago, extraordinary insights have been gained in the pathophysiology of DMD, and this has facilitated the development of numerous creative therapeutic approaches for the treatment of DMD. As dystrophin delivery to DMD muscle has the potential to be curative, gene therapy is one of the more alluring potential treatment modalities. Within this pursuit, Ad vectors are exceptionally promising, especially because third-generation vectors have the ability to deliver full-length dystrophin to mature muscle and can be produced as high titer stocks. It has been clearly demonstrated that Ad vector–mediated dystrophin delivery can provide both histological and functional benefits to transduced muscle, thereby establishing the feasibility of this therapeutic approach. However, basic research applying Ad vector technology to muscle gene transfer has highlighted two important remaining problems, the immune response induced by gene delivery and the inefficient transduction of muscle following systemic administration. It is of paramount importance to continue delineating the nature of the detrimental immune response triggered by the Ad vector and transgene. Controlling this inflammatory reaction will enhance the persistence of dystrophin expression and facilitate vector readministration. In addition to alleviating immune-mediated clearance of transduced muscle cells, it is necessary to develop strategies to improve muscle transduction following systemic administration of Ad vectors. Targeting Ad vectors to relatively muscle-specific receptors that are highly expressed at the sarcolemmal surface has the potential to overcome both the lack of muscle tropism and the concomitant inability of Ad to transduce muscle following systemic delivery. Progress in these areas has the potential to advance DMD research toward its ultimate goal—being of therapeutic benefit to patients.

REFERENCES

1. Horwitz MS. Adenoviruses. In: Knipe DM and Howley PM, eds. Fields Virology. Philadelphia: Lippincott Williams & Wilkins, 2001:2301–2326.
2. Shenk TE. Adenoviridae: the viruses and their replication. In: Knipe DM and Howley PM, eds. Fields Virology. Philadelphia: Lippincott Williams & Wilkins, 2001:2265–2300.
3. Bergelson JM, Cunningham JA, Droguett G, et al. Isolation of a common receptor for Coxsackie B viruses and adenoviruses 2 and 5. Science 1997; 275(5304):1320–1323.
4. Tomko RP, Xu R, Philipson L. HCAR and MCAR: the human and mouse cellular receptors for subgroup C adenoviruses and group B coxsackieviruses. Proc Natl Acad Sci USA 1997; 94(7):3352–3356.
5. Roelvink PW, Lizonova A, Lee JG, et al. The coxsackievirus-adenovirus receptor protein can function as a cellular attachment protein for adenovirus serotypes from subgroups A, C, D, E, and F. J Virol 1998; 72(10): 7909–7915.
6. Leon RP, Hedlund T, Meech SJ, et al. Adenoviral-mediated gene transfer in lymphocytes. Proc Natl Acad Sci USA 1998; 95(22):13159–13164.
7. Walters RW, van't Hof W, Yi SM, et al. Apical localization of the coxsackie-adenovirus receptor by glycosyl-phosphatidylinositol modification is sufficient for adenovirus-mediated gene transfer through the apical surface of human airway epithelia. J Virol 2001; 75(16):7703–7711.
8. Wang X, Bergelson JM. Coxsackievirus and adenovirus receptor cytoplasmic and transmembrane domains are not essential for coxsackievirus and adenovirus infection. J Virol 1999; 73(3):2559–2562.
9. Cohen CJ, Shieh JT, Pickles RJ, Okegawa T, Hsieh JT, Bergelson JM. The coxsackievirus and adenovirus receptor is a transmembrane component of the tight junction. Proc Natl Acad Sci USA 2001; 98(26):15191–15196.
10. Fechner H, Haack A, Wang H, et al. Expression of coxsackie adenovirus receptor and alphav-integrin does not correlate with adenovector targeting in vivo indicating anatomical vector barriers. Gene Ther 1999; 6(9):1520–1535.
11. Hong SS, Karayan L, Tournier J, Curiel DT, Boulanger PA. Adenovirus type 5 fiber knob binds to MHC class I alpha2 domain at the surface of human epithelial and B lymphoblastoid cells. EMBO J 1997; 16(9): 2294–2306.

12. Arnberg N, Kidd AH, Edlund K, Olfat F, Wadell G. Initial interactions of subgenus D adenoviruses with A549 cellular receptors: sialic acid versus alpha(v) integrins. J Virol 2000; 74(16):7691–7693.
13. Arnberg N, Edlund K, Kidd AH, Wadell G. Adenovirus type 37 uses sialic acid as a cellular receptor. J Virol 2000; 74(1):42–48.
14. Arnberg N, Kidd AH, Edlund K, Nilsson J, Pring-Akerblom P, Wadell G. Adenovirus type 37 binds to cell surface sialic acid through a charge-dependent interaction. Virology 2002; 302(1):33–43.
15. Arnberg N, Pring-Akerblom P, Wadell G. Adenovirus type 37 uses sialic acid as a cellular receptor on Chang C cells. J Virol 2002; 76(17):8834–8841.
16. Huang S, Kamata T, Takada Y, Ruggeri ZM, Nemerow GR. Adenovirus interaction with distinct integrins mediates separate events in cell entry and gene delivery to hematopoietic cells. J Virol 1996; 70(7):4502–4508.
17. Gaden F, Franqueville L, Hong SS, Legrand V, Figarella C, Boulanger P. Mechanism of restriction of normal and cystic fibrosis transmembrane conductance regulator-deficient human tracheal gland cells to adenovirus infection and ad-mediated gene transfer. Am J Respir Cell Mol Biol 2002; 27(5):628–640.
18. Dechecchi MC, Tamanini A, Bonizzato A, Cabrini G. Heparan sulfate glycosaminoglycans are involved in adenovirus type 5 and 2-host cell interactions. Virology 2000; 268(2):382–390.
19. Dechecchi MC, Melotti P, Bonizzato A, Santacatterina M, Chilosi M, Cabrini G. Heparan sulfate glycosaminoglycans are receptors sufficient to mediate the initial binding of adenovirus types 2 and 5. J Virol 2001; 75(18):8772–8780.
20. Kimura E, Maeda Y, Arima T, et al. Efficient repetitive gene delivery to skeletal muscle using recombinant adenovirus vector containing the Coxsackievirus and adenovirus receptor cDNA. Gene Ther 2001; 8(1):20–27.
21. Nalbantoglu J, Pari G, Karpati G, Holland PC. Expression of the primary coxsackie and adenovirus receptor is downregulated during skeletal muscle maturation and limits the efficacy of adenovirus-mediated gene delivery to muscle cells. Hum Gene Ther 1999; 10(6):1009–1019.
22. Einfeld DA, Schroeder R, Roelvink PW, et al. Reducing the native tropism of adenovirus vectors requires removal of both CAR and integrin interactions. J Virol 2001; 75(23):11284–11291.
23. Wickham TJ, Mathias P, Cheresh DA, Nemerow GR. Integrins alpha v beta 3 and alpha v beta 5 promote adenovirus internalization but not virus attachment. Cell 1993; 73(2):309–319.
24. Davison E, Kirby I, Whitehouse J, Hart I, Marshall JF, Santis G. Adenovirus type 5 uptake by lung adenocarcinoma cells in culture correlates with Ad5 fibre binding is mediated by alpha(v)beta1 integrin and can be modulated by changes in beta1 integrin function. J Gene Med 2001; 3(6):550–559.
25. Li E, Brown SL, Stupack DG, Puente XS, Cheresh DA, Nemerow GR. Integrin alpha(v)beta1 is an adenovirus coreceptor. J Virol 2001; 75(11):5405–5409.
26. Davison E, Diaz RM, Hart IR, Santis G, Marshall JF. Integrin alpha5beta1-mediated adenovirus infection is enhanced by the integrin-activating antibody TS2/16. J Virol 1997; 71(8):6204–6207.

27. Nakano MY, Boucke K, Suomalainen M, Stidwill RP, Greber UF. The first step of adenovirus type 2 disassembly occurs at the cell surface, independently of endocytosis and escape to the cytosol. J Virol 2000; 74(15):7085–7095.
28. Varga MJ, Weibull C, Everitt E. Infectious entry pathway of adenovirus type 2. J Virol 1991; 65(11):6061–6070.
29. Leopold PL, Ferris B, Grinberg I, Worgall S, Hackett NR, Crystal RG. Fluorescent virions: dynamic tracking of the pathway of adenoviral gene transfer vectors in living cells. Hum Gene Ther 1998; 9(3):367–378.
30. Wang K, Huang S, Kapoor-Munshi A, Nemerow G. Adenovirus internalization and infection require dynamin. J Virol 1998; 72(4):3455–3458.
31. Li E, Stupack D, Klemke R, Cheresh DA, Nemerow GR. Adenovirus endocytosis via alpha(v) integrins requires phosphoinositide-3-OH kinase. J Virol 1998; 72(3):2055–2061.
32. Li E, Stupack D, Bokoch GM, Nemerow GR. Adenovirus endocytosis requires actin cytoskeleton reorganization mediated by Rho family GTPases. J Virol 1998; 72(11):8806–8812.
33. Li E, Stupack DG, Brown SL, Klemke R, Schlaepfer DD, Nemerow GR. Association of p130CAS with phosphatidylinositol-3-OH kinase mediates adenovirus cell entry. J Biol Chem 2000; 275(19):14729–14735.
34. Chiu CY, Mathias P, Nemerow GR, Stewart PL. Structure of adenovirus complexed with its internalization receptor, alpha v beta5 integrin. J Virol 1999; 73(8):6759–6768.
35. Wickham TJ, Filardo EJ, Cheresh DA, Nemerow GR. Integrin alpha v beta 5 selectively promotes adenovirus mediated cell membrane permeabilization. J Cell Biol 1994; 127(1):257–264.
36. Wang K, Guan T, Cheresh DA, Nemerow GR. Regulation of adenovirus membrane penetration by the cytoplasmic tail of integrin beta5. J Virol 2000; 74(6):2731–2739.
37. Blumenthal R, Seth P, Willingham MC, Pastan I. pH-dependent lysis of liposomes by adenovirus. Biochemistry 1986; 25(8):2231–2237.
38. Seth P. Adenovirus-dependent release of choline from plasma membrane vesicles at an acidic pH is mediated by the penton base protein. J Virol 1994; 68(2):1204–1206.
39. Greber UF, Webster P, Weber J, Helenius A. The role of the adenovirus protease on virus entry into cells. EMBO J 1996; 15(8):1766–1777.
40. Cotten M, Weber JM. The adenovirus protease is required for virus entry into host-cells. Virology 1995; 213(2):494–502.
41. Greber UF, Singh I, Helenius A. Mechanisms of virus uncoating. Trends Microbiol 1994; 2(2):52–56.
42. Greber UF, Suomalainen M, Stidwill RP, Boucke K, Ebersold MW, Helenius A. The role of the nuclear pore complex in adenovirus DNA entry. EMBO J 1997; 16(19):5998–6007.
43. Wisnivesky JP, Leopold PL, Crystal RG. Specific binding of the adenovirus capsid to the nuclear envelope. Hum Gene Ther 1999; 10(13):2187–2195.
44. Saphire AC, Guan T, Schirmer EC, Nemerow GR, Gerace L. Nuclear import of adenovirus DNA in vitro involves the nuclear protein import pathway and hsc70. J Biol Chem 2000; 275(6):4298–4304.

45. Hay RT, Freeman A, Leith I, Monaghan A, Webster A. Molecular interactions during adenovirus DNA replication. In: Doerfler WBP, ed. The Molecular Repertoire of Adenoviruses. Berlin: Springer, 1995:31–48.
46. Ginsberg HS, Lundholm-Beauchamp U, Horswood RL, et al. Role of early region 3 (E3) in pathogenesis of adenovirus disease. Proc Natl Acad Sci USA 1989; 86(10):3823–3827.
47. Weigel S, Dobbelstein M. The nuclear export signal within the E4 or f6 protein of adenovirus type 5 supports virus replication and cytoplasmic accumulation of viral mRNA. J Virol 2000; 74(2):764–772.
48. Russell WC. Update on adenovirus and its vectors. J Gen Virol 2000; 81(Pt 11):2573–2604.
49. Greber UF, Willetts M, Webster P, Helenius A. Stepwise dismantling of adenovirus 2 during entry into cells. Cell 1993; 75(3):477–486.
50. Lai CM, Lai YK, Rakoczy PE. Adenovirus and adeno-associated virus vectors. DNA Cell Biol 2002; 21(12):895–913.
51. Graham FL, Smiley J, Russell WC, Nairn R. Characteristics of a human cell line transformed by DNA from human adenovirus type 5. J Gen Virol 1977; 36(1):59–74.
52. Ragot T, Vincent N, Chafey P, et al. Efficient adenovirus-mediated transfer of a human minidystrophin gene to skeletal muscle of mdx mice. Nature 1993; 361(6413):647–650.
53. Vincent N, Ragot T, Gilgenkrantz H, et al. Long-term correction of mouse dystrophic degeneration by adenovirus-mediated transfer of a minidystrophin gene. Nat Genet 1993; 5(2):130–134.
54. Deconinck N, Ragot T, Marechal G, Perricaudet M, Gillis JM. Functional protection of dystrophic mouse (mdx) muscles after adenovirus-mediated transfer of a dystrophin minigene. Proc Natl Acad Sci USA 1996; 93(8):3570–3574.
55. Yang L, Lochmuller H, Luo J, et al. Adenovirus-mediated dystrophin minigene transfer improves muscle strength in adult dystrophic (MDX) mice. Gene Ther 1998; 5(3):369–379.
56. Yuasa K, Miyagoe Y, Yamamoto K, Nabeshima Y, Dickson G, Takeda S. Effective restoration of dystrophin-associated proteins in vivo by adenovirus-mediated transfer of truncated dystrophin cDNAs. FEBS Lett 1998; 425(2):329–336.
57. Clemens PR, Krause TL, Chan S, Korb KE, Graham FL, Caskey CT. Recombinant truncated dystrophin minigenes: construction, expression, and adenoviral delivery. Hum Gene Ther 1995; 6(11):1477–1485.
58. Phelps SF, Hauser MA, Cole NM, et al. Expression of full-length and truncated dystrophin mini-genes in transgenic mdx mice. Hum Mol Genet 1995; 4(8):1251–1258.
59. Wells DJ, Wells KE, Asante EA, et al. Expression of human full-length and minidystrophin in transgenic mdx mice: implications for gene therapy of Duchenne muscular dystrophy. Hum Mol Genet 1995; 4(8):1245–1250.
60. Rafael JA, Cox GA, Corrado K, Jung D, Campbell KP, Chamberlain JS. Forced expression of dystrophin deletion constructs reveals structure-function correlations. J Cell Biol 1996; 134(1):93–102.

61. Yang Y, Nunes FA, Berencsi K, Furth EE, Gonczol E, Wilson JM. Cellular immunity to viral antigens limits E1-deleted adenoviruses for gene therapy. Proc Natl Acad Sci USA 1994; 91(10):4407–4411.
62. Acsadi G, Lochmuller H, Jani A, et al. Dystrophin expression in muscles of mdx mice after adenovirus-mediated in vivo gene transfer. Hum Gene Ther 1996; 7(2):129–140.
63. Gilgenkrantz H, Duboc D, Juillard V, et al. Transient expression of genes transferred in vivo into heart using first-generation adenoviral vectors: role of the immune response. Hum Gene Ther 1995; 6(10):1265–1274.
64. Tripathy SK, Black HB, Goldwasser E, Leiden JM. Immune responses to transgene-encoded proteins limit the stability of gene expression after injection of replication-defective adenovirus vectors. Nat Med 1996; 2(5):545–550.
65. Dai Y, Schwarz EM, Gu D, Zhang WW, Sarvetnick N, Verma IM. Cellular and humoral immune responses to adenoviral vectors containing factor IX gene: tolerization of factor IX and vector antigens allows for long-term expression. Proc Natl Acad Sci USA 1995; 92(5):1401–1405.
66. Zoltick PW, Chirmule N, Schnell MA, Gao GP, Hughes JV, Wilson JM. Biology of E1-deleted adenovirus vectors in nonhuman primate muscle. J Virol 2001; 75(11):5222–5229.
67. Yang Y, Su Q, Wilson JM. Role of viral antigens in destructive cellular immune responses to adenovirus vector-transduced cells in mouse lungs. J Virol 1996; 70(10):7209–7212.
68. Yang Y, Nunes FA, Berencsi K, Gonczol E, Engelhardt JF, Wilson JM. Inactivation of E2a in recombinant adenoviruses improves the prospect for gene therapy in cystic fibrosis. Nat Genet 1994; 7(3):362–369.
69. Engelhardt JF, Ye X, Doranz B, Wilson JM. Ablation of E2A in recombinant adenoviruses improves transgene persistence and decreases inflammatory response in mouse liver. Proc Natl Acad Sci USA 1994; 91(13):6196–6200.
70. Fang B, Wang H, Gordon G, et al. Lack of persistence of E1-recombinant adenoviral vectors containing a temperature-sensitive E2A mutation in immunocompetent mice and hemophilia B dogs. Gene Ther 1996; 3(3):217–222.
71. Zhou H, O'Neal W, Morral N, Beaudet AL. Development of a complementing cell line and a system for construction of adenovirus vectors with E1 and E2a deleted. J Virol 1996; 70(10):7030–7038.
72. Amalfitano A, Hauser MA, Hu H, Serra D, Begy CR, Chamberlain JS. Production and characterization of improved adenovirus vectors with the E1, E2b, and E3 genes deleted. J Virol 1998; 72(2):926–933.
73. Gorziglia MI, Kadan MJ, Yei S, et al. Elimination of both E1 and E2 from adenovirus vectors further improves prospects for in vivo human gene therapy. J Virol 1996; 70(6):4173–4178.
74. Hu H, Serra D, Amalfitano A. Persistence of an [E1-, polymerase-] adenovirus vector despite transduction of a neoantigen into immune-competent mice. Hum Gene Ther 1999; 10(3):355–364.
75. Gao GP, Yang Y, Wilson JM. Biology of adenovirus vectors with E1 and E4 deletions for liver-directed gene therapy. J Virol 1996; 70(12):8934–8943.
76. Kochanek S, Clemens PR, Mitani K, Chen HH, Chan S, Caskey CT. A new adenoviral vector: replacement of all viral coding sequences with 28 kb of

DNA independently expressing both full-length dystrophin and beta-galactosidase. Proc Natl Acad Sci USA 1996; 93(12):5731–5736.
77. Haecker SE, Stedman HH, Balice-Gordon RJ, et al. In vivo expression of full-length human dystrophin from adenoviral vectors deleted of all viral genes. Hum Gene Ther 1996; 7(15):1907–1914.
78. Kumar-Singh R, Chamberlain JS. Encapsidated adenovirus minichromosomes allow delivery and expression of a 14 kb dystrophin cDNA to muscle cells. Hum Mol Genet 1996; 5(7):913–921.
79. Parks RJ, Chen L, Anton M, Sankar U, Rudnicki MA, Graham FL. A helper-dependent adenovirus vector system: removal of helper virus by Cre-mediated excision of the viral packaging signal. Proc Natl Acad Sci USA 1996; 93(24):13565–13570.
80. Hardy S, Kitamura M, Harris-Stansil T, Dai Y, Phipps ML. Construction of adenovirus vectors through Cre-lox recombination. J Virol 1997; 71(3):1842–1849.
81. Umana P, Gerdes CA, Stone D, et al. Efficient FLPe recombinase enables scalable production of helper-dependent adenoviral vectors with negligible helper-virus contamination. Nat Biotechnol 2001; 19(6):582–585.
82. Barjot C, Hartigan-O'Connor D, Salvatori G, Scott JM, Chamberlain JS. Gutted adenoviral vector growth using E1/E2b/E3-deleted helper viruses. J Gene Med 2002; 4(5):480–489.
83. Sakhuja K, Reddy PS, Ganesh S, et al. Optimization of the generation and propagation of gutless adenoviral vectors. Hum Gene Ther 2003; 14(3):243–254.
84. Gilbert R, Nalbantoglu J, Howell JM, et al. Dystrophin expression in muscle following gene transfer with a fully deleted ("gutted") adenovirus is markedly improved by trans-acting adenoviral gene products. Hum Gene Ther 2001; 12(14):1741–1755.
85. DelloRusso C, Scott JM, Hartigan-O'Connor D, et al. Functional correction of adult mdx mouse muscle using gutted adenoviral vectors expressing full-length dystrophin. Proc Natl Acad Sci USA 2002; 99(20):12979–12984.
86. Gilchrist SC, Ontell MP, Kochanek S, Clemens PR. Immune response to full-length dystrophin delivered to Dmd muscle by a high-capacity adenoviral vector. Mol Ther 2002; 6(3):359–368.
87. Gilbert R, Liu A, Petrof B, Nalbantoglu J, Karpati G. Improved performance of a fully gutted adenovirus vector containing two full-length dystrophin cDNAs regulated by a strong promoter. Mol Ther 2002; 6(4):501–509.
88. Gilbert R, Dudley RW, Liu AB, Petrof BJ, Nalbantoglu J, Karpati G. Prolonged dystrophin expression and functional correction of mdx mouse muscle following gene transfer with a helper-dependent (gutted) adenovirus-encoding murine dystrophin. Hum Mol Genet 2003; 12(11):1287–1299.
89. Clemens PR, Kochanek S, Sunada Y, et al. In vivo muscle gene transfer of full-length dystrophin with an adenoviral vector that lacks all viral genes. Gene Ther 1996; 3(11):965–972.
90. Chen HH, Mack LM, Kelly R, Ontell M, Kochanek S, Clemens PR. Persistence in muscle of an adenoviral vector that lacks all viral genes. Proc Natl Acad Sci USA 1997; 94(5):1645–1650.

91. Chen HH, Mack LM, Choi SY, Ontell M, Kochanek S, Clemens PR. DNA from both high-capacity and first-generation adenoviral vectors remains intact in skeletal muscle. Hum Gene Ther 1999; 10(3):365–373.
92. Brough DE, Hsu C, Kulesa VA, et al. Activation of transgene expression by early region 4 is responsible for a high level of persistent transgene expression from adenovirus vectors in vivo. J Virol 1997; 71(12):9206–9213.
93. Armentano D, Zabner J, Sacks C, et al. Effect of the E4 region on the persistence of transgene expression from adenovirus vectors. J Virol 1997; 71(3):2408–2416.
94. Vilquin JT, Guerette B, Kinoshita I, et al. FK506 immunosuppression to control the immune reactions triggered by first-generation adenovirus-mediated gene transfer. Hum Gene Ther 1995; 6(11):1391–1401.
95. Petrof BJ, Lochmuller H, Massie B, et al. Impairment of force generation after adenovirus-mediated gene transfer to muscle is alleviated by adenoviral gene inactivation and host CD8+ T cell deficiency. Hum Gene Ther 1996; 7(15):1813–1826.
96. Lochmuller H, Petrof BJ, Pari G, et al. Transient immunosuppression by FK506 permits a sustained high-level dystrophin expression after adenovirus-mediated dystrophin minigene transfer to skeletal muscles of adult dystrophic (mdx) mice. Gene Ther 1996; 3(8):706–716.
97. Liu Q, Muruve DA. Molecular basis of the inflammatory response to adenovirus vectors. Gene Ther 2003; 10(11):935–940.
98. Zsengeller Z, Otake K, Hossain SA, Berclaz PY, Trapnell BC. Internalization of adenovirus by alveolar macrophages initiates early proinflammatory signaling during acute respiratory tract infection. J Virol 2000; 74(20):9655–9667.
99. Bruder JT, Kovesdi I. Adenovirus infection stimulates the Raf/MAPK signaling pathway and induces interleukin-8 expression. J Virol 1997; 71(1):398–404.
100. Bowen GP, Borgland SL, Lam M, Libermann TA, Wong NC, Muruve DA. Adenovirus vector-induced inflammation: capsid-dependent induction of the C-C chemokine RANTES requires NF-kappa B. Hum Gene Ther 2002; 13(3):367–379.
101. Liu Q, Zaiss AK, Colarusso P, et al. The role of capsid-endothelial interactions in the innate immune response to adenovirus vectors. Hum Gene Ther 2003; 14(7):627–643.
102. Muruve DA, Barnes MJ, Stillman IE, Libermann TA. Adenoviral gene therapy leads to rapid induction of multiple chemokines and acute neutrophil-dependent hepatic injury in vivo. Hum Gene Ther 1999; 10(6):965–976.
103. Schnell MA, Zhang Y, Tazelaar J, et al. Activation of innate immunity in nonhuman primates following intraportal administration of adenoviral vectors. Mol Ther 2001; 3(5 Pt 1):708–722.
104. Janeway Jr, CTPWMSM. T Cell-Mediated Immunity in Immunobiology: The Immune System in Health and Disease. New York: Garland Publishing, 2001:295–340.
105. Yang Y, Li Q, Ertl HC, Wilson JM. Cellular and humoral immune responses to viral antigens create barriers to lung-directed gene therapy with recombinant adenoviruses. J Virol 1995; 69(4):2004–2015.
106. Yang Y, Greenough K, Wilson JM. Transient immune blockade prevents formation of neutralizing antibody to recombinant adenovirus and allows repeated gene transfer to mouse liver. Gene Ther 1996; 3(5):412–420.

107. Jiang ZL, Reay D, Kreppel F, et al. Local high-capacity adenovirus-mediated mCTLA4Ig and mCD40Ig expression prolongs recombinant gene expression in skeletal muscle. Mol Ther 2001; 3(6):892–900.
108. Jiang Z, Feingold E, Kochanek S, Clemens PR. Systemic delivery of a high-capacity adenoviral vector expressing mouse CTLA4Ig improves skeletal muscle gene therapy. Mol Ther 2002; 6(3):369–376.
109. Guibinga GH, Lochmuller H, Massie B, Nalbantoglu J, Karpati G, Petrof BJ. Combinatorial blockade of calcineurin and CD28 signaling facilitates primary and secondary therapeutic gene transfer by adenovirus vectors in dystrophic (mdx) mouse muscles. J Virol 1998; 72(6):4601–4609.
110. Guerette B, Vilquin JT, Gingras M, Gravel C, Wood KJ, Tremblay JP. Prevention of immune reactions triggered by first-generation adenoviral vectors by monoclonal antibodies and CTLA4Ig. Hum Gene Ther 1996; 7(12):1455–1463.
111. Ohtsuka Y, Udaka K, Yamashiro Y, Yagita H, Okumura K. Dystrophin acts as a transplantation rejection antigen in dystrophin-deficient mice: implication for gene therapy. J Immunol 1998; 160(9):4635–4640.
112. Mack CA, Song WR, Carpenter H, et al. Circumvention of anti-adenovirus neutralizing immunity by administration of an adenoviral vector of an alternate serotype. Hum Gene Ther 1997; 8(1):99–109.
113. Zabner J, Chillon M, Grunst T, et al. A chimeric type 2 adenovirus vector with a type 17 fiber enhances gene transfer to human airway epithelia. J Virol 1999; 73(10):8689–8695.
114. Farina SF, Gao GP, Xiang ZQ, et al. Replication-defective vector based on a chimpanzee adenovirus. J Virol 2001; 75(23):11603–11613.
115. Hofmann C, Loser P, Cichon G, Arnold W, Both GW, Strauss M. Ovine adenovirus vectors overcome preexisting humoral immunity against human adenoviruses in vivo. J Virol 1999; 73(8):6930–6936.
116. Klonjkowski B, Gilardi-Hebenstreit P, Hadchouel J, et al. A recombinant E1-deleted canine adenoviral vector capable of transduction and expression of a transgene in human-derived cells and in vivo. Hum Gene Ther 1997; 8(17):2103–2115.
117. Kremer EJ, Boutin S, Chillon M, Danos O. Canine adenovirus vectors: an alternative for adenovirus-mediated gene transfer. J Virol 2000; 74(1):505–512.
118. Michou AI, Lehrmann H, Saltik M, Cotten M. Mutational analysis of the avian adenovirus CELO, which provides a basis for gene delivery vectors. J Virol 1999; 73(2):1399–1410.
119. Reddy PS, Idamakanti N, Chen Y, et al. Replication-defective bovine adenovirus type 3 as an expression vector. J Virol 1999; 73(11):9137–9144.
120. Hartigan-O'Connor D, Kirk CJ, Crawford R, Mule JJ, Chamberlain JS. Immune evasion by muscle-specific gene expression in dystrophic muscle. Mol Ther 2001; 4(6):525–533.
121. Gilbert R, Nalbantoglu J, Petrof BJ, et al. Adenovirus-mediated utrophin gene transfer mitigates the dystrophic phenotype of mdx mouse muscles. Hum Gene Ther 1999; 10(8):1299–1310.
122. Wakefield PM, Tinsley JM, Wood MJ, Gilbert R, Karpati G, Davies KE. Prevention of the dystrophic phenotype in dystrophin/utrophin-deficient muscle following adenovirus-mediated transfer of a utrophin minigene. Gene Ther 2000; 7(3):201–204.

123. Cerletti M, Negri T, Cozzi F, et al. Dystrophic phenotype of canine X-linked muscular dystrophy is mitigated by adenovirus-mediated utrophin gene transfer. Gene Ther 2003; 10(9):750–757.
124. Ebihara S, Guibinga GH, Gilbert R, et al. Differential effects of dystrophin and utrophin gene transfer in immunocompetent muscular dystrophy (mdx) mice. Physiol Genomics 2000; 3(3):133–144.
125. Spencer MJ, Montecino-Rodriguez E, Dorshkind K, Tidball JG. Helper [CD4(+)] and cytotoxic [CD8(+)] T cells promote the pathology of dystrophin-deficient muscle. Clin Immunol 2001; 98(2):235–243.
126. Yang EY, Kim HB, Shaaban AF, Milner R, Adzick NS, Flake AW. Persistent postnatal transgene expression in both muscle and liver after fetal injection of recombinant adenovirus. J Pediatr Surg 1999; 34(5):766–772.
127. Hoffman EP, Brown RH Jr, Kunkel LM. Dystrophin: the protein product of the Duchenne muscular dystrophy locus. Cell 1987; 51(6):919–928.
128. Acsadi G, Jani A, Huard J, et al. Cultured human myoblasts and myotubes show markedly different transducibility by replication-defective adenovirus recombinants. Gene Ther 1994; 1(5):338–340.
129. Acsadi G, Jani A, Massie B, et al. A differential efficiency of adenovirus-mediated in vivo gene transfer into skeletal muscle cells of different maturity. Hum Mol Genet 1994; 3(4):579–584.
130. Huard J, Lochmuller H, Acsadi G, et al. Differential short-term transduction efficiency of adult versus newborn mouse tissues by adenoviral recombinants. Exp Mol Pathol 1995; 62(2):131–143.
131. Quantin B, Perricaudet LD, Tajbakhsh S, Mandel JL. Adenovirus as an expression vector in muscle cells in vivo. Proc Natl Acad Sci USA 1992; 89(7):2581–2584.
132. van Deutekom JC, Hoffman EP, Huard J. Muscle maturation: implications for gene therapy. Mol Med Today 1998; 4(5):214–220.
133. Feero WG, Rosenblatt JD, Huard J, et al. Viral gene delivery to skeletal muscle: insights on maturation-dependent loss of fiber infectivity for adenovirus and herpes simplex type 1 viral vectors. Hum Gene Ther 1997; 8(4):371–380.
134. van Deutekom JC, Cao B, Pruchnic R, Wickham TJ, Kovesdi I, Huard J. Extended tropism of an adenoviral vector does not circumvent the maturation-dependent transducibility of mouse skeletal muscle. J Gene Med 1999; 1(6):393–399.
135. Bewley MC, Springer K, Zhang YB, Freimuth P, Flanagan JM. Structural analysis of the mechanism of adenovirus binding to its human cellular receptor, CAR. Science 1999; 286(5444):1579–1583.
136. Roelvink PW, Mi LG, Einfeld DA, Kovesdi I, Wickham TJ. Identification of a conserved receptor-binding site on the fiber proteins of CAR-recognizing adenoviridae. Science 1999; 286(5444):1568–1571.
137. Kirby I, Davison E, Beavil AJ, et al. Identification of contact residues and definition of the CAR-binding site of adenovirus type 5 fiber protein. J Virol 2000; 74(6):2804–2813.
138. Stewart PL, Burnett RM, Cyrklaff M, Fuller SD. Image reconstruction reveals the complex molecular organization of adenovirus. Cell 1991; 67(1):145–154.
139. Leissner P, Legrand V, Schlesinger Y, et al. Influence of adenoviral fiber mutations on viral encapsidation, infectivity and in vivo tropism. Gene Ther 2001; 8(1):49–57.

140. Kirby I, Davison E, Beavil AJ, et al. Mutations in the DG loop of adenovirus type 5 fiber knob protein abolish high-affinity binding to its cellular receptor CAR. J Virol 1999; 73(11):9508–9514.
141. Krasnykh V, Dmitriev I, Mikheeva G, Miller CR, Belousova N, Curiel DT. Characterization of an adenovirus vector containing a heterologous peptide epitope in the HI loop of the fiber knob. J Virol 1998; 72(3):1844–1852.
142. Dmitriev I, Krasnykh V, Miller CR, et al. An adenovirus vector with genetically modified fibers demonstrates expanded tropism via utilization of a coxsackievirus and adenovirus receptor-independent cell entry mechanism. J Virol 1998; 72(12):9706–9713.
143. Wickham TJ, Roelvink PW, Brough DE, Kovesdi I. Adenovirus targeted to heparan-containing receptors increases its gene delivery efficiency to multiple cell types. Nat Biotechnol 1996; 14(11):1570–1573.
144. Biermann V, Volpers C, Hussmann S, et al. Targeting of high-capacity adenoviral vectors. Hum Gene Ther 2001; 12(14):1757–1769.
145. Michael SI, Hong JS, Curiel DT, Engler JA. Addition of a short peptide ligand to the adenovirus fiber protein. Gene Ther 1995; 2(9):660–668.
146. Mizuguchi H, Koizumi N, Hosono T, et al. A simplified system for constructing recombinant adenoviral vectors containing heterologous peptides in the HI loop of their fiber knob. Gene Ther 2001; 8(9):730–735.
147. Michael SI, Huang CH, Romer MU, Wagner E, Hu PC, Curiel DT. Binding-incompetent adenovirus facilitates molecular conjugate-mediated gene transfer by the receptor-mediated endocytosis pathway. J Biol Chem 1993; 268(10):6866–6869.
148. Reynolds P, Dmitriev I, Curiel D. Insertion of an RGD motif into the HI loop of adenovirus fiber protein alters the distribution of transgene expression of the systemically administered vector. Gene Ther 1999; 6(7):1336–1339.
149. Wickham TJ, Tzeng E, Shears LL, et al. Increased in vitro and in vivo gene transfer by adenovirus vectors containing chimeric fiber proteins. J Virol 1997; 71(11):8221–8229.
150. Wickham TJ, Carrion ME, Kovesdi I. Targeting of adenovirus penton base to new receptors through replacement of its RGD motif with other receptor-specific peptide motifs. Gene Ther 1995; 2(10):750–756.
151. Vigne E, Mahfouz I, Dedieu JF, Brie A, Perricaudet M, Yeh P. RGD inclusion in the hexon monomer provides adenovirus type 5-based vectors with a fiber knob-independent pathway for infection. J Virol 1999; 73(6):5156–5161.
152. Dmitriev IP, Kashentseva EA, Curiel DT. Engineering of adenovirus vectors containing heterologous peptide sequences in the C terminus of capsid protein IX. J Virol 2002; 76(14):6893–6899.
153. Douglas JT, Miller CR, Kim M, et al. A system for the propagation of adenoviral vectors with genetically modified receptor specificities. Nat Biotechnol 1999; 17(5):470–475.
154. Einfeld DA, Brough DE, Roelvink PW, Kovesdi I, Wickham TJ. Construction of a pseudoreceptor that mediates transduction by adenoviruses expressing a ligand in fiber or penton base. J Virol 1999; 73(11):9130–9136.
155. Belousova N, Krendelchtchikova V, Curiel DT, Krasnykh V. Modulation of adenovirus vector tropism via incorporation of polypeptide ligands into the fiber protein. J Virol 2002; 76(17):8621–8631.

156. Douglas JT, Rogers BE, Rosenfeld ME, Michael SI, Feng M, Curiel DT. Targeted gene delivery by tropism-modified adenoviral vectors. Nat Biotechnol 1996; 14(11):1574–1578.
157. Goldman CK, Rogers BE, Douglas JT, et al. Targeted gene delivery to Kaposi's sarcoma cells via the fibroblast growth factor receptor. Cancer Res 1997; 57(8):1447–1451.
158. Wickham TJ, Segal DM, Roelvink PW, et al. Targeted adenovirus gene transfer to endothelial and smooth muscle cells by using bispecific antibodies. J Virol 1996; 70(10):6831–6838.
159. Wickham TJ, Lee GM, Titus JA, et al. Targeted adenovirus-mediated gene delivery to T cells via CD3. J Virol 1997; 71(10):7663–7669.
160. Harari OA, Wickham TJ, Stocker CJ, et al. Targeting an adenoviral gene vector to cytokine-activated vascular endothelium via E-selectin. Gene Ther 1999; 6(5):801–807.
161. Heideman DA, Snijders PJ, Craanen ME, et al. Selective gene delivery toward gastric and esophageal adenocarcinoma cells via EpCAM-targeted adenoviral vectors. Cancer Gene Ther 2001; 8(5):342–351.
162. van Beusechem VW, Grill J, Mastenbroek DC, et al. Efficient and selective gene transfer into primary human brain tumors by using single-chain antibody-targeted adenoviral vectors with native tropism abolished. J Virol 2002; 76(6):2753–2762.
163. Gu DL, Gonzalez AM, Printz MA, et al. Fibroblast growth factor 2 retargeted adenovirus has redirected cellular tropism: evidence for reduced toxicity and enhanced antitumor activity in mice. Cancer Res 1999; 59(11):2608–2614.
164. Printz MA, Gonzalez AM, Cunningham M, et al. Fibroblast growth factor 2-retargeted adenoviral vectors exhibit a modified biolocalization pattern and display reduced toxicity relative to native adenoviral vectors. Hum Gene Ther 2000; 11(1):191–204.
165. Reynolds PN, Zinn KR, Gavrilyuk VD, et al. A targetable, injectable adenoviral vector for selective gene delivery to pulmonary endothelium in vivo. Mol Ther 2000; 2(6):562–578.
166. Bouri K, Feero WG, Myerburg MM, et al. Polylysine modification of adenoviral fiber protein enhances muscle cell transduction. Hum Gene Ther 1999; 10(10):1633–1640.
167. Volpers C, Thirion C, Biermann V, et al. Antibody-mediated targeting of an adenovirus vector modified to contain a synthetic immunoglobulin g-binding domain in the capsid. J Virol 2003; 77(3):2093–2104.
168. Bilbao R, Reay DP, Hughes T, et al. Fetal muscle gene transfer is not enhanced by an RGD capsid modification to high-capacity adenoviral vectors. Gene Ther 2003; 10(21):1821–1829.

18

Retroviridae-Based Gene Transfer Vectors in Duchenne Muscular Dystrophy Therapy

Michael L. Roberts and George Dickson
School of Biological Science, Royal Holloway–University of London, Egham, Surrey, U.K.

Michael Themis
Division of Biomedical Sciences, Imperial College of Science, Technology and Medicine, London, U.K.

MOLECULAR BIOLOGY OF RETROVIRAL VECTORS AND THEIR APPLICATION IN DMD

Duchenne muscular dystrophy (DMD) is a fatal, X-linked muscle wasting disease characterized by extensive cycles of muscle degeneration that arise in male patients due to mutations in the gene encoding dystrophin. The dystrophin protein, expressed from a 14 kb mRNA, serves to maintain myofiber integrity during muscle contraction by linking the actin cytoskeleton to the extracellular matrix through the dystrophin-associated protein complex (DPC). The dystrophin protein attaches to the DPC complex at its N-terminal region and anchors to actin in the myofiber cytoskeleton at its C-terminal region; the intervening central rod domain is composed of many spectrin-like repeats that act in a buffering capacity during excessive muscle force. Many of these repeat elements are actually dispensable, as the dystrophin protein in Becker muscular dystrophy (BMD) patients is truncated in this region and is encoded for by shorter mini-dystrophin mRNAs. Many BMD patients survive far longer than those with DMD, having an almost normal life expectancy, and in a number of studies viral vectors expressing dystrophin mini-genes have been constructed and shown to be of potential therapeutic value for DMD patients. As one would expect, female carriers of DMD, who have one allele of the normal dystrophin gene, only express approximately 50% of normal dystrophin levels. However, a degree of dystrophin normalization occurs so that by later years dystrophin is expressed at more than 80% of myofibers. This has been proposed to be due to the combined effects of myofiber stabilization and muscle stem cells (satellite cells or myoblasts), a natural process which could be exploited in gene therapy of DMD if integrating vectors are used as the gene transfer vehicles. For example, in DMD patients, after myofiber degeneration and satellite stem cell activation, an integrating vector could be introduced to stably transduce rapidly dividing myoblasts to provide a permanent gene therapy for this debilitating disease. One such vector with medium insert capacity that has been used in a large number of gene transfer experiments and gene therapy protocols thus far is the retroviral vector. This vector has the potential to deliver a therapeutic mini-dystrophin gene and hence provide substantial benefits to DMD patients. In this chapter we will provide a brief introduction to the molecular biology of retroviruses and a more detailed analysis of the preclinical studies that have been carried out using this vector in *mdx* mice (the standard mouse model of muscular dystrophy). Finally, we will introduce some of the more modern concepts of retroviral-mediated gene therapy that may be of particular relevance in the successful treatment of DMD.

Retroviral particles typically comprise two identical copies of single-stranded, positive sense RNA as a genome, ranging between 7 and 10 kb, which is contained within a protein shell (capsid). The capsid is surrounded by a lipid membrane from which envelope glycoproteins extrude, resulting in a total particle size between 90 and 140 µm. It is the envelope proteins that confer retroviral specificity, as they are responsible for attachment to the target cell that allows for virus internalization. The envelope-dependent tropism of retroviruses is commonly categorized into three groups: ecotropic (infects murine cells only), xenotropic (infects all cell types except those of murine origin), and amphotropic (infects cells of both murine and nonmurine lineage). Subsequent to viral entry into the cell, the RNA genome is reverse transcribed into double-stranded cDNA by the retroviral reverse transcriptase (RT). Reverse transcribed cDNA then translocates to the nucleus and integrates into the host cell genome through the action of retroviral integrase. Therefore, retroviral-mediated transduction of target cells results in stable integration of the viral genome. This is perhaps the most attractive feature of the retrovirus as a gene transfer vehicle in DMD gene therapy, which requires permanent therapeutic transgene expression.

During the life cycle of the wild-type retrovirus, production of new particles arises subsequent to the transcription of integrated viral DNA (provirus). The core proteins assemble in the cytoplasm at the plasma membrane where the RNA genome is targeted to the capsid by the packaging signal (psi). The onco-retroviral genome is divided into three regions: gag, pol, and env encoding for capsid proteins, viral enzymes, and envelope proteins, respectively (Fig. 1A). The structural genes encoded by the gag (group-specific antigen) gene are expressed in the form of a polyprotein yielding four proteins: p10 (nucleocapsid), p12, p15 (matrix protein), and p30 (capsid protein). The polymerase (*pol*) gene, lying downstream of the *gag* gene, encodes the integrase, RT, and the protease enzymes. Finally, the envelope (*env*) gene, which is downstream of the *pol* gene, also encodes a polyprotein that is cleaved by viral protease to yield gp70 (surface glycoprotein) and p15E (transmembrane protein). The entire retroviral genome encoding these structural and enzymatic proteins is flanked by two long terminal repeats (LTRs). The LTRs are essential for the initiation of viral DNA synthesis, the integration of proviral DNA, and the regulation of viral gene expression. Finally, the psi located just upstream of the gag region is an essential *cis* element during retroviral particle production. The most commonly utilized retrovirus for gene transfer applications is based on an onco-retrovirus, the Moloney murine leukemia virus (MoMLV), which has one of the simplest genomes of all the retroviruses, thus making it ideal for modification and use as a gene transfer agent.

Retroviruses are made replication incompetent and suitable for gene transfer applications by the removal of the *gag*, *pol*, and *env* genes, which are subsequently replaced by an expression cassette containing the transgene of interest (Fig. 1A). However, the essential LTR and psi *cis*-elements are retained to allow transgene expression and packaging into viral capsids during vector production. As a result, retroviral vectors are still capable of transducing a cell and expressing the foreign gene, but further viral particles can no longer be produced due to the lack of the structural and enzymatic genes. To facilitate vector production, the *gag*, *pol*, and *env* genes are provided in *trans* and introduced into murine or human cell lines to make retroviral-packaging or retroviral-producing cells. These cell lines are then transiently or stably transfected with plasmid DNA encoding the retroviral vector genome containing the therapeutic transgene. Subsequent to transfection, the viral genome is expressed, packaged, and released by the cell as a replication-incompetent retrovirus (Fig. 1C). Retroviral vector is then harvested from the culture medium and purified by ultracentrifugation, generating vector of titers in the range from 10^6 to 10^7 cfu/mL (colony forming units; as determined by the ability of the vector to stably transduce target cells generating vector-containing cell colonies). This is quite a low yield when compared to the production of vectors based on other virus types. However, there are extensive efforts to increase vector production from

(A) Genome of Retrovirus

(I)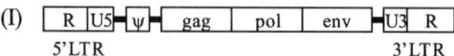

(II)

(B) Genome of Lentivirus

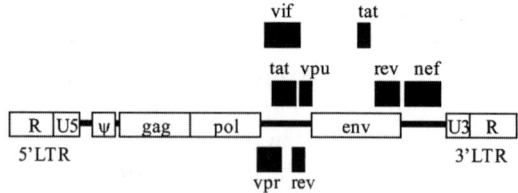

(C) Production of Retroviridae-Based Vectors

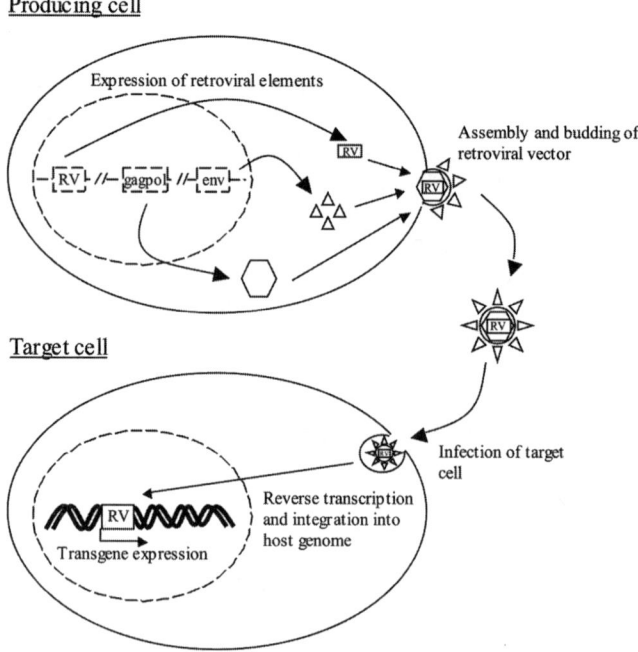

Figure 1 *(Caption on facing page)*

retroviral-producer cell lines by altering the temperature and pH at which the producer cells are cultured, by the addition of compounds that increase expression from the retroviral LTRs, e.g., sodium butyrate, or by the use of advanced cell culture facilities, e.g., the cell cube microcarrier suspension culture system and the packed or fluidized bed (1). Production of retroviral vector from stable cell lines is associated with a risk of the generation of replication competent retrovirus (RCR) that arises subsequent to the recombination of the different retroviral elements in the producer cells. To avoid this phenomenon the viral elements can be split onto at least three separate plasmids, so that one plasmid contains the therapeutic transgene-expressing viral genome, a second expresses the gag–pol polypeptide, and the third expresses the envelope protein. By doing this, three separate recombination events are necessary to generate RCR, a highly unlikely occurrence. Despite the separation of these elements onto separate plasmids, some risk of homologous recombination remains. This is because the *pol* and *env* genes are out of frame and share some common sequences, as do the psi and gag gene. To avoid this potential recombination, more recent generations of retroviral vectors contain envelope proteins derived from retroviruses isolated from a different species with dissimilar env sequences. The result of these modifications is the generation of a vector capable of highly efficient and stable transgene expression, more suited for the gene therapy of many dominantly

Figure 1 *(Facing page)* (**A**) Schematic showing the wild-type retrovirus genome (I) and that of the modified retroviral vector (II). The retroviral genome comprises three enzymatic and structural elements: gag, pol, and env flanked by a packaging signal (ψ) and two LTRs. Within the LTR there are repeat (R) regions common to both the 5′ and 3′ LTRs and unique (U) sequences present either in the 5′ (U5) or 3′ (U3) LTR only. Retroviral vectors are rendered replication incompetent by the removal of the gag, pol, and env regions, which are replaced with an expression cassette containing the therapeutic transgene. Normally the vector also contains a NeoR to allow selection of retrovirally transduced cells. The IRS allows polycistronic expression of both NeoR and transgene from the retroviral 5′ LTR. (**B**) Schematic illustrating the wild-type genome of the lentivirus. Lentiviruses comprise the basic retroviral genome, but are more complex, also expressing a number of accessory proteins illustrated by the shaded boxes. (**C**) Schematic showing production of retroviral producer cells that express RV genome, gag–pol, and env from three different expression cassettes. These expression cassettes can either be in the form of integrated or nonintegrated plasmid vectors, or in the form of other viral vector templates (e.g., adenoviral vectors). Subsequent to expression of all the retroviral elements, the vector assembles at the membrane and buds off with the host cell membrane fused with envelope components. After infection of the target cell, the RNA genome is reverse transcribed into cDNA and integrates into the genome, resulting in stable expression of the therapeutic transgene. *Abbreviations*: IRS, internal ribosome entry site; LTR, long terminal repeats; NeoR, neomycin resistance gene; RV, retroviral.

inherited monogenic disorders (such as DMD). However, onco-retroviral vectors do have some limitations. Firstly, they can only transduce rapidly dividing cells, as the reverse transcribed retroviral genome cannot enter the cell's nucleus unless the nuclear membrane is disrupted during mitosis. Secondly, subsequent to integration, the retroviral LTR that drives transgene expression is often silenced by promoter methylation, making gene expression transient in these cases. However, the most severe limitation of the use of retroviral vectors is the fact that they integrate into the host genome in a random manner. This raises the potential of insertional mutagenesis or the activation of certain oncogenes that may be adjacent to the strong retroviral promoter. Most of these problems can be overcome by the elegant manipulation of the viral genome by molecular biological techniques. However, not until some degree of site-specific integration is afforded to retroviral vectors will they be considered as the ideal gene therapy tool. In spite of this final limitation, retroviral vectors remain the most commonly used viruses in gene therapy clinical trials. In the following sections we will introduce and discuss the results of some studies that have utilized this virus with a view to developing an effective genetic therapy for the treatment of DMD.

RETROVIRAL-MEDIATED GENE DELIVERY TO MUSCLE CELLS: IN VITRO AND EX VIVO APPROACHES

In the early 1990s, a number of groups began to investigate whether retroviral vectors could transduce cells of myogenic lineage in a variety of different species. Initial studies on dog and rat primary cultures of myoblasts demonstrated a high efficiency of retroviral-mediated gene expression without any deleterious effects on myoblast differentiation (2). Indeed, genes initially expressed from the retroviral vector in myoblasts were continually expressed during the formation of mature myofibers. It was quickly demonstrated that a retroviral vector expressing a therapeutic dystrophin mini-gene could stably transduce primary cultures of *mdx* mouse myoblasts in vitro, which located directly to the sarcolemma and displayed an identical staining pattern to that displayed by normal dystrophin expressed in myoblasts isolated from wild-type mice (3). This result paved the way for studies aimed at using retroviral vectors for the gene therapy of muscular dystrophy, and a number of studies using retroviral vectors directly in the muscles of *mdx* mice were soon to follow. At the same time, in an effort to improve safety, muscle-specific retroviral-mediated expression was also being developed. In one study, promoter elements from the muscle creatinine kinase (MCK) gene were incorporated into the U3 region of the mouse MoMLV LTR to generate a virus that would express transgene only in mature muscle cells (4). The authors were able to show restricted gene expression using this construct as no retroviral-mediated gene expression occurred in immature proliferating primary cultures of human myoblasts or a mouse myogenic cell line, but was only activated upon myoblast fusion to form mature myotubes. Moreover, introduction of the retrovirally transduced human primary myoblast cells into the quadriceps muscle of immunosupressed mice resulted in expression of transgene only after the transplanted cells had fused with existing myofibers. This ability of the retrovirally-modified primary human myoblasts to successfully fuse with murine myofibers in vivo, at the same time conferring transgene expression, has been extensively explored in a number of studies, as it raises the possibility of ex vivo gene therapy for muscle-based disorders. It had previously been demonstrated that a proportion of proliferating myoblasts from patients with DMD could be isolated, transduced with retrovirus in vitro, and reimplanted into regenerating muscles of immunodeficient mice (5). However, a subsequent study demonstrated that myoblasts might not act as the most efficient vehicles for gene replacement. Myoblasts isolated from isogenic littermates expressing β-galactosidase from an adenoviral vector survived only for one month after implantation in the muscle (6). Although the authors debated that fused myofibers died from necrosis in a fashion unrelated to immune rejection, it is tempting to speculate that the myofibers were indeed targeted for immune-mediated destruction because of the adenoviral vector elements they were originally infected with. Nevertheless, the authors did demonstrate that a substantial proportion of myoblasts were lost 48 hours postinjection, thereby demonstrating the inefficiency of myoblast-mediated gene transfer. It is possible to overcome this inefficiency if stem cells are used as the donors. In one study, a myogenic stem cell line (PD50A) was isolated from *mdx* mouse muscle and transduced with retroviral vector expressing β-galactosidase (7). Transduced stem cells were then reimplanted into dystrophic muscle of *mdx* mice, and the efficiency of β-galactosidase expression was measured over time. Myofibers expressing transgene were detected for up to 14 months following implantation, and there was no evidence of tumor formation. Detailed analysis revealed that after one week the implanted cells took position on the periphery of the muscle, and they fused to form myofibers after eight weeks. The stem cell status of these transduced cells was confirmed by rederiving β-galactosidase–expressing myoblasts from transplanted muscle after one year and successfully establishing primary cultures. The results from this study hold great promise for the retroviral-mediated ex vivo gene therapy of DMD. If, as this study suggests, myogenic stem cells can be isolated from patients with DMD, transduced with retroviral vector expressing dystrophin gene constructs, and reimplanted, then the chances of immune rejection may be low. For this approach to succeed, either the efficiency of myogenic stem cell isolation from DMD patients has to be assessed or the use of stem cells derived from bone marrow or other sources, tested (see section on Cell-Based Strategies of Muscle-Directed Retroviral Delivery). In any event, there remain a number of opportunities for the application of retroviral vector–mediated gene transfer in stem cell therapy for muscular dystrophy, and future studies using ex vivo protocols may benefit from adopting the use of these pluripotent cells.

EFFICACY OF MUSCLE-DIRECTED RETROVIRAL DELIVERY IN VIVO

The ability of retroviral vectors to mediate dystrophin mini-gene expression in the muscles of *mdx* mice in vivo was first demonstrated in 1993 (8). In this study, the expression of a 6.3 kb Becker mini-dystrophin from a retroviral vector in the muscles of treated animals was shown to occur for nine months in some 6% of myofibers, provided muscle degeneration (and subsequent regeneration) was first enhanced by pretreatment with $BaCl_2$. However, further study revealed that the efficacy of retroviral vector–mediated expression of transgenes depended on the strain of mouse used, as some strains displayed less than 1% transduction following retroviral vector treatment (9). It was proposed that this was due to existing immunity to murine retroviruses present in many different populations of laboratory mice, and therefore may not be an issue when treating humans. Despite this, most studies do show a low efficiency of retroviral vector–mediated gene expression in vivo when muscle degeneration is not stimulated prior to vector administration. There are several reasons for this low efficacy of transduction. First, there is the problem of vector production. Retroviral vectors are produced by cells grown in tissue culture flasks and are harvested from the medium used to grow the cells. Large numbers of cells are required to generate sufficient titers of virus for use in vivo, and often the concentration of these vectors is low, requiring extensive ultracentrifugation. This process is unwieldy and only results in the purification of retroviral vectors to titers in the region of 10^6 cfu/mL. However, it is now possible to further increase titers up to 10-fold by pseudotyping (the process of altering retroviral tropism by switching the *env* gene). Retroviral vector pseudotyped with the VSV-G viral *env* gene can be purified to higher titers because this envelope protein withstands higher centrifugation forces than the amphotropic envelope protein (10). Also, VSV-G pseudotyped viral vector transduces target cells with higher efficiency and has a broader tropic range. This approach has been particularly effective in gene transfer protocols utilizing lentiviral vectors (see section on The Development of Lentiviral Vectors for DMD Gene Therapy), but its application to onco-retroviral vectors has still not been fully realized in muscle-directed gene therapy (despite the fact that a number of studies have demonstrated its potential in the treatment of hematopoietic disorders). Another problem previously associated with retroviral transduction in vivo is the short half-life of retrovirus viral particles. This was originally thought to be due to complement-mediated particle lysis, where human C1q interacts directly with murine retroviral particles and stimulates activation of the classical complement cascade (11). Despite observations that the development of retroviral producer cells based on human cell lines largely overcomes this problem, the short half-life (five to eight hours) of viral particles in vivo still remains a confounding issue. More recently, another immune-related problem resulting from muscle-directed retroviral gene transfer has been identified. Subsequent to intramuscular administration of a retroviral vector encoding the human immunodeficiency virus (HIV) IIIB env and rev genes, vector sequences were detected in the lymph nodes (a site not previously examined) (12). Although this result had beneficial implications to the study in question, it raised serious concerns over the potential efficiency of muscle-based retroviral vector gene therapy protocols. If intramuscularly injected retroviral vector can locate to the lymph nodes, then it is conceivable that a substantial antiretroviral immune response could subsequently be activated.

In spite of these problems, the accumulative evidence obtained from studies of the efficacy of retroviral transduction of muscle cells in vivo suggested that a proportion of viral particles do indeed stably transduce muscle satellite stem cells, and that this is enough to induce some degree of myofiber normalization and muscle remodeling. However, the efficiency of transduction still remains low. Attention has therefore switched to the development of techniques that allow the production and concentration of therapeutic retroviral vector at the pathologic site, i.e., in the diseased muscle, to allow more efficient transduction of the cells most in need of correction. In the following sections we shall discuss some of the approaches that have been adopted to achieve this goal and hence increase the efficiency of muscle-directed retroviral gene transfer.

CELL-BASED STRATEGIES OF MUSCLE-DIRECTED RETROVIRAL DELIVERY

As an alternative to the direct administration of vector preparations, retroviral producer cells can also be directly implanted into dystrophic muscle. This approach has been mainly adopted to circumvent the low efficiency of retroviral-mediated gene expression that arises because of the low vector titers achieved during the production of conventional retroviral vectors. In one study, mitotically inactive cells producing a retroviral vector expressing the 6.3 kb Becker mini-dystrophin gene were implanted into the tibialis anterior (TA) muscle of nude/*mdx* mice, and the efficiency of transgene expression and its functionality were measured at various times subsequent to administration (13). To increase the efficiency of retroviral-mediated transduction of myocytes, each muscle was first injected with $BaCl_2$ (which promotes muscle degeneration and increases the proportion of rapidly dividing myoblasts). The proportion of muscle fibers expressing the mini-dystrophin gene ranged from 6% to 19%, a significant increase from that observed previously in studies where retroviral vector preparations expressing the mini-dystrophin gene had been directly injected into tibialis anterior (TA) muscle. Having shown the efficiency of this protocol in immunosuppressed mice, immunocompetent *mdx* mice were then subjected to an immunosuppressive regime using FK506 and treated with retroviral producer cells in an identical manner. When mitosis in retroviral producer cells was inhibited with mitomycin C, the proportion of mini-dystrophin expressing fibers was found to be similar to that present in the nude/*mdx* mice. Also, the functionality of mini-dystrophin was demonstrated by its ability to restore expression of some elements of the dystrophin-associated protein complex (DPC).

However, there remain a few severe limitations in adopting this approach in the clinic. Firstly, it is unlikely that a clinical protocol will be approved that requires extensive artificial degeneration of muscle prior to retroviral administration in patients with a disease in which the major symptom is also that of muscle degeneration. Although the results from this study implied that a significant proportion of satellite stem cells were transduced with the vector, as manifested by the appearance of dystrophin-positive clusters of myofibers, without the induction of muscle degeneration, the authors suggest that the required threshold of stem cell transduction to allow muscle remodeling may be difficult to achieve during treatment. Secondly, if producer cells are able to divide, the immune system can quickly eliminate them after the immunosuppressive treatment is removed. It is unlikely that the proliferative capacity of every single cell can be inhibited permanently; therefore, the beneficial effects of this approach may be short lived. Thirdly, and most importantly, there is significant evidence to suggest that retroviral producer cells can generate palpable tumors in treated mice if they are not first treated with antimitotic agents (9). This in itself is enough to cause serious concerns over safety and the subsequent adoption of this approach in the clinic. It is largely for this reason that the use of retroviral vector producer cells in the treatment of DMD has not been taken forward, despite the high efficiency of vector transduction observed. Nevertheless, these studies have shown that if retroviral vector production is allowed to occur in situ, efficient and stable transduction of stem cells will occur resulting in a high percentage of dystrophin-expressing myofibers. With this in mind, alternative approaches allowing for in situ production of retroviral vector have been developed and will be discussed in the Modern Approaches to Muscle-Directed Retroviral Delivery section.

In modern times, with the emergence of stem cells as therapeutic tools, intravenous transplantation of bone marrow stem cells from healthy individuals may serve to act as a stable source of dystrophin-expressing muscle satellite stem cells, provided sufficient numbers of cells locate to the muscle (14). Such an approach would obviate the need for retroviral-mediated transduction ex vivo; however, as alluded to earlier, retroviral transduction of the patient's own stem cells may represent a more efficient strategy. This represents the most promising treatment regime for DMD thus far, provided a safe site of retroviral vector integration is selected prior to the readministration of modified stem cells to the patient. Intravenous transplantation of whole bone marrow and hematopoietic and muscle-derived stem cells from wild-type C57BL/10 mice have been shown to reconstitute lethally irradiated *mdx* recipients with all myeloid cell lineages, thus demonstrating the feasibility of adopting a bone marrow transplant approach for the treatment of DMD. In terms of therapeutic value, up to 10% of muscle fibers from the TA muscle in recipient mice were found to express dystrophin derived from these donors after three months (14). In a separate study, a similar level of dystrophin expression (12%) in *mdx* mice, intra-arterially transplanted with muscle-derived cells, was only shown to occur subsequent to severe muscle damage in muscle groups near the injected artery (15). Although stem cell–mediated therapy of DMD holds great promise, a recent study has demonstrated the extremely low efficiency of this technique in the *mdx^{4cv}* mouse model (16). The *mdx^{4cv}* model has a stop codon mutation in exon 53 of the dystrophin gene, preventing the formation of revertant dystrophin-expressing fibers that arise after exon skipping and allowing the expression of truncated functional forms of dystrophin. Less than 1% of muscle fibers were found to express dystrophin at any given time, over 10 months, in *mdx^{4cv}* mice injected with whole bone marrow cells. The cumulative data from these studies would suggest that stem cell–mediated recruitment of dystrophin-expressing myoblasts to dystrophic muscle might only occur through revertant fibers. If this were proven, then the application of this therapy in the treatment of DMD will be extremely limited.

It has also been proposed that circulating monocytes may be able to deliver dystrophin constructs to the site of muscle degeneration provided they can be induced to produce retroviral vector (17). During the degeneration of skeletal muscle, large numbers of monocytes and macrophages that act to clear muscle cell debris infiltrate the damaged tissue. Using a hybrid HSV-1 amplicon/retroviral vector system, Parrish et al. (18) were able to convert a monocyte/macrophage cell line into retroviral producing cells releasing retroviral vectors capable of transducing dividing myoblasts. However, the overall efficiency of this technique was found to be extremely low as less than 0.1% of myoblasts were transduced by retroviral vectors produced from macrophages. This was likely a consequence of the toxicity that the HSV-1 vector conferred on the producer monocytes coupled with the low level of HSV-1–mediated monocyte infection (approximately 1% of monocytes were proposed to be producer cells). Therefore, other means of achieving this goal have been explored. Given the high efficiency of adenoviral-mediated human monocyte/macrophage infection, it has also been proposed to use adenoviruses as templates in retroviral vector production (see section on Modern Approaches to Muscle-Directed Retroviral Delivery) with a similar monocyte-mediated targeting approach. In preliminary studies, monocyte/macrophages infected with hybrid adeno-retroviral vectors expressing green fluorescent protein (GFP) were able to produce enough retroviral vectors capable of transducing proliferating cultures of primary myoblasts from the *mdx* mouse (19). A fourfold increase was observed in GFP expression in myotubes cocultured with macrophages producing retroviral vector over those infected with adenoviral vector only. However, retroviral vector production was also found to be extremely inefficient in monocyte/macrophages when using the adeno-retroviral vector system, presumably because adenoviral infection of macrophages results in the release of cytokines, which may attenuate expression of the retroviral LTR (20–22). It will be necessary to optimize this method by employing retroviral elements with hybrid CMV/LTR promoters and adenoviral vectors with increased deletions and lower cytotoxicity before examining its feasibility in vivo.

MODERN APPROACHES TO MUSCLE-DIRECTED RETROVIRAL DELIVERY

In an attempt to circumvent the problems associated with inefficient in vivo retroviral vector delivery in muscle and the safety concerns over introducing retroviral vector producer cells into diseased muscle, hybrid adeno-retroviral vectors have been used in preclinical studies in the *mdx* mouse model. Generation of functional retroviral vectors using adenoviral vector templates is a two-step process. Target cells are first infected with adenoviruses expressing retrovirus structural genes and provirus sequences (Fig. 1C). Adenovirus-infected cells then produce and release functional retroviral vectors which then transduce neighboring cells, resulting in the stable integration of the therapeutic gene. These vectors were initially developed and tested in murine models of cancer. The first hybrid adeno-retroviral system consisted of two adenoviral vectors, one expressing the retroviral genome with reporter gene and a second expressing a gag–pol–env polyprotein (23,24). Despite the observation that adenoviral-infected cells were capable of producing retroviral vectors, the overall efficiency of production was low, but encouragingly, the ability of adenoviral templates to mediate retroviral vector production in vivo was demonstrated.

Further studies revealed that by splitting the gag–pol–env element onto two separate adenoviral vectors, the efficiency of retroviral vector production could be improved (25). Thus one adenovirus expressed the retroviral genome, another expressed the gag–pol polyprotein, and the third expressed the envelope protein. Not only was retroviral vector production increased, but the safety was also improved and the resultant retroviral vectors could be pseudotyped just by changing the adenoviral vector element that expressed the *env* gene. Subsequently, a number of groups used this system to assess the ability of different cell types to produce retroviral vector, and to test which elements of retroviral vector production were rate limiting (26,27). It was found by this system that too much expression of the gag products is inhibitory to retroviral vector production (27). Using adenovirus templates to produce retroviral vector in this manner offers an opportunity to produce retroviral vector in situ from autologous cells, thereby reducing complement-mediated lysis and increasing the efficiency of retroviral vector transduction at the target site. The following aspect of DMD pathology makes it an ideal target for gene therapy using in situ delivery of retroviral vectors. Muscle fibers not expressing dystrophin degenerate and are subsequently replaced by proliferating myoblast stem cells during regeneration. If existing muscle fibers were allowed to act as a platform for retroviral production, myoblasts that are proliferating during the course of muscle regeneration could be transduced by the newly produced retroviral vector in the surrounding milieu.

In pilot experiments using differentiated and undifferentiated C2C12 myocytes, three adenoviral vectors expressing gag–pol, 10A1-env, and a retroviral genome encoding eGFP transgene were coinfected into cultures in vitro and the efficacy of retroviral vector production was measured at different times (28). It was found that retroviral vector production occurred best in nonproliferating myocytes, and titers were achievable that were similar to those obtained using conventional stable-transduced retroviral producer cells. The observation that mature postmitotic myotubules were more efficient at producing functional retroviral vectors in vitro implied that this approach could be expanded in vivo, as the majority of myocytes in mature muscle exist as postmitotic myofibers. Further experiments using the same hybrid adeno-retroviral vector system, but with the eGFP transgene replaced with one encoding β-galactosidase, revealed that retroviral vector production mediated from adenoviral vector templates could also occur in situ at the site of pathological muscle in *mdx* mice (29). Initial experiments revealed that myocyte cultures derived from TA muscle originally injected with the hybrid vector cassettes were stably transduced with a retroviral vector provirus expressing β-galactosidase. Up to 50 colonies of stably transduced myocytes could be obtained from each hybrid vector injected TA muscle, and direct visualization of injected TA muscle sections revealed a five-fold increase in β-galactosidase expression compared to muscles injected with the adenoviral vector alone. The expression of β-galactosidase was transient when mice over four weeks of age were used. Presumably, this was due to a strong immune response to the adenoviral elements of the hybrid system and to the transgene sequence itself.

This is a problem which confounds the majority of gene therapy protocols based on adenoviral vectors, and is just beginning to be addressed with the development of fully gutted adenoviral vectors that contain only structural proteins. After having achieved efficient transgene expression by using reporter constructs, attention focused on the employment of hybrid adeno-retroviral vectors expressing therapeutic dystrophin constructs, in an attempt to correct the dystrophic pathology of *mdx* mice. TA muscles from mice at different ages were injected with hybrid adeno-retroviral vectors expressing a highly truncated microdystrophin construct, and its ability to reverse the dystrophic phenotype was assessed after one and three months. The most striking results were achieved in the muscles of mice that were injected at a very early age (six or seven days old); this approach was adopted to avoid the immune response observed in the studies using the β-galactosidase reporter construct. One month following injection, some mice expressed microdystrophin in nearly 70% of muscle fibers, which was further detected in the context of an integrated provirus in the muscle cell genomic DNA.

The functionality of the microdystrophin construct was demonstrated by its ability to attenuate muscle degeneration as assessed by the extent of centrally nucleated myofibers and the observed restoration of the DPC complex. This initial high efficiency of microdystrophin expression was most likely due to a combination of adenoviral- and retroviral-mediated transduction of muscle cells and may serve to allow rapid muscle remodeling of dystrophic tissue prior to the stable transduction of diseased tissue over time, mediated by the retroviral vector. Three months following injection, the microdystrophin construct was still expressed in the vast majority of myofibers in the TA muscle and the amount of integrated proviruses had increased from those observed at one month. At the same time there was a substantial decrease in expression of microdystrophin in the muscles injected with adenoviral vector alone.

The development of microdystrophin constructs has largely progressed so that adeno-associated viral (AAV) vectors can be used in the gene therapy of DMD (30). Recombinant AAV vectors have become the vectors of choice in most gene therapy protocols because of their ability to persist in a wide variety of human and animal tissues, particularly skeletal muscle, without eliciting an overt immune response. Owing to its small capsid size, AAV vectors accommodate less than 5 kb of exogenous DNA, making them far too small to package the 14 kb dystrophin cDNA. With this in mind, dystrophin microgenes have been constructed that can be accommodated into this small viral vector (see Chapter 18). Most of these constructs have been modeled on the truncated form of partially functional dystrophins found in BMD patients. Dystrophin microgenes are between 3.5 and 4.7 kb in size and contain extensive deletions in the spectrin-like repeats found in the central rod domain of dystrophin. The therapeutic value of these microgenes has been demonstrated by their ability to restore DPC complex expression at the sarcolemma, prevent muscle degeneration as assessed by their ability to effect a reduction in centrally nucleated myofibers in the muscles of *mdx* mice, and improve physiological function. Therefore, these microconstructs represent an ideal means to restore force-generating capacity in the muscles of DMD patients when using improved vectors with limited capacity, such as the AAV and the hybrid adeno-retrovirus, capable of efficient and long-term expression in diseased muscle.

The combined observations from studies using hybrid adeno-retroviral vectors have revitalized the hopes of employing retroviral vectors in gene therapy of muscular dystrophies. The hybrid vectors employed in these initial studies were based on first-generation adenoviral and second-generation retroviral vectors, and were designed with a view to test the feasibility of the hybrid vector approach in the treatment of DMD. We await the development of less immunogenic hybrid adeno-retroviral vectors. Such vectors should be based on adenoviruses with more deletions for expanded capacity, allowing the expression of mini-dystrophin genes based on the Becker dystrophin gene, and the incorporation of retroviral vectors with improved safety to permit myofiber-specific expression with reduced chances of recombination to generate the RCR and of activation of host cell oncogenes. Once these vectors have been constructed and tested in mouse models, the use of adeno-retroviral vectors in the treatment of DMD and other muscular dystrophies holds great promise.

THE DEVELOPMENT OF LENTIVIRAL VECTORS FOR DMD GENE THERAPY

Long-term gene expression in several affected muscles groups is an important prerequisite for permanent correction of DMD. Although onco-retroviruses show promising potential to achieve this, they are hampered by the need for nuclear envelope disruption during mitosis, the occurrence of promoter shutdown following proviral integration, and the limited size of the inserted foreign DNA. Lentivirus-derived retroviral vectors have an advantage over onco-retroviral vectors in that they are able to integrate their genetic cargo into the genome of nondividing cells, are relatively nonimmunogenic, and have the capacity to accommodate a variety of dystrophin truncations (31,32). The potential of lentivirus vectors to transduce nondividing cells was demonstrated by Naldini et al. (31) using HIV type 1–derived vectors. In addition, gene expression in vitro and in vivo was accomplished with vectors pseudotyped with the VSV-G envelope (33,34). Lentiviruses are a subgroup of the retrovirus family and share the structural and enzymatic genes coding for *gag*, *pol*, and *env* polyproteins common to all retroviruses (Fig. 1B). Modified lentivirus vectors have been developed for gene therapy as potential alternatives to HIV-1, notably to circumvent the use of a vector based on a natural human pathogen. These lentiviruses include those that are based on feline immunodeficiency virus (FIV), equine infectious anemia virus (EIAV), bovine immunodeficiency (BIV), and HIV-2. HIV-1 has been the most extensively characterized of the lentiviruses, and has therefore been the most successful vector system developed. The derivation of the HIV-1 vector has been extensively reviewed by Barker and Planelles (35) and by Quinonez and Sutton (36).

Similar to MoMLV vectors, the HIV genome has been "split" into *cis*- and *trans*-acting components. The *cis*-acting RNA, characterized as being devoid of viral coding sequences, is crucial to vector design and is often described as the virus backbone. It is this backbone that has been engineered to contain foreign or therapeutic genes that will integrate into the host cell genome. The *trans*-acting genes, which have been removed from the virus, are provided on plasmid vectors and are used to generate "defective" viral particles by the transfection of human embryonic kidney 293 T cells with the backbone-containing plasmid. The HIV genome is complex as it contains regulatory and accessory genes known to control not only viral gene expression, but also the movement of viral cDNA, after reverse transcription, into the nucleus of the infected host, the assembly of new viral particles, and the structure and function of the infected cell. These *trans*-acting viral elements encode the structural *gag*, *pol*, and *env* genes, regulatory *tat* and *rev* genes, and the accessory genes *vif*, *vpr*, *vpu*, and *nef* (Fig. 1B).

The Gag protein is the initial product of translated, unspliced mRNA that is then cleaved, giving rise to matrix (MA) p17, capsid (CA) p24, nucleocapsid (NC) p7 protein, and the p6 polyproline-rich protein. MA is involved in virus assembly and in the process of infection of nondividing cells; CA is a viral core protein also involved in virus assembly and maturation; NC associates closely with the viral RNA. The p6 protein is involved in virus release from the cell and the incorporation of the Vpr protein into the mature virus particle. A viral protease (PR) is required for Gag and Gag–pol cleavage to provide proteins for virus maturation. RT has RNA-dependent polymerase, RNase H, and DNA-dependent DNA polymerase activities to generate viral cDNA before being integrated into the host genome using the HIV-1 integrase (IN) enzyme.

The *tat* gene is important in the HIV life cycle, producing a regulatory protein that interacts with a *trans*-activation response element (TAR) located in the 5′ LTR region of nascent viral RNA. This interaction mediates viral transcription for early replication of the virus genome. Viral mRNAs are produced in two forms, either as unspliced mRNA for packaging into new virions, or spliced mRNAs for viral gene expression. Rev contains a nuclear export signal and interacts with a Rev-response element (RRE) on viral RNAs. This allows mRNA export with the help of cellular nuclear transport mechanisms. The viral Env protein is cleaved to form gp120, which naturally binds to CD4. The nonessential accessory genes *vif*, *vpr*, *vpu*, and *nef* are dispensable and their omission provides additional space for foreign gene insertion into the virus backbone.

Several modifications have been used to produce safe, high titer HIV-1–based lentivirus vectors for potential therapeutic use. First generation HIV-1 vectors, created by Naldini and coworkers (37), were based on the development of HIV-1 vectors in several laboratories. The early HIV-1 vectors were improved to create high titer virus by separating the *trans*- and *cis*-acting elements onto discrete plasmids and by modification of the vector backbone by deleting *vpu*. This system used the cytomegalovirus (CMV) immediate–early enhancer/promoter to drive the expression of viral components required to generate defective genome-encapsulated viral particles. Also by deleting the viral 3' LTR and replacing it with a cellular polyadenylation sequence, the likelihood of producing replication-competent lentivirus (RCL) by recombination between the plasmids carrying the *cis* and *trans* elements was reduced. An internal promoter was then used to drive transgene expression from the vector. To produce high viral titers, the VSV-G envelope was used to pseudotype HIV-1 particles from transiently transfected 293T cells as previously reported for MoMLV vectors (38).

As the theoretical risk of RCL still remains, due to homology between viral elements present on packaging constructs and the viral backbone, the second generation HIV-1 system was produced by removal of all accessory genes from the packaging vector (37,39). To reduce the risk of RCL further, an additional *trans*-acting packaging plasmid was used to express *rev*. Also, a chimeric LTR was used in the defective genome which allowed independence from *tat* control, after which alternative internal promoters were used to drive gene expression (40). Furthermore, the CMV immediate–early enhancer/promoter replaced the 5' U3 of the LTR. An additional safety consideration is the potential to activate host genes by the virus LTR near the site of provirus insertion. To reduce this risk, self-inactivating (SIN) vectors have been created. This was accomplished by introducing deletions in the 3' LTR, which naturally becomes part of the 5' LTR after reverse transcription to render both 5' and 3' LTRs inactive. Gene expression from the provirus is subsequently achieved using internal promoters. Augmented gene expression has since been accomplished by the addition of the woodchuck hepatitis virus post-transcriptional regulatory element (WPRE) at the 3' end of the vector (41).

Kafri et al. (42) have reported the potential of the HIV-1 system for gene delivery to muscle. These studies showed significant gene transfer with long-term gene expression in adult wild-type Fischer rats following hind-leg injection of VSV-G–pseudotyped HIV-1 particles carrying the GFP reporter gene, without sufficient cellular or humoral immune responses to inhibit repeat injection of the vector. Interestingly, little or no muscle gene expression was observed with MoMLV virus using the same pseudotype. Another potential advantage of lentiviruses is the ease by which different envelopes can be used for altered tissue tropism. Pseudotyping to improve specific gene transfer to muscle cells using lentiviruses has been demonstrated recently by MacKenzie et al. (43), who compared VSV-G-, Ebola-, and Mokola-pseudotyped HIV-1–based vectors carrying the β-galactosidase reporter gene for direct intramuscular injection in utero. In a similar study in neonatal mice, Kobinger et al. (44) extended the number of pseudotypes investigated to include rabies, MoMLV, and lymphocytic choriomeningitis (LCMV) envelope proteins. Not surprisingly, the intramuscular route of injection restricted expression primarily to the site of the injected muscles, while other muscle groups necessary for the treatment of DMD were poorly transduced or nontransduced.

Gene expression by HIV-1 vectors has also been maintained over long periods following intramuscular injection to fetal and adult mice and rats (42–45). Because gene transfer to postmitotic muscle may eventually lead to loss of dystrophin following muscle damage or repair, and because degeneration and regeneration would occur throughout life, gene transfer to muscle stem cells may be necessary. Lentiviral vectors have previously been reported to transduce hematopoietic stem cells (46,47). Recently, Kobinger et al. (44) has extended this in newborn *mdx* mice by using an ebola pseudotype. HIV-1 vector carrying dystrophin to muscle satellite cells was shown to be capable of regenerating functional skeletal muscle. Interestingly, only partial phenotypic correction was observed using the HIV-1–based vector, whereas more comprehensive muscle fiber correction was found using a MoMLV vector pseudotyped with this envelope. MoMLV appeared to transduce mature muscle fibers in addition to muscle satellite cells. In the adult *mdx* mouse, HIV-1 pseudotyped with the mokola envelope provided protection to injury but did not protect from deterioration in contractile forces following rounds of eccentric contractions.

With the development of safer forms of the HIV-1–based vector, several alternative lentivirus systems, and the ability to pseudotype vectors for improved muscle gene transfer, the permanent treatment of DMD is becoming closer to reality. Experiments using the *mdx* model mouse are beginning to show proof of principle that correction may be attainable even without immune responses to the vector or dystrophin transgene.

FUTURE PROSPECTS

The accumulated data on the use of retroviral vectors in preclinical studies suggest that this vector is well suited as a gene delivery vehicle for the treatment of DMD. Over the past decade, significant progress has been made in the application of these vectors to degenerating regions of dystrophic muscle. During this time, we have witnessed successful retroviral-mediated stable introduction of therapeutic dystrophin to myoblasts in vitro (raising the possibility of ex vivo gene therapy approaches), the direct application of retroviral vectors to dystrophic muscle in vivo, the development of improved cell-based means to produce vector at the pathologic site, and the ability of hybrid adeno-retroviral vectors to mediate efficient retroviral production in situ. Given the rapid advances in this field, it is only a matter of time before retroviral vectors are tested in the clinic for DMD. In recent months, safety considerations related to the future use of this vector in the clinic have come under renewed scrutiny. In the only real success story of gene therapy thus far, the retroviral-mediated cure of children suffering from X-linked severe combined immunodeficiency disorder (X-SCID), a setback has occurred. Several patients treated with autologous cells stably expressing the gamma chain receptor (γc) in T cells, mediated by ex vivo transduction by a retroviral vector, have gone on to develop leukemia as a direct result of retroviral vector integration (48). In two cases the vector sequences were found to integrate adjacent to the *LMO2* gene (previously associated with leukemia), thus promoting the rapid selective proliferation of these cells and the development of leukemia. It has been suggested that the adverse effects might be specific to the X-SCID trials due to cooperation between *LMO2* and γc, thus promoting selection of transduced T cells. In the treatment of fatal disorders such as DMD, the risk of adverse vector-mediated side effects has to be balanced against the ultimate fatality of the disease. It is unlikely that DMD patients treated with retroviral vector will develop leukemia, as it is the myogenic stem cells in the patient's muscles that will be targeted. Nevertheless, there remains the risk of development of myogenic-derived tumors, although the utilization of muscle promoters capable of regulating transgene expression only in differentiated myofibers may further reduce this risk. Until retroviral vectors with restrictive integrative capacity and improved safety are constructed, it is unlikely that they will be extensively adopted in the clinic. Rather, they will probably be reserved for the treatment of genetic disorders with the worst clinical prognosis. Given the rate at which gene transfer vector technology is proceeding, it is highly likely that safe retroviral vectors with specific integrative capacity will one day be developed.

For lentiviral-mediated gene correction, it remains clear that further vector development is required. Intense research is currently underway to further improve vector safety and to understand the mechanisms that give rise to adverse effects caused by integration into the host genome and neoplastic development. As in the case of retroviral vectors, such questions must be addressed before the use of lentiviruses in the clinic becomes widespread, with the knowledge that retroviruses gave rise to the early identification of several oncogenes and that proviral involvement in gene activation or inactivation is possible. The potential of such vectors in the treatment of genetic diseases has entered a new phase of research, and it is the question of safety that must now be addressed.

REFERENCES

1. McTaggart S, Al-Rubeai M. Retroviral vectors for human gene delivery. Biotech Adv 2002; 20:1–31.
2. Smith BF, Hoffman RK, Giger U, Wolfe JH. Genes transferred by retroviral vectors into normal and mutant myoblasts in primary cultures are expressed in myotubes. Mol Cell Biol 1990; 10:3268–3271.

3. Dunckley MG, Love DR, Davies KE, Walsh FS, Morris GE, Dickson G. Retroviral-mediated transfer of a dystrophin minigene into mdx mouse myoblasts in vitro. FEBS Lett 1992; 296:128–134.
4. Ferrari G, Salvatori G, Rossi C, Cossu G, Mavilio F. A retroviral vector containing a muscle-specific enhancer drives gene expression only in differentiated muscle fibers. Hum Gene Ther 1995; 6:733–742.
5. Salvatori G, Ferrari G, Mezzogiorno A, et al. Retroviral vector-mediated gene transfer into human primary myogenic cells leads to expression in muscle fibers in vivo. Hum Gene Ther 1993; 4:713–723.
6. Huard J, Acsadi G, Jani A, Massie B, Karpati G. Gene transfer into skeletal muscles by isogenic myoblasts. Hum Gene Ther 1994; 5:949–958.
7. Smith J, Schofield PN. Stable integration of an mdx skeletal muscle cell line into dystrophic (mdx) skeletal muscle: evidence for stem cell status. Cell Growth Differ 1997; 8:927–934.
8. Dunckley MG, Wells DJ, Walsh FS, Dickson G. Direct retroviral-mediated transfer of a dystrophin minigene into mdx mouse muscle in vivo. Hum Mol Genet 1993; 2:717–723.
9. Fassati A, Wells DJ, Walsh FS, Dickson G. Efficiency of in vivo gene transfer using murine retroviral vectors is strain dependent in mice. Hum Gene Ther 1995; 6:1177–1183.
10. Yee JK, Friedmann T, Burns JC. Generation of high-titer pseudotyped retroviral vectors with very broad host range. Meth Cell Biol 1994; 43: 99–112.
11. Cooper NR, Jensen FC, Welsh RM Jr, Oldstone MB. Lysis of RNA tumor viruses by human serum: direct antibody-independent triggering of the classical complement pathway. J Exp Med 1976; 144:970–984.
12. Kamantigue E, Edwards W III, Chada S, et al. Evidence for localization of biologically active recombinant retroviral vector to lymph nodes in mice injected intramuscularly. Gene Ther 1996; 3:128–136.
13. Fassati A, Wells DJ, Serpente PAS, et al. Genetic correction of dystrophin deficiency and skeletal muscle remodelling in adult mdx mouse via transplantation of retroviral producer cells. J Clin Invest 1997; 100:620–628.
14. Gussoni E, Soneoka Y, Strickland CD, et al. Dystrophin expression in the mdx mouse restored by stem cell transplantation. Nature 1997; 401:390–394.
15. Torrente Y, Tremblay JP, Pisati F, et al. Intraarterial injection of muscle-derived CD34(+)Sca-1(+) stem cells restores dystrophin in mdx mice. J Cell Biol 2001; 152:335–348.
16. Ferrari G, Stornaiuolo A, Mavilio F. Failure to correct murine muscular dystrophy. Nature 2001; 411:1014–1015.
17. Parrish EP, Cifuentes-Diaz C, et al. Targeting widespread sites of damage in dystrophic muscle: engrafted macrophages as potential shuttles. Gene Ther 1996; 3:13–20.
18. Parrish E, Peltekian E, Dickson G, Epstein AL, Garcia L. Cell engineering for muscle gene therapy: Extemporaneous production of retroviral vector packaging macrophages using defective herpes simplex virus type 1 vectors harbouring *gag, pol, env* genes. Cytotechnology 1999; 30:173–180.

19. Roberts ML, Patterson S, Dickson G. Integrating vector and stem cell-based strategies for gene therapy of Duchenne muscular dystrophy. Gene Ther Mol Biol 2001; 6:183–194.
20. Kristoffersen AK, Sindre H, Mandi Y, Rollag H, Degre M. Effect of adenovirus 2 on cellular gene activation in blood-derived monocytes and macrophages. APMIS 1997; 105:402–409.
21. Zhang Y, Chirmule N, Gao GP, et al. Acute cytokine response to systemic adenoviral vectors in mice is mediated by dendritic cells and macrophages. Mol Ther 2001; 3:697–707.
22. Kitamura M. Bystander macrophages silence transgene expression driven by the retroviral long terminal repeat. Biochem Biophys Res Commun 1999; 257:74–78.
23. Feng M, Jackson WH, Goldman CK, et al. Stable in vivo gene transduction via a novel adenoviral/retroviral chimeric vector. Nature Biotech 1997; 15:866–870.
24. Caplen NJ, Higginbotham JN, Scheel JR, et al. Adeno-retroviral chimeric viruses as in vivo transducing agents. Gene Ther 1999; 6:454–459.
25. Lin X. Construction of new retroviral producer cells from adenoviral and retroviral vectors. Gene Ther 1998; 5:1251–1258.
26. Ramsey WJ, Caplen NJ, Li Q, Higginbotham JN, Shah M, Blaese RM. Adenovirus vectors as transcomplementing templates for the production of replication defective retroviral vectors. Biochem Biophys Res Commun 1998; 246:912–919.
27. Duisit G, Salvetti A, Moullier P, Cosset FL. Functional characterization of adenoviral/retroviral chimeric vectors and their use for efficient screening of retroviral producer cell lines. Hum Gene Ther 1999; 10:189–200.
28. Roberts ML, Athanasopoulos T, Pohlschmidt M, Duisit G, Cosset FL, Dickson G. Post-mitotic, differentiated myotubes efficiently produce retroviral vector from adeno-retrovirus templates. Gene Ther 2001; 8:1580–1586.
29. Roberts ML, Wells DJ, Graham IR, et al. Stable micro-dystrophin gene transfer using an integrating adeno-retroviral hybrid vector ameliorates the dystrophic pathology in mdx mouse muscle. Hum Mol Genet 2002; 11:1719–1730.
30. Roberts ML, Dickson G. The future of Duchenne muscular dystrophy gene therapy: shrinking the dystrophin gene. Curr Opin Mol Ther 2002; 4:343–348.
31. Naldini L, Blomer U, Gallay P, et al. In vivo gene delivery and stable transduction of nondividing cells by a lentiviral vector. Science 1996; 272:263–267.
32. Naldini L, Verma IM. Lentiviral vectors. Adv Virus Res 2000; 55:599–609.
33. Naldini L, Blomer U, Gage FH, Trono D, Verma IM. Efficient transfer, integration, and sustained long-term expression of the transgene in adult rat brains injected with a lentiviral vector. Proc Natl Acad Sci USA 1996; 93:11382–11388.
34. Blomer U, Naldini L, Kafri T, Trono D, Verma IM, Gage FH. Highly efficient and sustained gene transfer in adult neurons with a lentivirus vector. J Virol 1997; 71:6641–6649.
35. Barker E, Planelles V. Vectors derived from the human immunodeficiency virus, HIV-1. Front Biosci 2003; 8:d491–d510.
36. Quinonez R, Sutton RE. Lentiviral vectors for gene delivery into cells. DNA Cell Biol 2002; 21:937–951.

37. Zufferey R, Nagy D, Mandel RJ, Naldini L, Trono D. Multiply attenuated lentiviral vector achieves efficient gene delivery in vivo. Nat Biotechnol 1997; 15:871–875.
38. Burns JC, Friedmann T, Driever W, Burrascano M, Yee JK. Vesicular stomatitis virus G glycoprotein pseudotyped retroviral vectors: concentration to very high titer and efficient gene transfer into mammalian and nonmammalian cells. Proc Natl Acad Sci USA 1993; 90:8033–8037.
39. Kim VN, Mitrophanous K, Kingsman SM, Kingsman AJ. Minimal requirement for a lentivirus vector based on human immunodeficiency virus type 1. J Virol 1998; 72:811–816.
40. Dull T, Zufferey R, Kelly M, et al. A third-generation lentivirus vector with a conditional packaging system. J Virol 1998; 72:8463–8471.
41. Zufferey R, Donello JE, Trono D, Hope TJ. Woodchuck hepatitis virus posttranscriptional regulatory element enhances expression of transgenes delivered by retroviral vectors. J Virol 1999; 73:2886–2892.
42. Kafri T, Blomer U, Peterson DA, Gage FH, Verma IM. Sustained expression of genes delivered directly into liver and muscle by lentiviral vectors. Nat Genet 1997; 17:314–317.
43. MacKenzie TC, Kobinger GP, Kootstra NA, et al. Efficient transduction of liver and muscle after in utero injection of lentiviral vectors with different pseudotypes. Mol Ther 2002; 6:349–358.
44. Kobinger GP, Louboutin JP, Barton ER, Sweeney HL, Wilson JM. Correction of the dystrophic phenotype by in vivo targeting of muscle progenitor cells. Hum Gene Ther 2003; 14:1441–1449.
45. Seppen J, Barry SC, Harder B, Osborne WR. Lentivirus administration to rat muscle provides efficient sustained expression of erythropoietin. Blood 2001; 98:594–596.
46. Hu J, Dunbar CE. Update on hematopoietic stem cell gene transfer using nonhuman primate models. Curr Opin Mol Ther 2002; 4:482–490.
47. Demaison C, Parsley K, Brouns G, et al. High-level transduction and gene expression in hematopoietic repopulating cells using a human immunodeficiency [correction of imunodeficiency] virus type 1-based lentiviral vector containing an internal spleen focus forming virus promoter. Hum Gene Ther 2002; 13:803–813.
48. Kaiser J. Seeking the cause of induced leukaemia's in X-SCID trial. Science 2003; 299:495.

19

Gene Therapy of Muscular Dystrophy Using Adeno-Associated Viral Vectors: Promises and Limitations

Michael J. Blankinship, Paul Gregorevic, and Jeffrey S. Chamberlain

Department of Neurology, Senator Paul D. Wellstone Muscular Dystrophy Cooperative Research Center, University of Washington School of Medicine, Seattle, Washington, U.S.A.

OVERVIEW

Gene therapy vectors based on adeno-associated virus (AAV) have garnered much attention for the potential treatment of Duchenne muscular dystrophy (DMD). These vectors are attractive due to their production characteristics, demonstrated muscle tropism, long lasting expression, and relatively low, but not absent, immunogenicity. In this chapter, we introduce some basic information on AAV and its recombinant vector (rAAV) derivatives and discuss their potential applications to gene therapy for DMD.

AAV: THE GENOME AND CAPSID

AAV is a member of the Parvoviridae viral family, commonly called parvoviruses. Parvoviridae includes two classes, the Densovirinae, which are native to insects, and the Parvovirinae, which are native to vertebrates (1). AAV is also classified as a Dependovirus, a group of nonautonomous parvoviruses whose replication requires coinfection with a second virus, such as adenovirus or herpes virus, to supply necessary helper functions in trans (2–4). AAV was identified in the 1960s as a contaminant in adenoviral preparations, and since then several unique serotypes have been identified (3,5–9). Though many individuals harbor detectable levels of AAV genomes in various tissues and are sero-positive against one or more of the serotypes, AAV has not been identified as the causative agent of any human pathology (10,11). Even though the vast majority of recombinant AAV (rAAV) genomes exist within cells as episomes, rAAV expression has lasted beyond four years in animal models (12,13).

AAV is a single stranded DNA virus. The wild-type genome is approximately 4.7 kilobases (kb) in length (14). The virus packages both DNA strands with equal fidelity (15,16). The genome is capped on both the 5′ and 3′ ends with inverted terminal repeats (ITRs) of approximately 150 base pairs (16,17). These ITRs form double stranded secondary structure, critical for stability, and are involved in priming genome replication through a "rolling hair pin" (18,19). The ITRs also function as a necessary and sufficient packaging signal and are generally the only regions from the wild-type genome included in rAAVs (19,20). AAV's genome codes for two open reading frames (ORFs) termed Rep and Cap (14). The Rep ORF, through splicing and the use of alternative promoters, produces various Rep proteins that are involved in viral replication and integration (20–22). The Cap reading frame codes for the three viral coat proteins, VP1, VP2, and VP3, which make up the capsid in an approximate ratio of 1:1:10. The capsid is proteinaceous, nonenveloped, and has T1 icosahedral symmetry with a diameter in the 20- to 25-nm range (23,24). Though phosphorylated, the capsid proteins appear to be devoid of other modifications such as glycosylation. The crystal structure of the commonly used AAV2 serotype capsid has been solved (23).

AAV SEROTYPES

Nine different serotypes of AAV have been reported, which have been grouped into multiple clades, although there are likely more (5,7–9,25,26). Some serotypes are highly similar, such as AAV1 and AAV6, whose capsid proteins share over 99% amino acid identity (7). They can also be very divergent, such as AAV2 and AAV5 (27,28). Vectors based on all of these serotypes have been developed; however, vectors based on AAV2 are by far the most common and well characterized. rAAV2 vectors have been used in several human clinical trials with no reports of serious adverse events (29–31). Despite the common usage of rAAV2 vectors, vectors based on the capsids of alternate serotypes often demonstrate greater levels of transduction in many tissues (32–34). For example, transduction of the musculature, to treat diseases such as DMD, is far more efficient (up to 500-fold) with rAAV1, rAAV5, or rAAV6 vectors than with the more commonly used rAAV2

(32,35,36). Capsids of several of the more recently described serotypes, such as AAV7 and AAV8, may also demonstrate high levels of muscle transduction (8). This feature could translate into important advantages in production and safety by enabling a lower required vector dose merely by utilizing the optimal serotype.

rAAV CLONING AND PRODUCTION

rAAV genomes are produced by flanking the expression cassette of interest with the AAV ITRs (Fig. 1A). The ITR sequence allows for genome replication by Rep and acts as a signal for packaging into the AAV capsids (19). The ITR sequence from AAV2 is most commonly used. Conveniently, the ITR sequence of AAV2 can be cross-packaged into the capsids of most other commonly used serotypes; AAV5 is an exception (33,37,38). Cross-packaging allows for the rapid generation of pseudotyped vectors with the same AAV2 ITR genome, but with the transduction characteristics of the capsid from another serotype. One of the major disadvantages of rAAV vectors is their relatively small packaging capacity (14). Though recombinant genomes can be significantly smaller than the 4.7-kb wild-type genome, packaging efficiency decreases greatly if the genome is larger than approximately 5 kb (38). For expression of a protein product, this approximately 5-kb recombinant genome must include the AAV ITRs, a promoter, an open reading frame (ORF), and a polyadenylation signal. This size limitation presents a significant challenge for using rAAV vectors in the treatment of DMD due to the enormous size of both the dystrophin gene and cDNA (see below).

As AAV is a nonautonomous virus, its production as a vector requires helper functions to be provided in trans. Originally, this was accomplished with a transfection/infection protocol. In this protocol, producer cells (such as HEK293) were cotransfected with two plasmids, one containing the AAV Rep/Cap ORFs and the other containing the ITR flanked expression cassette, followed by infection with a replication defective adenovirus to supply necessary helper functions. This protocol has been commonly replaced with a three-plasmid cotransfection technique. Here, the essential adenoviral products are encoded on a third plasmid which is included in the cotransfection (39). A refinement of the three-plasmid system is available for several AAV serotypes; here the adenoviral functions and the Rep/Cap ORFs are included on a single plasmid, enabling a two-plasmid cotransfection (40,41).

Though rAAV can be purified by density gradient centrifugation, many of the serotypes may also be purified by ion-exchange or affinity chromatography (Fig. 1B) (32,34,42,43). Column chromatography has an advantage over density centrifugation techniques as it lends itself to large-scale production. However, in any given vector production a large percentage of the capsids will assemble without packaging a genome. Density centrifugation can remove these empty capsids while current chromatography

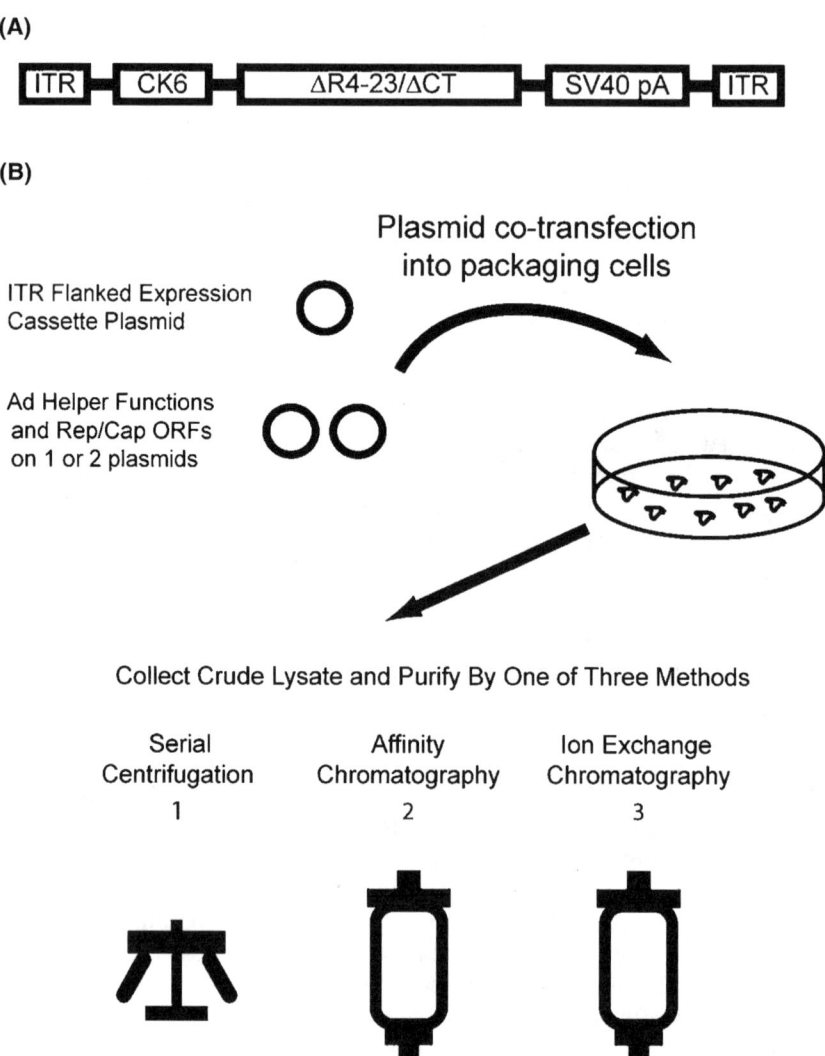

Figure 1 rAAV cloning and production. (A) Schematic illustration of a rAAV expression cassette. The ITRs flank a promoter, in this case CK6, driving expression of a transgene, in this case the microdystrophin cDNA ΔR4-23/ΔCT, followed by a polyadenylation signal derived from SV40. (B) Illustration showing common methods of rAAV production. Plasmids containing the vector genome, AAV ORFs, and helper functions are transfected into producer cells. These cells are then collected and lysed. The rAAV is purified by serial centrifugation, or by passing the crude lysate over an affinity or ion-exchange column. *Abbreviations*: rAAV, recombinant AAV; AAV, adeno-associated virus; ITRs, inverted terminal repeats; ORFs, open reading frames.

techniques do not (44). Affinity chromatography can be used only if a binding ligand for the serotype of choice is available. AAV2 binds heparin sulfate with high affinity and can be purified on heparin columns (45). However, many other serotypes bind heparin much more weakly, leading to large losses during purification (46). An exception to this is AAV6, which can also be purified on a heparin column, though the very similar AAV1 does not bind heparin (32,34). AAV5 and AAV4 bind sialic acid, allowing for purification over a sialic acid rich column (47–50).

Production of rAAV for the treatment of DMD will require large quantities of virus (12). Though such a use is likely several years away, preclinical studies in rodents, and especially larger animals, such as the dog and primates, will require increasing quantities of vector as research gets closer to the ultimate goal of whole body transduction of the human musculature.

SAFETY OF rAAV VECTORS

The encouragingly low immune response triggered by rAAV in animal studies indicates that rAAV may have a significant advantage over other vectors, such as adenovirus, in terms of safety (12,51,52). These animal studies, coupled with the fact that AAV has not been identified as the causative agent of any human pathology, raise the hope that rAAV vectors may eventually be a beneficial and safe vector for use in the clinic. The primary safety concerns for any vector are acute local and/or systemic toxicity, induction of a cellular or humoral immune response against the vector or transgene, mutations arising from insertion of the vector genome into the patient's genome, and the potential for disadvantageous integration into the patient's germ line cells.

The potential for acute toxicity of rAAV in patients is of great concern in light of an adverse reaction leading to the death of a patient administered an adenoviral vector (53). However, to date very little evidence for rAAV vectors causing direct toxicity exists in either animal studies or human clinical trials. In mouse models, doses up to approximately 5×10^{14} vector genomes (vg)/kg were well tolerated with little evidence of acute toxicity (51). Blood cell counts and various blood chemistries did not change significantly from baseline. In human studies, doses up to approximately 10^{12} vg/kg of rAAV were well tolerated with little evidence of toxicity (12,29,30). Patient blood chemistries such as alkaline phosphatase and creatine kinase levels did not deviate significantly from preadministration levels. Additionally, the concentration of various white blood cells did not increase or decrease appreciably. In these studies the vectors were administered intravenously, intramuscularly, and directly to the lining of the respiratory tract. While the human data come from a relatively small number of patients and with rather focused vector delivery, taken in combination with the vast body of animal data, it would seem that rAAV vectors may be associated with little acute toxicity.

Pre-existing antibodies to AAV are relatively common in the general population (10). This fact may complicate therapies with rAAV vectors either through neutralizing antibodies preventing transduction, or by priming the immune system to destroy transduced cells. Clinical experience with patients possessing pre-existing anti-AAV antibodies demonstrates that these antibodies do not block transduction following intramuscular injections (12). However, they may be more problematic with intravascular delivery protocols, as intramuscular injections likely deliver a local concentration of vector too high for pre-existing antibodies to neutralize. It is also clear that patients without pre-existing anti-AAV antibodies can develop a neutralizing response following vector administration, complicating re-administration of the vector (12).

In gene replacement therapies, development of an immune response to the therapeutic gene product is an additional concern. This problem could be compounded in patients whose mutation eliminates expression of the endogenous protein. Thus, DMD patients whose muscles do not express any dystrophin may be more likely to develop an immune response to vector-delivered dystrophin than would patients whose muscles express low levels or truncated forms of dystrophin. Patients with different types of mutations may also respond differently to gene transfer. For example, point mutations or partial gene deletions can lead to expression of low levels of portions of the dystrophin protein, potentially inducing immune tolerance only against those portions of the protein that are expressed. It remains unclear whether revertant dystrophin-positive fibers might lead to immune tolerance against those portions of dystrophin expressed in revertant fibers, which depends on the nature of the mutation (54). Patients with large deletions in the dystrophin gene may develop an immune response to an exogenous dystrophin protein containing protein domains normally encoded by deleted exons. It is possible that the smaller isoforms of dystrophin, expressed in nonmuscle tissues of most DMD patients, may attenuate the immune system to portions of the protein. The proper choice of promoter/enhancers to limit expression of the protein in antigen presenting cells, such as dendritic cells, may also reduce immune responses (51,55,56). Finally, many groups are working on nondystrophin-based gene therapy for DMD, utilizing proteins already expressed in the patient (see below).

rAAV vectors display only low frequencies of genomic integration, although vector integration events have not been found in muscle tissue to date (57,58). While the overall frequency of rAAV integration appears to be low, these vectors have been reported to preferentially integrate into areas of actively expressed genes (57). This preference for active chromatin may increase the chance of insertion into a gene that plays an important role in the targeted cell. Such insertions could have the effect of either knocking out a critical gene or activating a gene, either constitutively or under a subset of inappropriate conditions. This event would likely have little consequence if it merely killed the cell involved, as the overall rate of integration seems to be low. However, if the insertional mutation contributed to malignant transformation, this would be of great concern. It is now apparent that integration of gene therapy vectors is capable of contributing to cancer formation in light of recent observations in an X-linked SCID trial (59–61). However, the age of the patients, the nature of the vector, the clonal expansion of the transduced cells, and the nature of the delivered transgene all may have contributed to these adverse events. It is unclear how relevant this observation will be to other gene therapy protocols, but it is important to design vectors with safety in mind. With rAAV vectors this will include driving transgene expression with promoter/enhancers that will be active only in the tissue of interest, lowering the chances of ectopic expression or activating genes in nontarget tissues. For DMD, dystrophin expression should be limited to postmitotic myocytes and myofibers.

Germline transmission of rAAV vectors is a special case of the genomic integration discussed above. In a gene therapy trial for hemophilia A using rAAV vectors, genomes were detectable in the semen of patients following vector administration (12). However, genomes were not present in all patients or at all time points. Also, the presence of vg dropped to undetectable levels a few weeks after gene transfer. These observations indicate that the vector genomes were present in the semen as a transient component and not as an integrated genome. While the relevant human data are sparse, the risk of stable integration events leading to germ line transfer appear acceptably low with rAAV vectors (62–64).

ENGINEERING OF MICRODYSTROPHINS

Dystrophin is the largest gene in nature, spanning approximately 2.4 Mb on the human X chromosome. It is a complicated gene with seven promoters and unique first exons plus an additional 78 exons, and the primary transcript displays alternative splicing (65). In muscle, the dystrophin gene gives rise to a 14-kb mRNA and a 427 kDa protein (66). Consequently, gene replacement strategies for DMD face a serious challenge: the gene and even the cDNA are too large to be packaged by most commonly used gene therapy vectors. The dystrophin cDNA itself is approximately three times larger than the AAV genome. However, engineering of the gene has resulted in small cDNA encoding truncated, yet highly functional, dystrophins that can be expressed from AAV vectors (67–71). Some of the inspiration for this engineering comes from the allelic disorder, Becker muscular dystrophy (BMD) (72,73). BMD also results from mutations in the dystrophin gene, but is characterized by a milder dystrophy. This reduced severity is due to the fact that in BMD, dystrophin is present but at levels lower than normal or, frequently, is expressed as a truncated form that retains partial functionality. One mildly affected patient remains ambulatory in his 70s despite an in-frame deletion of exons 17–48 (74).

As described in Chapters 2 and 3, dystrophin links the actin cytoskeleton to the extracellular matrix (ECM) via the dystroglycan complex (DGC) (75–79). The amino-terminal portion of dystrophin attaches to the actin cytoskeleton (80–83). The middle of the dystrophin protein, termed the rod domain, is comprised of 24 spectrin-like repeats with four proline rich regions of minimally ordered secondary structure termed "hinges" (83–85). The rod domain is followed by the dystroglycan-binding domain, composed of a WW domain, and a cysteine-rich (CR) region, the latter of which includes a "ZZ" zinc-finger motif (84,86–92). Dystroglycan and other DGC members associate with the ECM through an interaction with laminin. Additionally, dystrophin has a fourth region, the carboxy-terminal (CT) region, located immediately following the CR region. The CT region forms interactions with the syntrophins and dystrobrevins (93–96). These proteins are thought to play a signaling role through interaction with molecules such as neuronal nitric oxide synthase (nNOS; see Chapter 3) (70). To retain functionality, a dystrophin molecule must be capable of anchoring to the cytoskeleton and the DGC to enable transmission of force from within myofibers to the ECM.

Several labs have reported studies using dystrophin genes encoding "mini-dystrophins" (Fig. 2). These mini-dystrophins are based on the protein expressed from the exons 17–48 deletion associated with very mild BMD, which lacks the rod domain region spanning hinge 2 through a portion of spectrin-like repeat 19 (71,74). This mutation has also been extended slightly to delete repeat 19 in its entirety (67). In transgenic mouse experiments, this mini-dystrophin appears to be identical in function to the full-length isoform, identifying one region of dystrophin that tolerates functional truncations (67,71). This mini-dystrophin contains eight of the 24 repeats and three of the four hinge domains and is small enough to fit into gene therapy vectors such as adenovirus and lentivirus, but is still too large for AAV (Fig. 2). Removal of the amino-terminal region of dystrophin has been shown to result in detrimental effects on both the stability and the mechanical properties of dystrophin (76,77,100,101). Though few patients have been identified with mutations in the CT domain, one patient with a deletion of the entire CT region displayed a very mild BMD phenotype (102). Transgenic *mdx* mice expressing a dystrophin lacking the CT region did not display any obvious muscle pathology, and assembly of the DGC was not significantly impaired (70).

Mini-genes lacking sequences that encode the CT domain and 16 of the 24 spectrin-like repeats are significantly smaller than full-length clones, but remain too large for inclusion in rAAV vectors (Fig. 2). All attempts to

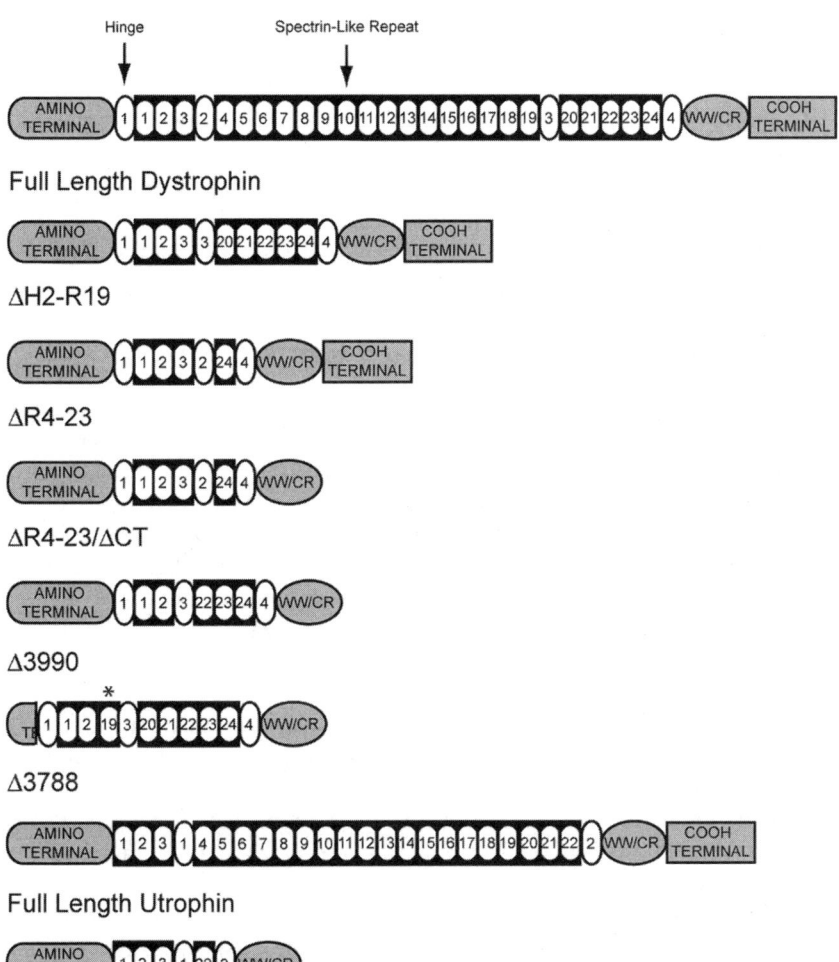

Figure 2 The domain structure of dystrophin and utrophin based proteins. This diagram shows the various domains and their arrangement in full-length dystrophin as well as in the mini-dystrophin, ΔH2-R19, and in the microdystrophins, ΔR4-23, ΔR4-23/ΔCT, Δ3990, and Δ3778. Asterisk in Δ3778 denotes a partial repeat 19. Domain arrangement in utrophin and the microutrophin, μU-ΔR4-21/ΔCT, is also shown. *Source*: Modified from Refs. 32, 67, 69, 100, 101, 119.

truncate the dystroglycan-binding domain have completely inactivated dystrophin, and truncations of the N-terminal actin binding domain have adversely affected dystrophin stability and/or function (88,95,96). Further truncations of these domains therefore seems unlikely to be clinically useful.

These observations suggested the rod domain as the most promising area for further shrinkage of dystrophin. Indeed, several laboratories have described highly truncated "microdystrophins" that lack the CT domain and the vast majority of the spectrin-like repeats (Fig. 2) (67–69). Though the smallest microdystrophins were nonfunctional, many were capable of significantly preventing the onset of dystrophy when expressed in *mdx* mouse muscles. These various microdystrophins are approximately one-third the size of the full-length protein and small enough to be encoded by rAAV vectors (51,67,68).

DYSTROPHIN REPLACEMENT IN ANIMAL MODELS OF DMD

The functionality of various microdystrophins has been studied in *mdx* mice, in both transgenic mice and following rAAV mediated gene delivery. Microdystrophins were effective in preventing dystrophy when expressed from birth and can at least partially reverse many aspects of the dystrophic pathology when expressed in adult and old animals with an established dystrophy. The route of delivery in these studies addresses slightly different questions. In transgenic studies, the microdystrophin is expressed from late embryonic development onwards, and the question whether these constructs can *prevent* the onset of dystrophy in the *mdx* mouse is addressed. When expression cassettes are delivered via rAAV vectors, the experiments more directly address the question whether the microdystrophins can halt and/or reverse the dystrophic phenotype after a degree of dystrophic pathology has already become established.

Though all of the reported microdystrophins have been shown to correctly localize to the sarcolemma and stabilize expression of most DGC members (except for nNOS), not all of the constructs can prevent the onset of dystrophy (Fig. 2). Constructs with no spectrin-like repeats were nonfunctional (67). Constructs with one or three spectrin-like repeats reduced the severity of the dystrophic phenotype only modestly (68). It appears that at least four spectrin-like repeats are needed for a high degree of functionality. The best of the four repeat microdystrophins linked the second hinge domain up to the 24th spectrin-like repeat (ΔR4-23) (67,68). Although the specific force generated by ΔR4-23 transgenic mice was higher than in *mdx* animals, it was somewhat lower than in wild-type mice. Interestingly, other variations of four spectrin-like repeat microdystrophins were less effective in ameliorating the *mdx* dystrophy (67). These data suggest that the different repeats are not functionally interchangeable and possess different properties. These properties presumably include differences in their affinity for actin binding, their elasticity and strength, and the nature of their cooperative interactions with adjacent repeats and hinges. It should be noted that in the transgenic animal experiments described here, the microdystrophin constructs included the CT domain.

A variety of microdystrophin clones have also been tested after delivery to *mdx* mouse muscles using rAAV. Such constructs included a series of five and six repeat microdystrophins, an eight repeat/amino-terminally deleted construct, and three four repeat constructs (67,69,97,98). All constructs tested in AAV have also lacked sequences encoding the CT domain. The six repeat construct fused repeat 3 to repeat 22, and lacked an internal hinge (Δ4173); one five repeat construct fused repeat 2 to hinge 3, which was then joined to repeat 22 (Δ3990), while the second five repeat construct joined repeat 2 to repeat 22 and lacked an internal hinge (Δ3849) (69,97). Injection of these constructs into *mdx* muscles restored expression of most DGC members to the sarcolemmal membrane (69). Fibers expressing these microdystrophins displayed intact sarcolemmal membranes and were less likely to contain centrally nucleated fibers (69). When injected into 10-day-old mouse pups the effect was more pronounced. This was likely due to the fact that dystrophic pathology begins at week 3 in the *mdx* mouse, and the microdystrophin was able to prevent the onset of pathology. In the older, 50-day-old animals, the dystrophin expression was only able to halve the number of centrally nucleated fibers two months postinjection, and this number increased to about two-thirds of *mdx* levels at four months postinjection. In a subsequent study, the Δ3990 five repeat construct (Fig. 2) was shown to improve the mechanical performance of the *mdx* musculature (97).

The Δ3788 construct (Fig. 2) differs from those previously mentioned in that it contains a large deletion in the amino-terminal domain (98). Δ3788 is deleted for exons 3–9 in the amino-terminus, and fuses spectrin-like repeat 2 to repeat 19. When this construct was delivered to the TA muscles of immune compromised nude/*mdx* mice, expression of most of the DGC was again restored to the sarcolemmal membrane. Further, the Δ3788 positive myofibers had a very low level of central nucleation, on par with wild-type animals, suggesting that the construct could protect from degeneration. However, it is unclear how effective this construct will be at reversing rather than preventing dystrophic pathology, as this construct was delivered to 12-day-old mouse pups which had not yet developed a pathology.

Four repeat microdystrophins have been delivered via rAAV, recorded in five published studies (51,67,68,103,104). The first is delivered via a rAAV2 vector containing the muscle specific CK6 promoter driving expression of either ΔR4-23/ΔCT, ΔR2-21/ΔCT, or ΔR2-21 + H3/ΔCT (Fig. 2) (67). Five months postinjection the *gastocnemius* muscles were examined for microdystrophin and DGC member expression, central nucleation, and fiber diameter characteristics. The percentage of centrally nucleated fibers in dystrophin-positive fibers was reduced to approximately 15% (ΔR4-23/ΔCT), 25% (ΔR2-21/ΔCT), and 55% (ΔR2-21 + H3/ΔCT) compared to approximately 1% and 65% in age matched wild-type and *mdx* animals, respectively (67). A later study examined the mechanical properties of *mdx* muscles following systemic delivery of a rAAV6 vector containing a

CK6:ΔR4-23/ΔCT expression cassette (51). Here, treated TA muscles demonstrated significantly improved absolute and specific forces after eccentric lengthening contractions eight weeks postinjection. Complete transduction of a muscle with a microdystrophin is not required to have a measurable effect on the dystrophic phenotype. As little as 20% to 30% transduction of a muscle has been reported to lead to an increase in mechanical properties of *mdx* muscles (104). Additionally, the degree of correction conferred to a dystrophic muscle is influenced by the age of the muscle. *mdx* mice injected with a rAAV2 vector encoding a microdystrophin transgene at 10 days had lower overall dystrophin expression (20% positive myofibers) than mice injected at five weeks (50% positive myofibers), though the contractile properties of both groups were very similar to wild-type controls when assayed at 24 weeks postinjection (104). Similarly, rAAV5 vectors expressing the ΔR4-23/ΔCT microdystrophin displayed better correction of the dystrophic pathology when injected into seven-week-old mice than when injected into nine-month-old mice (105). Though more studies exploring these observations will be needed, they suggest that early treatment of a mildly dystrophic musculature may be more effective than a later treatment of muscles with a more advanced pathology.

rAAV DELIVERY OF NONDYSTROPHIN GENES FOR THE TREATMENT OF DMD

The primary biochemical deficiency in DMD is lack of a functional dystrophin protein, and successful treatment of this disease will likely necessitate delivery of a dystrophin gene (see Chapter 2). However, other genes are being considered for genetic therapies of DMD using rAAV vectors. These alternate genes offer a means of relieving some of the severity of DMD by bypassing the primary defect and focusing on secondary pathological abnormalities. Many of these techniques may even act synergistically with dystrophin replacement, leading to a more effective treatment than either alone. This consideration is especially important because rAAV will likely be able to deliver only truncated forms of dystrophin.

One reason to consider delivery of alternate transgenes is the possibility that DMD patients, lacking endogenous full-length dystrophin, will view exogenous dystrophin as a foreign protein and mount an immune reaction against the expressing cells. Utrophin has been shown to functionally replace dystrophin in animal models of muscular dystrophy (106,107). This observation raises the possibility of using a rAAV vector expressing a microutrophin construct instead of a microdystrophin construct. The domain structures of a microutrophin and the full-length utrophin are shown in Figure 2. A chimeric molecule containing portions of dystrophin and utrophin may also prove to be an alternate approach. Here, utrophin domains could be substituted for potentially immunogenic dystrophin domains, leading to a less immunogenic transgene retaining the maximum amount of dystrophin functionality. Overexpression of α7-integrin has also been reported to functionally replace dystrophin to some degree, raising another possibility of a "self" protein for rAAV mediated delivery (108).

Gene repair strategies represent an alternative method of restoring dystrophin expression which does not involve the delivery of a traditional expression cassette (109–111). This approach is attractive, as it would restore dystrophin in a manner incorporating the proper control by native enhancers and promoters (see Chapter 15). Many of the these strategies involve the use of small DNA or DNA/RNA hybrid oligonucleotides to repair point mutations or frameshifting mutations resulting from small insertions or deletions (110,111). Delivery of small oligos does not require the use of rAAV as a delivery vehicle (112). However, DNA repair through larger nucleotides could benefit from delivery via rAAV. In this situation, a DNA molecule corresponding to a wild-type version of the genetic lesion, with flanking sequence for targeting to the correct genomic location via homologous base pairing, is delivered by the rAAV vector in place of a traditional expression cassette (113–115). Following delivery, the repair molecule is targeted to the lesion by the flanking regions, and the lesion is then repaired via recombination or DNA repair mechanisms, as yet to be fully understood. Though an attractive approach, gene repair via rAAV delivery does have some inherent difficulties. One difficulty is that individual mutations will have to be determined for each patient so that the proper repair molecule can be generated. Also, the size of lesions that can be repaired is limited. rAAV can only package a limited amount of DNA that must include the region to be repaired as well as enough flanking homology to target the DNA repair molecule to the proper location. Though less developed than gene replacement technology and yet to be used for in vivo dystrophin repair via rAAV, this is a potentially promising field of inquiry. A somewhat related approach was recently described by Danos and coworkers (116). In that study, the authors used rAAV1 vectors to deliver a gene construct expressing antisense oligonucleotides against the splice sequences flanking murine dystrophin intron 23. Recipient muscles accumulated transcripts largely lacking exon 23, which contains the *mdx* mutations, leading to expression of nearly normal levels of dystrophin.

Some of the most prominent characteristics of DMD are the loss of muscle mass and muscle fibers, as well as their replacement with fat and fibrous tissue. One potential method for increasing the amount of muscle present is to make the remaining muscle fibers undergo hypertrophy without hyperplasia. One gene being studied intensely for this purpose is insulin-like growth factor-1 (IGF-1). IGF-1 is a small signaling peptide involved in muscle growth and maintenance and has been shown to increase the size of individual muscle fibers and whole muscles when overexpressed as a transgene or following rAAV2 vector delivery in wild-type mice (117,118).

IGF-1 overexpression in *mdx* mice has been shown to have a beneficial effect on the force producing capacity of the dystrophic muscle (99,119). Another protein of interest is myostatin, which negatively regulates the size and number of muscle fibers (120). Inhibitors of myostatin function could result in hypertrophy and hyperplasia, increasing the size and, importantly, the number of total myofibers in a previously diseased muscle. A rAAV vector could potentially be used to deliver a gene cassette that could block myostatin expression, such as a siRNA cassette. Alternately a myostatin inhibitor such as follistatin could be delivered by rAAV (120). Mice have been engineered that lack normal levels of myostatin, and these animals show a tremendous amount of muscle hypertrophy (120,121). *Mdx* mice without normal myostatin levels were reported to demonstrate an ameliorated dystrophy (122,123). However, neither IGF-1 nor decreased levels of myostatin could directly increase the mechanical integrity of the sarcolemmal membrane in the absence of dystrophin, suggesting that codelivery of two rAAV6 vectors, one expressing microdystrophin and the other expressing IGF-1 or a myostatin inhibitor, might lead to improved effects in dystrophic muscle (99).

DELIVERY OF rAAV VECTORS

Methods for systemic delivery of various vectors are reviewed in Chapter 20. Here we will briefly discuss a few of the most recent advances related to rAAV vector delivery. An ideal delivery method for rAAV would be simple, safe, and result in the transduction of the entire musculature with a single treatment. Transduction of the majority of the musculature even in a small animal model, such as the *mdx* mouse, has been challenging (124,125). One technique that achieves nearly body-wide muscle transduction in the mouse is injection of rAAV into the intraperitoneal (IP) space, either in utero or shortly after birth (32,126–128). This technique leads to reasonably widespread and sustained transgene expression and is a useful experimental tool. However, the IP delivery route seems unlikely to be clinically relevant as the permissiveness of transduction is thought to be due to the relatively "leaky" state of the vasculature and the relatively small amounts of intervening connective tissue in young mice. The efficiency of this method decreases significantly after birth and may not be effective in neonate humans, which are relatively mature compared to mice at the same developmental stage.

Although the heart and diaphragm are severely affected in DMD, they have been extremely difficult to transduce in animal models of DMD (36,102,125,129–131). Various techniques employing direct injection of these muscles have met with modest success in the *mdx* mouse. Scaling direct injection of the heart and diaphragm from the mouse to humans is likely to be difficult for the reasons discussed above. Other techniques include vascular isolation of these tissues followed by vector infusion with either hydrostatic pressure and/or inducers of vascular permeability in attempts to increase the efficiency of gene transfer. Such techniques have met with varying degrees of success, but are typically invasive and frequently use cofactors with potential toxicity; it is unclear how well dystrophic patients will tolerate such procedures. Recently, techniques have been developed for efficient transduction of the diaphragm in the *mdx* mouse. One of these techniques involves making an incision in the abdominal wall and retracting the liver to expose the diaphragm. A gel containing rAAV is then "painted" onto the surface of the diaphragm and the incision is then closed (36). A second technique involves injection of rAAV vectors directly into the intrathoracic space via a blind injection between the ribs (32). Both techniques are relatively efficient at diaphragm transduction, while the intrathoracic technique also targets many of the intercostal muscles. These approaches are most effective when using an AAV serotype with a high degree of tropism for muscle, such as rAAV1 and rAAV6.

The vasculature supplies myofibers with oxygen and other vital nutrients and lies in close contact with all muscles. It is thus an attractive route of delivery. Encouragingly, a recent report describes a technique capable of achieving body-wide transduction of the striated musculature, including the heart and diaphragm, following a single intravascular injection of rAAV6 vectors (51). This technique delivers a high vector dose (up to 4×10^{14} vg/kg) in a volume equivalent to approximately 15% to 20% of the blood volume. With some vector doses the efficiency of this method was greatly enhanced by the inclusion of vascular endothelial growth factor (VEGF). VEGF is a potent, though short-lived, inducer of vascular permeability (132–134). VEGF has less toxic effects than many vascular permeabilizers, such as histamine, and was well tolerated by all animals in the study (51,124,134). In addition to delivery of a marker transgene to wild-type animals, the investigators delivered the microdystrophin, ΔR4-23/ΔCT, body-wide to all *mdx* mouse striated muscles. Figure 3 summarizes the procedure used and the extent of transduction observed (51). Delivery of the ΔR4-23/ΔCT was capable of protecting the otherwise dystrophic *mdx* muscles from contraction induced injury and resulted in a reduction of serum creatine kinase levels. The procedure also appeared to be safe, as no significant changes in blood chemistries, such as ALT and AST levels, nor any deaths attributable to the vector were observed (51).

This technique is highly encouraging, but numerous additional studies are required, particularly in large animal models, to determine if the results in mice can be safely scaled-up to larger mammals. As the vector is delivered intravascularly, it will have access to tissues other than the striated musculature. Therefore, the immunology and toxicity of both the vector and any transgene must be fully elucidated, and the potential for mutagenesis from vector integration into chromosomes must be explored. Additionally, this technique, or any systemic delivery technique, raises the possibility of germline transgene transmission. Though germline transmission is not

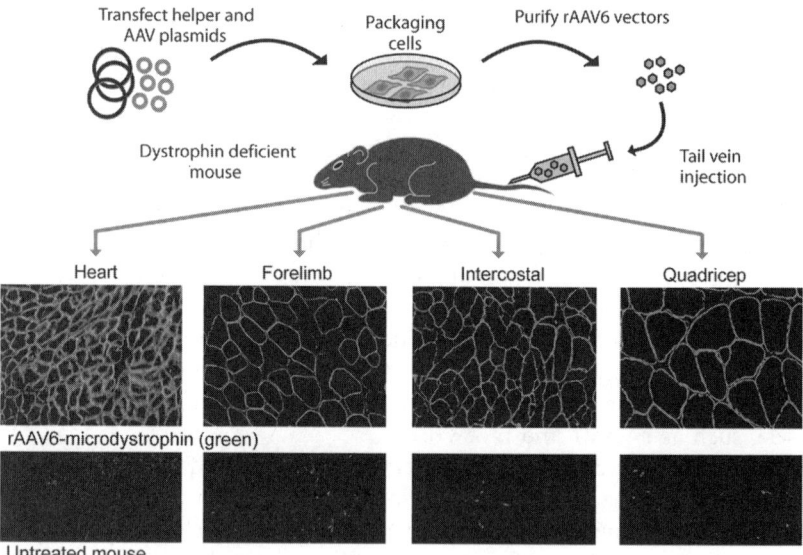

Figure 3 Systemic delivery of rAAV via the vasculature. This figure graphically outlines the steps leading to systemic transduction of murine musculature with a recently reported technique (51). In this example, the ΔR4-23/ΔCT vector is produced through a two-plasmid cotransfection (67). Following purification, the vector is delivered to the musculature of an *mdx* mouse with a single intravascular injection into the lateral tail vein. Six weeks postinjection, high and very uniform expression of the ΔR4-23/ΔCT transgene is seen in muscles throughout the treated *mdx* mouse leading to greater than 90% transduction of muscle fibers in all muscles examined; shown here are representative fields from heart, forelimb (*carpi radialis*), intercostals, and quadriceps. ΔR4-23/ΔCT expression was detected by immunofluorescence (*white*) with a polyclonal rabbit antidystrophin antibody. *Abbreviations*: AAV, adeno-associated virus; rAAV, recombinant AAV.

necessarily a safety concern per se, in the current political and scientific climate such a possibility must be explored and if present, its magnitude must be understood.

TRANSDUCTION OF MYOGENIC PRECURSOR CELLS BY rAAV VECTORS

While AAV vectors are highly efficient in transducing muscle fibers in vivo, their utility for gene transfer into dividing mononuclear cells in vitro and in vivo is limited due to the predominantly episomal nature of the viral genome in transduced cells. AAV2 vectors transduce many types of cells in culture at high efficiency, although for reasons that are unclear AAV6 poorly transduces most tissue culture cells. AAV6 vectors transduce many cell types, such as 293 or HT1080 cells, nearly 100,000 times less efficiently than do AAV2 vectors (135) (Allen JM, personal communication). In our experience, myoblasts, myocytes, and myotubes are the only cells efficiently transduced by AAV6 in vitro. In myogenic cultures, AAV6 and AAV2 work equally well, despite the two orders of magnitude better transduction of myofibers achieved with AAV6 following intramuscular injection (32). These observations suggest a possible critical ECM component needed for transduction by AAV6 that is lacking in cell cultures. We have performed pilot studies in which AAV6 vectors were injected intramuscularly prior to isolation of myonuclear cells for culturing in vitro. At the time of harvest, gene expression was detectable in varying percentages of muscle SP cells and myoblasts, but no further gene expression was detected after several cell doublings in vitro (En Kimura, JSC, unpublished observations). These observations suggest that transduction of muscle satellite cells or other presumptive myogenic stem cells by AAV vectors would not contribute significantly to gene expression following muscle regeneration. Studies in liver also show rapid loss of episomal AAV genomes upon cell division (57).

CONCLUSIONS

Whether rAAV vectors will ever be used in the clinic to treat DMD patients cannot be predicted. However, rAAV vectors are one of the most promising candidates for gene therapy treatments of this disease. It remains to be determined if bench and clinical research in the coming years will validate this optimism by creating effective therapeutic expression cassettes that can be delivered via rAAV, optimizing techniques to produce adequate amounts of vector for human use, and developing safe delivery protocols capable of transducing enough of the musculature to have a therapeutic effect.

ACKNOWLEDGMENTS

We thank James Allen, David Russell, Dusty Miller, and Christine Halbert for helpful discussions. Supported by grants from the U.S. National Institutes of Health and the Muscular Dystrophy Association (U.S.A.).

REFERENCES

1. Siegl G, Bates RC, Berns KI, et al. Characteristics and taxonomy of Parvoviridae. Intervirology 1985; 23:61–73.
2. Buller RM, Janik JE, Sebring ED, Rose JA. Herpes simplex virus types 1 and 2 completely help adenovirus-associated virus replication. J Virol 1981; 40:241–247.

3. Atchison RW, Casto BC, Hammon WM. Adenovirus-associated defective virus particles. Science 1965; 149:754–756.
4. Muzyczka N. Use of adeno-associated virus as a general transduction vector for mammalian cells. Curr Top Microbiol Immunol 1992; 158:97–129.
5. Xiao W, Chirmule N, Berta SC, McCullough B, Gao G, Wilson JM. Gene therapy vectors based on adeno-associated virus type 1. J Virol 1999; 73:3994–4003.
6. Chiorini JA, Kim F, Yang L, Kotin RM. Cloning and characterization of adeno-associated virus type 5. J Virol 1999:1309–1319.
7. Rutledge EA, Halbert CL, Russell DW. Infectious clones and vectors derived from adeno-associated virus (AAV) serotypes other than AAV type 2. J Virol 1998; 72:309–319.
8. Gao GP, Alvira MR, Wang L, Calcedo R, Johnston J, Wilson JM. Novel adeno-associated viruses from rhesus monkeys as vectors for human gene therapy. Proc Natl Acad Sci USA 2002; 99:11854–11859.
9. Chiorini JA, Yang L, Liu Y, Safer B, Kotin RM. Cloning of adeno-associated virus type 4 (AAV4) and generation of recombinant AAV4 particles. J Virol 1997; 71:6823–6833.
10. Chirmule N, Propert K, Magosin S, Qian Y, Qian R, Wilson J. Immune responses to adenovirus and adeno-associated virus in humans. Gene Ther 1999; 6:1574–1583.
11. Blacklow NR, Hoggan MD, Kapikian AZ, Austin JB, Rowe WP. Epidemiology of adenovirus-associated virus infection in a nursery population. Am J Epidemiol 1968; 88:368–378.
12. Manno CS, Chew AJ, Hutchison S, et al. AAV-mediated factor IX gene transfer to skeletal muscle in patients with severe hemophilia B. Blood 2003; 101:2963–2972.
13. Herzog RW, Yang EY, Couto LB, et al. Long-term correction of canine hemophilia B by gene transfer of blood coagulation factor IX mediated by adeno-associated viral vector. Nat Med 1999; 5:56–63.
14. Srivastava A, Lusby EW, Berns KI. Nucleotide sequence and organization of the adeno-associated virus 2 genome. J Virol 1983; 45:555–564.
15. Berns KI, Adler S. Separation of two types of adeno-associated virus particles containing complementary polynucleotide chains. J Virol 1972; 9:394–396.
16. Straus SE, Sebring ED, Rose JA. Concatemers of alternating plus and minus strands are intermediates in adenovirus-associated virus DNA synthesis. Proc Natl Acad Sci USA 1976; 73:742–746.
17. Lusby E, Fife KH, Berns KI. Nucleotide sequence of the inverted terminal repetition in adeno-associated virus DNA. J Virol 1980; 34:402–409.
18. Tattersall P, Ward DC. Rolling hairpin model for replication of parvovirus and linear chromosomal DNA. Nature 1976; 263:106–109.
19. Xiao X, Xiao W, Li J, Samulski RJ. A novel 165-base-pair terminal repeat sequence is the sole cis requirement for the adeno-associated virus life cycle. J Virol 1997; 71:941–948.
20. Berns KI, Linden RM. The cryptic life style of adeno-associated virus. Bioessays 1995; 17:237–245.
21. Urcelay E, Ward P, Wiener SM, Safer B, Kotin RM. Asymmetric replication in vitro from a human sequence element is dependent on adeno-associated virus Rep protein. J Virol 1995; 69:2038–2046.

22. Weitzman MD, Kyostio SR, Kotin RM, Owens RA. Adeno-associated virus (AAV) Rep proteins mediate complex formation between AAV DNA and its integration site in human DNA. Proc Natl Acad Sci USA 1994; 91:5808–5812.
23. Xie Q, Bu W, Bhatia S, et al. The atomic structure of adeno-associated virus (AAV-2), a vector for human gene therapy. Proc Natl Acad Sci USA 2002; 99:10405–10410.
24. Green MR, Roeder RG. Definition of a novel promoter for the major adenovirus-associated virus mRNA. Cell 1980; 22:231–242.
25. Muramatsu S, Mizukami H, Young NS, Brown KE. Nucleotide sequencing and generation of an infectious clone of adeno-associated virus 3. Virology 1996; 221:208–217.
26. Chiorini JA, Kim F, Yang L, Kotin RM. Cloning and characterization of adeno-associated virus type 5. J Virol 1999; 73:1309–1319.
27. Bantel-Schaal U, Delius H, Schmidt R, zur Hausen H. Human adeno-associated virus type 5 is only distantly related to other known primate helper-dependent parvoviruses. J Virol 1999; 73:939–947.
28. Gao G, Vandenberghe LH, Alvira MR, et al. Clades of adeno-associated viruses are widely disseminated in human tissues. J Virol 2004; 78:6381–6388.
29. Moss RB, Rodman D, Spencer LT, et al. Repeated adeno-associated virus serotype 2 aerosol-mediated cystic fibrosis transmembrane regulator gene transfer to the lungs of patients with cystic fibrosis: a multicenter, double-blind, placebo-controlled trial. Chest 2004; 125:509–521.
30. Wagner JA, Nepomuceno IB, Messner AH, et al. A phase II, double-blind, randomized, placebo-controlled clinical trial of tgAAVCF using maxillary sinus delivery in patients with cystic fibrosis with antrostomies. Hum Gene Ther 2002; 13:1349–1359.
31. Kay MA, Manno CS, Ragni MV, et al. Evidence for gene transfer and expression of factor IX in haemophilia B patients treated with an AAV vector. Nat Genet 2000; 24:257–261.
32. Blankinship MJ, Gregorevic P, Allen JM, et al. Efficient transduction of skeletal muscle using vectors based on adeno-associated virus serotype 6. Mol Ther 2004; 10:671–678.
33. Grimm D, Zhou S, Nakai H, et al. Preclinical in vivo evaluation of pseudotyped adeno-associated virus vectors for liver gene therapy. Blood 2003; 102:2412–2419.
34. Halbert CL, Allen JM, Miller AD. Adeno-associated virus type 6 (AAV6) vectors mediate efficient transduction of airway epithelial cells in mouse lungs compared to that of AAV2 vectors. J Virol 2001; 75:6615–6624.
35. Chao H, Monahan PE, Liu Y, Samulski RJ, Walsh CE. Sustained and complete phenotype correction of hemophilia B mice following intramuscular injection of AAV1 serotype vectors. Mol Ther 2001; 4:217–222.
36. Mah C, Fraites TJ Jr, Cresawn KO, Zolotukhin I, Lewis MA, Byrne BJ. A new method for recombinant adeno-associated virus vector delivery to murine diaphragm. Mol Ther 2004; 9:458–463.
37. Rabinowitz JE, Rolling F, Li C, et al. Cross-packaging of a single adeno-associated virus (AAV) type 2 vector genome into multiple AAV serotypes enables transduction with broad specificity. J Virol 2002; 76:791–801.

38. Hermonat PL, Quirk JG, Bishop BM, Han L. The packaging capacity of adeno-associated virus (AAV) and the potential for wild-type-plus AAV gene therapy vectors. FEBS Lett 1997; 407:78–84.
39. Xiao X, Li J, Samulski RJ. Production of high-titer recombinant adeno-associated virus vectors in the absence of helper adenovirus. J Virol 1998; 72:2224–2232.
40. Grimm D, Kleinschmidt JA. Progress in adeno-associated virus type 2 vector production: promises and prospects for clinical use. Hum Gene Ther 1999; 10:2445–2450.
41. Grimm D, Kern A, Rittner K, Kleinschmidt JA. Novel tools for production and purification of recombinant adenoassociated virus vectors. Hum Gene Ther 1998; 9:2745–2760.
42. Davidoff AM, Ng CY, Sleep S, et al. Purification of recombinant adeno-associated virus type 8 vectors by ion exchange chromatography generates clinical grade vector stock. J Virol Methods 2004; 121:209–215.
43. Kaludov N, Handelman B, Chiorini JA. Scalable purification of adeno-associated virus type 2, 4, or 5 using ion-exchange chromatography. Hum Gene Ther 2002; 13:1235–1243.
44. Sommer JM, Smith PH, Parthasarathy S, et al. Quantification of adeno-associated virus particles and empty capsids by optical density measurement. Mol Ther 2003; 7:122–128.
45. Clark KR, Liu X, McGrath JP, Johnson PR. Highly purified recombinant adeno-associated virus vectors are biologically active and free of detectable helper and wild-type viruses. Hum Gene Ther 1999; 10:1031–1039.
46. Rabinowitz JE, Bowles DE, Faust SM, Ledford JG, Cunningham SE, Samulski RJ. Cross-dressing the virion: the transcapsidation of adeno-associated virus serotypes functionally defines subgroups. J Virol 2004; 78:4421–4432.
47. Walters RW, Yi SM, Keshavjee S, et al. Binding of adeno-associated virus type 5 to 2,3-linked sialic acid is required for gene transfer. J Biol Chem 2001; 276:20610–20616.
48. Kaludov N, Brown KE, Walters RW, Zabner J, Chiorini JA. Adeno-associated virus serotype 4 (AAV4) and AAV5 both require sialic acid binding for hemagglutination and efficient transduction but differ in sialic acid linkage specificity. J Virol 2001; 75:6884–6893.
49. Walters RW, Pilewski JM, Chiorini JA, Zabner J. Secreted and transmembrane mucins inhibit gene transfer with AAV4 more efficiently than AAV5. J Biol Chem 2002; 277:23709–23713.
50. Auricchio A, O'Connor E, Hildinger M, Wilson JM. A single-step affinity column for purification of serotype-5 based adeno-associated viral vectors. Mol Ther 2001; 4:372–374.
51. Gregorevic P, Blankinship MJ, Allen JM, et al. Systemic delivery of genes to striated muscles using adeno-associated viral vectors. Nat Med 2004; 10:828–834.
52. Arruda VR, Schuettrumpf J, Herzog RW, et al. Safety and efficacy of factor IX gene transfer to skeletal muscle in murine and canine hemophilia B models by adeno-associated viral vector serotype 1. Blood 2004; 103:85–92.
53. Raper SE, Chirmule N, Lee FS, et al. Fatal systemic inflammatory response syndrome in a ornithine transcarbamylase deficient patient following adenoviral gene transfer. Mol Genet Metab 2003; 80:148–158.

54. Zammit PS, Partridge TA. Sizing up muscular dystrophy. Nat Med 2002; 8:1355–1356.
55. Hartigan-O'Connor D, Kirk CJ, Crawford R, Mule JJ, Chamberlain JS. Immune evasion by muscle-specific gene expression in dystrophic muscle. Mol Ther 2001; 4:525–533.
56. Yuasa K, Sakamoto M, Miyagoe-Suzuki Y, et al. Adeno-associated virus vector-mediated gene transfer into dystrophin-deficient skeletal muscles evokes enhanced immune response against the transgene product. Gene Ther 2002; 9:1576–1588.
57. Nakai H, Montini E, Fuess S, Storm TA, Grompe M, Kay MA. AAV serotype 2 vectors preferentially integrate into active genes in mice. Nat Genet 2003; 34:297–302.
58. Ponnazhagan S, Erikson D, Kearns WG, et al. Lack of site-specific integration of the recombinant adeno-associated virus 2 genomes in human cells. Hum Gene Ther 1997; 8:275–284.
59. Hacein-Bey-Abina S, Von Kalle C, Schmidt M, et al. LMO2-associated clonal T cell proliferation in two patients after gene therapy for SCID-X1. Science 2003; 302:415–419.
60. Hacein-Bey-Abina S, von Kalle C, Schmidt M, et al. A serious adverse event after successful gene therapy for X-linked severe combined immunodeficiency. N Engl J Med 2003; 348:255–256.
61. Check E. Gene therapy put on hold as third child develops cancer. Nature 2005; 433:561.
62. Arruda VR, Fields PA, Milner R, et al. Lack of germline transmission of vector sequences following systemic administration of recombinant AAV-2 vector in males. Mol Ther 2001; 4:586–592.
63. Pachori AS, Melo LG, Zhang L, Loda M, Pratt RE, Dzau VJ. Potential for germ line transmission after intramyocardial gene delivery by adeno-associated virus. Biochem Biophys Res Commun 2004; 313:528–533.
64. Couto L, Parker A, Gordon JW. Direct exposure of mouse spermatozoa to very high concentrations of a serotype-2 adeno-associated virus gene therapy vector fails to lead to germ cell transduction. Hum Gene Ther 2004; 15:287–291.
65. Feener CA, Koenig M, Kunkel LM. Alternative splicing of human dystrophin mRNA generates isoforms at the carboxy terminus. Nature 1989; 338:509–511.
66. Koenig M, Hoffman EP, Bertelson CJ, Monaco AP, Feener C, Kunkel LM. Complete cloning of the Duchenne muscular dystrophy (DMD) cDNA and preliminary genomic organization of the DMD gene in normal and affected individuals. Cell 1987; 50:509–517.
67. Harper SQ, Hauser MA, DelloRusso C, et al. Modular flexibility of dystrophin: implications for gene therapy of Duchenne muscular dystrophy. Nat Med 2002; 8:253–261.
68. Sakamoto M, Yuasa K, Yoshimura M, et al. Micro-dystrophin cDNA ameliorates dystrophic phenotypes when introduced into mdx mice as a transgene. Biochem Biophys Res Commun 2002; 293:1265–1272.
69. Wang B, Li J, Xiao X. Adeno-associated virus vector carrying human minidystrophin genes effectively ameliorates muscular dystrophy in mdx mouse model. Proc Natl Acad Sci USA 2000; 97:13714–13719.

70. Crawford GE, Faulkner JA, Crosbie RH, Campbell KP, Froehner SC, Chamberlain JS. Assembly of the dystrophin-associated protein complex does not require the dystrophin COOH-terminal domain. J Cell Biol 2000; 150:1399–1410.
71. Phelps SF, Hauser MA, Cole NM, et al. Expression of full-length and truncated dystrophin mini-genes in transgenic mdx mice. Hum Mol Genet 1995; 4:1251–1258.
72. Koenig M, Beggs AH, Moyer M, et al. The molecular basis for Duchenne versus Becker muscular dystrophy: correlation of severity with type of deletion. Am J Hum Genet 1989; 45:498–506.
73. Hoffman EP, Brown RH Jr, Kunkel LM. Dystrophin: the protein product of the Duchenne muscular dystrophy locus. Cell 1987; 51:919–928.
74. England SB, Nicholson LV, Johnson MA, et al. Very mild muscular dystrophy associated with the deletion of 46% of dystrophin. Nature 1990; 343:180–182.
75. Pasternak C, Wong S, Elson EL. Mechanical function of dystrophin in muscle cells. J Cell Biol 1995; 128:355–361.
76. Cox GA, Sunada Y, Campbell KP, Chamberlain JS. Dp71 can restore the dystrophin-associated glycoprotein complex in muscle but fails to prevent dystrophy. Nat Genet 1994; 8:333–339.
77. Greenberg DS, Sunada Y, Campbell KP, Yaffe D, Nudel U. Exogenous Dp71 restores the levels of dystrophin associated proteins but does not alleviate muscle damage in mdx mice. Nat Genet 1994; 8:340–344.
78. Ervasti JM, Campbell KP. A role for the dystrophin–glycoprotein complex as a transmembrane linker between laminin and actin. J Cell Biol 1993; 122:809–823.
79. Petrof BJ, Shrager JB, Stedman HH, Kelly AM, Sweeney HL. Dystrophin protects the sarcolemma from stresses developed during muscle contraction. Proc Natl Acad Sci USA 1993; 90:3710–3714.
80. Hemmings L, Kuhlman PA, Critchley DR. Analysis of the actin-binding domain of alpha-actinin by mutagenesis and demonstration that dystrophin contains a functionally homologous domain. J Cell Biol 1992; 116:1369–1380.
81. Corrado K, Mills PL, Chamberlain JS. Deletion analysis of the dystrophin-actin binding domain. FEBS Lett 1994; 344:255–260.
82. Way M, Pope B, Cross RA, Kendrick-Jones J, Weeds AG. Expression of the N-terminal domain of dystrophin in *E. coli* and demonstration of binding to F-actin. FEBS Lett 1992; 301:243–245.
83. Roberts RG, Coffey AJ, Bobrow M, Bentley DR. Exon structure of the human dystrophin gene. Genomics 1993; 16:536–538.
84. Koenig M, Monaco AP, Kunkel LM. The complete sequence of dystrophin predicts a rod-shaped cytoskeletal protein. Cell 1988; 53:219–226.
85. Koenig M, Kunkel LM. Detailed analysis of the repeat domain of dystrophin reveals four potential hinge segments that may confer flexibility. J Biol Chem 1990; 265:4560–4566.
86. Broderick MJ, Winder SJ. Towards a complete atomic structure of spectrin family proteins. J Struct Biol 2002; 137:184–193.
87. Ponting CP, Blake DJ, Davies KE, Kendrick-Jones J, Winder SJ. ZZ and TAZ: new putative zinc fingers in dystrophin and other proteins. Trends Biochem Sci 1996; 21:11–13.

88. Ishikawa-Sakurai M, Yoshida M, Imamura M, Davies KE, Ozawa E. ZZ domain is essentially required for the physiological binding of dystrophin and utrophin to beta-dystroglycan. Hum Mol Genet 2004; 13:693–702.
89. Huang X, Poy F, Zhang R, Joachimiak A, Sudol M, Eck MJ. Structure of a WW domain containing fragment of dystrophin in complex with beta-dystroglycan. Nat Struct Biol 2000; 7:634–638.
90. Rafael JA, Cox GA, Corrado K, Jung D, Campbell KP, Chamberlain JS. Forced expression of dystrophin deletion constructs reveals structure–function correlations. J Cell Biol 1996; 134:93–102.
91. Suzuki A, Yoshida M, Yamamoto H, Ozawa E. Glycoprotein-binding site of dystrophin is confined to the cysteine-rich domain and the first half of the carboxy-terminal domain. FEBS Lett 1992; 308:154–160.
92. Jung D, Yang B, Meyer J, Chamberlain JS, Campbell KP. Identification and characterization of the dystrophin anchoring site on beta-dystroglycan. J Biol Chem 1995; 270:27305–27310.
93. Sadoulet-Puccio HM, Rajala M, Kunkel LM. Dystrobrevin and dystrophin: an interaction through coiled-coil motifs. Proc Natl Acad Sci USA 1997; 94:12413–12418.
94. Peters MF, O'Brien KF, Sadoulet-Puccio HM, Kunkel LM, Adams ME, Froehner SC. beta-dystrobrevin, a new member of the dystrophin family. Identification, cloning, and protein associations. J Biol Chem 1997; 272:31561–31569.
95. Yang B, Jung D, Rafael JA, Chamberlain JS, Campbell KP. Identification of alpha-syntrophin binding to syntrophin triplet, dystrophin, and utrophin. J Biol Chem 1995; 270:4975–4978.
96. Suzuki A, Yoshida M, Ozawa E. Mammalian alpha 1- and beta 1-syntrophin bind to the alternative splice-prone region of the dystrophin COOH terminus. J Cell Biol 1995; 128:373–381.
97. Watchko J, O'Day T, Wang B, et al. Adeno-associated virus vector-mediated minidystrophin gene therapy improves dystrophic muscle contractile function in mdx mice. Hum Gene Ther 2002; 13:1451–1460.
98. Fabb SA, Wells DJ, Serpente P, Dickson G. Adeno-associated virus vector gene transfer and sarcolemmal expression of a 144 kDa micro-dystrophin effectively restores the dystrophin-associated protein complex and inhibits myofibre degeneration in nude/mdx mice. Hum Mol Genet 2002; 11:733–741.
99. Abmayr S, Gregorevic P, Allen JM, Chamberlain JS. Phenotypic improvement of dystrophic muscles by rAAV/micro-dystrophin vectors is augmented by Igf-1 co-delivery. Mol Ther 2005; 12:441–450.
100. Warner LE, DelloRusso C, Crawford RW, et al. Expression of Dp260 in muscle tethers the actin cytoskeleton to the dystrophin–glycoprotein complex and partially prevents dystrophy. Hum Mol Genet 2002; 11:1095–1105.
101. Corrado K, Rafael JA, Mills PL, et al. Transgenic mdx mice expressing dystrophin with a deletion in the actin-binding domain display a "mild Becker" phenotype. J Cell Biol 1996; 134:873–884.
102. McCabe ER, Towbin J, Chamberlain J, et al. Complementary DNA probes for the Duchenne muscular dystrophy locus demonstrate a previously

undetectable deletion in a patient with dystrophic myopathy, glycerol kinase deficiency, and congenital adrenal hypoplasia. J Clin Invest 1989; 83:95–99.
103. Yue Y, Li Z, Harper SQ, Davisson RL, Chamberlain JS, Duan D. Microdystrophin gene therapy of cardiomyopathy restores dystrophin–glycoprotein complex and improves sarcolemma integrity in the mdx mouse heart. Circulation 2003; 108:1626–1632.
104. Yoshimura M, Sakamoto M, Ikemoto M, et al. AAV vector-mediated microdystrophin expression in a relatively small percentage of mdx myofibers improved the mdx phenotype. Mol Ther 2004; 10:821–828.
105. Liu M, Yue Y, Harper SQ, Grange RW, Chamberlain JS, Duan D. Adeno-Associated virus-mediated microdystrophin expression protects young mdx muscle from contraction-induced injury. Mol Ther. In press.
106. Tinsley JM, Potter AC, Phelps SR, Fisher R, Trickett JI, Davies KE. Amelioration of the dystrophic phenotype of mdx mice using a truncated utrophin transgene. Nature 1996; 384:349–353.
107. Deconinck N, Tinsley J, De Backer F, et al. Expression of truncated utrophin leads to major functional improvements in dystrophin-deficient muscles of mice. Nat Med 1997; 3:1216–1221.
108. Burkin DJ, Wallace GQ, Nicol KJ, Kaufman DJ, Kaufman SJ. Enhanced expression of the alpha 7 beta 1 integrin reduces muscular dystrophy and restores viability in dystrophic mice. J Cell Biol 2001; 152:1207–1218.
109. Liu L, Parekh-Olmedo H, Kmiec EB. The development and regulation of gene repair. Nat Rev Genet 2003; 4:679–689.
110. Kmiec EB. Targeted gene repair in the arena. J Clin Invest 2003; 112:632–636.
111. Bertoni C, Rando TA. Dystrophin gene repair in mdx muscle precursor cells in vitro and in vivo mediated by RNA-DNA chimeric oligonucleotides. Hum Gene Ther 2002; 13:707–718.
112. Rando TA. Oligonucleotide-mediated gene therapy for muscular dystrophies. Neuromuscul Disord 2002; 12(suppl 1):S55–S60.
113. Cathomen T. AAV vectors for gene correction. Curr Opin Mol Ther 2004; 6:360–366.
114. Hirata R, Chamberlain J, Dong R, Russell DW. Targeted transgene insertion into human chromosomes by adeno-associated virus vectors. Nat Biotechnol 2002; 20:735–738.
115. Chamberlain JR, Schwarze U, Wang PR, et al. Gene targeting in stem cells from individuals with osteogenesis imperfecta. Science 2004; 303:1198–1201.
116. Goyenvalle A, Vulin A, Fougerousse F, et al. Rescue of dystrophic muscle through U7 snRNA-mediated exon skipping. Science 2004; 306:1796–1799.
117. Musaro A, McCullagh K, Paul A, et al. Localized Igf-1 transgene expression sustains hypertrophy and regeneration in senescent skeletal muscle. Nat Genet 2001; 27:195–200.
118. Barton-Davis ER, Shoturma DI, Musaro A, Rosenthal N, Sweeney HL. Viral mediated expression of insulin-like growth factor I blocks the aging-related loss of skeletal muscle function. Proc Natl Acad Sci USA 1998; 95:15603–15607.
119. Barton ER, Morris L, Musaro A, Rosenthal N, Sweeney HL. Muscle-specific expression of insulin-like growth factor I counters muscle decline in mdx mice. J Cell Biol 2002; 157:137–148.

120. Lee SJ, McPherron AC. Regulation of myostatin activity and muscle growth. Proc Natl Acad Sci USA 2001; 98:9306–9311.
121. Zhu X, Hadhazy M, Wehling M, Tidball JG, McNally EM. Dominant negative myostatin produces hypertrophy without hyperplasia in muscle. FEBS Lett 2000; 474:71–75.
122. Wagner KR, McPherron AC, Winik N, Lee SJ. Loss of myostatin attenuates severity of muscular dystrophy in mdx mice. Ann Neurol 2002; 52:832–836.
123. Bogdanovich S, Krag TO, Barton ER, et al. Functional improvement of dystrophic muscle by myostatin blockade. Nature 2002; 420:418–421.
124. Greelish JP, Su LT, Lankford EB, et al. Stable restoration of the sarcoglycan complex in dystrophic muscle perfused with histamine and a recombinant adeno-associated viral vector. Nat Med 1999; 5:439–443.
125. Bridges CR, Burkman JM, Malekan R, et al. Global cardiac-specific transgene expression using cardiopulmonary bypass with cardiac isolation. Ann Thorac Surg 2002; 73:1939–1946.
126. Huard J, Lochmuller H, Acsadi G, et al. Differential short-term transduction efficiency of adult versus newborn mouse tissues by adenoviral recombinants. Exp Mol Pathol 1995; 62:131–143.
127. Gregory LG, Waddington SN, Holder MV, et al. Highly efficient EIAV-mediated in utero gene transfer and expression in the major muscle groups affected by Duchenne muscular dystrophy. Gene Ther 2004; 11:1117–1125.
128. Coutelle C, Themis M, Waddington S, et al. The hopes and fears of in utero gene therapy for genetic disease–a review. Placenta 2003; 24(suppl B):S114–S121.
129. Liu F, Nishikawa M, Clemens PR, Huang L. Transfer of full-length Dmd to the diaphragm muscle of Dmd(mdx/mdx) mice through systemic administration of plasmid DNA. Mol Ther 2001; 4:45–51.
130. Petrof BJ, Acsadi G, Jani A, et al. Efficiency and functional consequences of adenovirus-mediated in vivo gene transfer to normal and dystrophic (mdx) mouse diaphragm. Am J Respir Cell Mol Biol 1995; 13:508–517.
131. Huard J, Lochmuller H, Acsadi G, Jani A, Massie B, Karpati G. The route of administration is a major determinant of the transduction efficiency of rat tissues by adenoviral recombinants. Gene Ther 1995; 2:107–115.
132. Roberts WG, Palade GE. Increased microvascular permeability and endothelial fenestration induced by vascular endothelial growth factor. J Cell Sci 1995; 108(Pt 6):2369–2379.
133. Senger DR, Perruzzi CA, Feder J, Dvorak HF. A highly conserved vascular permeability factor secreted by a variety of human and rodent tumor cell lines. Cancer Res 1986; 46:5629–5632.
134. Eppler SM, Combs DL, Henry TD, et al. A target-mediated model to describe the pharmacokinetics and hemodynamic effects of recombinant human vascular endothelial growth factor in humans. Clin Pharmacol Ther 2002; 72:20–32.
135. Allen JM, Halbert CL, Miller AD. Improved adeno-associated virus vector production with transfection of a single helper adenovirus gene, E4orf6. Mol Ther 2000; 1:88–95.

20

Regional and Systemic Gene Delivery Using Viral Vectors

Leonard T. Su and Hansell H. Stedman
Department of Surgery, University of Pennsylvania, Philadelphia, Pennsylvania, U.S.A.

INTRODUCTION

Muscular dystrophy is a systemic disease. Methods outlined in this chapter have shown great potential in restoring near-normal histology to muscle fibers and in improving the function of whole muscles in in vivo assays following the use of virus-based vectors for gene delivery. Most of these studies focus on local delivery, assaying the efficacy of the vectors at the level of individual muscles in small animal models. A limitation of these model becomes evident when attempts are made to deliver these vectors regionally or systemically. This process is further compounded when studies are extended into large animal models. In the clinical setting, treatment that can safely confer significant benefit, both as perceived by the patient and as measured through standardized strength testing, must be the ultimate goal. This translation from local to systemic delivery, from "benchtop to bedside," may be one of the greatest challenges faced in gene therapy for muscular dystrophy. The complete reversal of histopathological signs of muscular dystrophy in several murine models following germline gene transfer has prompted consideration of a wide range of strategies for achieving systemic gene transfer. In this chapter, we focus specifically on strategies pertaining to the use of virus-based vectors to directly transduce striated muscle in situ, thereby complementing advances in vector development described in other chapters.

DIRECT INTRAMUSCULAR INJECTION

The most common approach to study in situ gene transfer using virus-based vectors begins with the direct intramuscular (IM) injection. Direct syringe injection allows for diffusion of vector particles into the interstitium surrounding the site. Connective tissue limits such diffusion to a radius of few millimeters surrounding the site of injection (1–3). In a small animal model this does not present itself as a limitation given the size of the target muscle, usually the tibialis anterior, whose cross-sectional area falls well within the radius of diffusion. IM injections of dystrophin-expressing vectors, especially in neonatal *mdx* mice, have been shown to restore normal or near-normal histology in the entire cross-sections of injected muscle (4). Furthermore, analyses of the muscle function show that IM injections can restore a protective effect from force-induced damage, as well as a significant improvement in force generating capacity (5). However, the limitation to vector diffusion becomes evident in nominally larger animals such as the hamster, rat, or mature mouse, if studies address muscles with a marginally larger cross-sectional radius or delivery to multiple muscle groups. In large animal studies, limitations of direct IM injection become increasingly unwieldy, requiring a geometrically higher number of injections for a single muscle. The problems of simple volumetric scaling are illustrated by the experience with intramuscularly injected preparations of adeno-associated virus (AAV) vectors encoding factor IX, where a single injection in the mouse provided serum levels higher than did 60 separate injections in the dog (6,7). Although our personal experience with older patients with muscular dystrophy suggests that maintenance of strength in a limited number of muscles in the forearm would be perceived as a substantive clinical benefit, much of the current research in this area focuses on the prospects of expanded gene delivery to the musculature of entire limbs and ultimately the respiratory apparatus and heart.

Several studies have shown the feasibility and efficacy of wide-scale regional delivery in the isolated rodent hindlimb and in global cardiac delivery (see below). These illustrate not only the potential of systemic vector delivery but also the challenges in eventually developing clinically applicable protocols for it.

REGIONAL DELIVERY

Intravascular Approach

Limitations: The Endothelial Barrier to Intravascular Delivery

The seemingly straightforward alternative to direct IM injection is the intravascular approach. Skeletal muscle is richly invested by its capillary network, allowing for widespread homogenous distribution of oxygen and glucose throughout the muscle during times of maximal substrate utilization. A similar pattern of distribution of vector throughout the muscle would appear to circumvent the dependence on diffusion through the interstitium from an injection site. This approach also has the apparent advantage of single injections into easily accessible vessels. Despite these considerations, simple intravascular injections of a variety of vectors have shown disappointingly poor transduction of skeletal muscle.

Specifically, simple IV injection of recombinant adenoviruses via the tail vein in young rodents results in transduction of a large variety of tissues, particularly hepatocytes, but yields low-efficiency transduction of skeletal muscle (1,8). This affinity for the liver, displayed by a variety of vectors, allows therapeutic levels of transduction in hepatocytes for various inherited metabolic diseases (9). Furthermore, while IV injection seemed promising in skeletal muscle of neonates, transduction in adult muscle fibers was notably less efficient (1).

Conceptually, intraarterial injection has the advantage of more specifically targeting end vascular beds (e.g., muscle groups) while avoiding first-pass elimination by the liver. However, intraarterial delivery similarly is affected by the nonspecific volume of distribution and inefficient transduction of skeletal muscle. Proximal arterial injections, such as left intraventricular or intraaortic infusion of marker adenovirus, result in measurable transduction of a variety of tissues but extremely inefficient transduction of cardiac and skeletal muscle (10). Injecting more distally for more specific targeting of end vascular beds, such as injections into coronary arterial circulation via surgical or catheter-based approaches, has met with varying degrees of efficiency of delivery to cardiac myocytes. Directed injection into arteries supplying skeletal muscle beds (e.g., femoral artery) shows little to no muscle fiber transduction in mature animals, even under modestly increased hydrostatic pressure (11). Closer analysis of these infusions shows that uptake of vector is limited to the microvasculature surrounding the muscle fibers, indicating that the barrier preventing passage of vector into the muscle fiber lies in the continuous endothelium of the microvasculature. Evidence exists that mature skeletal muscle fibers can be transduced following direct IM injection. Data from these direct IM injections suggest that, in the absence of the endothelial barrier, vector delivery and gene transfer are limited primarily by lateral diffusion through the interstitium. More direct evidence of the endothelial barrier to delivery, in the case of adenoviral vectors, has been shown in vitro, where a confluent human umbilical vein endothelial cell monolayer leads to a highly significant decrease in adenovirus gene transfer to cultured cardiac myocytes, which in the absence of this barrier are efficiently infected by the same vector (12). Finally, the high levels of hepatocyte transduction after intravascular administration suggest that a critical architectural difference between the liver and most other organ systems is the fenestration of the hepatic endothelium.

Transendothelial Transport

There are no naturally occurring viruses whose life cycle depends on efficient penetration of the continuous endothelium of skeletal muscle. Thus development of a virus-based vector system with a naturally occurring biological mechanism for crossing this barrier seems unlikely. Transendothelial transport of particles and solutes is classically modeled as a three-component process with contributions from three mechanistic pathways: diffusion, such as small lipid-soluble molecules diffusing through endothelial cell plasma membranes; facilitated transport, as seen with vesicles; and convection in which the flow of molecules is determined by the flow of solvent (13–15). For macromolecules approaching the size of albumin (50 kDa), transcellular permeability is essentially zero, with paracellular convective flow predominating. Major determinants of this transcapillary convective flow have been defined classically by Starling's hypothesis with differences in hydrostatic (δ_p) and osmotic (δ_π) pressures between the capillary and interstitium as the main driving forces for solvent flow. Further expansion of these principles leads to the Kedem–Katchalsky equation for solvent flow: $J_v = L_p(\delta_p - \delta_\pi)$, where solvent or volume flow, J_v, is determined by L_p, a constant of hydraulic conductivity or filtration, and δ, the reflection coefficient ranging from 0 (freely permeable) to 1 (impermeable). Manipulation of one or more of these parameters may allow for increased flow and, therefore, solute transport across the endothelial barrier (16,17).

A closer look at the architecture of the endothelium itself suggests potential methods for breaching it. Paracellular permeability is restricted in a tissue-specific manner by intercellular adherens and tight junctions (18–20). A variety of ligands can rapidly and reversibly modulate junctional permeability (21–27). Some of the protein–protein interactions and signal transduction events have been recently elucidated in detail, but there are significant gaps in our understanding. It has long been recognized that both adherens and tight junctions are anchored to the actin-based cytoskeleton, and that they respond to alterations in the contractile state of the nonmuscle class II myosins. A range of inflammatory mediators induce rapid changes in cytoskeletal architecture and in the phosphorylation states or intracellular distribution of myosin and several integral junctional proteins (27,28). There has been recent confirmation and extension of classical studies (29–31) in which the inflammatory mediators histamine, bradykinin, and serotonin rapidly induced alterations in endothelial cell morphology, temporally associated with the extravasation of tracer macromolecules and microscopically visible particles. Even in the absence of such gross morphological changes, histamine-induced alterations in permeability are associated with rapid changes in the phosphorylation state of junctional proteins (27). Engagement of specific receptors on the endothelial cell surface is thought to initiate a signal transduction cascade which is propagated, and ultimately reversed, by alterations in cytosolic calcium concentration and the activities of cyclic nucleotide-regulated kinases (27,32). The rapid reversibility of mediator effects on endothelial permeability suggests the possibility of their use to augment vector transport from the bloodstream to the interstitium, providing indirect access to parenchymal cells from the vascular space.

Breaching the Endothelial Barrier

Large Volume Infusion, Modifying Starling Forces

Cho et al. (33), in their work, focus on increasing the driving pressure for transcapillary flow out of the intravascular space. They studied the effect of large volume infusion on the Starling forces by cannulating the femoral artery and occluding venous outflow from the femoral vein, and predicted that large volumes would induce an increase in hydrostatic pressure and a decrease in osmotic pressure gradients. A comparison between large volume infusions of 20 to 25 mL/kg and standard volume infusions (1–1.5 mL/kg) showed a significant increase in whole muscle wet to dry weight ratios. Histologically they observed an increase in the endomysial space between muscle fibers, consistent with fluid extravasation and edema. Also in the large volume group there was a significant increase in the amount of extravasated macromolecular tracer particles of a size approximate to that of adenovirus. All of this suggests that the large volume group did indeed alter transcapillary flow, albeit without a direct measurement of the actual increase in the hydrostatic pressure, δ_p, or in the osmotic pressure, δ_π.

Interestingly, when a recombinant adenovirus containing the *LacZ* reporter gene was administered intraarterially under the same conditions, both standard and large volume groups were unsuccessful in achieving significant transgene expression. The aoouthors therefore focused on the possibility of low levels of the Coxsackie adenovirus receptor (CAR) expression in mature myocytes causing this lack of *LacZ* expression. They sought to determine if induced myocyte regeneration could increase CAR levels in immature fibers. Specifically, several days prior to the intraarterial delivery experiments, they directly injected the muscles of the hindlimbs (gastrocnemius, tibialis anterior, and soleus) by IM injection with the notexin which can produce transient degeneration of mature myofibers with subsequent rapid muscle regeneration. In the face of these pretreatments with notexin, the large volume and not the standard volume group showed *LacZ* expression over a large uniformly distributed cross-section in the pretreated muscles. However, a fairly wide variability between animals was noted, from 0% to 36% of muscle fibers transduced throughout the three muscles studied. Similar findings could be seen in *mdx* mouse hindlimbs in pretreated muscles with up to 44% of fibers expressing *LacZ*. It is noteworthy that 0.65% of the gastrocnemius muscle fibers expressed *LacZ* in un-pretreated animals, suggesting that spontaneous muscle regeneration in the *mdx* animal allowed immature fibers to be transduced (33).

Inflammatory Mediators: Histamine and Endothelial Permeability

Work in our laboratory sought to effect changes in microvascular permeability at the paracellular junctions, thereby increasing transcapillary volume flow and, by convection, vector flow. Starting with an adenovirus vector expressing *LacZ* under the control of the constitutive cytomegolovirus (CMV) promoter, we noted virtually no muscle staining with X-gal following rat femoral artery infusions alone (Fig. 1, panels A–C; reproduced from Ref. 11). As stated earlier, all *LacZ* expression was confined to the microvasculature, suggesting that no adenovirus had traversed the endothelium. However, by achieving circulatory isolation of the hindlimb through the use of surgically placed tourniquets, followed by vasodilatation using papavarine, permeabilization of the endothelial sheet could be achieved with histamine. Under these conditions, nearly universal and homogenous expression was achieved throughout the entire hindlimb seen both on whole-mount staining and on microscopic cross-sections (Fig. 1, panels E–K). Interestingly, the photomicrographs revealed that the vessel walls themselves remained unstained despite strong staining of neighboring muscle fibers. Finally, this approach was extended to the heterotopically transplanted heart, where anastamosis to the femoral artery distal to the level of the tourniquets enabled global *LacZ* expression, showing that endothelial permeability in the cardiac circulation could be achieved and that cardiac myocytes could be efficiently transduced under these conditions (Fig. 1, panel L) (11).

Figure 1 (*Facing page*) Gene transfer across the endothelial barrier: Use of histamine and papaverine to transiently increase permeability. **(A–C)** Pattern of gene transfer in the absence of inflammatory mediators demonstrates integrity of microvascular barrier to adenovirus transport. **(D)** For contrasting appearance, whole mount stained leg of adult rat following intramuscular injection of AdCMVlacZ, showing focal uptake of virus by a few fibers in the immediate vicinity of needle tract ($\times 50$). **(E–K)** Highly efficient gene transfer to adult skeletal muscle fibers following forced exudation in the presence of histamine and papaverine. **(L)** Heterotopically transplanted heart following isolated perfusion with histamine and papaverine analogous to that used for isolated limb ($100\times$). **(M)** Quadriceps muscle from BIO 14.6 hamster perfused with 7×10^{11} particles of AAVCMVd-sarcoglycan without use of histamine or papaverine ($\times 100$). **(N–Q)** Rescue of the sarcoglycan complex in muscles throughout the adult BIO 14.6 hamster hindlimb following perfusion with histamine, papaverine and rAAV. *Key to muscles*: **(N)** biceps femoris ($\times 200$), **(O)** quadriceps ($\times 100$), **(P)** semimembranosus ($\times 200$), **(Q)** gastrocnemius ($\times 100$).

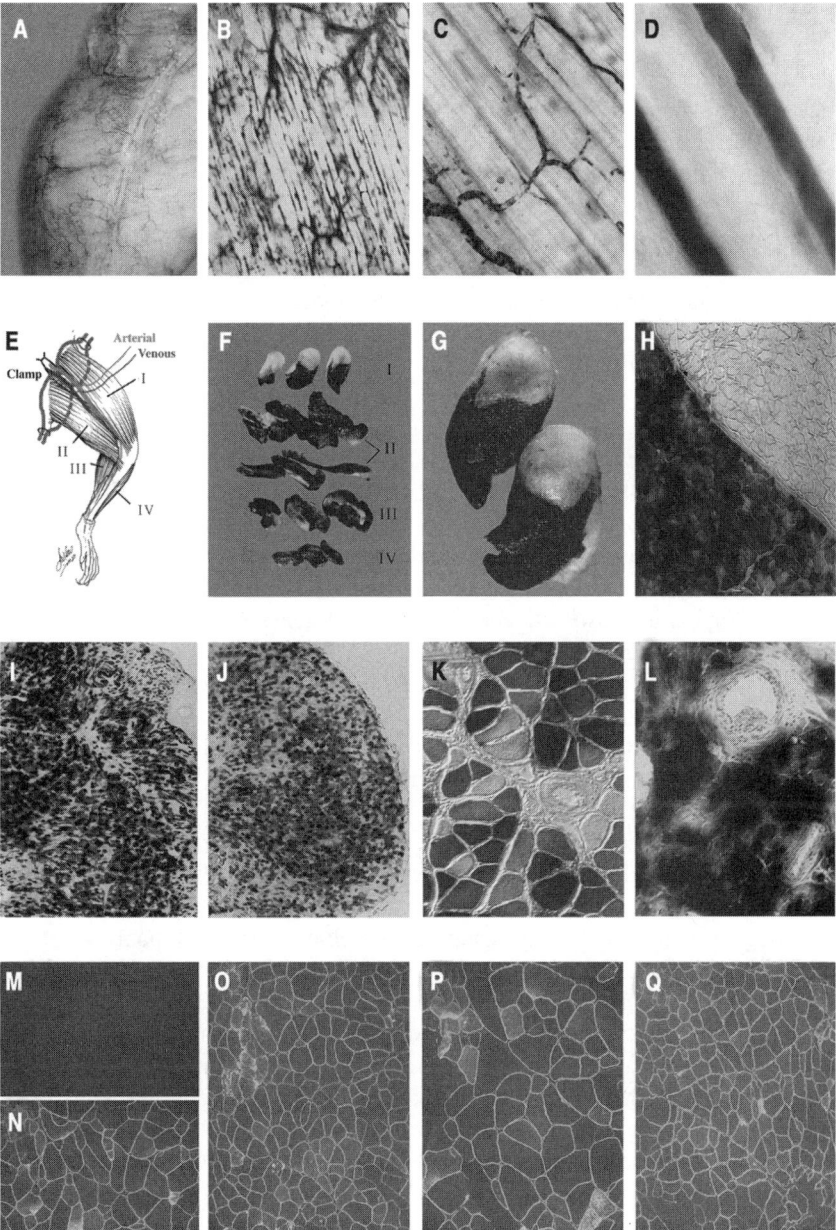

Figure 1 (*Caption on facing page*).

Turning attention to the Bio 14.6 hamster as a model for delta-sarcoglycanopathy, one of the recessively inherited limb-girdle muscular dystrophies, a recombinant adeno-associated virus (rAAV) containing a delta-sarcoglycan cDNA within a CMV transcriptional cassette was constructed and used. This vector, when directly injected intramuscularly into Bio 14.6 hamster muscle, rescued sarcoglycan complex expression in the sarcolemma and conferred a protective effect against eccentric contraction-induced myofiber injury as seen in vital dye uptake assays. This rAAV, even at high (1×10^{11} particles per gram of tissue) titers, failed to penetrate the endothelial barrier when intra-arterially injected into the Bio 14.6 (Fig. 1, panel M). The circulatory isolation technique and pretreatment with papavarine and histamine, previously used in the rat, resulted in dose-dependent, wide-scale restoration of the sarcoglycan complex throughout the hindlimb (Fig. 1, panels N–Q) (11). A mosaic-form pattern of fibers with sarcoplasmic delta-sarcoglycan against a background of fibers staining exclusively in the sarcolemma indicates that delivery yielded a high multiplicity of infection in the best-perfused fibers, thereby achieving supranormal delta-sarcoglycan gene expression. Importantly, these experiments were conducted in adult hamsters to ensure the passage of the neonatal window for immunological nonresponsiveness to viral antigens, and to model the histological barriers that might impede gene transfer in the clinical setting where symptomatic patients have already experienced myodegeneration and endomysial fibrosis (34). In addition, more recent studies have applied this approach to therapeutic gene transfer in a canine model for hemophilia B, demonstrating scale independence (Arruda, Stedman, et al., in press).

Regional Delivery to Cardiac Myocytes

The ultrastructural similarities between cardiac and skeletal muscles reflect the large number of genes that are coexpressed in these striated muscles. Although skeletal myopathy results in the characteristic clinical symptoms and signs associated with most forms of muscular dystrophy, underlying cardiomyopathy is more the rule than the exception. In Duchenne muscular dystrophy, for instance, it is estimated that cardiomyopathy is the ultimate cause of death in a significant percentage of cases. In clinically mild Becker muscular dystrophy, echocardiographic signs of cardiomyopathy may be the first detectable signs of disease (35). In several genes initially identified on the basis of their etiologic role in skeletal myopathy, additional mutations have been found that result in isolated cardiomyopathy (36). These positional cloning and candidate gene approaches have contributed substantially to the scientific armamentarium for addressing the more general and epidemic disease, congestive heart failure. The study of gene transfer to skeletal muscle is complementary to this process, both benefiting from and contributing to parallel advances in cardiac gene therapy. Although the heart represents a sarcomeric muscle mass as little as 2% to that of the aggregate skeletal muscle mass, the risk of even transient periprocedural contractile dysfunction is greatly amplified.

By direct analogy to the chronologic progression of studies in skeletal muscle, the earliest reports of gene transfer to the heart described regional transduction in small animals following direct IM injections into the ventricular wall (3). Coronary infusion of vector at cardiac catheterization was evaluated as a logical extension of standard procedure in interventional cardiology. Initial reports showed impressive staining of whole-mounted tissue preparations, but provided little direct evidence for transduction of cardiac myocytes in situ. We next focus on the combined works of Ikeda et al. (37) and Hoshijima et al. (38), because they relate to the principles of endothelial barrier permeability as outlined above, and represent experiments performed in the Bio 14.6 hamster, a model for muscular dystrophy and cardiomyopathy. These authors used an approach based initially on aortic root administration that involved a short (10 second) cross-clamping of the aorta and pulmonary artery (39). Efficiency of delivery was highly variable using this method, even when mediated with histamine. Ikeda et al. (37) modified this technique by inducing hypothermia, cooling the rat to 18°C to 25°C, and then occluding the aorta and pulmonary artery, followed by the use of a cardioplegic solution containing histamine, and the solution being allowed to remain in site for three to five minutes. Marker adenovirus or recombinant AdV expressing delta-sarcoglycan was then administered. Cross-clamping was released; the animal was then resuscitated and rewarmed. This use of hypothermia and cardioplegic arrest allows prolongation of exposure to endothelial permeability mediators (histamine) and the virus itself. This technique achieved homogenous *LacZ* staining in cross-sections of the heart with 77% of myocardial nuclei positive (vs. 0–19% in a non–hypothermia-cardioplegia group). Similarly in the Bio 14.6 hamster these investigators observed diffuse staining of d-Sarcoglycan on cross-sectional immunohistochemistry in 50% to 60% of myocytes. Similar observations were reported for rAAV vectors expressing marker *LacZ* or a pseudophosphorylated mutant of human phospholamban in the Bio 14.6 hamster. Transduction with the latter construct resulted in measurable improvement in cardiac function, suggesting a potential therapeutic modality for heart failure.

The evolution of this technique illustrates the challenge of regional gene delivery to the heart when using the vascular space as a conduit. Use of aortic occlusion alone, where one might expect an increase in hydrostatic pressure as the heart pumps isovolumetrically against the clamps, only nominally increases the efficiency of gene delivery. However, strict vascular isolation to prevent coronary venous admixture with the central circulation requires occlusion of the vena cavae and venting of the right heart (40). Without this, most of the vector will ultimately be taken up by the liver, as seen with the constitutively expressed marker gene in the report by Ikeda et al. (37). The use of histamine to facilitate vector transport to the interstitium provides a reproducible method for augmenting the efficiency of gene transfer to the myocardium, translating the challenge to that of managing the biodistribution of histamine. Complete containment of histamine in this context is easiest to visualize in the setting of an open surgical procedure, not in the setting of an interventional radiological procedure where the Thebesian venous drainage to the right atrium would escape retrieval by a catheter in the coronary sinus. A number of alternatives will have to be comparatively evaluated in scale-up studies before a clinically feasible approach can be optimized for patients with congestive heart failure.

FUTURE DIRECTIONS: APPLICATIONS OF THE CURRENT TECHNOLOGY

The methods described in the above-mentioned studies individually have the ability to effect widespread regional vector delivery to skeletal and cardiac muscle. The above studies also identify some of the hurdles that need to be overcome in future translational studies. Hindlimb studies from Cho et al. (33) and Greelish et al. (11) rely on vascular outflow control, a concept that is easily achieved in the isolated limb, but far more difficult to perform in other regions of major clinical significance in muscular dystrophy (e.g., muscles of respiration or proximal muscles involved in posture control and locomotion). Such regions generally have a very rich blood supply with numerous and anatomically variable venous outflow vessels. Occlusion of individual vessels surgically or radiologically is impractical. In the case of the findings of Cho et al., prior local injection of notexin or other similar substances to induce adenoviral transduction reprises the original problem of IM injections and its concomitant requirements. On the other hand, the methods of Greelish et al. require the presence of histamine, a potent inflammatory mediator with systemic toxicity. The vascular isolation by surgically placed tourniquets avoids such systemic toxicity, and isolated limb perfusions are performed clinically in humans, for example, to administer high-dose chemotherapeutic agents to a limb for treatment of malignant melanoma. Modifying this technique for proximal muscle or central muscle groups will be challenging in the face of the risk from a systemic leak should the vascular isolation not be complete. Alternatively, the hemodynamic consequences of histamine infusion could be countered by providing mechanical support through an extracorporeal pump-oxygenator. The reliance of efficient cardiac gene delivery on the histamine effect suggests that either the vector infusion should be performed in the setting of complete cardiac circulatory isolation (40) or with a plan for sustained cardiopulmonary support as in postcardiotomy ECMO (41).

Translational studies in the large animal will focus on safety as well as efficacy. These studies will allow for improvements in the physical techniques, surgical and/or radiological, for gene delivery, as well as refinements in intra- and postprocedural care with formalized respiratory, anesthesia, and intensive care support. Human clinical trials at all phases will, of course, be guided by such large animal studies and may ultimately require significant alterations in protocol during extrapolation from the proof-of-concept studies in the small animal to avoid or minimize systemic toxicity. Hence there will be a high premium on the development of procedures that offer well-defined potential for therapeutic benefit at the lowest possible risk to the patient. Muscular dystrophy is a systemic disease. Severe forms of the disease are universally lethal and may ultimately require whole-body systemic therapy using relatively invasive techniques, as long as the risks are justified by the potential for therapeutic gain. For clinical investigators contemplating even the simplest of studies using the vectors described, another risk must be carefully considered and revealed in the informed consent process: that of immune sensitization to the vector capsid, precluding the individual patient's participation in a later phase of the research program. These interrelated issues are at the focus of current translational research programs in cardiac, regional, and systemic "gene delivery."

REFERENCES

1. Stratford-Perricaude LD, Makeh I, Perricaudet M, Briand P. Widespread long-term gene transfer to mouse skeletal muscles and heart. J Clin Invest 1992; 90:626–630.
2. French BA, Mazur W, Geske RS, Bolli R. Direct in vivo gene transfer into porcine myocardium using replication-deficient adenoviral vectors. Circulation 1994; 90:2414–2424.
3. Guzman RJ, Lemarchand P, Crystal RG, Epstein SE, Finkel T. Efficient gene transfer into myocardium by direct injection of adenovirus vectors. Circ Res 1993; 73:1202–1207.
4. Ragot T, Vincent N, Chafey P, et al. Efficient adenovirus-mediated transfer of a human minidystrophin gene to skeletal muscle of mdx mice. Nature 1993; 361:647–650.
5. Deconinck N, Ragot T, Marechal G, Perricaudet M, Gillis JM. Functional protection of dystrophic mouse (mdx) muscles after adenovirus-mediated transfer of a dystrophin minigene. Proc Natl Acad Sci USA 1996; 93:3570–3574.
6. Herzog RW, Hagstrom JN, Kung SH, et al. Stable gene transfer and expression of human blood coagulation factor IX after intramuscular injection of recombinant adeno-associated virus. Proc Natl Acad Sci USA 1997; 94:5804–5809.
7. Herzog RW, Yang EY, Couto LB, et al. Long-term correction of canine hemophilia B by gene transfer of blood coagulation factor IX mediated by adeno-associated viral vector (see comments). Nat Med 1999; 5:56–63.
8. Huard J, Lochmuller H, Acsadi G, Jani A, Massie B, Karpati G. The route of administration is a major determinant of the transduction efficiency of rat tissues by adenoviral recombinants. Gene Ther 1995; 2:107–115.

9. Kay MA, Woo SL. Gene therapy for metabolic disorders. Trends Genet 1994; 10:253–257.
10. Fechner H, Haack A, Wang H, et al. Expression of Coxsackie adenovirus receptor and alphav-integrin does not correlate with adenovector targeting in vivo indicating anatomical vector barriers. Gene Ther 1999; 6:1520–1535.
11. Greelish JP, Su LT, Lankford EB, et al. Stable restoration of the sarcoglycan complex in dystrophic muscle perfused with histamine and a recombinant adeno-associated viral vector. Nat Med 1999; 5:439–443.
12. Nevo N, Chossat N, Gosgnach W, Logeart D, Mercadier JJ, Michel JB. Increasing endothelial cell permeability improves the efficiency of myocyte adenoviral vector infection. J Gene Med 2001; 3:42–50.
13. Starling E. On the absorption of fluids from the connective tissue spaces. J Physiol 1896; 19:312.
14. Pappenheimer RJ, Renkin EM, Borrero LM. Filtration, diffusion and molecular sieving through peripheral capillary membranes. A contribution to the pore theory of capillary permeability. Am J Physiol 1951; 167:13–28.
15. Clough G. Relationship between microvascular permeability and ultrastructure. Prog Biophys Mol Biol 1991; 55:47–69.
16. Kedem O, Katchalsky A. Thermodynamic analysis of the permeability of biological membranes to non-electrolytes. Biochim Biophys Acta 1989; 1000:413–430.
17. Kargol M, Kargol A. Mechanistic formalism for membrane transport generated by osmotic and mechanical pressure. Gen Physiol Biophys 2003; 22:51–68.
18. Dejana E. Endothelial adherens junctions: implications in the control of vascular permeability and angiogenesis. J Clin Invest 1996; 98:1949–1953.
19. Lampugnani MG, Dejana E. Interendothelial junctions: structure, signalling and functional roles. Curr Opin Cell Biol 1997; 9:674–682.
20. Tsukita S, Furuse M. Pores in the wall: claudins constitute tight junction strands containing aqueous pores. J Cell Biol 2000; 149:13–16.
21. Curry FE. Modulation of venular microvessel permeability by calcium influx into endothelial cells. FASEB J 1992; 6:2456.
22. Johns A, Lategan TW, Lodge NJ, Ryan US, Van Breemen C, Adams DJ. Calcium entry through receptor-operated channels in bovine pulmonary artery endothelial cells. Tissue Cell 1987; 19:733–745.
23. Joris I, Majno G, Lorey EJ, Lewis RA. The mechanism of vascular leakage induced by leukotriene E(4) endothelial contraction. Am J Pathol 1987; 126:19.
24. Keck PJ, Hauser SD, Krivi G, et al. Vascular permeability factor, an endothelial cell mitogen related to PDGF. Science 1989; 246:1309–1312.
25. Kurose I, Miura S, Fukumura D, Tsuchiya M. Mechanism of endothelin-induced macromolecular leakage in microvascular beds of rat mesentery. Eur J Pharm 1993; 250:85–94.
26. Northover AM, Northover BJ. The effects of histamine, 5 hydroxytryptamine and bradykinin on rat mesenteric blood vessels. J Pathol 1969; 98:265–275.
27. Andriopoulou P, Navarro P, Zanetti A, Lampugnani MG, Dejana E. Histamine induces tyrosine phosphorylation of endothelial cell-to-cell adherens junctions. Arterioscler Thromb Vasc Biol 1999; 19:2286–2297.
28. Gardner TW, Lesher T, Khin S, Vu C, Barber AJ, Brennan WA Jr. Histamine reduces ZO-1 tight-junction protein expression in cultured retinal microvascular endothelial cells. Biochem J 1996; 320:717–721.

29. McDonald DM, Thurston G, Baluk P. Endothelial gaps as sites for plasma leakage in inflammation. Microcirculation 1999; 6:7–22.
30. Majno G, Palade GE. Studies on inflammation. I. The effect of histamine and serotonin on vascular permeability: an electron microscopic study. J Biophys Biochem Cytol 1961; 11:571–597.
31. Majno G, Palade GE, Schhoeft GI. Studies on inflammation. II. The site of action of histamine an serotonin along the vascular tree: a topographic study. J Biophys Biochem Cytol 1961; 11:607–626.
32. Yuan SY. Signal transduction pathways in enhanced microvascular permeability (in process citation). Microcirculation 2000; 7:395–403.
33. Cho WK, Ebihara S, Nalbantoglu J, et al. Modulation of Starling forces and muscle fiber maturity permits adenovirus-mediated gene transfer to adult dystrophic (mdx) mice by the intravascular route. Hum Gene Ther 2000; 11:701–714.
34. DeMatteo R, Chu G, Chang E, Barker C, Markmann J. Long-lasting adenovirus transgene expression in mice through neonatal intrathymic tolerance induction without the use of immunosuppression. J Virol 1997; 71:5330–5335.
35. Melacini P, Fanin M, Danieli GA, et al. Myocardial involvement is very frequent among patients affected with subclinical Becker's muscular dystrophy. Circulation 1996; 94:3168–3175.
36. Towbin JA, Bowles NE. The failing heart. Nature 2002; 415:227–233.
37. Ikeda Y, Gu Y, Iwanaga Y, et al. Restoration of deficient membrane proteins in the cardiomyopathic hamster by in vivo cardiac gene transfer. Circulation 2002; 105:502–508.
38. Hoshijima M, Ikeda Y, Iwanaga Y, et al. Chronic suppression of heart-failure progression by a pseudophosphorylated mutant of phospholamban via in vivo cardiac rAAV gene delivery. Nat Med 2002; 8:864–871.
39. Hajjar RJ, Schmidt U, Matsui T, et al. Modulation of ventricular function through gene transfer in vivo. Proc Natl Acad Sci USA 1998; 95:5251–5256.
40. Bridges CR, Burkman JM, Malekan R, et al. Global cardiac-specific transgene expression using cardiopulmonary bypass with cardiac isolation. Ann Thorac Surg 2002; 73:1939–1946.
41. Jaggers JJ, Forbess JM, Shah AS, et al. Extracorporeal membrane oxygenation for infant postcardiotomy support: significance of shunt management. Ann Thorac Surg 2000; 69:1476–1483.

Index

α-sarcoglycan (α-SG) protein, 299
AAV vectors, 210
AAV-based gene transfer, 210
Acetylcholine receptor (AChR), 253
Actin filaments, 31
   dystrophin binding and, 36, 252
Acute gastric dilation, late stage DMD complication, 15
Adaptive immunity, 373
Adeno-associated virus (AAV), 413
   genome and capsid, 413
   genome codes, 414
   serotypes, 414, 415
   types,
      dependovirus, 413
      densovirinae, 413
      parvovirinae, 413
   vectors, 404
Adeno-retroviral system, 402
Adenoviral capsid structure, 364
Adenoviral vectors, 209, 368
Adenoviral-mediated gene therapy, 363
Adenoviruses (Ad), 363
   albuterol, 234
   capsid components, 372
   infection pathway, 365
   internalization, 366
Allopurinol, 214
Ambulation, 154, 179, 183

[Ambulation]
   loss of, 6
   prolong, 133, 158, 213, 228
   steroids effect on, 127
Aminoglycoside antibiotic gentamicin, 211
Anabolic agents
   anabolic corticosteroids, 234
   β_2 adrenoceptor agonists, 233
   for muscle strength increase, 233
Anabolic hormones, 232
Animal models, in development of therapies for DMD, 202, 203
Ankle deformity, correction of, 158
Antidystrophin antibodies, 357
Anti-inflammatory agents, to stabilize mast cells, 236
Antineuronal cell adhesion molecule (NCAM), 378
Antisense oligonucleotides (AONs), 320
   clinical applications, 325
   mechanism of action, 320
   modifications, 323
   specificity of, 326
   structure, 320
   systemic delivery, 324
   toxicity of, 326
   transient efficacy, 325
Antisense-mediated exon skipping, 321

AON-mediated gene therapy, 322
Apneic episodes, 164
Apoptotic death, 61, 63
Aquatic therapy, 5
Arginine–glycine–aspartic acid (RGD) motif, 366
Arrhythmias, 8
Atrophy, 22, 23, 41

Basal lamina, protective ability of, 37
Becker mini-dystrophin, 398, 399
Becker muscular dystrophy (BMD), 2, 33, 202, 322
β-dystroglycan, 201
β-globin gene splicing, in nuclear extracts, 320
β2-syntrophin, 253
BiPAP machine, 164
BMD vs. DMD, 11, 78, 151, 202
BM-derived cells, 302, 308
BMD. *See* Becker muscular dystrophy
Bone deformities, 22
Bone marrow precursors, 297
Bone marrow transplantation model of cell delivery, 298
Bovine immunodeficiency (BIV), 405
Bowel movements, 9

CAR. *See* Coxsackie adenovirus receptor
CMD. *See* Congenital muscular dystrophy
CMV. *See* Cytomegalovirus
cis-acting components, 406
Calcineurin, 260
Calcium channel blockers, 139
Calcium ions. *See* Muscle degeneration, inducer
Calf muscle hypertrophy, 22
Calmodulin, 65, 228
Calpain, 45, 65
Calponin homology (CH) domains, 252
Capsid, 392, 393, 404, 406
Capsomeres, 364
Caregiver burden, 229
Carrier detection, 82

Casting, 183
Cell delivery
  of functional donor cells, 298
  intraarterial, 298
  intramuscular, 298
  intravenous, 298, 299
  for muscular dystrophy, 295, 298
Cell transplants, 206
Cellular energy buffer, 234
Cellular response, 373
Chimeraplasts. *See* Chimeric RNA/DNA oligonucleotides
Chimeric RNA/DNA oligonucleotides (RDO), 327
  applications, 329
  clinical application, 335
  mechanism of action, 327, 328
  oligonucleotide uptake and translocation, 334
  point mutation correction, 329
  RDO-mediated gene repair, 329
  RNA splicing, 332
  systemic delivery, 334, 335
Chromosomal DNA (cDNA), 368
Circulatory isolation technique, 446
Clenbuterol, 233
Clinical therapeutic agent, for DMD treatment, 363
Compartment syndrome, 187
Congenital muscular dystrophy (CMD), 32
Contraction–relaxation cycle, 42
Contractures, 13, 154, 179, 189
  principal therapy modalities, 156
Corticosteroids, 16, 130, 213
Coxsackie adenovirus receptor (CAR), 209, 366, 443
Creatine kinase, 227
Cryptic splice site, 333
C-terminal region of gene, 252
Cushingoid features, 229
C-xmd canine model, of DMD, 308
Cyclosporin, 138
Cysteine-rich (CR) region, 420
Cystic fibrosis transmembrane conductance regulator (CFTR), 237
Cytomegalovirus (CMV), 407
  promoter, 444

Index

[Cytomegalovirus (CMV)]
  retinitis, 320
Cytoskeletal protein, 295
Cytotoxic T cell (CT) GalNac
  transferase, 263

DAPC. *See* Dystrophin associated
  protein complex
DIF. *See* Desmin intermediate filaments
DGC. *See* Dystroglycan complex
DGGE. *See* Denaturing gradient gel
  electrophoresis
Deflazacort, 229, 230
Deletion pattern, nonrandom, 93
Denaturing gradient gel electrophoresis
  (DGGE), 81
Density gradient centrifugation, for
  purification of rAAV, 415
Dermal fibroblasts, 310
Desmin intermediate filaments
  (DIF), 38
Direct intramuscular (IM) injection, 440
DMD/BMD, Diagnostic flowchart, 84
DNA duplex molecules, 327
Donor cell selection, 301, 302
Donor-derived dystrophin, 300
Donor-derived nuclei, 302
Dorsiflexion, 181, 186
Downstream utrophin enhancer
  (DUE), 262
Dual-energy X-ray absorptiometry, 234
Duchenne muscular dystrophy (DMD)
  biopsies, 228
  cardiac complications in, 166
  cardiomyopathy in, 160
  clinical stages, 4
  disease progression, 154
  dystrophic histopathology, 232
  exercise role of, 167–169
  genetic diagnosis, 80, 83, 91
  laboratory diagnosis—algorithm,
    10, 106
  laboratory studies vs. clinical
    treatments, potential problems,
    214–216
  noncorticosteroid trials, 135–140
  orthopedic management in, 179

[Duchenne muscular dystrophy (DMD)]
  pharmacological therapeutic
    approaches, 211
  structural defects in, 33–38
  therapeutic approaches, 203
  wheel-chaired confinement. *See* Spinal
    deformity
Dysphagia, 167
Dystroglycan complex (DGC), 420
Dystrophic phenotype, 232
Dystrophin
  deficiency, 56, 213
  effects, 15, 24
  gene, deletions and duplications,
    92, 93, 99
  immunostaining, 113
  structure, 57
  synthesis location, 29
Dystrophin-associated protein complex
  (DAPC), 252
Dystrophin bolt, 30–32
  defects, 36–38
Dystrophin delivery, first-generation Ad
  vectors, 370
Dystrophin expression, restoration of,
  330
Dystrophin gene structure of, 252
Dystrophin microgenes, 404
Dystrophin mini-gene, 396, 398
Dystrophin muscle enhancer (DME),
  262
Dystrophin protein, 24
Dystrophin replacement, in animal
  models, 422
Dystrophin-associated proteins (DAP),
  27
Dystrophin–glycoprotein complex
  (DGC), 228
Dystrophin-positive cells, 353
Dystrophin-positive fibers, 344
Dystrophin-related protein (DRP)
  utrophin, 252

EIAV. *See* Equine infectious anemia
  virus
ERF. *See* ETS2 repressor factor
ERS. *See* Exon recognition sequences

E-Box element, 259
Elbow flexion contractures, 4, 166
Electroblotting, 118
Electroporation, for uptake of injected pDNA, 347
Endocytosis, 367
Endothelial progenitors, 297
Enhancer elements, 262
Equine infectious anemia virus (EIAV), 209, 405
Equinus. *See* Toe walking.
ERF-like molecules, 258
ETS2 repressor factor (ERF), 258
Eukaryotic promoters, 256
Exon 23/intron 23 splice junction, 322
Exon recognition sequences (ERS), 322
Exonic splicing enhancer sequences (ESEs), 205
Expression profiling, for muscular dystrophy study, 233
Extensor digitorum longus (EDL) muscle fiber, 283
Extracellular matrix (ECM), 420
Extracorporeal pump-oxygenator, 448

FIV. *See* Feline immunodeficiency virus
Facioscapulohumeral muscular dystrophy, 234
F-actin, 252
Feline immunodeficiency virus (FIV), 405
Feline muscular dystrophy, 204
Fetal muscle biopsies, 227
Fiber protein, 364
Fibroblast growth factor-6 (FGF-6), 280
Forced vital capacity (FVC), 8, 159, 192
Fractures, 183

Gag gene
  capsid (CA) p24, 406
  encodes, 395
  matrix (MA) p17, 406
  nucleocapsid (NC) p7 protein, 406
  p6 polyproline-rich protein, 406
Gene correction
  activity, 328
  efficiency, 328

Gene editing, 326
  by chimeric oligonucleotides, 320
  by nonchimeric oligonucleotides, 320
Gene expression analyses, 233
Gene expression required, for treatment of DMD, 344
Gene therapy
  adeno-associated viral vectors, 413, 418, 419, 429
  DMD, 205
  gene repair, 205, 326, 336, 425
  gene transfer, 206
  splicing, 205
  theoretical basis, 30
Gene transfer, different viral vectors for, 207–210
  efficiency, 347
  physical methods, 211
Gene transfer vehicle, in DMD gene therapy, 392
Genetically engineered murine models, for DMD, 232
Germline
  gene therapy, 206
  mosaicism, 100
  transmission, of rAAV, 419
Globular knob domain, 364
Glucocorticoids, 229, 230
Golden retriever muscular dystrophy (GRMD) dog, 204
Gowers' sign, 3, 78, 153
Grb2 pathways, 228
Green fluorescent protein (GFP), 402
GRMD. *See* Golden retriever muscular dystrophy dog
Growth-associated binding protein (GABP), 257
Growth factors, as regenerative therapy, 283–285
Gyrate atrophy, 235

H1-receptor antagonist (oxatomide), 236
Hematopoietic muscle cell, 307
Hemoangioblastic markers (CD34, Flk-1, and c-kit), 307
Hepatocyte growth factor (HGF) receptor, 283, 297

Index

Heregulin, 266
  Erk and, 257
Herpes simplex virus (HSV), 210
Herpesvirus vectors, 210
Hexons, 364
Hip extensor muscles, weakness of, 3, 151
HIV genome, components, 406
HIV-1 vectors,
  first generation, 406
  gene expression, 408
  second generation, 407
Homologous recombination technology, 336, 337
Horseradish peroxidase (HRP), 113
Host immune response, by Ad vector–mediated gene delivery, 372
Host immunosuppression, 301
Hot spots, 325
HSV-1, 401
Human Ad serotypes, 364
Human leukocyte antigen (HLA) class I humanized mouse model, 358
Huntington's disease, 235
Hydraulic conductivity, 442
Hypokalemia, 9

Icosahedrons, 364
IGF-I, 237
Immunity, adaptive, 373
Immunogenicity, 370
Immunostaining, of dystrophin, 113
Inflammatory mediators, endothelial permeability, 444
  histamine, 444
Insulin-like growth factor binding protein-5 (IGFBP-5) protease, 282
Insulin-like growth factors (IGF-1 and IGF-2), 280, 425
Intestinal motility, 9
Intramuscular transplants, of myoblasts, 299, 300
Intravascular delivery, of naked DNA, 343
Intravascular procedure, safety of, 352

Intron/exon structure, 252
Inverted terminal repeat (ITR) sequences, 368

J-bands, 95
Junction fragments, 95
Junctional permeability, 442

Kedem–Katchalsky equation, for solvent flow, 442
Keratinocyte stem cells, 310
Knee buckling, 151
Knee extension lag, 184
Knee–ankle–foot arthoses, 185, 189

LCMV. See Lymphocytic choriomeningitis
Lentiviral vectors, 209, 398
  for DMD gene therapy, 405–408
Lentiviruses, 409
  advantages of, 405, 407
Leupeptin, 213
Limb–girdle muscles, use, 23
Limb–girdle muscular dystrophy model, 299
Line of gravity, 178
Linkage analysis, 101
Long terminal repeats, 393
Luciferase expression, 350
Lumbar lordosis, 178
Lymphoblastoid human cells, 322
Lymphocytic choriomeningitis (LCMV), 407

MAPK. See Mitogen-activated protein kinases
MCK. See Muscle creatinine kinase
MDSC. See Muscle-derived stem cells
MHC. See Major histocompatibility complex
MPC. See Mesodermal progenitor cells
MSC. See Mesenchymal stem cells
Major histocompatibility complex (MHC), 366

M-cadherin, 297
mdx mouse studies, 353
  dystrophin expression in, 353
  stable mDys expression in, 353, 355–357
Mental retardation, cause of, 24
Mesangioblasts, 307
Mesenchymal stem cells (MSC), 286, 309
Mesodermal progenitor cells (MPC), 309
Microdystrophin, 404, 419–422
Mini-dystrophins, 420
Mismatch repair activity, of gene, 328
Missense mutations, 94
Mitogen-activated protein kinases (MAPK) signaling pathways, 62
Mobility, improving functional for DMD, 169
Moloney murine leukemia virus (MoMLV), 201, 393
Monocytes, 401
Multipotent stem cell populations, 304
Muscle biopsy, 106
Muscle cell, 396, 399, 404, 407
  apoptosis, 65
  for DMD therapy, 296, 303
  survival, 61
Muscle creatinine kinase (MCK), 396
Muscle degeneration, inducer, 41
Muscle-derived stem cells (MDSC), 304
Muscle-directed retro viral delivery, cell-based strategies of, 399–402
  limitations of, 400
Muscle fiber atrophy, type II, 235
Muscle fibers
  essential function, 22
  surface layers, 30
Muscle injury severity, indication, 23
Muscle protein synthesis, 234
Muscle score, decline of, 5
Muscle side population (SP) cells, 302
Muscle-specific muscle creatine kinase (MCK) promoter, 357
Muscle-specific transcription factors, 309
Muscle wasting, 2, 151, 205, 295, 391
Mutagenesis, site-directed, 326, 327
Myoblast transplantation, 282
Myogenesis, 259

Myogenic cells, 206
  precursor, 428, 429
  myeloid progenitors, 297
Myopathy, 41
Myostatin, 214, 284
Myotonic dystrophy, 236

NFAT. *See* Nuclear factor-activated T cell
NMD. *See* Nonsense mediated decay
NPC. *See* Nuclear pore complex
Naked DNA transport and uptake, mechanisms of, 352, 353
Naked plasmid DNA (pDNA), 344
  advantages, 346, 347
  injection in muscles, 347
Neck flexor strength, 8
Negative regulator, of muscle growth, 214
Neoantigen, 373
Neuromuscular junction (NMJ), 253
Neuronal nitric oxide synthase (nNOS), 64, 228
Nonrandom deletion pattern, 93
Nonsense mediated decay (NMD), 33
Nontranscribed strand (ODN2), of gene, 333
Nonviral (plasmid) vectors, 211, 345
Normal muscles vs. DMD muscles, 34
Nuclear factor-activated T cell (NFAT), 257, 260
Nuclear pore complex (NPC), 367
Nutritional/metabolic supplements, in DMD, 234
  coenzyme Q10 (ubiquinone), 235, 236
  creatine, 234, 235
  glutamine, 236

2-O-methyl oligoribonucleotides, 322
ORF. *See* Open reading frames
Oligonucleotide-mediated gene therapy, for DMD, 320
Oligonucleotides, as gene therapy vectors, 319
Onco-retroviral genome, 393
Onco-retroviral vectors, 395, 396, 398, 405

Index

Onco-retrovirus, 393
Open reading frames (ORFs), for genome codes, 414
Orthopedic management, in DMD, 179
Osteoporosis, 132, 183
Out-of-frame mutation, 35
Oxazolone derivative, of prednisolone, 229

pDNA. *See* Plasmid DNA
Paired-domain transcription factor Pax7, 296
Paracellular permeability, 442
Parvoviridae viral family, 413
PCr/Pi ratio, 236
Penton base, 364
Phosphocreatine (PCr), 235
Piriformis syndrome, 190
Plasmid DNA (pDNA) delivery, 345
Plasmid DNA size, effect on gene expression, 350
Platelet-derived growth factor-BB (PDGF-BB), 280
Point mutation detection, 102
Polyadenylation site, of pCILuc, 351
Polyethylenimine (PEI), 345
Polymerase chain reaction (PCR) products, 334
Postnatal gene transfer studies, 344
Postnatal skeletal muscle, 296
Prednisone, 229, 230
Prednisone monotherapy, 127
Pre-mRNA splicing, 320
Prenatal diagnosis, 83, 97
Preplate technique, 303
Protease inhibitors, 213
PTC therapeutics, 212

RCL. *See* Replication-competent lentivirus
RCR. *See* Replication competent retrovirus
RLD. *See* Restrictive lung disease
RT. *See* Reverse transcriptase
RRE. *See* Rev-response element
Radiation-resistant muscle cell, 286

Reading-frame theory, 80
Recombinant AAV (rAAV) genomes, 414, 415
  cloning and production, 414, 415
  nondystrophin gene delivery, 424
Recombinant AAV vectors, 404
  delivery of, 426, 427
  safety of, 417
Regenerative therapy, of muscle fibers, 279
Regional gene delivery, 439, 440
  intravascular approach, 440
  transendothelial transport, 442
Replication competent retrovirus (RCR), 395
Replication-competent lentivirus (RCL), 407
Resting tachycardia, 9
Restrictive lung disease (RLD), 159
Retroviral LTR, 396, 402
Retroviral particles, 392, 398
Retroviral transduction, 398, 399, 400
Retroviral vectors, 207
  for gene therapy, 319
  gene transfer experiments, 392
  generation of, 395, 402, 405
  in treatment of DMD, 400
  molecular biology of, 391–396
  production of, 393, 394, 397, 400
Retroviral-mediated gene therapy, 392, 396–398
Retroviral-mediated transduction, 392, 399, 400, 404
Reverse transcriptase (RT), 392
Rev-response element (RRE), 406
RGD–αv integrin interaction, 378
RNA/DNA chimeric molecules, 327
Rod domain, of dystrophin and utrophin, 253

SCID. *See* Severe combined immunodeficiency
snRNA. *See* Small nuclear RNA
Satellite cells, 281, 297
Scoliosis, 13, 22, 132, 158–160, 179, 191, 192, 194–197, 358
Second-generation vectors, 370, 371

Self-inactivating (SIN) vectors, 407
Serotypes, 364, 368, 374
Serum creatine kinase (CK), 23, 38, 78, 427
Serum response element (SRE), 262
Severe combined immunodeficiency (SCID), 207
Shaft domain, 364
Short fragment homologous recombination (SFHR), 335, 336
Side population (SP) cells, 286
Signaling proteins, 61, 64
Single stranded oligodeoxyribonucleotides, 332
Site-directed mutagenesis, 326, 327
Skeletal muscle regeneration
  effect of the environment on, 282
  from muscle precursor cells, 281, 282
Skeletal muscle size regulation mechanism, 280
Skin source for cell-mediated therapy, 309, 310
Sleep apnea, 4
Small compound evaluation, methodologies of, 266
Small nuclear RNAs (snRNAs), 325
Somatic gene therapy, 206
Southern blot analysis, 80, 83
Spectrin super family, of proteins, 251
Spinal deformity, 159, 191
Spinal stabilization, 194
Stable displacement loops (D-loops), 328
Stanozolol, 234
Starling forces, 443
Starling's hypothesis, 442
"Stem cell–like" muscle precursor cells, 281
Stem cell antigen-1 (Sca-1), 303
Stem cells in skeletal muscles, 285, 286
  See also Mesangioblasts
Steroid therapy, 127, 132
Stop codons (UGA, UAG, UAA), 237
Stop mutations, 211
Stuffer DNA, 210, 351
Sustained-release albuterol, 234
Synaptic regulation, via N-box, 257
Synaptically expressed genes, 256
Synthetic vectors, 345

TAL. *See* Tendo-achilles lengthening
TFR. *See* Triplex-forming oligonucleotides (TFR), 336
TFS. *See* Transverse fixation system
Tachycardia, resting, 9
Talipes equinovarus, 188
Targeting adenoviral vectors, to muscle, 375–377
  native tropism, 376
  rerouting vector, 376
Targeting moieties, 377
Tarsal medullostomy, 188
Tendo-achilles lengthening (TAL), 158
TGF-β signaling, 283
Third-generation vectors, 371, 372
Tibialis posticus, 186
Toe walking, 151, 180
Trans-acting components, 406
Transcribed (ODN1), of gene, 333
Transcriptional modifier, 130
Transendothelial transport, 442
Trans-splicing (SMaRT) oligonucleotides, 336
Transverse fixation system (TFS), 38
Trendelenburg gait pattern, 153
Trimeric amino acid, 213
Trimeric fiber protein, 364
Triplex-forming oligonucleotides (TFR), 336
T-waves, abnormal, 165

UAA (A) stop codon mutation, 237
Ultracentrifugation, 393, 398
Utrophin, 253
  activity, 262
  dystrophin autosomal homologue, 130, 212
  expression control, 255
  mRNA stability, 262
  overexpression, in muscle, 253, 254
  post-transcriptional regulation, 262
  promoter studies of, 255
  regulation of, 263
  types of, 252
Utrophin A promoter, 256
Utrophin B promoter, 260

Index

Utrophin exon, 255
Utrophin–based therapeutic strategies, 263–265
Utrophin-based upregulation strategy, 252
Utrophin-null mutant mice, 253

Vectors, First-generation, 368, 369
Verbal working memory skills, 4
Viral protease (PR), 406
Viral vectors, for gene transfer, 207, 208, 347
Viral-derived delivery systems, 345
Virus-mediated gene therapy, 319
Vitravene™, 320
VSV-G envelope, 405, 407

Weight gain, 131, 133
Western blot analysis,
    detecting muscular dystrophies by, 79
    dystrophin quantitation by, 114
Wheel-chaired confined, due to DMD. *See* Spinal deformity
Wheelchair dependency, 5, 155
Woodchuck hepatitis virus posttranscriptional regulatory element (WPRE), 407

X-linked recessive disease, 227, 295
X-linked SCID treatments, 209

"ZZ" zinc-finger motif, 420